W9-BZK-902

1995
YEAR BOOK OF
NUCLEAR MEDICINE®

Statement of Purpose

The YEAR BOOK Service

The YEAR BOOK series was devised in 1901 by practicing health professionals who observed that the literature of medicine and related disciplines had become so voluminous that no one individual could read and place in perspective every potential advance in a major specialty. In the final decade of the 20th century, this recognition is more acutely true than it was in 1901.

More than merely a series of books, YEAR BOOK volumes are the tangible results of a unique service designed to accomplish the following:

- to *survey* a wide range of journals of proven value
- to *select* from those journals papers representing significant advances and statements of important clinical principles
- to provide *abstracts* of those articles that are readable, convenient summaries of their key points
- to provide *commentary* about those articles to place them in perspective

These publications grow out of a unique process that calls on the talents of outstanding authorities in clinical and fundamental disciplines, trained literature specialists, and professional writers, all supported by the resources of Mosby, the world's preeminent publisher for the health professions.

The Literature Base

Mosby subscribes to nearly 1,000 journals published worldwide, covering the full range of the health professions. On an annual basis, the publisher examines usage patterns and polls its expert authorities to add new journals to the literature base and to delete journals that are no longer useful as potential YEAR BOOK sources.

The Literature Survey

The publisher's team of literature specialists, all of whom are trained and experienced health professionals, examines every original, peer-reviewed article in each journal issue. More than 250,000 articles per year are scanned systematically, including title, text, illustrations, tables, and references. Each scan is compared, article by article, to the search strategies that the publisher has developed in consultation with the 270 outside experts who form the pool of YEAR BOOK editors. A given article may be reviewed by any number of editors, from one to a dozen or more, regardless of the discipline for which the paper was originally published. In turn, each editor who receives the article reviews it to determine whether or not the article should be included in the YEAR BOOK. This decision is based on the article's inherent quality, its probable usefulness to readers of that YEAR BOOK, and the editor's goal to represent a balanced picture of a given field in each volume of the YEAR BOOK. In addition, the editor indicates when to include figures and tables from the article to help the YEAR BOOK reader better understand the information.

Of the quarter million articles scanned each year, only 5% are selected for detailed analysis within the YEAR BOOK series, thereby assuring readers of the high value of every selection.

The Abstract

The publisher's abstracting staff is headed by a physician-writer and includes individuals with training in the life sciences, medicine, and other areas, plus extensive experience in writing for the health professions and related industries. Each selected article is assigned to a specific writer on this abstracting staff. The abstracter, guided in many cases by notations supplied by the expert editor, writes a structured, condensed summary designed so that the reader can rapidly acquire the essential information contained in the article.

The Commentary

The YEAR BOOK editorial boards, sometimes assisted by guest commentators, write comments that place each article in perspective for the reader. This provides the reader with the equivalent of a personal consultation with a leading international authority—an opportunity to better understand the value of the article and to benefit from the authority's thought processes in assessing the article.

Additional Editorial Features

The editorial boards of each YEAR BOOK organize the abstracts and comments to provide a logical and satisfying sequence of information. To enhance the organization, editors also provide introductions to sections or individual chapters, comments linking a number of abstracts, citations to additional literature, and other features.

The published YEAR BOOK contains enhanced bibliographic citations for each selected article, including extended listings of multiple authors and identification of author affiliations. Each YEAR BOOK contains a Table of Contents specific to that year's volume. From year to year, the Table of Contents for a given YEAR BOOK will vary depending on developments within the field.

Every YEAR BOOK contains a list of the journals from which papers have been selected. This list represents a subset of the nearly 1,000 journals surveyed by the publisher and occasionally reflects a particularly pertinent article from a journal that is not surveyed on a routine basis.

Finally, each volume contains a comprehensive subject index and an index to authors of each selected paper.

The 1995 Year Book Series

Year Book of Allergy and Clinical Immunology: Drs. Rosenwasser, Borish, Gelfand, Leung, Nelson, and Szefler

Year Book of Anesthesiology and Pain Management: Drs. Tinker, Abram, Chestnut, Roizen, Rothenberg, and Wood

Year Book of Cardiology®: Drs. Schlant, Collins, Engle, Gersh, Kaplan, and Waldo

Year Book of Chiropractic: Dr. Lawrence

Year Book of Critical Care Medicine®: Dr. Parrillo

Year Book of Dentistry®: Drs. Meskin, Berry, Currier, Kennedy, Leinfelder, Roser, and Zakariasen

Year Book of Dermatologic Surgery: Drs. Swanson, Glogau, and Salasche

Year Book of Dermatology®: Drs. Sober and Fitzpatrick

Year Book of Diagnostic Radiology®: Drs. Federle, Clark, Gross, Latchaw, Madewell, Maynard, and Young

Year Book of Digestive Diseases®: Drs. Greenberger and Moody

Year Book of Drug Therapy®: Drs. Lasagna and Weintraub

Year Book of Emergency Medicine®: Drs. Davidson, Dronen, King, Niemann, Roberts, and Wagner

Year Book of Endocrinology®: Drs. Bagdade, Braverman, Horton, Kannan, Landsberg, Molitch, Morley, Nathan, Odell, Poehlman, Rogol, and Ryan

Year Book of Family Practice®: Drs. Berg, Bowman, Davidson, Dietrich, and Scherger

Year Book of Geriatrics and Gerontology®: Drs. Beck, Burton, Goldstein, Reuben, Small, and Whitehouse

Year Book of Hand Surgery®: Drs. Amadio and Hentz

Year Book of Hematology®: Drs. Spivak, Bell, Ness, Quesenberry, and Wiernik

Year Book of Infectious Diseases®: Drs. Keusch, Barza, Bennish, Gelfand, Klempner, Snydman, and Skolnik

Year Book of Infertility and Reproductive Endocrinology®: Drs. Mishell, Lobo, and Sokol

Year Book of Medicine®: Drs. Bone, Cline, Epstein, Greenberger, Malawista, Mandell, O'Rourke, and Utiger

Year Book of Neonatal and Perinatal Medicine®: Drs. Fanaroff and Klaus

Year Book of Nephrology®: Drs. Coe, Curtis, Favus, Henderson, Kashgarian, and Luke

Year Book of Neurology and Neurosurgery®: Drs. Bradley and Wilkins

Year Book of Neuroradiology: Drs. Osborn, Eskridge, Grossman, Hudgens, and Ross

Year Book of Nuclear Medicine®: Drs. Gottschalk, Blaufox, McAfee, Zaret, and Zubal

Year Book of Obstetrics and Gynecology®: Drs. Mishell, Kirschbaum, and Morrow

Year Book of Occupational and Environmental Medicine®: Drs. Emmett, Frank, Gochfeld, and Hessl

Year Book of Oncology®: Drs. Simone, Bosl, Glatstein, Longo, Ozols, and Steele

Year Book of Ophthalmology®: Drs. Cohen, Augsburger, Benson, Eagle, Flanagan, Laibson, Nelson, Rapuano, Sergott, Tasman, Tipperman, and Wilson

Year Book of Orthopedics®: Drs. Sledge, Cofield, Dobyns, Griffin, Springfield, Swiontkowski, Wiesel, and Wilson

Year Book of Otolaryngology–Head and Neck Surgery®: Drs. Paparella and Holt

Year Book of Pain: Drs. Gebhart, Haddox, Jacox, Janjan, Marcus, Rudy, and Shapiro

Year Book of Pathology and Laboratory Medicine®: Drs. Mills, Bruns, Gaffey, and Stoler

Year Book of Pediatrics®: Dr. Stockman

Year Book of Plastic, Reconstructive, and Aesthetic Surgery: Drs. Miller, Cohen, McKinney, Robson, Ruberg, and Whitaker

Year Book of Podiatric Medicine and Surgery®: Dr. Kominsky

Year Book of Psychiatry and Applied Mental Health®: Drs. Talbott, Ballanger, Breier, Frances, Meltzer, Schowalter, and Tasman

Year Book of Pulmonary Disease®: Drs. Bone and Petty

Year Book of Rheumatology®: Drs. Sergent, LeRoy, Meenan, Panush, and Reichlin

Year Book of Sports Medicine®: Drs. Shephard, Drinkwater, Eichner, Torg, Col. Anderson, and Mr. George

Year Book of Surgery®: Drs. Copeland, Bland, Deitch, Eberlein, Howard, Luce, Seeger, Souba, and Sugarbaker

Year Book of Thoracic and Cardiovascular Surgery: Drs. Ginsberg, Lofland, and Wechsler

Year Book of Transplantation®: Drs. Sollinger, Eckhoff, Hullett, Knechtle, Longo, Mentzer, and Pirsch

Year Book of Ultrasound®: Drs. Merritt, Babcock, Carroll, Fagan, Finberg, and Fleischer

Year Book of Urology®: Drs. Howards and deKernion

Year Book of Vascular Surgery®: Dr. Porter

Editor-in-Chief

Alexander Gottschalk, M.D.

Professor of Radiology, Department of Radiology, Michigan State University, East Lansing, Michigan

Associate Editors

M. Donald Blaufox, M.D., Ph.D.

Chairman, Department of Nuclear Medicine, Albert Einstein College of Medicine and Montefiore Medical Center, Bronx, New York

John G. McAfee, M.D.

Chief, Radiopharmaceutical Research Section, National Institutes of Health Clinical Center, Bethesda, Maryland

Barry L. Zaret, M.D.

Robert W. Berliner Professor of Medicine, Professor of Diagnostic Radiology, and Chief, Section of Cardiovascular Medicine, Yale University School of Medicine, New Haven, Connecticut

I. George Zubal, Ph.D.

Associate Professor of Diagnostic Radiology, Section of Nuclear Medicine, Department of Diagnostic Radiology, Yale University School of Medicine, New Haven, Connecticut

Editor Emeritus

Paul B. Hoffer, M.D.

Professor of Diagnostic Radiology; Director, Section of Nuclear Medicine, Department of Diagnostic Radiology, Yale University School of Medicine, New Haven, Connecticut

1995

The Year Book of NUCLEAR MEDICINE®

Editor-in-Chief
Alexander Gottschalk, M.D.

Associate Editors
M. Donald Blaufox, M.D., Ph.D.
John G. McAfee, M.D.
Barry L. Zaret, M.D.
I. George Zubal, Ph.D.

Editor Emeritus
Paul B. Hoffer, M.D.

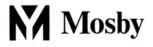 Mosby

St. Louis   Baltimore   Boston   Carlsbad   Chicago   Naples   New York   Philadelphia   Portland
London   Madrid   Mexico City   Singapore   Sydney   Tokyo   Toronto   Wiesbaden

Vice President and Publisher, Continuity Publishing: Kenneth H. Killion
Director, Editorial Development: Gretchen C. Murphy
Manager, Continuity–EDP: Maria Nevinger
Developmental Editor: Kris Baumgartner
Acquisitions Editor: Jennifer Roche
Illustrations and Permissions Coordinator: Lois M. Ruebensam
Director of Editorial Services: Edith M. Podrazik, R.N.
Senior Information Specialist: Terri Santo, R.N.
Information Specialist: Nancy Dunne, R.N.
Senior Medical Writer: David A. Cramer, M.D.
Senior Project Manager, Production: Max F. Perez
Project Manager, Editing: Tamara L. Smith
Senior Production Editor: Wendi Schnaufer
Freelance Services Supervisor: Barbara M. Kelly
Vice President, Professional Sales and Marketing: George M. Parker
Marketing and Circulation Manager: Barry J. Bowlus
Marketing Coordinator: Lynn Stevenson

1995 EDITION
Copyright © April 1995 by Mosby–Year Book, Inc.

All rights reserved. No part of this publication may be reproduced, stored in a retrieval system, or transmitted, in any form or by any means, electronic, mechanical, photocopying, recording, or otherwise, without prior written permission from the publisher.

Permission to photocopy or reproduce solely for internal or personal use is permitted for libraries or other users registered with the Copyright Clearance Center, provided that the base fee of $4.00 per chapter plus $.10 per page is paid directly to the Copyright Clearance Center, 21 Congress Street, Salem, MA 01970. This consent does not extend to other kinds of copying, such as copying for general distribution, for advertising or promotional purposes, for creating new collected works, or for resale.

Printed in the United States of America
Composition by International Computaprint Corporation
Printing/binding by Maple-Vail

Mosby–Year Book, Inc.
11830 Westline Industrial Drive
St. Louis, MO 63146

Editorial Office:
Mosby–Year Book, Inc.
200 North LaSalle St.
Chicago, IL 60601

International Standard Serial Number: 0084-3903
International Standard Book Number: 0-8151-4513-6

Table of Contents

MOSBY DOCUMENT EXPRESS xi

JOURNALS REPRESENTED xiii

PUBLISHER'S PREFACE xv

INTRODUCTION xvii

Emeritus Editor's Essay

    Therapeutic Nuclear Medicine, by RICHARD A. HOLMES,
      M.D. xix

  1. Pulmonary 1

  2. Hematology and Oncology 41

  3. Infection and Inflammation 79

  4. Musculoskeletal 109

  5. Endocrine 153

  6. Renal 177

  7. Gastrointestinal 205

  8. Vascular 239

  9. Central Nervous System 251

10. Cardiovascular 283

11. Correlative Imaging 349

12. Radiopharmaceutical 387

13. Physics and Dosimetry 421

    SUBJECT INDEX 449

    AUTHOR INDEX 525

Mosby Document Express

Copies of the full text of the original source documents of articles abstracted or referenced in this publication are available by calling Mosby Document Express, toll-free, at 1 (800) 55-MOSBY.

With Mosby Document Express, you have convenient, 24-hour-a-day access to literally every article on which this publication is based. In fact, through Mosby Document Express, virtually any medical or scientific article can be located and delivered by FAX, overnight delivery service, international airmail, electronic transmission of bitmapped images (via Internet), or regular mail. The average cost of a complete, delivered copy of an article, including up to $4 in copyright clearance charges and first-class mail delivery, is $12.

For inquiries and pricing information, please call the toll-free number shown above. To expedite your order for material appearing in this publication, please be prepared with the code shown next to the bibliographic citation for each abstract.

Journals Represented

Mosby subscribes to and surveys nearly 1,000 U.S. and foreign medical and allied health journals. From these journals, the Editors select the articles to be abstracted. Journals represented in this YEAR BOOK are listed below.

Acta Radiologica
American Heart Journal
American Journal of Cardiology
American Journal of Gastroenterology
American Journal of Nephrology
American Journal of Physical Medicine & Rehabilitation
American Journal of Roentgenology
American Journal of Sports Medicine
American Journal of Surgery
American Surgeon
Annals of Internal Medicine
Annals of Surgery
Annals of Thoracic Surgery
Archives of Internal Medicine
Archives of Neurology
Archives of Orthopaedic and Trauma Surgery
Archives of Physical Medicine and Rehabilitation
Arthritis and Rheumatism
Australasian Radiology
Australian and New Zealand Journal of Medicine
British Journal of Radiology
Canadian Association of Radiologists Journal
Canadian Journal of Surgery
Cancer
Chest
Circulation
Clinical Infectious Diseases
Clinical Nuclear Medicine
Clinical Radiology
Digestion
Digestive Diseases and Sciences
European Heart Journal
European Journal of Cancer
European Journal of Nuclear Medicine
European Neurology
European Respiratory Journal
Foot and Ankle
Frontiers in Neuroendocrinology
Gut
Health Physics
IEEE Transactions on Medical Imaging
Injury
Investigative Radiology
Journal of Assisted Reproduction and Genetics
Journal of Bone and Joint Surgery (American Volume)
Journal of Bone and Joint Surgery (British Volume)
Journal of Burn Care and Rehabilitation
Journal of Clinical Endocrinology and Metabolism
Journal of Hand Surgery (British)
Journal of Labelled Compounds and Radiopharmaceuticals

Journal of Neurology, Neurosurgery and Psychiatry
Journal of Nuclear Cardiology
Journal of Nuclear Medicine
Journal of Pediatric Gastroenterology and Nutrition
Journal of Pediatric Orthopedics
Journal of Pediatric Surgery
Journal of Rheumatology
Journal of Trauma
Journal of Urology
Journal of the American College of Cardiology
Journal of the American College of Surgeons
Journal of the American Medical Association
Kidney International
Lancet
Magnetic Resonance Imaging
Medical Physics
Nephron
Neurosurgery
Nuclear Medicine Communications
Orthopedic Review
Pediatric Nephrology
Pharmacotherapy
Physics in Medicine and Biology
Postgraduate Medical Journal
RadioGraphics
Radiology
Seminars in Nuclear Medicine
Skeletal Radiology
Stroke
Thyroid
Transplantation Proceedings
World Journal of Surgery

Standard Abbreviations

The following terms are abbreviated in this edition: acquired immunodeficiency syndrome (AIDS), cardiopulmonary resuscitation (CPR), central nervous system (CNS), cerebrospinal fluid (CSF), computed tomography (CT), deoxyribonucleic acid (DNA), electrocardiography (ECG), gadolinium-diethylenetriamine-pentaacetic acid (Gd-DTPA), health maintenance organization (HMO), human immunodeficiency virus (HIV), intensive care unit (ICU), intramuscular (IM), intravenous (IV), magnetic resonance (MR) imaging (MRI), nuclear magnetic resonance (NMR), positron emission tomography (PET), ribonucleic acid (RNA), and single-photon emission CT (SPECT).

Publisher's Preface

Publication of the 1994 YEAR BOOK OF NUCLEAR MEDICINE marked the end of an outstanding period of editorship by Paul B. Hoffer, M.D. During his 14 years as Editor-in-Chief, Dr. Hoffer made certain that the readers of the YEAR BOOK were provided with discerning and informative literature and editorial commentary of the highest caliber. We extend our sincere thanks to Dr. Hoffer for his everpresent commitment to the YEAR BOOK OF NUCLEAR MEDICINE.

Leaving with Dr. Hoffer are John C. Gore, Ph.D; Zachary Rattner, M.D.; Alan Waxman, M.D.; William C. Eckelman, Ph.D.; and Manuel L. Brown, M.D. We wish to thank them for their ongoing dedication to the YEAR BOOK OF NUCLEAR MEDICINE. Their participation will be greatly missed.

Alexander Gottschalk, M.D., who has been an Associate Editor for the YEAR BOOK OF NUCLEAR MEDICINE for the past 14 years, has assumed the responsibility of being Editor-in-Chief for the 1995 YEAR BOOK OF NUCLEAR MEDICINE and future editions. He has assembled a first-rate editorial team consisting of Donald M. Blaufox, M.D., Ph.D.; John G. McAfee, M.D.; Barry L. Zaret, M.D.; and I. George Zubal, Ph.D. This team continues the tradition of distinguished editorial direction for the YEAR BOOK.

Introduction

Those of you who read the introduction to the 1994 YEAR BOOK OF NUCLEAR MEDICINE found out that, for personal reasons, Dr. Paul B. Hoffer decided to make 1994 his last year as Editor. He thus becomes our only living Editor Emeritus and only the second past Editor this YEAR BOOK has had. It has been my pleasure to have been on Paul's Editorial Board during the entire 13 years he guided this effort, so I can tell you firsthand that he did it with dedication, intellect, hard work, overview, and class. In my opinion, the entire international nuclear medicine community is in his debt for the outstanding job he did. Therefore, on your behalf, I say simply, "Thanks, Paul." I also told Paul that if, at some future time, he wanted to get his hands back into this business, we will always find a way to make it happen.

This year's Editorial Board has one new name: Dr. John G. McAfee. John, as virtually all of you know, brings to this task decades of experience as both an investigator and clinician, and we look forward to his insights. Don Blaufox will expand his efforts this year, whereas Barry Zaret, George Zubal, and I continue on. I am also folding our MRI efforts into a correlative imaging section, which will be my responsibility. It will start as an eclectic collection of abstracts that has some MRI, some CT, and some other modalities that all relate in some way to nuclear medicine. If you like it—or if you don't, let me know. In fact, if you have any *constructive* criticism you wish to share with me or the Editorial Board, send it in. We may not use your idea, but we promise to consider it carefully.

One of the innovations that Paul Hoffer developed in this YEAR BOOK was the James L. Quinn, III, essay. The late Jim Quinn, the first YEAR BOOK OF NUCLEAR MEDICINE Editor, was a close personal friend of mine and a sort of academic godfather to Paul Hoffer when he was my resident. I knew Jim well enough to know he would have been delighted at the change we made with this volume—to rename the essay the Emeritus Editor's Essay, honoring both Jim and Paul for their efforts. This year, Dr. Richard A. Holmes has written an overview of nuclear therapy. Therapy is a topic that we often allude to, and occasionally pick out abstracts for, but never put in one place, because the organization of the YEAR BOOK is geared to cover, in large part, diagnostic work. Dick has ably filled this void with this year's Emeritus Editor's Essay. If you have ideas for future essays you would like to read, send them in to our publisher. We may be able to grant your request.

Alexander Gottschalk, M.D.

Emeritus Editor's Essay

honoring

James L. Quinn, III, M.D.   and   Paul B. Hoffer, M.D.
editor, 1966 to 1980   editor, 1981 to 1994

Therapeutic Nuclear Medicine

RICHARD A. HOLMES, M.D.

Vice President of Research and Development, Du Pont-Merck Radiopharmaceuticals, Billerica, Massachusetts

Introduction

Although nuclear medicine has evolved into a diagnostic imaging specialty, it has long indulged in unsealed radioisotope therapy, using almost exclusively 2 radioisotopes. Iodine-131 (physical half-life, 8.08 days; beta emission, .606 MeV, .335 MeV; gamma emission, .365 MeV) is the principal therapy for most forms of hyperthyroidism and thyroid cancer. For thyroid cancer after exterpation surgery, iodine-131 is used to treat functional metastatic thyroid cancer and local thyroid cancer recurrence. Other radioiodine isotopes, such as iodine 132 and iodine-125, have also been used therapeutically, with similar results (iodine-132) or variable responses (iodine-125). Phosphorus-32 phosphate, or orthophosphate (physical half-life, 14.3 days; beta emission, 1.71 MeV; gamma emission, none), is an effective therapy used to diminish red blood cell proliferation in polycythemia ruba vera; however, it is problematic as an ancillary therapy for the leukemias, the lymphomas, and multiple myeloma. As a method for palliating metastatic bone cancer pain, its clinical effectiveness has been muted by its bone marrow depression. As phosphorus-32 colloid, the radiopharmaceutical has been used for cavitary instillation in malignant effusions, inflammatory synovitis–arthritis, and intraperitoneally with chemotherapy to treat advanced recurrent ovarian carcinoma. Successful and effective therapy depends on the appropriateness of the radiopharmaceutical dose, the correctness of the administration technique, the residence time of the radioisotope at the site of the instillation, and the limited metabolism and general distribution of the radiotherapy.

In the past decade, several unique radiopharmaceuticals have evolved and been added to the unsealed therapeutic radioisotope armamentarium. The compounds have embraced a host of ligands and mechanisms of localization while introducing a bevy of radioisotopes with particulate emissions and high specific activity needed for radiotherapy. To classify this heterogenous list of compounds, we have chosen to characterize them by their general structure and, in the case of antibodies and protein receptors, their function. Table 1 categorizes these unsealed therapeutic

---

TABLE 1.—Unsealed Therapeutic Radioisotopes

- Radioactive Small Molecules (e.g., radioisotopes and chelates)
- Radiolabeled Particles (e.g., colloids, microspheres, macroaggregates)
- Radioimmunotherapy (e.g., monoclonal antibodies, antibody fragments)
- Radiolabeled Peptide–Receptor System (e.g., somatostatin, bombesin)

(Courtesy of R.A. Holmes, M.D.)

radioisotopes into 4 groups: radioactive small molecules, radiolabeled particles, radioimmunotherapy, and radiopeptide-receptors. In assessing each group, we will consider their structure, radiopharmacokinetics, and clinical application, and we will speculate on future developments in each category.

Radiolabeled Small Molecules

This grouping includes a number of chelates and one therapeutic ionic molecule. Most have not attained routine approval from the Food and Drug Administration (FDA) but are in phase III evaluation. They generally fall into 2 therapeutic areas: palliation of metastatic bone cancer pain and metaiodobenzylguanidine therapy of malignant pheochromocytoma/neuroblastoma.

Palliation of Metastatic Bone Cancer Pain

Common human cancers of the lung, breast, and prostate frequently metastisize to bone, where their proliferation is commonly associated with progressive pain. In its early state, the pain is controllable with oral analgesics, but with continued proliferation, greater amounts of analgesics and other therapies (e.g., hormone therapy or chemotherapy) may be required. If the bony lesions and pain are diffuse, progressive generalized irradiation would provide optimum therapy, but permanent bone marrow depression is the limiting factor. As stated earlier, ionic phosphorus-32 has been used to treat the systemic pain, but like external-beam irradiation, it too was associated with unacceptable marrow toxicity. From the work of Pecher (1), who studies the biological activity of both radiocalcium and radiostrontium, and the latter's use in treating metastatic bone cancer, Schmidt and Firusian (2) first used strontium-89 chloride (physical half-life, 50.5 days; beta emission, 1.48 MeV; gamma emission, none) in 1974 to treat incurable pain in patients with neoplastic osseous infiltration. As an analogue of the calcium, strontium exchanges with hydroxyapatite calcium and concentrates in osteoblastic bony lesions. The radiopharmaceutical remained clinically dormant until 1977, when Ralph G. Robinson, M.D., received Investigational New Drug (IND) approval from the FDA to administer strontium-89 chloride for relief of metastatic bone pain. The strontium-89 chloride was obtained from Amersham International, which subsequently used Dr. Robinson's clinical results (3) and the findings of others to submit a new drug application (NDA) that led to FDA approval in 1993. Indicated in patients with cancer who failed to respond to conventional therapy, strontium-89 is usually administered in a dose of 4 mCi given intravenously. Reduction in bone pain begins during the second week following administration. On average, 10% of the treated group will become pain free, whereas others will experience varying degrees of pain reduction, which are objectively demonstrated by a decrease in the number of administered analgesics. Metastron (Medi Physics Amersham, Chicago, IL), the commercial name for strontium-89 chloride, has been compared with regional external-beam irradiation (4). The results have shown comparability, and its lower cost makes strontium-89 chloride a good alternative. Bone marrow suppression following administration of strontium-89 chloride is transient, usually hitting the thrombocytopenic nadir 8 or more weeks post administration and then returning to baseline in 2 to 3 months. The pain reduction of strontium-89 chloride lasts an average 3 to 4 months, and it probably relates to its slow osseous pharmacokinetics and its long physical half-life.

In a time almost paralleling the evolution of that of the strontium-89 chloride, Deutch and associates (5) developed rhenium-186 hydroxyethylenediphosphonic acid (HEDP) chelate (physical half-life, 90.6 hours; beta emission, 1.07 MeV; gamma emission, .137 MeV, .122 MeV) to treat bone cancer pain. Rhenium-186 HEDP clears the blood rapidly and avidly concentrates in osteoblastic bone lesions. It localizes by bridging the rhenium-186 to hydroxyapatite with the phosphonate ligand. Initial clinical studies by Maxon et al. (6) demonstrated reasonable efficacy and transient bone marrow depression. Mallinckrodt Radiopharmaceuticals began a multi-institutional phase III study, which has led to an NDA submission. Clinical results indicate comparable pain relief (65% to 75%), transient bone marrow depression, and a higher treatment dose (35 mCi).

A second short-lived therapeutic radiopharmaceutical for palliation of bone cancer pain, samarium-153 ethylenediaminetetramethylene phosphoric acid (EDTMP) (physical half-life, 46.3 hours; beta emission, .819 MeV, .71 MeV, .64 MeV; gamma emission, .103 MeV), was discovered and developed at the University of Missouri (7). It appears that a combination of mechanisms is involved in the osseous localization of samarium. Cationic samarium forms an insoluble hydroxide salt with hydroxyapatite, in addition to bridging to hydroxyapatite through the phosphonate ligand. Early animal and clinical studies established its safety (8, 9), and Cytogen has sponsored a multicenter phase III study leading to an NDA submission. Its high bone uptake may allow therapeutic bone cancer reduction, in addition to its analgesic effect, which is comparable to that shown with strontium-89 chloride and rhenium-186 HEDP. Thrombocytopenia was transient, and like the other agents, early hyperacute pain ("flare reaction") was seen (3 to 4 days) in some patients (1%) after administration.

A third chelate, stannum-117m DTPA (physical half-life, 13.6 days; beta emission, internal conversion; gamma emission, .159 MeV), developed at Brookhaven (10) and recently licensed by Diatech, is just entering clinical evaluation to treat metastatic bone cancer pain. Because it has relatively low-energy conversion electrons, it is hoped that bone marrow toxicity will be less than the others, although all have shown only transient depression. It will also be some time before the chelate therapies are available for routine use.

I-131 Metaiodobenzylguanidine Therapy of Adrenergic Tumors

Early studies to develop radiolabeled agents that would concentrate in adrenergic tumors, such as phechromotocytomas and neuroblastomas, failed until the Michigan group led by Wieland and Beierwalters (11) developed iodine-131 meta-iodobenzylguanidine (MIBG), a structural analogue of the drug guanethidine and similar to norepinephrine that is elaborated by these tumors. Initial use of MIBG was diagnostic, because it was functionally concentrated in catecholamine storage granules in the sympathetic nerve endings; however, unlike norepinephrine, which clears the nerve endings (exocytosis) in hours, MIBG is retained for several days. Therapy with MIBG became a serious consideration when the detection of pheochromocytomas by diagnostic MIBG revealed a 46% incidence of metastasis to the liver, bone, lymph nodes, and/or lung in the first 176 patients studied with iodine-131 MIBG at the University of Michigan (12). This far exceeded the 10% incidence of malignant pheochromocytoma that was previously presumed typical (13), and it resulted in the development of the therapeutic protocol shown in Table 2. Although the outcome of this therapy has not been spectacular, some favorable results have been obtained. Iodine-131 MIBG does permit a more sensitive way of staging neuroblastoma. However, therapeutically, we can only expect a short prolongation of life at best. The disease is invariably fatal, and ablation of the tumor is not possible (11). Although other tumors, such as carcinoids, nonsecreting paraganglioma, medullary thyroid cancer, chemodectomas, choriocarcinoma, and a Merkel cell skin cancer, have been demonstrated by iodine-131 MIBG imaging, none but the carcinoids have been treated, again with mixed results (14).

Given the wide array of currently available particulate radioisotopes and the recent advances in radiochemistry, future developments in unsealed radioisotope therapy using small molecules should be possible. Two directions seem likely: developing radiopharmaceuticals for specific malignancies, such as Kaposi's sarcoma in AIDS, or devising radiopharmaceuticals to treat benign diseases, such as the progressive pain of inflammatory arthritis. Although conceptually intriguing, current government regulations could make the second alternative difficult, if not impossible to pursue.

TABLE 2.—[I-131] MIBG Treatment of
Malignant Pheochromocytoma

- [I-131] MIBG—iv 3 doses* at 3-month intervals
- Chemotherapy—3-week cycle** × 1 year

*100–250 mCi; < 5 mg MIBG.
**cyclophosphamide, vincristine, dicarbazine
(Courtesy of R.A. Holmes, M.D.)

Radiolabeled Particles

Radioactive particles used for therapy vary in their composition and size, ranging from microcolloids to larger macroaggregates. They are administered either intravascularly (usually intra-arterially) or by direct instillation into either specific body cavities or cystic lesions, where the resultant high concentration (dose) may exert a therapeutic effect. When radiocolloids (gold-198 colloid: physical half-life, 2.7 days; beta emission, .96 MeV; gamma emission, .41 MeV; phosphorus-32 colloid) are injected into malignant pleural and peritoneal effusions, they frequently limit the rate of reaccumulation. Phosphorus-32 colloid, combined with cisplatinum administered intraperitoneally, has also been effective in treating recurrent ovarian carcinoma and in cystic brain tumor by reducing tumor hypersecretion after direct instillation of the radiocolloid. Radioparticles, such as ytterium-90 (physical half-life, 2.7 days; beta emissions, 2.2 MeV; gamma emission, none) and phosphorus-32 microspheres, have been used to treat metastatic liver cancer; rhenium-186-hydroxyethylenediphosphonic acid (HEDP) (physical half-life, 90.6 hours; beta emission, 1.07 MeV; gamma emissions, .137 MeV, .122 MeV) is one of many chelates used to treat inflammatory arthritis (radiation synovectomy).

Treatment of Metastatic Liver Cancer

The spread of cancer from the bowel, genitourinary tract, or lung is hematogenous, and metastatic hepatic growth results, in part, from hepatic arterial blood supply. Therapy for this malignant complication is difficult, because the normal liver is relatively radiosensitive and the size of the liver makes it hard to direct therapy exclusively to the lesion while sparing normal liver. Optimum therapy would require direct administration to the lesion and tracer retention without significant metabolism and systemic distribution. Administration of radiocolloids into the hepatic artery (e.g., gold-198 and phosphorus-32) was not encouraging because of limited lesion retention, radiocolloid metabolism, and systemic distribution. Glass microspheres incorporating phosphorus-32 and ytterium-90 were developed, and because they showed minimal leaching of the radioisotope, they are being studied as potential therapeutic agents for metastatic liver cancer (15). Based on hepatic dosimetry, ytterium-90 glass microspheres appear to be the optimum radiopharmaceutical for this type of therapy (16, 17). Early results have produced guarded optimism.

Radiation Synovectomy

Rheumatoid arthritis (RA) is a chronic progressive disease involving the joint synovial membrane that proliferates, causing pannus formation and destruction of the articular cartilage. As many as 1% to 3% of the United States population has RA, and more than half of those affected have involvement of the knee joint. Therapies consist of analgesic and anti-inflammatory drugs, steroids, and antimetabolites. When medical therapy fails to control synovial proliferation, inflammation, and pain (particularly in the knee), surgical synevectomy is the preferred treatment. Surgical synovectomy removes the inflamed synovium, relieving the pain and eliminating further destruction of the joint. Because it is technically impossible to completely remove all of the synovia surgically, other approaches, such as chemical synovectomy (e.g., osmic acid, alkylating agents) and radiation synovectomy (ytterium-90; gold-198; erbium-169: physical half-life, 9.5 days; beta emission, .34 MeV; gamma emission, .03 MeV; rhenium-186; radiocolloids or radioparticles) (18), have also been tried. In recent years, Sledge and associates (19) used dysprosium-105-ferric hydroxide macroaggregates (FHMA) (physical half-life, 2.3 hours: beta emission, 1.30 MeV; gamma emissions, .05, .1, .5 MeV) to treat knees with stage II RA with excellent results. Its efficacy is the result of its optimum synovial penetration (Table 3) and limited joint leakage, which is reflected by very low liver uptake (.17%). Patients so treated have remained either symptom free or with reduced discomfort and decreased synovial proliferation for more than 2 years. Because of the short physical half-life of dysprosium-165, other radioisotopes, such as rhenium-186 and samarium-153, are now being studied.

Although the knee has been the principal joint treated with radiation synovectomy, smaller joints of the hands, wrists, and ankles have also responded to this form of therapy (18). In addition to RA, radiation synovectomy has been successfully used to treat the pain and discomfort of hemophiliac arthropathy, pigmented villonodular synovitis, and seronegative arthridities (18).

In certain situations, radioparticle therapy may be advantageous. We can expect that radioparticle therapy will use alpha-emitters, such as astatine-211 (physical half-life, 7.2 hours; alpha energy, 6.8 MeV) and bismuth-212 (physical half-life, 1 hour; alpha energy, 7.8 MeV), and the beta-emitters, such as copper-67 (physical half-life, 61.9 hours; beta emission, .58 MeV; gamma emission, .185 MeV), palladium-109 (physical half-life, 13.5 hours; beta emission, 1.03 MeV; gamma emission, .088

TABLE 3.—Optimum Synovial Penetration

Radioisotope	Beta Energy (MeV)	Tissue Penetration (mm)
Ytterium-90	0.34	11.0
Samarium-153	0.819	2.7
Gold-198	0.96	3.6
Rhenium-186	1.07	3.7
Erbium-169	0.34	1.0
Dysprosium-165	1.30	5.7

(Courtesy of R.A. Holmes, M.D.)

MeV), and rhenium-188 (physical half-life, 17 hours; beta emission, 2.12 MeV; gamma emission, .155 MeV). It is likely that these newer therapeutic radioisotopes will replace those presently available and that because of their physical characteristics (e.g., half-life, energy, and tissue penetration), the particulate radiopharmaceutical will be individualized for the clinical problem.

Radioimmunotherapy

The basis of radioimmunotherapy (RIT) is the availability of a specific radiolabeled antibody against tumor-specific and/or tumor-associated antigens. The antibodies are immunoglobulins, usually of the IgG class (MW 150,000 daltons), made by host plasma cells and precursor B lymphocytes. They circulate throughout the blood and lymph and bind to the specific antigen against which they were produced, forming an antibody-antigen complex. They may be polyclonal where the antigenic stimulus is heterogenous (i.e., reacts with different determinants on the antigen) or monoclonal (MoAb) where the antigenic stimulus is homogenous (i.e., reacts with a single antigenic focus.) The immunoglobulin molecule can selectively be cleaved into fragments by the proteolytic enzymes papain and pepsin. These fragments retain discrete properties, such as antigen binding (Fab fragments) and complement fixation (Fc fragment, MW 50,000 dalton).

Polyclonal antibodies, which are widely used for many immunochemical procedures, were the first radiolabeled antibodies used for tumor therapy. They were bound to iodine-131 using the radiolabeling technique devised by Pressman and Korngold (20). This has become a standard method for documenting specific immune uptake while correcting for nonspecific extra cellular uptake. Iodine-131–labeled antiferritin polyclonal antibody has been used in patients with primary hepatic cell cancer (hepatoma) with varying response that apparently is the result of large tumor volume (> 2,300 cm³) and a low mean tumor-to-liver ratio (21). In patients with refractory Hodgkin's disease, the radioiodinated antiferritin MoAb produced more positive objective response (21). Bone marrow toxicity with thrombocytopenia (< 100,00/dL) was observed in 50% of the study patients, and a small number required platelet transfusion. Allergic reactions to repeated cycles of antibody therapy were avoided by using different host species with each cycle of therapy (e.g., first rabbit, second pig, third monkey).

In 1975, Kohler and Milstein (22) developed the mouse spleen–myeloma hybridoma technique to generate monoclonal antibodies. Theoretically, the advantages of hybridoma MoAbs are their high specificity, their compositional homogeniety, and their ability to produce unlimited quantities of antibody. In practice, however, the yield of most MoAb-producing clones frequently is lower than anticipated. Production can be improved by using non–immunoglobulin-producing myeloma cells and better immunogenic antigens (specific epitopes). Because a limitation of immunotherapy using xenogeneic antibodies (i.e., mouse, rabbit) is the tendency for an immune response against repeated therapeutic antibodies to develop (e.g., development of human antimouse antibody [HAMA]) this may in part be overcome if chimeric mouse/human antibodies can be constructed, which decrease the amount of foreign protein but maintain antitumor specificity. Studies using the iodine-131 chimeric B 72.3 (human IgG4) in metastatic colorectal cancer demonstrated longer plasma retention, slower tumor localization, and the absence of immune response after repeated injections (23).

Because the objective of RIT is to exploit the tumor specificity of monclonal antibodies by conjugating an agent with the ability to selectively destroy the cancer cell, it is important to select an appropriate radioisotope. Iodine-131 is the most commonly used radioisotope for RIT, even though it dehalogenates in vivo, emits a medium-energy gamma photon, and has a maximum beta-particle range of approximately 200 cell diameters (24). Optimally, beta-emitters, such as rhenium-186 and -188, ytterium-90, copper-67, or palladium-109, should be used for their high local radiation deposition and their ability to chelate to the MoAb. All can emit radiation to either sub- or multicellular ranges, and they can be selected specifically for certain cancers and cancer size. Alpha-emitters such as astatine-211 have been considered, but astatine-211 is a questionable therapeutic radiolabel because of its unstable protein binding and its low protein-bound specific activity. Lower-energy electron emitters (i.e., conversion electrons, Auger electrons, Coster-Kronig electrons), such as bromine-77 (physical half-life, 57 hours, Auger electron [L], 1.3 KeV; Coster-Kronig electron [LM], .04–.08 KeV), rhuthenium-907 (physical half-life 2.88 days; Auger electron [L], 2.2 KeV; Auger electron [M], 15.5–17.8 KeV), and mercury-197 (physical half-life 2.7 days, Auger electron [L], 12.0 KeV), can irradiate tissue at the cellular and subcellular levels. This may be of particular importance when the therapeutic MoAb is internalized in the cancer cell.

Although therapeutic trials of MoAb have been actively pursued for many years, their success has been limited and the number of clinical studies comparatively small. Malignant melanoma has been the most widely studied cancer, because it causes 65% of all the skin cancer deaths with metastases to the lungs, liver, and brain. It is resistent to chemotherapy and external-beam irradiation. A melanoma-associated antigen, p97, has been isolated, and radioiodinated murine anti-p97 IgG has been detected by imaging in 88% of melanomas. Subsequently, anti-p97 Fab fragments were used for RIT (25). Additional MoAb against epitopes of the melanoma-associated antigen have been isolated and radiolabeled, but all have shown only limited success to date.

Recent FDA approval of the indium-111–labeled murine B72.3 antibody, which reacts with a tumor-associated glycoprotein (TAG-72) expressed by several epithelial-derived cancers (colon, breast, lung, ovary, stomach, prostate) for immunoscintigraphy (Oncoscin, Cytogen Corporation, Princeton, NJ), has renewed interest in using iodine-131–labeled B72.3 antibody for immunotherapy. Preliminary phase I–II studies are under way in several laboratories, but to date, use of neither the whole antibody nor antibody fragments has shown much success.

Optimism for the use of radioimmunotherapy has existed for more than a decade, but to date, it has been generally disappointing. As a specific therapeutic "magic bullet," RIT has many favorable characteristics: specific antigen-antibody affinity, attachment of a radioisotope without altering its binding affinity, low nontumor activity, and adequate tumor retention time. In contrast, problems occur when the antibody conjugate has limited access to the tumor because of its size, the tumor cells have low antigenic expression, the tumor lacks specific antigens, and immune complex formation fails in the target area as a result of the presence of circulating antigen and conjugate degeneration. The latter may result in the release of radioisotope and allergic reactions on repeat administrations. This, in turn, results in lower tumor uptake and ineffective therapy. Although research continues in the area of radioimmunotherapy, it is unlikely to provide more than a selective therapeutic adjuvant in special clinical situations.

Peptide Receptor System

It has long been observed that humoral factors can effect the growth and regression of human tumors. Studies have shown that the cancer cell is composed of a myriad of receptor sites that bind these peptides, which in turn stimulate tumor-cell proliferation or inhibition. Many of the tumor receptors originate embryologically from the neural crest cells and take on the *a*mine *p*recursor *u*ptake and *d*ecarboxylation (APUD) characteristics of neuroendocrine secretors. One such tumor receptor is the somatostatin receptor, which is found on a variety of human tumors. These include pituitary tumors, endocrine pancreatic tumors (e.g., insulinoma, glucagonoma, gastrinomas, and vipomas), carcinoids, paragangliomas, small-cell lung cancer, thyroid medullary carcinoma, pheochromocytomas, meningiomas, astrocytomas, neuroblastomas, and some breast tumors. Chronic treatment with somatostatin or a somatostatin analogue (tyrosine-3-octreotide [Tyr-3-octreotide]) has resulted in the control of hormonal hypersecretion and tumor shrinkage in patients with acromegaly, insulinomas, and metastatic carcinoid and growth inhibition in experimental transplanted chondrosarcoma and pancreatic carcinomas. The somatostatin tumor receptors are demonstrated on human tumors by classic biochemical binding techniques and in vitro autoradiography. By using a bifunctional chelate (DTPA), iodine-123 has been coupled to the somatostatin analogue Tyr-3-octreotide and used to image somatostatin receptor–positive tumors. In a series of patients with somatostatin receptor–positive tumors, Lamberts et al. (26) were able to image both primary tumors mentioned previously and metastases. Because of the availability of more favorable radiopharmacokinetics, these authors, using indium-111 DTPA-octreotide in a larger series of somatostatin receptor–positive tumors, were able to detect more tumors more rapidly and with less liver uptake. Coupled with therapeutic amounts of the somatostatin analogue, indium-111 DTPA-octreotide has been used to assess its effect on somatostatin receptor–positive tumors (26).

Receptor-mediated endocytosis (internalization) usually occurs when polypeptide hormones bind to high-affinity receptors on cell surfaces. Imaging of somatostatin receptor–positive tumors, such as metastatic carcinoid tumors, can be accomplished 48 hours post injection, suggesting internalization, because tumor surface uptake elutes well before this time. It is thus likely that a radiolabeled beta-emitting radioisotope coupled to a somatostatin analogue could provide a means of treating certain human cancers. To date, no direct clinical application of this therapeutic hypothesis has occurred. However, cold octreotide given in doses of 300 μg per day has been used therapeutically with success in growth hormone–secreting pituitary tumors, primary and metastatic endocrine pancreatic tumors, and metastatic carcinoid.

The therapeutic potential of polypeptide receptor agents is generally high, because a variety of compounds, including growth factors, have been isolated and shown to have high receptor affinity on tumor cells. Although the radiolabeling of small proteins is complex, methods using bifunctional chelates are well studied and adaptable to chelating a number of beta- and alpha-emitting radioisotopes. Techniques for direct conjugation of the protein to the metalloisotope are being developed and should become available for this form of therapy in the future.

Future Expectations

Unsealed-source radiotherapy uses many methods to deliver concentrated radiation to target locations. Although the number of ways to accomplish delivery and localization is impressive, clinical success, to date, has often been disappointing. It seems obvious that future efforts will concentrate on immune and protein receptor techniques. Although one can only speculate on the outcome of receptor therapy at this time, it would appear that with the number and variety of peptide receptors and continued improvement in radiolabeling chemistry, we are justified in retaining enthusiasm for future developments. Our nuclear armory may still produce the therapeutic "magic bullet."

References

1. Pecher C: Biological investigations with radioactive calcium and strontium: Preliminary report on the use of radioactive strontium in the treatment of metastatic bone cancer. *Univ Cal Pub Pharmacol* 2:117–149, 1942.
2. Schmidt CG, Firusian N: 89-Sr for the treatment of incurable pain in patient with neoplastic osseous infiltration. *Int J Clin Pharmacol Res* 9:199–205, 1974.
3. Robinson RG, Spicer JA, Preston DE, et al: Treatment of metastatic bone pain with strontium-89. *Nucl Med Biol* 14:219–222, 1987.
4. Porter AT, McEwan AJB, Powe JE, et al: Results of a randomized phase-III trial to evaluate the efficacy of strontium-89 adjuvant to local field external beam irradiation in the management of endocrine resistant metastatic prostate cancer. *Int J Radiat Oncol Biol Phys* 25:805–813, 1993.
5. Mathieu L, Chevalier P, Galy G, et al: Preparation of 186-rhenium labelled

HEDP and its possible use in the treatment of osseous neoplasma. *Int J Appl Radiat Isot* 30:725–727, 1979.

6. Maxon HR, Schroder LE, Thomas SR, et al: Re-186 (Sn) HEDP for treatment of painful occeous metastases: Initial clinical experience in 20 patients with hormone-resistant prostate cancer. *Radiology* 176:155–159, 1990.

7. Goeckler WF, Edwards B, Volkert WA, et al: Skeletal localization of Samarium-153 chelates: Potential therapeutic bone agents. *J Nucl Med* 28:495–504, 1987.

8. Lattimer JC, Corwin LA, Stapleton J, et al: Clinical and clinicopathologic effects of Samarium 153-EDTMP administered intravenously in normal dogs. *J Nucl Med* 31:586–593, 1990.

9. Farhangi M, Holmes RA, Volkert WA, et al: Samarium-153 EDTMP: Pharmacokinetic, toxicity and pain response using an escalating dose schedule in treatment of metastatic bone cancer. *J Nucl Med* 33:1451–1458, 1992.

10. Atkins HL, Mausner LF, Strivastava SC, et al: Biodistribution of Sn-117m (4+) DTPA for palliative therapy of painful osseous metastasis. *Radiology* 186:279–283, 1993.

11. Beierwalters WH, Wieland DM, Yu T, et al: Adrenal imaging agents: Rationale, synthesis, formulation and metabolism. *Semin Nucl Med* 8:5–16, 1978.

12. Beierwalters WH: Applications of [131I]m-iodobenzlguanidine([131I]MIBG). *Nucl Med Biol* 14:184–189, 1987.

13. Mangner WM, Dufford RW Jr: Hypertension secondary to pheochromocytoma. *Bull N Y Acad Med* 58:139–143, 1983.

14. Shapiro B, Von Moll L, McEwan A, et al: I-131 metaiodobenzlguanidine (MIBG) uptake by a wide range of neuroendocrine tumors other than pheochromocytoma and neuroblastoma. *J Nucl Med* 27:908–916, 1986.

15. Ehrhardt GJ, Day DE: Therapeutic use of 90Y microspheres. *Nucl Med Biol* 14:233–242, 1987.

16. Herba MJ, Illescas FF, Thirlwell MP: Hepatic malignancies: Improved treatment with intraarterial Y-90. *Radiology* 169:311–314, 1988.

17. Russell JL, Carden JL, Herron HL: Dosimetry calculations for radioactive ytterium-90 used for treatment of liver cancer. *Endocurie Therapy/Hyperthermia Oncology* 4:171–186, 1988.

18. Zuckerman JD, Sledge CB, Shortkroff S, et al: Treatment of rheumatoid arthritis using radiopharmaceuticals. *Nucl Med Biol* 14:211–218, 1987.

19. Sledge CB: Treatment of rheumatoid synovitis of the knee with intraarticular injection of dysprosium-165 ferric hydroxide macroaggregates. *Arthritis Rheum* 29:153–158, 1986.

20. Pressman D, Korngold L: The in vivo localization of anti-Wagner osteogenic sarcoma antibodies. *Cancer* 6:7619–7621, 1953.

21. Order SE, Stillwagon GB, Klein JL, et al: Iodine-131 antiferrin, a new treatment modality in hepatoma: A Radiation Therapy Oncology Group Study. *J Clin Oncol* 3:1573–1580, 1985.

22. Kohler G, Milstein C: Continuous culture of fused cells secreting antibody of proven defined specificity. *Nature* 256:495–500, 1975.

23. Meredith RF, Khazaeli MB, Platt WE, et al: Phase I trial of iodine-131-chimeric B 72.3 (human IgG4) in metastatic colorectal cancer. *J Nucl Med* 33:23–29, 1992.

24. Zalutsky MR: Antibody-mediated radiotherapy: Future prospects in antibodies in radiodiagnosis and therapy. Boca Raton, FL, CRC Press, 1988, pp 215–224.

25. Larson SM, Carrasqiullo JA, Korhn KA, et al: Localization of 131I-labeled p97-specific Fab fragments in human melanoma as a basis for radiotherapy. *J Clin Invest* 72:2101–2107, 1983.

26. Lamberts SWJ, Krenning EP, Reubi JC: The role of somatostatin and its analog in the diagnosis and treatment of tumors. *Endocr Rev* 12:212–224, 1993.

1 Pulmonary

Introduction

This has been a particularly productive year for investigators publishing articles on pulmonary embolism. The revised Prospective Investigation of Pulmonary Embolism Diagnosis (PIOPED) criteria have been presented. Chronic perfusion defects/silent emboli in deep venous thrombosis have been studied. An algorithm that bypasses pulmonary angiography has been developed, patient stratification has been suggested, and improvements in technique are available. Studies that relate to understanding of referring physicians' scan reports also have been done.

Alexander Gottschalk, M.D.

Frequent Asymptomatic Pulmonary Embolism in Patients With Deep Venous Thrombosis

Moser KM, Fedullo PF, LittleJohn JK, Crawford R (Univ of California, San Diego; Burroughs Wellcome Co, Research Triangle Park, NC)
JAMA 271:223–225, 1994   124-95-1–1

Introduction.—It is generally accepted that venous thromboembolism represents a single process, yet the treatment and diagnostic implications of the concept are not generally applied. These include needs to evaluate the lower extremity veins of patients with pulmonary embolism and to look for pulmonary embolism in patients with deep vein thrombosis. As part of a dosing study of tissue-type plasminogen activator, a high frequency of pulmonary embolism was found in patients with deep vein thrombosis.

Methods.—An open, multicenter, dose-ranging study was designed to examine the safety and pharmacokinetic characteristics of intravenous tissue-type plasminogen activator in deep vein thrombosis and pulmonary embolism. Seven patients with pulmonary embolism and 44 with deep vein thrombosis were studied. All the latter underwent perfusion-ventilation lung scans, chest radiography, and venography before and after therapy with tissue-type plasminogen activator and IV heparin. The study was terminated for technical rather than medical reasons.

Results.—Forty-three percent of the patients with deep vein thrombosis were found to have a preinfusion lung scan score of 5 or greater, and all met the Prospective Investigation of Pulmonary Embolism Diagnosis (PIOPED) criteria for high probability. Thirty-four patients in the deep vein thrombosis group had no symptoms of pulmonary embolism and underwent both preinfusion and postinfusion scans; 38% of them had preinfusion scan scores of 5 or higher (i.e., high probability). The mean scan score for these patients declined from 4.3 to 2.7 after infusion.

Conclusion.—Nearly 40% of the patients who are admitted for treatment of deep vein thrombosis have lung scan evidence of asymptomatic pulmonary embolism. These findings underscore the need to consider venous thromboembolism as a single disorder. If lung scanning is not done in a patient with deep venous thrombosis until symptoms of pulmonary embolism develop, it often generates discussion about the apparent failure of heparin therapy and the need for other interventions. The authors routinely perform a lung scan as part of the initial evaluation for patients with deep vein thrombosis.

▶ This is a very important paper. As far as is known, this concept was first articulated by Drs. Dorfman, Cronan, and Tupper approximately 7 years ago (1). However, they placed their findings in the radiologic literature rather than in a place where individuals who ordered lung scans could see it. These data expand the indication for ordering the ventilation-perfusion scan. They also point out that the more you know about the legs of a patient with pulmonary embolism, the better off you are. This will be a recurrent theme in the following group of articles.

We have one nagging concern regarding these data: The authors suggest that these patients all have silent emboli; we are not so sure. The data we have (from the old USPET trial of the '70s) indicate that slightly less than half these individuals could well have a chronic perfusion deficit from a previous pulmonary embolism and not an acute pulmonary embolism. Even so, more than half of these patients probably have silent pulmonary emboli, because perfusion scans in this group improved after therapy. It would take little effort for the authors to ascertain which of these patients had a history of previous pulmonary embolism; we hope they do this. We know from data from the PIOPED trial (2) that one of the most likely sources of misdiagnosis of a high probability for pulmonary embolism is the chronic perfusion defect in patients with a previous pulmonary embolism.—A. Gottschalk, M.D.

References

1. Dorfman GS, et al: *Am J Radiol* 148:263, 1987.
2. The PIOPED Investigators: *JAMA* 263:2753, 1990.

Quantitative Plasma D-Dimer Levels Among Patients Undergoing Pulmonary Angiography for Suspected Pulmonary Embolism
Goldhaber SZ, Simons GR, Elliott CG, Haire WD, Toltzis R, Blacklow SC, Doolittle MH, Weinberg DS (Harvard Med School, Boston; LDS Hosp, Salt Lake

City, Utah; Univ of Nebraska, Omaha; et al)
JAMA 270:2819–2822, 1993   124-95-1–2

Introduction.—It would be very helpful to have a blood test for pulmonary embolism (PE) that possesses a high negative predictive value comparable to the serum creatine kinase that is used to exclude acute myocardial infarction. D-dimer is a degradatory product of endogenous fibrinolysis, which is seen when cross-linked fibrin clots are lysed. There are indications that plasma levels of D-dimer, which are estimated by enzyme-linked immunosorbent assay, are usually elevated in patients with acute PE.

Objective and Methods.—The negative predictive value of a D-dimer level less than 500 ng/mL was examined in 173 patients with suspected acute PE who underwent diagnostic pulmonary arteriography. The plasma D-dimer level, quantified by monoclonal antibody assay, was compared in a blinded manner with the results from a pulmonary angiography.

Results.—Angiography results were abnormal in 45 patients. Most demographic and clinical features were similar in patients with and without PE. Only 3 of 35 patients whose D-dimer value was less than 500 ng/mL had abnormal angiograms, for a negative predictive value of 91.4%. A level greater than 500 ng/mL was 93% sensitive for acute PE, but it was only 25% specific and had a positive predictive value of only 30%. Sensitivity was about the same at levels of 300–600 ng/mL, but it was more specific at a cutoff level of 600 ng/mL. There were 10 patients with D-dimer levels less than 500 ng/mL who had low-probability lung scans. All had normal angiograms.

Conclusion.—A plasma D-dimer level of less than 500 ng/mL strongly indicates that the pulmonary angiogram will be negative despite symptoms suggestive of acute PE.

▶ A simple test that would further confirm a low probability ventilation-perfusion (V/Q) scan diagnosis would be very useful. As you may know, well-known and well-respected pulmonolgists (Dr. Russell Hull, for example) have suggested that the low-probability V/Q scan is not reliable enough for clinical work. They further indicate that it should be abandoned and that anything that is not high probability should be considered nondiagnostic. I do not agree, and I think that the low-probability study, particularly with the revised criteria suggested by the Prospective Investigation of Pulmonary Embolism Diagnosis (PIOPED) group, is usable and is as reliable as the high-probability examination.

However, most of the referring physicians I talk with would be happier if there were an additional simple study that could be used to confirm the V/Q scan result. For me, a key aspect of this article is that the 10 patients with low-probability V/Q scans and D-dimer levels less than the cutoff point had no pulmonary emboli on angiography. Unfortunately, 2 of my residents tried a similar protocol in a small series of patients in one of our community hospitals, and they did not do so well. Nevertheless, my overall aggregate results are that only 1 of 15 patients with a low-probability V/Q scan and normal D-dimer levels showed a pulmonary embolism. This result approaches the precision of the pulmonary angiogram, which is about 5%. This is exciting, but a large prospective trial is needed to see whether it really works.

The interested reader may also want to obtain an article by the McMaster group on D-dimer levels in inpatients with clinically suspected pulmonary embolism (1).—A. Gottschalk, M.D.

Reference

1. Ginsberg JS, et al: *Chest* 104:1679, 1993.

Contribution of D-Dimer Plasma Measurement and Lower-Limb Venous Ultrasound to the Diagnosis of Pulmonary Embolism: A Decision Analysis Model
Perrier A, Bounameaux H, Morabia A, de Moerloose P, Slosman D, Unger P-F, Junod A (Univ Hosp, Geneva)
Am Heart J 127:624–635, 1994   124-95-1-3

Introduction.—Pulmonary embolism (PE) causes as many as 50,000 deaths in the United States each year. Pulmonary angiography is required for diagnosis in a large proportion of patients. Because this procedure is invasive and costly, and is associated with considerable morbidity, alternative diagnostic methods have been sought. The potential value of 2 tests in the diagnostic workup for PE—measurement of plasma levels of D-dimer and lower-limb venous ultrasound—were assessed.

Methods.—The 2 diagnostic tests were compared using a decision analysis model. The decision tree describes 5 possible strategies for managing patients in the emergency department who have suspected PE and abnormal lung scan results. These strategies are no treatment, treatment without further testing, angiography, D-dimer with or without ultrasound, and with or without ultrasound angiography. Based on previous research, the expected proportion of deep vein thrombosis (DVT) revealed by ultrasound in patients with PE was assumed to be 60%.

Results.—Those D-dimer measurements of less than 500 µg/L could be used with reliability to exclude PE in patients with an abnormal but not high-probability—and, therefore, inconclusive—lung scan. In patients with a high clinical suspicion of PE, however, a D-dimer measurement of less than 500 µg/L does not exclude PE. When D-dimer measurements were greater than 500 µg/L, this strategy had no positive predictive value for PE and should be followed by ultrasound, which may replace angiography when DVT is revealed. When ultrasound is negative, pulmonary angiography should be performed.

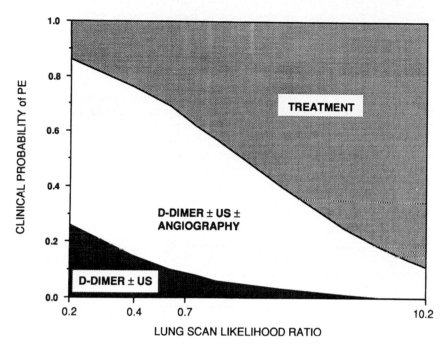

Fig 1–1.—Baseline analysis for all lung scan results. This diagram is a two-way sensitivity analysis. It shows the ranking of the 3 best strategies according to clinical probability of PE and lung scan result. (Courtesy of Perrier A, Bounameaux H, Morabia A, et al: *Am Heart J* 127:624–635, 1994.)

Conclusion.—The Prospective Investigation of Pulmonary Embolism Diagnosis, published in 1990, found that approximately half the patients with suspected PE will require pulmonary angiography for diagnosis. It has been calculated that the combination of D-dimer measurement and ultrasound might reduce the need for angiography by one third in patients whose lung scans are inconclusive and those who have an intermediate clinical probability of PE (pPE). Patients with very low-probability lung scans would be treated according to the strategy including DD with or without ultrasound up to a slightly higher pPE. A high-probability lung scan remains diagnostic of PE, except in the rare instance of a patient with a very low pPE (Fig 1–1).

▶ Dr. Junod's group has been worrying about this problem for some time. This article offers much useful data, some of which have been abstracted for you. In addition, it is a beautiful introduction to the thesis developed by Dr. Dalen, which is explained in the article that follows.—A. Gottschalk, M.D.

When Can Treatment Be Withheld in Patients With Suspected Pulmonary Embolism?
Dalen JE
Arch Intern Med 153:1415–1418, 1993   124-95-1–4

Background.—Pulmonary angiography and contrast venography, the most accurate tests for the diagnosis of pulmonary embolism and deep venous thrombosis (DVT), are expensive and invasive. Two noninvasive tests for DVT, impedance plethysmography (IPG) and ultrasonography, are accurate; however, the ventilation-perfusion (V/Q) lung scan is far less useful for diagnosing pulmonary embolism. A high incidence of concurrent proximal DVT has been found in patients with acute pulmonary embolism. As a result, patients with a nondiagnostic V/Q scan and positive results on IPG or ultrasonography can be treated with anticoagulants. However, the need for angiography in patients with suspected pulmonary embolism who have a nondiagnostic V/Q scan and negative results on IPG or ultrasonography of the legs is controversial. A clinical management strategy designed to avoid the use of pulmonary angiography in such patients was presented (table).

Rationale.—In a previously published study of 248 patients with suspected DVT, anticoagulants were withheld because the IPG was normal. Deep venous thrombosis was diagnosed in only 1 patient during follow-up, and no patient had pulmonary embolism. The results were similar in a study of 139 pregnant women with negative serial IPGs and a 3-month postpartum follow-up and in a study of 289 patients with normal IPGs on serial testing and 6 months of follow-up. A similarly favorable outcome might be expected if anti-coagulant treatment were withheld in patients with suspected pulmonary embolism who have nondiagnostic lung scans and negative IPGs or ultrasonography of the legs. One previous study tested this hypothesis and found 10 episodes (1 fatal) of venous thromboembolism among 801 patients with negative IPGs.

Conclusion.—Data indicate that patients with suspected venous thromboembolism and no evidence of proximal DVT have a low risk of

Indications for Treatment of Suspected Pulmonary Embolism

| | Impedance Plethysmography or Ultrasonogram | |
Ventilation/Perfusion	Positive	Negative
High probability	Treat	Treat
Nondiagnostic	Treat	No treatment,* serial leg examinations
Normal	Treat	No treatment

*Pulmonary angiography may be indicated if clinical suspicion of pulmonary embolism is very high.
(Courtesy of Dalen JE: *Arch Intern Med* 153:1415–1418, 1993.)

subsequent venous thromboembolism. Therefore, withholding antigoagulation therapy is an acceptable alternative to performing pulmonary angiography in such patients. Repeated IPG or ultrasonography at 5 and 10 days seems appropriate, because some patients in the studies cited had a positive IPG after negative findings at baseline. The proposed clinical management strategy is cost-effective and would avoid a costly, invasive test in thousands of patients.

▶ I suspect this will be a widely read and widely followed article, and I suggest that you read it in its entirety. We practiced at an institution where pulmonary angiography was frequently done by experienced angiographers. Angiography is an extremely accurate and effective test that provides answers right away. We suspect that, in most institutions, it is cheaper than the 5-serial leg studies suggested by Dr. Hull's group (1–5), who are quoted so often in the original article on which this abstract is based.

However, it is also true that frequent use of pulmonary angiography is rare in most institutions in this country. Consequently, Dr. Dalen's scheme to avoid pulmonary angiograms is likely to be extremely well received. However, there are some aspects that I find a little unusual. For example, why do a leg investigation with a high probability V/Q scan when you are going to treat the patient regardless of the outcome? We suspect this was included because many pulmonologists control the IPG studies and may do them before the patient needs a lung scan. A similar question could be asked about the normal V/Q scan. Why not stop there? We would add that the Prospective Investigation of Pulmonary Embolism Diagnosis (PIOPED) data suggest that a very low-probability V/Q scan (one with a gestalt probability of approximately 5%), when associated with a low clinical suspicion of pulmonary embolism, also is extremely reliable. Finally, will tests such as D-dimer obviate the need for serial leg testing? Obviously, data to support or reject this idea must be collected. As always, there are still problems to be solved in the diagnosis of pulmonary embolism.—A. Gottschalk, M.D.

References

1. Hull R, et al: *Circulation* 64:622, 1981.
2. Hull R, et al, in Colman RW, et al (eds): *Hemostasis and Thrombosis.* Philadelphia, JB Lippincott Co, 1987, pp 1220–1239.
3. Hull RD, et al: *Chest* 97:23, 1990.
4. Hull RD, et al: *Arch Intern Med* 149:2549, 1989.
5. Hull RD, et al: *Ann Intern Med* 94 (part 1):439, 1990.

Ventilation-Perfusion Scintigraphy in the PIOPED Study. Part II. Evaluation of the Scintigraphic Criteria and Interpretations
Gottschalk A, Sostman HD, Coleman RE, Juni JE, Thrall J, McKusick KA, Froelich JW, Alavi A (Michigan State Univ, East Lansing; Duke Univ, Durham, North Carolina; William Beaumont Hosp, Royal Oak, Mich; et al)
J Nucl Med 34:1119–1126, 1993   124-95-1–5

Introduction.—The computerized consensus descriptions from the ventilation-perfusion (V/Q) scan data obtained in the Prospective Investigation of Pulmonary Embolism Diagnosis (PIOPED) study were reviewed. The validity of the PIOPED interpretive criteria for categorical definition and for probability estimates of pulmonary embolism (PE) was retrospectively evaluated.

Methods.—Each criterion used for categorical probability evaluation was analyzed by comparing the components of the detailed descriptions of the V/Q scans produced by the members of the PIOPED Nuclear Medicine Working Group with the descriptions of the angiographic findings produced by the PIOPED Angiography Working Group.

Results.—Among the criteria for low probability, any perfusion defect that was seen with a larger chest radiographic abnormality and the finding of small or few matched segmental perfusion defects with a normal chest radiograph were considered appropriate. However, an unacceptably high rate of PE occurred in patients with this designation who had a single, moderate, mismatched segmental perfusion defect with a normal chest radiograph. Among the criteria for intermediate probability, multiple matched V/Q abnormalities were inappropriately stringent. Among the criteria for high probability, whole lung perfusion defects were appropriate. However, because 29% of the patients with 2 segmental mismatches on the V/Q scans did not have PE, this criterion may be too stringent.

Discussion.—Three alterations to the PIOPED criteria for PE probability classification are recommended (table). Scans demonstrating a single, moderate, segmental mismatch should be classified as intermediate, rather than low probability. Extensive matched V/Q defects should be classified as low rather than of intermediate probability. The finding of 2.5 rather than 2 large mismatched defects more accurately categorizes high probability, the presence of less than 2.5 large mismatched defects should be classified as intermediate probability.

▶ For those of you who are wondering how dumb the PIOPED Nuclear Medicine Working Group could be to call a moderate-sized (i.e., subsegmental) mismatch a low probability for PE, let me point out that the definitive paper by Rosen and associates (1), which clearly showed that a subsegmental mismatch was best called intermediate, appeared in 1986. However, the PIOPED criteria were developed in 1983–1984 and were cast in concrete toward the end of 1984 using the best data available. What we did not know turned out to hurt us a lot. We did know, however, that we had to computerize all our findings (as did the PIOPED angiographers), so that the re-

Revised PIOPED V/Q Scan Criteria

High Probability (≥80%)

≥2 Large mismatched segmental perfusion defects or the arithmetic equivalent in moderate or large + moderate defects*.

Intermediate Probability (20%–79%)

One moderate to two large mismatched segmental perfusion defects or the arithmetic equivalent in moderate or large + moderate defects*.

Single matched ventilation-perfusion defect with clear chest radiograph†.

Difficult to categorize as low or high, or not described as low or high.

Low Probability (≤19%)

Nonsegmental perfusion defects (e.g., cardiomegaly, enlarged aorta, enlarged hila, elevated diaphragm).

Any perfusion defect with a substantially larger chest radiographic abnormality.

Perfusion defects matched by ventilation abnormality† provided that there are: (1) clear chest radiograph and (2) some areas of normal perfusion in the lungs.

Any number of small perfusion defects with a normal chest radiograph.

Normal

No perfusion defects or perfusion outlines exactly the shape of the lungs seen on the chest radiograph (note that hilar and aortic impressions may be seen and the chest radiograph and/or ventilation study may be abnormal).

---

* Two large, mismatched perfusion defects are borderline for "high probability." Individual readers may correctly interpret individual scans with this pattern as "high probability." In general, it is recommended that more than this degree of mismatch be present for the "high probability" category.

† Very extensive matched defects can be categorized as "low probability." Single V/Q matches are borderline for "low probability," and, thus, should be categorized as "intermediate" in most circumstances by most readers, although individual readers may correctly interpret individual scans with this pattern as "low probability."

(Courtesy of Gottschalk A, Sostman HD, Coleman RE, et al: *J Nucl Med* 34:1119–1126, 1993.)

vised criteria presented in this abstract could be obtained. A companion article to this article (2) tells those who are interested how this was done.

At this time I would like to pay tribue to one of my co-authors of this paper, Dr. H. Dirk Sostman. After assembling most of the data, writing drafts about his findings, and lecturing based on the results, I was about out of gas, simply plain tired of working with this material. Dirk put in a new tank of premium, and this publication was the result. We could never have done it without him.

The revised criteria seemed to represent an improvement. At the June 1994 Society of Nuclear Medicine meeting, the Duke group presented 2 papers indicating that these criteria performed better than did the original criteria (3, 4).

If you read on, you will see that in some patients a single moderate mismatch not only is unsatisfactory for low probability, but it can be a low high probability with appropriate stratification.—A. Gottschalk, M.D.

References

1. Rosen JM, et al: *J Nucl Med* 27:361, 1986.
2. Gottschalk A, et al: *J Nucl Med* 34:1109, 1993
3. Sostman HD, et al: *J Nucl Med* 35:25, 1994.
4. Sostman HD, et al: *J Nucl Med* 35:25, 1994.

Stratification of Patients According to Prior Cardiopulmonary Disease and Probability Assessment Based on the Number of Mismatched Segmental Equivalent Perfusion Defects: Approaches to Strengthen the Diagnostic Value of Ventilation/Perfusion Lung Scans in Acute Pulmonary Embolism

Stein PD, Gottschalk A, Henry JW, Shivkumar K (Henry Ford Heart and Vascular Inst, Detroit; Michigan State Univ, East Lansing)
Chest 104:1461–1467, 1993   124-95-1–6

Purpose.—To improve the probability estimates of acute pulmonary embolism (PE) based on the number of mismatched segmental perfusion defects on ventilation-perfusion lung scans, a table of positive predictive values and specificities was used as opposed to assigning categorical diagnoses of high, intermediate, or low probability. In addition, patients were stratified according to the presence or absence of previous cardiopulmonary disease to determine whether the ventilation-perfusion scan evaluation of PE among both clinical categories of patients would be enhanced.

Patients and Methods.—Ventilation-perfusion scans from 378 patients with acute PE and 672 patients in whom suspected PE was excluded were assessed. Data obtained from the collaborative study of the Prospective Investigation of Pulmonary Embolism Diagnosis (PIOPED) were used.

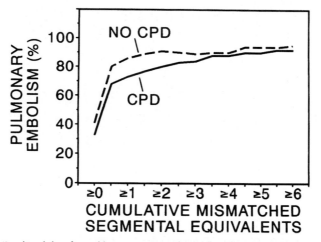

Fig 1–2.—Combined data from obligatory angiography group and physician requested angiography group showing predictive value of pulmonary embolism relative to the cumulative number of mismatched segmental equivalents. *Broken line* indicates patients with no prior cardiopulmonary disease (NO CPD). *Solid line* indicates patients with any prior cardiopulmonary disease (CPD). Significant differences occurred with ≥ .5 and ≥ 1 segmental equivalents (P < .02) and with ≥ 1.5 segmental equivalents (P < .05). (Courtesy of Stein PD, Gottschalk A, Henry JW, et al: *Chest* 104:1461–1467, 1993.)

Results.—All PIOPED patients in whom the diagnoses of PE or no PE was made by pulmonary angiogram were studied. In patients *without* previous cardiopulmonary disease, 1 or more mismatched segmental equivalents (Fig 1–2) indicated PE in 102 of 118 (86%) compared with 113 or 155 (73%) with previous cardiopulmonary disease. Two or more mismatched segmental equivalents were needed to indicate an 80% or greater probability of PE in those with previous cardiopulmonary disease (table). Stratification of patients according to previous or no previous history of cardiopulmonary disease enhanced the ability of the scan reader to assign an accurate positive predictive value and specificity to individual patients.

Conclusion.—Fewer mismatched segmental equivalent defects were required to indicate high probability of PE in those without previous cardiopulmonary disease compared with the PIOPED criteria. In some patients with no cardiopulmonary disease, intermediate probability would have been diagnosed using revised PIOPED criteria. However, when patients are stratified according to the presence or absence of previous cardiopulmonary disease, these indeterminate probability readings can be eliminated and a correct high-probability diagnosis can be made.

▶ At the risk of blowing our own horn too much, we think these data have significant diagnostic implications. In this case, stratification into different patient groups allows a more liberal use of diagnostic criteria with higher positive predictive value for those patients without previous cardiopulmonary disease. Incidentally, this stratification is done on clinical grounds,

Number of Mismatched Segmental Equivalent Defects and Positive Predictive Value Among All Patients With and Without Prior Cardiopulmonary Disease

Segmental Equivalents	Patients With No Prior Cardiopulmonary Disease (n = 421) PPV No. PE/No. PTS (%)	CI, %	Patients With Prior Cardiopulmonary Disease (n = 629) PPV No. PE/No. PTS (%)	CI, %	All Patients (n = 1,050) PPV No. PE/No. PTS (%)	CI, %
≥0.0	173/421 (41)	37–45	205/629 (33)†	29–37	378/1050 (36)	34–38
≥0.5	123/154 (80)	74–86	130/192 (68)‡	62–74	253/346 (73)	69–77
≥1.0	102/118 (86)	80–92	113/155 (73)‡	65–81	215/273 (79)	75–83
≥1.5	91/102 (89)	83–95	99/128 (77)§	69–85	190/230 (83)	79–87
≥2.0	79/87 (91)	85–97	91/114 (80)	72–88	170/201 (85)	79–91
≥2.5	72/80 (90)	84–96	87/105 (83)	75–91	159/185 (86)	80–92
≥3.0	65/73 (89)	81–97	81/97 (84)	76–92	146/170 (86)	80–92
≥3.5	60/67 (90)	82–98	77/88 (88)	82–94	137/155 (88)	82–94
≥4.0	57/63 (90)	82–98	74/84 (88)	80–96	131/147 (89)	83–95
≥4.5	50/53 (94)	88–100	70/78 (90)	84–96	120/131 (92)	88–96
≥5.0	49/52 (94)	88–100	65/72 (90)	82–98	114/124 (92)	88–96
≥5.5	47/50 (94)	88–100	61/66 (92)	86–98	108/116 (93)	89–97
≥6.0	42/44 (95)	89–100	59/64 (92)	86–98	101/108 (94)	90–98
≥6.5	40/42 (95)	89–100	56/61 (92)	86–98	96/103 (93)	87–99
≥7.0	38/40 (95)	89–100	51/56 (91)	83–99	89/96 (93)	87–99
≥7.5	34/36 (94)	86–100	43/47 (91)	83–99	77/83 (93)	87–99

Note: Obligatory angiography and physician-requested angiography. CI represents 95% confidence interval.
Abbreviations: PPV, positive predictive value; *PTS,* patients.
† P < .01.
‡ P < .02.
§ P < .05—No cardiopulmonary disease vs. any cardiopulmonary disease.
(Courtesy of Stein PD, Gottschalk A, Henry JW, et al: *Chest* 104:1461–1467, 1993.)

which are easily within the ability of a bright medical student and do not require a master pulmonologist.—A. Gottschalk, M.D.

Mismatched Vascular Defects: An Easy Alternative to Mismatched Segmental Equivalent Defects for the Interpretation of Ventilation/ Perfusion Lung Scans in Pulmonary Embolism
Stein PD, Henry JW, Gottschalk A (Henry Ford Heart and Vascular Inst, Detroit; Michigan State Univ, East Lansing)
Chest 104:1468–1471, 1993   124-95-1-7

Introduction.—Interpretation of ventilation-perfusion (V/Q) lung scans of patients with suspected pulmonary embolism (PE) requires that mismatched segmental defects of moderate size (25% to 75% of a segment) be distinguished from those of large size (more than 75% of a segment). The size of segmental defects is often underestimated, even by experienced readers of radionuclide lung scans. The hypothesis that V/Q lung scans could be evaluated on the basis of the total number of mismatched vascular defects, irrespective of segmental defect size, was evaluated.

Methods.—Lung scan data were obtained from the Prospective Investigation of Pulmonary Embolism Diagnosis (PIOPED). Acute PE was diagnosed in 383 patients and excluded in 681. The number of mismatched vascular defects was taken to be the number of large and/or moderate-sized mismatched defects.

Results.—The predictive value for PE of the cumulative number of mismatched large segments and the predictive value of the number of

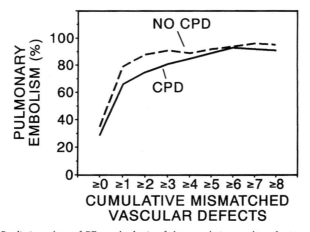

Fig 1–3.—Predictive values of PE on the basis of the cumulative number of mismatched vascular defects among patients without prior cardiopulmonary disease (NO CPD) and those with prior cardiopulmonary disease (CPD). Differences between the groups occurred with 1 or more mismatched vascular defects (*P* < .02) and 2 or more defects (*P* < .01). (Courtesy of Stein PD, Henry JW, Gottschalk A: *Chest* 104:1468–1471, 1993.)

Predictive Value of PE in Relation to the Cumulative Number of Mismatched Vascular Defects (Large and/or Moderate Size Segmental Perfusion Defects)

Cumulative No. of Defects	All Patients (n = 1064)		CI, %	No Prior CPD (n = 421)		CI, %	Any Prior CPD (n = 629)		CI, %
		(%)			(%)			(%)	
≥0	383/1064	(36)	34-38	173/421	(41)	37-45	205/629	(33) *	29-37
≥1	255/350	(73)	69-77	123/154	(80)	74-86	130/190	(68) †	62-74
≥2	200/244	(82)	78-86	94/106	(89)	83-95	105/136	(77) †	69-85
≥3	170/201	(85)	79-91	79/87	(91)	85-97	90/112	(80)	72-88
≥4	149/172	(87)	81-93	67/75	(89)	81-97	81/96	(84)	76-92
≥5	130/144	(90)	o4-96	55/60	(92)	84-100	75/84	(89)	83-95
≥6	116/124	(94)	90-98	49/52	(94)	88-100	67/72	(93)	87-99
≥7	103/110	(94)	90-98	43/45	(96)	90-100	60/65	(92)	86-98
≥8	93/100	(93)	87-99	41/43	(95)	89-100	52/57	(91)	83-99

Note: Among all patients (obligatory angiography and physician-requested angiography).
Abbreviations: CPD, cardiopulmonary disease; CI, 95% confidence interval.
* P < .01 for prior CPD vs. no CPD.
†P < .05.
(Courtesy of Stein PD, Henry JW, Gottschalk A: Chest 104:1468-1471, 1993.)

cumulative mismatched segments of moderate size were found to be nearly identical, suggesting that moderate and large defects are of equivalent diagnostic value. When lung scans that were evaluated on the basis of the number of mismatched vascular defects were compared with V/Q scans that were evaluated on the basis of the number of mismatched segmental equivalents, the maximum likelihood estimates of the areas under the receiver operating characteristic curves were similar (.8512 and .853, respectively). The predictive value of the number of mismatched vascular defects was enhanced when patients were stratified according to the presence or absence of previous cardiopulmonary disease (Fig 1–3).

Conclusion.—The total number of mismatched vascular defects, whether of large or moderate size, yields a diagnostic assessment of PE that is as accurate as one based on the number of mismatched segmental equivalents (table). Because the reader does not have to distinguish defects of moderate size from those of large size, an easier and more objective interpretation can be obtained.

▶ Personally, I have not had a problem using segmental equivalence. I do not think it is difficult to sort lesions into small (less than 25% of a segment), moderate (25% to 75% of the segment), or large (greater than 75% of a segment) segmental perfusion defects. However, in the 1994 YEAR BOOK OF NUCLEAR MEDICINE (1), we abstracted data that indicate that some observers have a problem with sizing perfusion defects.

The data we assembled in this paper indicate that you do not have to go through the trouble of sizing perfusion defects—unless, of course, you want to. I think everyone recognizes that small lesions (rat bites) do not represent embolism, and that anything else—in other words, subsegmental or segmental—represents an embolic-type lesion. These data show that you can make your analysis on the basis of whether a vascular lesion is present within each individual segment. We hope this makes it easier to read V/Q scans.—A. Gottschalk, M.D.

Reference

1. 1994 YEAR BOOK OF NUCLEAR MEDICINE, pp 97–99.

Reporting Ventilation-Perfusion Lung Scintigraphy: Impact on Subsequent Use of Anticoagulation Therapy
Kaboli P, Buscombe JR, Ell PJ (Univ College, London)
Postgrad Med J 69:851–855, 1993   124-95-1–8

Background.—Ventilation and perfusion lung scintigraphy has long been established as a safe, noninvasive means of detecting pulmonary embolism. However, as with other diagnostic procedures, a need to reevaluate the clinical efficacy of this test has recently arisen. Ways in which the findings of ventilation-perfusion scintigraphy affected subsequent anticoagulant therapy were studied, and whether these findings had any bearing on patient mortality was evaluated.

Patients and Findings. —Two hundred forty-four patients undergoing ventilation-perfusion lung scintigraphy were retrospectively reviewed. Although lung scintigrams were available for all patients, case record notes were found for only 203 patients. When the 203 patients with case notes were compared with all 244 patients, no difference in the character of the reports was noted. In terms of the pulmonary embolism, a normal or low probability was given in 91 of 203 reports, and a high probability was described in 46 of 203 reports. Medium probability or indeterminate results, which, without further information, are often of little help to the clinician, were given in only 9 of the 203 reports. In the remaining 57 studies, a more complex report that did not include probability reporting was given. In 28 of the 46 high-probability patients, clinical management was altered as a result of the scintigraphic finding. However, in patients with normal or low probability, clinical management was changed in only 5 of the 91 patients. Six deaths occurred, 1 of which was the result of pulmonary embolism. This patient died despite anticoagulation therapy after a high-probability finding at ventilation-perfusion scintigraphy. The other 5 deaths were the result of other causes.

Conclusion. —Studies that reported a normal or low probability of pulmonary embolism resulted in less change in clinical management than studies that reported a high probability. The low mortality from correctly identified embolic disease indicates that ventilation-perfusion lung scintigraphy is not only a safe procedure, but it can also be useful in reducing patient mortality.

▶ Although we understand part of these results, we are toubled by other parts. These English authors seem to agree with most North American trials indicating that a high clinical suspicion with a high-probability ventilation-perfusion scan is enough to anticoagulate a patient. However, we do not understand why it seems necessary to link normal and low probabilities.

In our experience, the normal scan is a very useful result, and the very low-probability study (estimated to have a probability of 5% or less) is also useful. Putting these both together with higher scan probabilities (e.g., in the 20% range) could easily cause the referring physician to have much less faith in these readings. These data suggest that this might have happened. Read on for further information.—A. Gottschalk, M.D.

Lung Scan Reports: Interpretation by Clinicians
Gray HW, McKillop JH, Bessent RG (Royal Infirmary, Glasgow, Scotland)
Nucl Med Commun 14:989–994, 1993   124-95-1–9

Results of Physicians' Interpretations of Lung Scan Reports

Physician interpretation of lung scan reports	Lung scan reports			
	Normal	Low probability	Indeterminate	High probability
PE highly unlikely – group 1 only	65 (34)	10 (5)	0	0
PE unlikely – group 2	35 (18)	58 (30)	0	0
PE uncertain – group 3	94 (48)	126 (65)	188 (97)	34 (18)
PE likely – group 4 only	0	0	6 (3)	156 (82)
Totals	194 (100)	194 (100)	194 (100)	194 (100)

Note: Numbers represent the positive selections in each scan group. Numbers in parentheses represent the percentages of selections in each scan group.
(Courtesy of Gray HW, McKillop JH, Bessent RG: Nucl Med Commun 14:989–994, 1993.)

Background.—Given the increasing emphasis on clinical audit, nuclear medicine providers must determine how well useful clinical information is communicated to the physician, particularly with respect to ventilation-perfusion (V/Q) lung scanning for pulmonary embolism (PE). Physicians' understanding of reports issued was assessed using the verbal probability scale, which currently is the most widely used method of reporting V/Q imaging.

Participants and Methods.—A questionnaire was sent to 217 consultant physicians in Scotland, all of whom were likely to encounter PE within the scope of their practice. A list of 18 expressions of likelihood of PE was included. Each participant was asked to choose which of these best described their interpretation of each of 4 lung scan reports, including normal, low probability of PE, indeterminate, and high probability of PE. Post-test questions on clinical management were also included in the survey.

Results.—Of the 217 questionnaires sent, 194 replies were received. Of those participating, only 34% understood that a normal lung scan made the possibility of PE highly unlikely. In addition, 65% reported that a low-probability scan was comparable to an uncertain diagnosis (table). The answers to the post-test management question verified this pattern of interpretation. After a normal lung scan report, 31% of the physicians were uncertain about the diagnosis. Moreover, this uncertainty increased to 37% for low-probability scan reports.

Conclusion.—These findings underscore that informed guidance must be provided to clinical staff after V/Q imaging. A more easily understood style of lung scan reporting is also needed. Such changes would undoubtedly aid in improving clinical management of patients.

▶ These are distressing data. I hope, although I am not totally convinced, that we have done a better job in North America in educating our referring physicians. These data also go a long way toward explaining the outcome analysis by Kaboli, Buscombe, and Ell (Abstract 124-95-1–8), which assumes there is a comparable understanding between physicians in Scotland and England.—A. Gottschalk, M.D.

Acute Pulmonary Embolism: Artificial Neural Network Approach for Diagnosis

Tourassi GD, Floyd CE, Sostman HD, Coleman RE (Duke Univ, Durham, NC)
Radiology 189:555–558, 1993   124-95-1–10

Background.—Ventilation-perfusion scanning, which is the initial study done to assess patients with suspected pulmonary embolism (PE), is safe and well tolerated, but it is limited in its efficacy for diagnosing PE. Improving the diagnostic yield of current methods may have a major effect. An artificial neural network was investigated as a computer-aided diagnostic tool for predicting PE from radiographic findings.

Methods and Findings.—The data base was composed of cases taken from the collaborative study of the Prospective Investigation of Pulmonary Embolism Diagnosis (PIOPED). Scan findings from 383 patients with PE and 681 without PE on pulmonary angiograms were used to train and test the artificial neural network using the jackknife method. A receiver-operating-characteristic analysis was then applied to compare

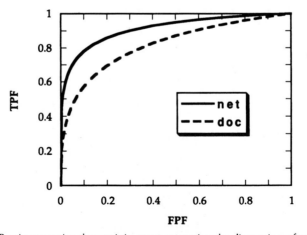

Fig 1–4.—Receiver-operating-characteristic curves comparing the diagnostic performance of the neural network (*net*) (evaluated with the jackknife method) with that of the physicians (*doc*). (Courtesy of Tourassi GD, Floyd CE, Sostman HD, et al: *Radiology* 189:555–558, 1993.)

the performance of the network with that of the physicians involved in the PIOPED study. The artificial neural network performed significantly better than the performance of physicians involved in the PIOPED study (Fig 1-4).

Conclusion.—An artificial neural network can form the basis of a computer-aided diagnostic system to assist physicians in diagnosing PE. A prospective study is under way to determine whether this computer aid can improve physicians' performance.

▶ This exciting tool can potentially help all who are interested in diagnosing PE. To use this network, every observer would have to enter the data to be analyzed in a consistent way. For example, these data were entered from the PIOPED scan description form (1). This consistency would already probably help your group give more consistent ventilation-perfusion scan results. Although we know that the artificial neural network performed as well as or better than the PIOPED observers, we don't know whether the network is in any way dependent on the incidence of such phenomena as pulmonary embolism, and intermediate scan patterns. We would like to believe that the network really recognizes all these variables, but I am not sure whether that is true. In other words, can artificial neural networks work effectively in small community centers, where those in the patient population may be vastly different?

Paul Stein's group at Henry Ford has also applied the artificial neural network to the clinical side of the diagnosis of PE. The group applied a neural network to the clinical diagnosis of acute PE (2) and concluded that the neural network could predict the clinical likelihood of PE with an accuracy comparable to that of an experienced pulmonologist. In short, it may be that future applications will allow us to be both more consistent and to immediately tie into the clinical probability estimate of PE, thereby enabling us to provide a better consultation.—A. Gottschalk, M.D.

References

1. Gottschalk A, et al: *J Nucl Med* 34:1109, 1993.
2. Patil S, et al: *Chest* 104:1685, 1993.

Detailed Analysis of Patients With Matched Ventilation-Perfusion Defects and Chest Radiographic Opacities
Worsley DF, Kim CK, Alavi A, Palevsky HI (Hosp of the Univ of Pennsylvania, Philadelphia)
J Nucl Med 34:1851–1853, 1993   124-95-1-11

Background.—The ventilation-perfusion (V/Q) lung scan is widely used to evaluate patients who are suspected of having pulmonary embolism (PE). Those with matching V/Q defects and corresponding opacities on chest radiography continue to be a diagnostic dilemma, because

Regional Distribution of PE in Lung Zones With Matching V/Q
Defects and Chest Radiographic Opacities

	PE+ (no. of zones)	PE− (no. of zones)	Prevalence of PE
Upper zone	4	32	11%
Middle zone	6	46	12%
Lower zone	61	126	33%
Total	71	204	26%

(Courtesy of Worsley DF, Kim CK, Alavi A, et al: *J Nucl Med* 34:1851–1853, 1993.)

of the difficulty of distinguishing between pulmonary infarction and other parenchymal disorders.

Objective and Methods.—The prevalence of PE in patients with triple matches was determined in a retrospective series of patients enrolled in the Pulmonary Embolism Diagnosis study. Chest radiographs were acquired within 24 hours of V/Q lung scanning and pulmonary angiography. All the patients had angiograms that, in the view of 2 readers from another center, were diagnostic in lung zones that had matching V/Q defects and opacities on chest radiographs.

Findings.—Of 1,487 patients with diagnostic V/Q scans, 247 (17%) had matching V/Q defects and radiographic opacities in at least 1 lung zone. Diagnostic angiograms were obtained in 275 lung zones in 233 of these patients. The overall prevalence of PE in lung zones with triple matches was 26%; PE was most frequent in triple matches in the lower lung zones (table). The majority of triple matches involved less than half of a given lung zone.

Conclusion.—Patients with matching V/Q defects and chest radiographic opacities in the lower lung zones have an intermediate probability of having PE, whereas those with matches in the upper and middle lung zones have a low probability.

▶ These data look too good to be true, and, unfortunately, I have some concerns for which I would require answers before I would use these data. The essence of my worry is that in PIOPED, the angiographer was permitted to stop when an embolus was discovered. In short, he was not required to examine the entire lung, let alone both lungs.

Note that the article specifically states that 233 patients had 275 lung zones examined by angiography. Because each patient—and let us generously assume the angiographer examined only 1 lung—has to have 3 zones in each lung, the possible total number of lung zones we would have liked to have seen examined was 699. In other words, only 39% of the possible data base has an angiographic correlation.

Furthermore, when passing a pulmonary catheter, it is easy to go into the lower lobe first; that creates a situation in which we may well be selectively biasing the detection of emboli in the lower lobes. Unfortunately, that is what these authors found. We don't know how many of these patients had triple matches in other lung zones that were not examined, and we don't know how many of these patients had only solitary triple matches that were precisely examined by the angiogram. If I had answers to these concerns, these data would be more useful.—A. Gottschalk, M.D.

The Limitations of Posterior View Ventilation Scanning in the Diagnosis of Pulmonary Embolism
Morrell NW, Nijran KS, Jones BE, Biggs T, Seed WA (Charing Cross and Westminster Med School, London)
Nucl Med Commun 14:983–988, 1993   124-95-1–12

Background.—In the diagnosis of pulmonary embolism, many facilities use a single-breath posterior-view xenon-133 ventilation scan for comparison with multiple-view perfusion images. However, it has been suggested that some ventilation defects may be overlooked with the posterior view, resulting in overdiagnosis of a ventilation-perfusion mismatch simply because the lung is not sufficiently imaged. The reliability of the posterior view ventilation scan in the detection of lobar and segmental defects was determined.

Participants and Methods.—Twenty healthy volunteers with normal lung function were studied. All participants underwent fiberoptic bronchoscopy after local anesthesia. Occluding balloon catheters were placed in lobar and segmental bronchi during the procedure to create defects of known anatomical location and size. During the occlusions, participants breathed ^{81m}Kr with air. Images were obtained in the posterior, posterior/oblique, and lateral positions. Three experienced nuclear medicine physicians then classified the posterior view images as normal or abnormal. If images were considered abnormal, physicians were asked to identify the lobe or segment involved.

Results.—Segmental defects were overlooked in 28% of the scan readings and were identified but erroneously located in 50% of the readings. Only 22% of the readings had correctly located these defects. Also, lobar defects were overlooked in 17% of the readings. In the posterior scan, with a defect involving the entire lingual, all observers reported a normal reading. Defects of the right and left lower lobes were underestimated.

Conclusion.—Ventilation scanning techniques that evaluate the distribution of ventilation using only the posterior view cannot reliably detect segmental and lobar defects and may increase the rate of false positive results in the diagnosis of pulmonary embolism.

▶ I think this is an excellent experimental design. However, I am not sure that I agree with all of the study's details or conclusions. The idea that lesions are either incorrectly located or missed on the posterior view of the xenon-133 (^{133}Xe) study because they are missed on these studies with ^{81}Kr troubles me. The lesions found using ^{133}Xe are predominantly on the washout views as areas of slow washout or hot spots. Instead of testing for this finding, this study looks for areas of decreased activity on the Kr image. On the other hand, I firmly believe that the posterior-view standard ^{133}Xe ventilation study can be improved by adding posterior oblique views to the equilibrium and the washout phases. Consequently, although I do not agree with the idea of a Xe/Kr relationship, I agree with the authors' conclusion. You can do better with ^{133}Xe if you add posterior oblique views to the study.—A. Gottschalk, M.D.

Technetium-99m Labeled Micro Aerosol "Pertechnegas": A New Agent for Ventilation Imaging in Suspected Pulmonary Emboli
Ashburn WL, Belezzuoli EV, Dillon WA, Mensh BD, Hoogland D, Yeung DW, Coade GE (Univ of California, San Diego; Baylor College of Medicine, Houston; Cheyenne Med Equipment, Inc, Agoura, Calif)
Clin Nucl Med 18:1045–1052, 1993   124-95-1–13

Background.—Technetium-99m (^{99m}Tc)-labeled microaerosol "Pertechnegas," a new agent used for ventilation imaging in patients with suspected pulmonary emboli, was evaluated. An advantage of Pertechnegas is that the radioactive ^{99m}Tc pertechnetate is rapidly cleared from the lungs at a somewhat predictable rate. Therefore, it may be potentially more useful in lung ventilation imaging than standard aerolized DTPA and, possibly, Technegas. Preliminary findings were reported.

Methods.—Four patients with suspected pulmonary emboli were studied. Approximately 1 mCi (37 MBq) of ^{99m}Tc Pertechnegas was inhaled in 5 breaths or less. Planar images in multiple projections were recorded for preset counts, and a final posterior image was obtained to assess residual lung background activity. Perfusion imaging in the identical projections was immediately performed after ventilation imaging with 4 mCi (148 MBq) of ^{99m}Tc macroaggregated albumin (MAA).

Results.—Normal ventilation and perfusion were noted in 2 patients (Fig 1–5). In the other 2 patients, segmental mismatched defects that were consistent with a diagnosis of pulmonary emboli were clearly demonstrated. The subsequent appearance of ^{99m}Tc pertechnetate in other organs did not hinder interpretation of either the ventilation or perfusion images. In all patients, residual pertechnetate background lung activity was less than 10% of the initial ^{99m}Tc MAA counts at the end of the last ventilation image.

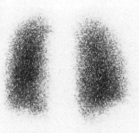
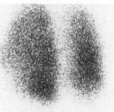

POST1 〈V〉   LPO 〈V〉

RPO 〈V〉   ANT 〈V〉

Fig 1–5.—*Abbreviations: POST1* (V), posterior view; *LPO* (V), left posterior oblique; *RPO* (V), right posterior oblique; *ANT* (V), anterior projection. Normal distribution of Pertechnegas in a man, 56, with a low pretest probability of pulmonary emboli. Only 5 tidal counts were required to produce adequate counts for ventilation (V) imaging. (Courtesy of Ashburn WL, Belezzuoli EV, Dillon WA, et al: *Clin Nucl Med* 18:1045-1052, 1993.)

Conclusion.—The advantages of Pertechnegas included less residual ventilation image activity superimposed on the MAA perfusion images, decreased demand for patient cooperation (because of fewer required breaths), and an absence of deposition of activity in the central airways. Pertechnegas is an ideal agent for conventional lung ventilation imaging.

▶ This is an interesting new wrinkle for the Tetley Generator. It is too bad there aren't more of them available in this country.—A. Gottschalk, M.D.

Ascending Aortic Dissection Causing Unilateral Absence of Perfusion on Lung Scanning

Worsley DF, Coupland DB, Lentle BC, Chipperfield P, Marsh JI (Vancouver Gen Hosp, BC, Canada; St Paul's Hosp, Vancouver, BC, Canada)
Clin Nucl Med 18:941–944, 1993   124-95-1-14

Objective.—Ascending aortic dissection occurred in a patient 8 years after aortic valve replacement, an uncommon finding that must be considered in the differential diagnosis of patients with a history of aortic valve surgery who are seen with a sudden onset of cardiorespiratory symptoms and unilateral absence of perfusion to the right lung.

Case Report.—Man, 71, was seen with a sudden onset of hypotension, hypoxia, and posterior chest pain. Except for the presence of previous aortic valve replacement, his cardiovascular and respiratory examinations were within normal limits. Perfusion to the entire right lung was absent, although perfusion to the left lung and ventilation images of that lung were normal (Fig 1–6). The tentative diagnosis was acute pulmonary thromboembolism. Pulmonary angiography revealed a type A dissection of the ascending aorta. The patient became hypotensive after angiography and required emergency resection of the aortic dissection. Surgical findings confirmed the angiographic findings. Except for hypoxic encephalopathy that quickly resolved, the patient had no further complications and was discharged 2 weeks after admission.

Discussion.—This is the second reported case of acute dissection of the aorta that caused complete pulmonary occlusion of the right pulmonary artery as detected by perfusion lung imaging. Vascular occlusion by pulmonary embolism and extrinsic compression by carcinoma of the lung are the 2 most common causes of a unilateral absence of perfusion. The right pulmonary artery is susceptible to extrinsic compression after aortic dissection because of the anatomical relationship of the aorta and pulmonary artery. Acute aortic dissection must be confirmed with angiography, because anticoagulation is contraindicated in these patients.

▶ As those of you who have been regular readers of the YEAR BOOK OF NUCLEAR MEDICINE know, our first editor, the late James L. Quinn, loved unusual cases that caused unilateral pulmonary whiteout. This case is a dandy, and I know Jim would have selected it for you. We present it in his memory.—A. Gottschalk, M.D.

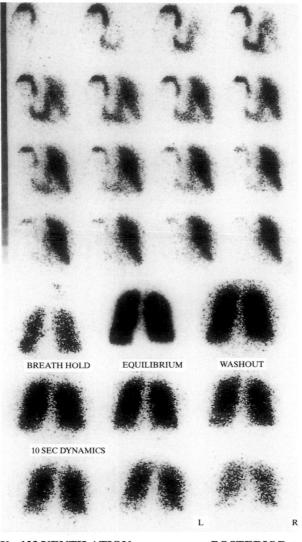

BREATH HOLD   EQUILIBRIUM   WASHOUT

10 SEC DYNAMICS

L   R

Xe-133 VENTILATION   POSTERIOR

Fig 1–6.—Xenon-133 and technetium-99m macroaggregated albumin lung scan demonstrating absent perfusion to the right lung. **Top 4 rows,** 2-second anterior dynamic images and (**bottom 3 rows**) xenon-133 posterior ventilation images. (Courtesy of Worsley DF, Coupland DB, Lentle BC, et al: *Clin Nucl Med* 18:941–944, 1993.)

Diagnostic Efficacy of PET-FDG Imaging in Solitary Pulmonary Nodules: Potential Role in Evaluation and Management

Dewan NA, Gupta NC, Redepenning LS, Phalen JJ, Frick MP (Creighton Univ, Omaha, Neb)

Chest 104:997–1002, 1993   124-95-1–15

Results in 30 Patients With Solitary Pulmonary Nodules

Patient No./ Age, yr/Sex	Nodule Size, cm	PET Scan	DUR	Histologic Features	Biopsy Mode
Benign					
1/39/M	1.5	Neg	0.47	Granuloma	Thoracotomy
2/74/M	1.0	Neg	0.15	Hamartoma	Thoracotomy
3/68/M	2.5	Neg	0.82	Carcinoid	Thoracotomy
4/57/F	1.8	Neg	0.40	Nonspecific inflammation	Bronchoscopy
5/64/M	1.0	Neg	0.92	Organizing pneumonia	Thoracotomy
6/68/M	1.0	Neg	0.42	Histoplasmosis	Thoracotomy
7/38/M	2.0	Neg	0.75	Stable nodule size over 3 yr	...
8/63/M	1.5	Neg	0.27	Necrotizing granuloma	Thoracotomy
9/41/F	2 × 1.5	Pos+	1.92	Caseating granuloma with histoplasma	Thoracotomy
10/51/M	2	Pos+	3.38	Caseating granuloma with histoplasma	Thoracotomy

Introduction.—The benign or malignant nature of a substantial proportion of solitary pulmonary nodules cannot be determined with plain chest radiography or CT. Although nodules that are larger than 3 cm have a high probability of malignancy, smaller lesions are especially difficult to analyze. The ability of the PET scan with 2-[F-18]-fluoro-2-deoxy-

Malignant					
11/72/M	2	Pos	8.17	Melanoma	TTNA
12/72/M	1.5	Pos	11.77	Adenocarcinoma	Thoracotomy
13/65/M	1.0	Neg++	1.67	Scar adenocarcinoma	Thoracotomy
14/62/M	1.5	Pos	6.79	Squamous cell carcinoma	Thoracotomy
15/73/M	1.0	Pos	3.23	Scar adenocarcinoma	Thoracotomy
16/69/M	2.0	Pos	5.86	Adenocarcinoma	Thoracotomy
17/41/F	1.5	Pos	5.65	Scar adenocarcinoma	Thoracotomy
18/81/F	1.2 × 2	Pos	3.26	Scar adenocarcinoma	Thoracotomy
19/63/M	1	Pos	2.61	Adenocarcinoma	Thoracotomy
20/76/M	0.6	Pos	6.11	Adenocarcinoma	Thoracotomy
21/74/F	1.5 × 2	Pos	2.3	Small-cell carcinoma	TTNA
22/89/M	1 × 2	Pos	3.88	Adenocarcinoma	TTNA
23/69/M	2 × 2.75	Pos	2.83	Non-small-cell carcinoma	TTNA
24/84/F	1.8 × 2.2	Pos	6.88	Squamous cell carcinoma	TTNA
25/73/M	2.0	Pos	11.71	Small-cell carcinoma	TTNA
26/64/M	2.0	Pos	6.07	Melanoma	TTNA
27/72/F	2.0	Pos	4.27	Bronchoalveolar adenocarcinoma	Thoracotomy
28/77/M	3.0	Pos	4.81	Non-small-cell carcinoma	TTNA
29/72/M	1.4 × 2.2	Pos	5.74	Adenocarcinoma	Thoracotomy
30/50/F	1.5 × 2	Pos	7.30	Adenocarcinoma	Thoracotomy

Abbreviations: +, false positive; ++, false negative; TTNA, transthoracic needle aspiration.
(Courtesy of Dewan NA, Gupta NC, Redepenning LS, et al: *Chest* 104:997–1002, 1993.)

D-glucose (FDG) to differentiate benign from malignant pulmonary nodules less than 3 cm in diameter was assessed.

Patients and Methods.—Thirty patients with solitary pulmonary nodules 3 cm or less in diameter were studied. All nodules were judged to be indeterminate on the basis of chest radiographs and CT scans. The final diagnosis was established by histologic examination of tissue obtained by thoracotomy, bronchoscopy, or fine-needle aspiration biopsy. Scanning was performed 1 hour after intravenous administration of 10 mCi of F-18-FDG. Two independent observers examined the images, focusing on the appearance of a relatively bright area of increased FDG uptake within the lung nodule. Semiquantitative analysis was performed by computation of the differential uptake ratio.

Results.—Twenty patients had malignant nodules and 10 had benign nodules. Nineteen of the 20 malignant pulmonary nodules and 8 of the 10 benign nodules were correctly identified with PET scanning. Uptake of FDG was not increased in a patient with a 1-cm scar adenocarcinoma. The 2 false positive cases both had caseating granulomas with active inflammation and *Histoplasma* organisms. Differential uptake ratio values were significantly greater for malignant nodules (mean, 5.55) than for benign nodules (mean, .95) (table).

Conclusion.—Sensitivity was 95% and specificity was 80% for the identification of benign and malignant solitary nodules with PET and FDG. The positive and negative predictive value for solitary pulmonary nodules was 90% and 89%, respectively. A negative PET study could potentially save a patient from thoracotomy and other invasive diagnostic studies, whereas a positive study could be used to directly refer the patient for thoracotomy.

▶ These are interesting data because they provide another example of the high accuracy of PET-FDG scanning for tumor diagnosis. However, these data also leave me wondering how to use the results effectively.

As the authors point out, needle biopsy of pulmonary nodules works in more than 90% of nodules larger than 2 cm. It is also widely available. Therefore, it would seem that PET scanning for pulmonary nodules would be most useful for smaller lesions. However, it is the smaller lesions that cause the most trouble in PET scanning.

These data were collected, as we understand it, by qualitative visual analysis of the scans. The authors note that they may be able to do better using numerical uptake ratios; however, this requires further work. We hope the authors will continue these investigations, and we will keep you posted in future YEAR BOOKS.—A. Gottschalk, M.D.

Evaluation of Suspected Malignant Pulmonary Lesions With [201]Tl Single Photon Emission Computed Tomography
Tonami N, Yokoyama K, Shuke N, Taki J, Kinuya S, Miyauchi T, Michigishi T,

Aburano T, Hisada K, Watanabe Y, Takashima T, Nonomura A (Kanazawa Univ, Japan)
Nucl Med Commun 14:602–610, 1993   124-95-1–16

Introduction.—Pulmonary lesions that are suspected of being lung cancer on chest radiographs or chest CTs must be confirmed noninvasively. The development of SPECT led to a reassessment of thallium-201 (^{201}Tl) scintigraphy as a means to differentiate pulmonary lesions.

Methods.—The participants included 170 patients with suspected lung cancer, all of whom had lesions greater than 20 mm on the longest diameter on the surgical specimen. Twenty-three patients had benign lesions and 147 had histologically proven untreated malignant pulmonary lesions, including 140 primary lung cancers. Tomographic scans were obtained at 15 minutes (early) and 3 hours (delayed) post injection, using a dual-headed rotating gamma camera with low-energy, high-resolution collimators and a system resolution of 15 mm (full width at half maximum).

Results.—Delayed ^{201}Tl SPECT visualized all 147 malignant pulmonary lesions and 16 of the 23 benign pulmonary lesions. In general, delayed images were clearer than early images (Fig 1–7). The delayed ratio of lesion to controlateral normal lung was 2.35 in all malignant pulmonary lesions and 2.06 in the 16 benign lesions visualized. The adenocarcinoma and small-cell carcinoma groups had the highest delayed ratio (2.4). The only significant difference in delayed ratio was between the adenocarcinoma and large-cell carcinoma groups. In malignant lesions, the retention index was 25, whereas in benign lesions it was 6, a significant difference. The highest retention index (38) was in the large-cell carcinoma group. The retention index did not differ significantly among different histology groups in malignant lesions.

Conclusion.—Findings indicate that malignancy can be ruled out if pulmonary lesions greater than 20 mm in diameter have no abnormal accumulation of ^{201}Tl on delayed SPECT. Semiquantitative analysis for smaller lesions is not very reliable mainly because of the partial volume effect. The retention index and the combination of early and delayed SPECT appears to help differentiate malignant from benign lesions with abnormal accumulation. The use of ^{201}Tl SPECT should help to reduce the number of unnecessary thoracotomies.

▶ A lot of work was done; however, using these authors' criteria, this test was useful in only 7 of 170 patients (4%). Consequently, we suspect that this technique will not catch on clinically.—A. Gottschalk, M.D.

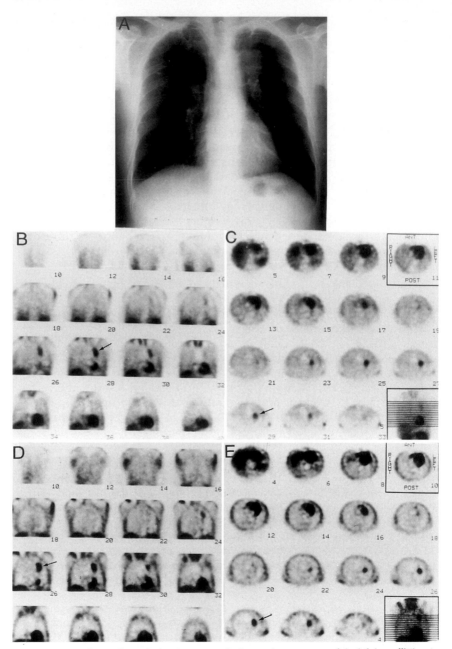

Fig 1–7.—A, chest radiograph showing a mass shadow at the upper part of the left lung. ^{201}Tl early (**B**) and coronal (**C**) transverse scans demonstrate an abnormal accumulation corresponding to the pulmonary lesion (*arrow*). Delayed (**D**) coronal and (**E**) transverse scans show more increased accumulation (*arrow*). No abnormal accumulation in the mediastinum was noted. (Courtesy of Tonami N, Yokoyama K, Shuke N, et al: *Nucl Med Commun* 14:602–610, 1993.)

Radioiodine Uptake by Squamous-Cell Carcinoma of the Lung

Misaki T, Takeuchi R, Miyamoto S, Kasagi K, Matsui Y, Konishi J (Kyoto Univ, Japan)
J Nucl Med 35:474–475, 1994   124-95-1-17

Objective.—The case of a patient with 2 primary neoplasms—a papillary thyroid adenocarcinoma and a squamous cell carcinoma of the lung—was presented. The latter tumor masqueraded as an iodine-concentrating metastasis from the thyroid cancer on post-therapy radioiodine imaging.

Case Report.—Man, 71, underwent total thyroidectomy and bilateral neck dissection for advanced papillary carcinoma. He had previously refused therapy, despite a 3-year history of a large neck mass. When thyroglobulin (Tg), a tumor marker for differentiated thyroid cancer, was found to be abnormally high after surgery, the patient was treated with 2 doses of ^{131}I in an attempt to reduce esophageal residue of the disease. His clinical symptoms diminished, but the esophageal invasion persisted on scintigraphy (Fig 1–8) and Tg remained elevated. Fifteen months after surgery, the patient noticed dyspnea and had a productive cough. His symptoms suggested lung metastasis from the thyroid tumor. However, biopsy material obtained at bronchoscopy revealed squamous cell car-

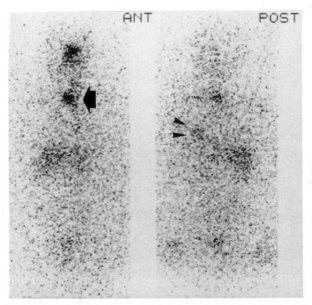

Fig 1–8.—Whole-body scan 6 days after a second therapeutic dose (4.44 GBq) of ^{131}I revealed fairly strong radioactivity at the esophageal invasion in the anterior view (*thick arrow*) and moderate spotty uptake at the left lower lung field in the posterior view (*arrows*). (Courtesy of Nisaki T, Takeuchi R, Miyamoto S, et al: *J Nucl Med* 35:474–475, 1994.)

cinoma of the lung. The patient has received radiotherapy and repeated courses of combined chemotherapy.

Conclusion.—This case illustrates a rare but important differential diagnosis from lung metastasis of thyroid cancer in ¹³¹I scintigraphy. Only 3 cases of iodine- or technetium-concentrating lung adenocarcinoma appear to have been reported. If such uptake proves common, it may lead to a new application of radioiodine imaging in pulmonary oncology.

▶ This is an unusual case. Because most thyroid pulmonary metastases are round and most lung cancers are not, we recommend a plain chest film as the first step in telling them apart. The authors have suggested the possibility of using iodine as a tracer to detect lung cancers. Years ago, we (and others) found a greater-than-95% pulmonary cancer detection rate with gallium-67 citrate. Note that the key problem in lung cancer detection usually is determining how many mediastinal metastases are present. Whether the primary tumor is, in fact, a cancer is usually determined by invasive diagnostic techniques. In this case, the discovery was made by bronchoscopy.—A. Gottschalk, M.D.

Late Pulmonary Scintigraphic Defects After Uneventful Recovery From Simple Focal Pneumonia of Childhood
Kenney IJ, Lenney W, Lutkin JE, Gordon I (Royal Alexandra Hosp for Sick Children, Brighton, England; Royal Sussex County Hosp, Brighton, England; Hosp for Sick Children, London)
Br J Radiol 66:1031–1034, 1993   124-95-1–18

Introduction.—Children with simple focal pneumonia are expected to recover without permanent changes. However, 2 recent studies found pulmonary scintigraphic abnormalities many years after foreign-body aspiration in childhood. Whether similar changes might be apparent after recovery from pneumonia without foreign-body aspiration was determined.

Methods.—Fourteen children with clinical pneumonia and focal consolidation on their chest radiograph (CXR) were examined approximately 12 months later. None of the children had previous abnormal radiographs or admissions for pneumonia. At follow-up, ventilation and perfusion lung scans and a CXR were obtained. Perfusion studies alone were obtained in 2 cases; the remaining 12 patients had both ⁸¹ᵐKr ventilation and technetium-99m perfusion studies. Scans and CXRs were independently assessed by 2 experienced pediatric radiologists. Cases that were considered abnormal or equivocal were reviewed clinically.

Results.—The patients consisted of 9 boys and 5 girls with a mean age of 4 years when first seen. All had a normal clinical examination at follow-up and had no significant respiratory symptoms. At 1 year, 5 patients were considered to have abnormalities on the ventilation-perfu-

Site of Presenting Infection, Results of Follow-Up CXR and Ventilation-Perfusion Scans, and Any Identified Organism

Case	Initial infection	Follow-up CXR	Observer 1	Observer 2	Agreed result	Organism
1	LLL	normal	v/q LLL	v/q LLL	v/q LLL	none
2	LLL	normal	normal	normal	normal	none
3	LLL	normal	normal	normal	normal	Mycoplasma
4	LLL	right LL	v/q LLL	normal	normal	Mycoplasma
5	LLL	normal	v RLL	v/q RLL	v/q RLL *	none
6	LLL	normal	v/q LLL	normal	v/q LLL	none
7	RML	normal	normal	normal	normal	none
8	LLL	normal	normal	normal	normal	Flu A
9	RLL	normal	q LLL	normal	q LLL * †	none
10	RUL	normal	normal	normal	normal †	none
11	RUL	normal	v RUL	normal	normal	none
12	LLL	normal	normal	normal	normal	none
13	RML	normal	normal	v LLL	normal	Haemophilus
14	RML	normal	normal	v LLL	v/q LLL *	none

Abbreviations: LLL, left lower lobe; RML, right middle lobe; RLL, right lower lobe; RUL, right upper lobe; v, ventilation defect; q, perfusion defect.
* Lung scan abnormality not corresponding to site of initial infection.
† Only perfusion scan available.
(Courtesy of Kenney IJ, Lenney W, Lutkin JE, et al: Br J Radiol 66:1031–1034, 1993.)

sion lung scan (table). Three defects had no correlation with the site of the previous pneumonia (Fig 1-9), and 2 occurred at the site. One patient with a normal lung scan had a CXR that showed a small focus of consolidation on the side opposite the previous pneumonia.

Conclusion.—Long-term sequelae of simple focal pneumonia are considered rare in children. However, these results suggest that lung scan defects are as common in the medium term in such cases as in those in-

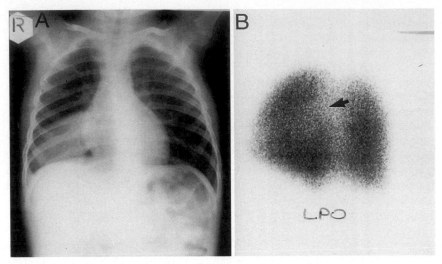

Fig 1–9.—A, segmental consolidation in the right lower lobe. **B,** left posterior oblique perfusion image with a defect (*arrow*) in the apical segment of the left lower lobe. (Courtesy of Kenney IJ, Lenney W, Lutkin JE, et al: *Br J Radiol* 66:1031–1034, 1993.)

volving foreign body aspiration and removal. The etiology of these defects is uncertain. The findings also show a considerable subjective element in the interpretation of ventilation-perfusion scans. Only 8 of 14 patients yielded agreement as to normal vs. abnormal.

▶ These are interesting and somewhat scary data. We hope other pediatric centers will repeat this work so that we can get some larger numbers to analyze. After all we have said and all that has been published about the difficulty in obtaining agreement between 2 observers who look at the same lung scan, we were not surprised at the subjective interpretation problem these 2 experts discovered.—A. Gottschalk, M.D.

Abnormalities on Ventilation/Perfusion Lung Scans Induced by Bronchoalveolar Lavage
Chen CC, Andrich MP, Shelhamer J (NIH, Bethesda, Md)
J Nucl Med 34:1854–1858, 1993   124-95-1–19

Background.—Patients who are seriously ill or immunocompromised may require bronchoscopy with bronchoalveolar lavage (BAL) and ventilation-perfusion (V/Q) lung scanning performed close together. When BAL is done before V/Q scanning, abnormalities caused by lavage can interfere with scan interpretation. Other changes on radionuclide V/Q scans may also occur.

Methods and Findings.—Ten healthy volunteers had V/Q scanning at various times after lavage to determine whether BAL significantly affects

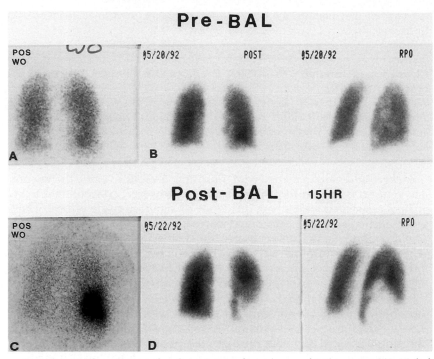

Fig 1–10.—Paired ventilation and perfusion images obtained pre- and 15 hours post BAL. Marked abnormalities after BAL involve multiple segments of the right lower lobe. The chest radiograph was normal. Posterior washout ventilation images (**A** and **C**); posterior and right posterior oblique perfusion images (**B** and **D**). (Courtesy of Chen CC, Andrich MP, Shelhamer J: *J Nucl Med* 34:1854–1858, 1993.)

V/Q lung scan and chest radiograph findings. Abnormal lung scans were obtained in 6 patients. These showed matched ventilation/perfusion defects and were interpreted as having intermediate, low, and very low probability for pulmonary emboli in 3, 1, and 2 patients, respectively. Defects varied from multisegmental to subsegmental in size (Fig 1–10). Chest radiographs were normal in all but 1 patient. The degree and frequency of defects tended to decrease over time. Twenty-four hours after bronchoalveolar lavage, only 1 of 4 volunteers had a minimally abnormal scan.

Conclusion.—Ventilation-perfusion lung scanning should be delayed at least 24 hours after BAL to avoid problems in interpreting defects that may be the result of lavage. In addition, chest radiographs cannot be used to determine when post-BAL scans can be safely obtained. They are often normal despite the V/Q defects seen on scans.

▶ This interesting observation could keep you from making a needless intermediate reading. I have never knowingly come across this situation, but I have known for years that V/Q scans that are done shortly after tapping a large plural effusion will continue to show abnormalities. This is probably a variation of that finding; the "drowned" lung takes a while to recover.—A. Gottschalk, M.D.

Clearance of Inhaled ^{99m}Tc-DTPA Predicts the Clinical Course of Fibrosing Alveolitis

Wells AU, Hansell DM, Harrison NK, Lawrence R, Black CM, du Bois RM (Royal Brompton Natl Heart & Lung Hosp, London; Royal Marsden Hosp, London; Royal Free Hosp, London)
Eur Respir J 6:797–802, 1993   1 24-95-1–20

Background.—In patients with fibrosing alveolitis, early therapeutic intervention is known to prolong survival. However, conventional treatment is associated with a high incidence of significant side effects. Thus, a diagnostic technique that could correctly predict progressive disease would be an important advance in managing fibrosing alveolitis. Whether the speed of clearance of technetium-99m (^{99m}Tc) DTPA from the lung can predict disease progression in fibrosing alveolitis, as determined by changes in respiratory function tests (RFTs), was assessed.

Patients and Methods.—Technetium-labeled DTPA clearance tests were performed in 82 nonsmoking patients with fibrosing alveolitis. Of these, 53 had progressive systemic sclerosis and 29 had lone cryptogenic fibrosing alveolitis. At initial measurement, patients were categorized as having normal or abnormal clearance. A further subdivision was made in those patients undergoing a second measurement of clearance approximately 12 months later. Categories were based on clearance trends and included persistently abnormal clearance, abnormal clearance reverting to normal, persistently normal clearance, and normal clearance reverting to abnormal. All patients were evaluated with RFTs within 4 weeks of the initial and repeat clearance measurements. These were repeated at regular intervals during a minimum of 6 months follow-up after the first clearance scan in all patients and 6 months after the second scan in those who underwent a second measurement.

Results.—At initial measurement, normal ^{99m}Tc-DTPA clearance was predictive of stable disease, whereas rapid clearance identified patients who were at risk for deterioration. In patients with rapid clearance, a decrease in RFT was noted, whereas patients with normal clearance did not show change at RFT. Repeat clearance measurements permitted the identification of both a subgroup of patients who were at higher risk and had persistently abnormal clearance and a smaller subgroup of patients in whom reversion of clearance to normal was associated with a sustained improvement in respiratory function indices. Treatment differences between subgroups did not alter these findings.

Conclusion.—In patients with fibrosing alveolitis, the speed of ^{99m}Tc-DTPA clearance can differentiate between stable and progressive disease. This finding is clinically important, particularly with respect to the selection and timing of follow-up and treatment.

► This looks like exciting stuff. These data should allow effective and inexpensive stratification of these patients relative to the cost of the imaging and pulmonary function studies that these patients now undergo on a regular basis.—A. Gottschalk, M.D.

Perfusion Lung Scintigraphy in Primary Pulmonary Hypertension
Ogawa Y, Nishimura T, Hayashida K, Uehara T, Shimonagata T (Natl Cardiovascular Ctr, Suita, Osaka, Japan)
Br J Radiol 66:677–680, 1993   124-95-1–21

Objective.—In primary pulmonary hypertension (PPH), a decrease in the peripheral pulmonary arterial bed leads to an extreme increase in pulmonary arterial pressure, ultimately resulting in heart failure and death. The pulmonary perfusion scintigraphic findings in PPH are thought to reflect the pulmonary arterial bed and, therefore, may relate to cardiac function and prognosis. The scintigraphic patterns were compared with the hemodynamic findings and survival time of patients with PPH.

Patients.—The patients included 11 females and 4 males with a mean age of 34.7 years. Perfusion scintigraphy was performed after IV injection of 5 mCi of technetium-99m macroaggregated albumin; the studies were performed at a mean of 25 months after onset of symptoms. All patients had a high pulmonary arterial pressure, with a mean greater than 25 mm Hg, as measured by cardiac catheterization. Patients were followed for up to 8 years.

Findings.—On evaluation by experienced nuclear medicine physicians, the perfusion lung scintigraphic findings were classified into 2 groups. Eight patients had a pattern of multiple, small, ill-defined defects, whereas the other 7 had a normal pattern. The mean pulmonary arterial pressure was 54 mm Hg in patients with the mottled pattern vs. 42 mm Hg in those with the normal pattern. There were no significant variations between groups in right ventricular ejection fraction, partial pressure of oxygen in the arterial blood, or alveoloarterial oxygen difference. Two-year survival was 0% in patients with the mottled pattern vs. 57% in those with the normal pattern.

Conclusion.—Although small and retrospective, this study suggests that the prognosis is poor for patients with PPH and a mottled pattern on perfusion lung scintigraphy. As the disease progresses, advanced obstructive changes in the peripheral pulmonary arteries may result in multiple perfusion defects.

► These data present an interesting but frightening hypothesis regarding a small group of patients. It would be useful if the San Diego group continued this analysis using their much larger patient registry.—A. Gottschalk, M.D.

Pulmonary Angiography With MR Imaging: Preliminary Clinical Experience

Grist TM, Sostman HD, MacFall JR, Foo TK, Spritzer CE, Witty L, Newman GE, Debatin JF, Tapson V, Saltzman HA (Univ of Wisconsin Hosps and Clinics, Madison; Duke Univ, Durham, NC; GE Med Systems, Milwaukee, Wis)
Radiology 189:523–530, 1993   124-95-1–22

Introduction.—An accurate, noninvasive method for direct imaging of the pulmonary vasculature would greatly enhance the evaluation of patients with suspected pulmonary embolism (PE). Technical obstacles have hindered the development of pulmonary MR angiography. An up-to-date technique of MRI of the pulmonary vasculature was used for evaluation of patients with suspected PE.

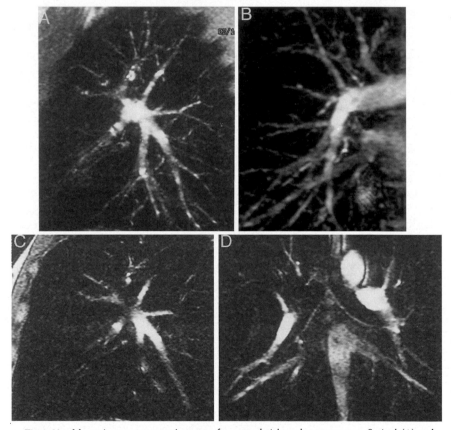

Fig 1–11.—Magnetic resonance angiograms of a normal right pulmonary artery. Sagittal (**A**) and coronal (**C**) MR pulmonary angiographic projection images obtained in a subject with normal pulmonary arteries are shown with examples (**B** and **D**) of the single-section images from which the projections are derived (e.g., **B** is included in **A**, and **D** is included in **C**). (Courtesy of Grist TM, Sostman HD, MacFall JR, et al: *Radiology* 189:523–530, 1993.)

Methods.—In a prospective study, 20 patients with clinically suspected PE underwent pulmonary vascular MR angiography. The procedure, done using a multisection, two-dimensional, time-of-flight technique, was performed in 14 patients before conventional pulmonary angiography and in 6 patients who were considered to have PE on the basis of findings of other studies. The images were reprojected to form projection pulmonary angiograms by means of a maximum-intensity-pixel projection algorithm (Fig 1–11). Thirteen patients had MR venography at the same time as MR pulmonary angiography.

Results.—Evaluable images were obtained in 11 patients. Twelve of the 20 patients proved to have acute PE. The sensitivity of MR angiography was 92% to 100%, depending on the reader, whereas the specificity was 63%. Together, the results of MR venography and pulmonary angiography correctly identified all 12 patients who required treatment for venous thromboembolism.

Conclusion.—The initial clinical experience with MR pulmonary angiography for evaluation of possible PE was reported. Specificity could be improved by enhancing sensitivity to slow flow and increasing spatial resolution; these advances must be achieved before MR pulmonary angiography can be recommended for routine clinical use.

▶ We included this article to ensure that you keep up to date regarding the non-nuclear, noninvasive world of PE diagnosis. Similar progress is very rapidly being made for diagnosis of PE with spiral CT.—A. Gottschalk, M.D.

Call Mosby Document Express at **1 (800) 55-MOSBY** to obtain copies of the original source documents of articles featured or referenced in the YEAR BOOK series.

2 Hematology and Oncology

Introduction

For many years, PET imaging with F-18-fluorodeoxyglucose has proven very effective in differentiating slow-growing from malignant brain tumors. More recently, this technique has achieved extremely high tumor-to-background ratios in a host of different primary, recurrent, and metastatic malignancies in other organs, which are unmatched by any single-photon radiopharmaceutical. Should more regional cyclotron-PET centers be established to make this approach more widely available to cancer patients?

Resistance to chemotherapy and radiation is one of the major causes of treatment failure in cancer. A major cause of this failure is the presence of a 170-kd membrane of glycoprotein called Pgp, which pumps toxic substances, including many chemotherapy agents, out of tumor cells (1). It is also called the multidrug resistance molecule (MDR). It is normally present in the endothelium of the testis and nervous system and in many secretory glands and organs, hematopoietic stem cells, and biliary tract and renal tubules, serving to protect these cells against poisons.

Cells with intrinsic or acquired drug resistance to chemotherapy can be made more sensitive by administering a variety of reversal agents that competitively block the Pgp pump mechanism (2). These agents tend to be small, cationic, somewhat lipophilic molecules similar to many chemotherapy agents. They include R-verapamil (d-verapamil has less cardiac toxicity than the racemic drug), cyclosporine, trifluoperazine, tamoxifen, and many other drugs. To block the Pgp effect, they must often be administered in large doses that are close to toxicity.

Piwnica-Worms and colleagues (3) have shown that the cellular concentration of technetium-99m sestamibi is influenced by the presence and density of Pgp molecules. In suspensions of cells that exhibit high MDR, the concentration of sestamibi was greatly increased by verapamil or cyclosporine. It is still not known whether these agents will improve the sestamibi tumor–background concentration ratios in vivo.

The search continues for reversal agents of lower toxicity and other radioactive agents that increase their tumor concentration with the reversal agents. Overexpression of Pgp tends to occur in acute lymphoblastic leukemia; gastric, colon, and endometrial cancer; neuroblastoma; and malignant myeloma, but not in malignant melanoma or ovarian cancer (1). At the NIH, transfected mice have been produced with overexpression of the MDR genes in bone marrow cells to selectively decrease the myelosuppression from chemotherapy. Can this technique ever be applied to patients with cancer?

In recent years, neutropenia resulting from large therapeutic doses of chemotherapeutic agents has been eliminated or minimized by administering the growth factors granulocyte-macrophage colony-stimulating factor or granulocyte colony-stimulating factor (G-CSF). The latter is preferred because it is less toxic and the thrombocytopenia is less. However, neither stimulates the proliferation of platelets. Stem cell factor does, but it is too toxic for human use.

After 30 years of searching for the real thrombopoietin, the success story came in 4 papers and a news report in 1994 (4). Developed both by Genentech Inc. and ZymoGenetics, Inc., it is hoped that it will be widely used in combination with G-CSF for balanced proliferation of neutrophils and platelets for high-dose chemotherapy and bone marrow transplants.

Should this approach be tried for high-dose iodine-131 sodium iodide radiation therapy for papillary or follicular thyroid carcinoma, radioimmunotherapy with monoclonal antibodies, or other therapeutic radiopharmaceuticals?

John G. McAfee, M.D.

References

1. Patel NH, Rothenberg ML: *Invest New Drugs* 12:1, 1994.
2. Raderer M, Scheithauer W: *Cancer* 72:3553, 1993.
3. 1994 YEAR BOOK OF NUCLEAR MEDICINE p 327.
4. Metcalf D: *Nature* 369:519, 1994.

Impact of Technetium-99M-Sestamibi Localization on Operative Time and Success of Operations for Primary Hyperparathyroidism
Casas AT, Burke GJ, Mansberger AR Jr, Wei JP (Med College of Georgia, Augusta)
Am Surg 60:12–17, 1994   124-95-2-1

Objective.—In patients with primary hyperparathyroidism, intraoperative identification of abnormal parathyroid glands during initial neck exploration may be a challenging problem. Extensive neck and mediastinal dissection is sometimes required. Technetium-99m sestamibi and iodine-123 radionuclide subtraction imaging was evaluated for preoperative localization of abnormal parathyroid glands.

Methods.—A total of 42 patients who underwent neck exploration for primary hyperparathyroidism were studied. In half, surgery was done with no preoperative radionuclide scanning. In the other half, radionuclide technetium-99m sestamibi localization was done before surgery. The 2 groups were comparable in mean age, mean intact parathyroid hormone levels, mean total calcium, and mean ionized calcium. They were compared for operative time and the success rate of their initial operations for primary hyperparathyroidism.

Results.—On pathologic examination, 15 patients in the control group had solitary adenomas and 6 had diffuse hyperplasia. In the technetium-99m sestamibi group, 16 had solitary adenomas, 4 had diffuse hyperplasia, and 1 had multiple adenomas. In both groups, the mean number of parathyroid glands identified and biopsied per patient was approximately 3, and the mean diameter of the resected adenomas was about 20 mm. There was no difference in the number of patients requiring thymectomy, thyroid resection, retroesophageal exploration, mediastinal exploration, or carotid sheath exploration. The initial operation was successful in 90% of the controls and 100% of those in the technetium-99m sestamibi group. The mean operative times were 180 vs. 135 minutes.

Conclusion.—In patients undergoing initial neck exploration for primary hyperparathyroidism, preoperative parathyroid localization with technetium-99m sestamibi can reduce operative time and may improve success rates. Prospective, randomized studies are needed to confirm the value of preoperative localization.

▶ Many practitioners now think that technetium-99m sestamibi is better than thallium-201 for subtraction imaging in combination with iodine-123 iodide or technetium-99m pertechnetate. Moreover, delayed images at 2 hours or more with sestamibi often show adenomas better after the thyroid activity has decreased.

As exemplified in the comments that accompany this paper, some surgeons believe that at the initial surgery, all 4 parathyroids should be explored routinely, because adenomas often are not solitary, and smaller ones may be missed by any external imaging procedure. Hence, they believe that imaging before the first surgery is unnecessary. However, preoperative imaging sometimes finds adenomas in unusual locations. There seems to be general agreement that in this radionuclide study, CT and MRI are indicated in persistent hyperparathyroidism after surgery.

A few centers are using handheld miniature scintillation probes to pinpoint the adenomas during surgery after administering sestamibi.—J.G. McAfee, M.D.

Thallium-201 Versus Technetium-99m-MIBI SPECT in Evaluation of Childhood Brain Tumors: A Within-Subject Comparison

O'Tuama LA, Treves ST, Larar JN, Packard AB, Kwan AJ, Barnes PD, Scott RM, PMcL Black , Madsen JR, Goumnerova LC, Sallan SE, Tarbell NJ (Children's Hosp, Boston; Harvard Med School, Boston)

J Nucl Med 34:1045–1051, 1993   124-95-2-2

Background.—In children with brain tumors, recurrence and focal cerebral necrosis cannot be differentiated by CT or MRI. Such diagnostic uncertainty can seriously affect treatment planning. In a previous study, thallium-201 (^{201}Tl) SPECT was found to be highly specific for locating metabolic activity in childhood brain tumors. The relative diagnostic accuracy of ^{201}Tl and a technetium-based tumor-avid agent was determined.

Patients and Methods.—Nineteen children, aged 1 to 18 years, were studied. All had brain tumors diagnosed on the basis of clinical or histologic findings. Using ^{201}Tl at 37 to 111 MBq, SPECT was obtained and followed immediately by an IV administration of technetium-99m methoxyisobutylisonitrile (MIBI) at 370 to 740 MBq.

Results.—Both tracers were similar, because each was almost entirely excluded from cerebral tissues inside the normal blood-brain barrier. The only distinguishing characteristic was a consistent and prominent uptake of MIBI by the normal choroid plexus, which occurred despite pretreatment with oral potassium perchlorate, 6 mg/kg, 30 minutes before the tracer was given. Thallium uptake was also noted in the area of the choroid plexus, but to a lesser degree than MIBI. In 6 true positive studies, a moderate-to-intense focal uptake was noted for both tracers at the site of tumor activity. A greater signal-to-noise ratio with MIBI resulted in more clearly defined lesion boundaries. Preliminary evaluation revealed approximately 67% sensitivity for Tl and MIBI. Specificity was approximately 91% and 100% for Tl and MIBI, respectively. Two tumors, a medulloblastoma and a dysgerminoma, were Tl and MIBI nonavid. A semiquantitative evaluation of tracer uptake, using a ratio of radioactivity in tumor-containing areas compared with uninvolved brain, showed a mean value of 7.88 ± 7.7 for Tl and 27.1 ± 36.41 for MIBI.

Conclusion.—The spectrum of tumor avidity is comparable for both Tl and MIBI. However, further studies are needed to determine possible differences in tracer distribution because it may have important implications for grading.

▶ The results in the preliminary study are not too encouraging; 6 true positive and either 2 or 3 false negative results for brain tumors seen with either agent. With a sensitivity of detection of only 67% to 75%, this imaging would be of questionable value in decision-making when CT or MRI findings are equivocal. However, these results may improve in a larger series of patients. The images obtained with technetium-99m sestamibi are obviously superior to those obtained with [201]Tl.—J.G. McAfee, M.D.

The Role of Thallium-201 Single Photon Emission Tomography in the Investigation and Characterisation of Brain Tumours in Man and Their Response to Treatment

Yoshii Y, Satou M, Yamamoto T, Yamada Y, Hyodo A, Nose T, Ishikawa H, Hatakeyama R (Univ of Tsukuba, Tsukuba-shi, Ibaraki, Japan)
Eur J Nucl Med 20:39–45, 1993   124-95-2–3

Background.—Planar thallium-201 imaging reportedly has potential for the characterization of brain tumors. Brain tumor type and treatment response were determined in relation to thallium-201 uptake, which is caused by increased sodium potassium adenosine triphosphatase activity in viable tumor cell membranes.

Patients and Methods.—Fifty-eight patients with diagnosed intracranial lesions were studied. Thallium-201 SPECT imaging was performed in all patients. In addition, statistical comparisons of the early and delayed thallium-201 indices were undertaken in 56 patients. Indices were expressed as the ratio of the tumor to the contralateral cerebral hemisphere uptake. The retention index (RI) of thallium-201 in the tumor tissue, which is calculated from early and delayed scans, was also assessed. Finally, the diagnostic value was compared between high uptake

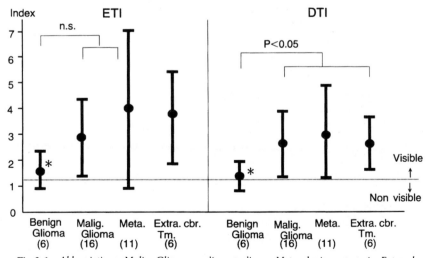

Fig 2–1.—*Abbreviations: Malig. Glioma*, malignant glioma; *Meta.*, brain metastasis; *Extra cbr. Tm.*, extracerebral tumor; *ETI* and *DTI*, early and delayed thallium-201 indices, respectively. Early and delayed thallium-201 indices in viable tumors. The *dotted line* marks the separation between "positive" (visible) and "negative" scan findings. (Courtesy of Yoshii Y, Satou M, Yamamoto T, et al: *Eur J Nucl Med* 20:39–45, 1993.)

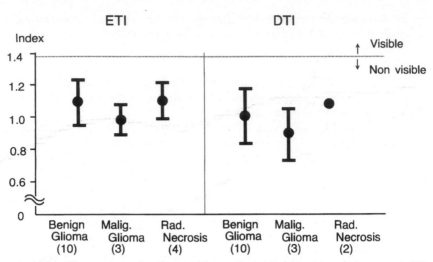

Fig 2–2.—*Abbreviations: Malig. Glioma,* malignant glioma; *Rad. Necrosis,* radiation necrosis; *ETI* and *DTI,* early and delayed thallium-201 indices, respectively. Early and delayed thallium-201 indices in the stabilized tumors and cases of radiation necrosis. Note the poor thallium-201 uptake values and the negative scans with thallium-201 SPECT. (Courtesy of Yoshii Y, Satou M, Yamamoto T, et al: *Eur J Nucl Med* 20:39–45, 1993.)

of thallium-201 and Gd-DTPA enhancement on MRI scans in 56 patients.

Results.—A high thallium-201 uptake was noted in viable malignant gliomas, brain metastases, meningiomas, and malignant teratoma. However, thallium-201 indices failed to differentiate the viable malignant gliomas from brain metastases and extracerebral tumors (Fig 2–1). In addition, such differentiation was not demonstrated in stabilized tumors (Fig 2–2). The percentage of RI tended to be high in the viable brain metastases and extracerebral tumors. In stabilized tumors and cases of radiation necrosis, the RI was not as high. Although visualized by Gd-DTPA–enhanced MRI, thallium-201 SPECT failed to identify a viable ring-enhanced tumor with a thin rim and small tumors measuring less than 1.5 cm in diameter.

The retention index values in Figure 2–3 were obtained from a region of interest (ROI) of the tumor in the slice with the highest tumor in a semi-oval ROI over the whole contralateral hemisphere on the same slice.

Conclusion.—Despite the aforementioned underestimation, thallium-201 SPECT may be effective in determining the malignant viability of tumors.

▶ Thallium-201 SPECT imaging undoubtedly demonstrates the majority of intracranial tumors well. However, much of the initial enthusiasm regarding the ability of this technique to differentiate tumor types has waned. Figures 2–1 to 2–3 show considerable overlap in tumor-to-normal brain ratios and

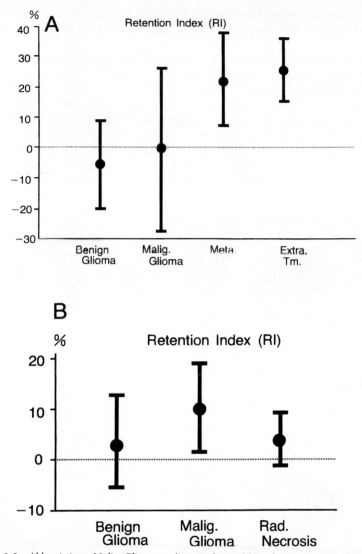

Fig 2–3.—*Abbreviations: Malig. Glioma,* malignant glioma; *Meta.,* brain metastasis; *Extra. Tm.,* extracerebral tumor; *Rad. Necrosis,* radiation necrosis. **A,** retention index of thallium-201 in viable tumors. **B,** RI of thallium-201 in stabilized tumors and cases of radiation necrosis. Although not statistically significant, there was a tendency toward a high retention index in viable brain metastases and extracerebral tumors. (Courtesy of Yoshii Y, Satou M, Yamamoto T, et al: *Eur J Nucl Med* 20:39-45, 1993.)

retention indexes with relatively large standard deviations. Even the values in radiation necrosis are similar to tumor values, presumably because of passive diffusion of thallium-201 into necrotic areas and the breakdown of the blood-brain barrier.—J.G. McAfee, M.D.

Clinical Evaluation of Thallium-201 SPECT in Supratentorial Gliomas: Relationship to Histologic Grade, Prognosis and Proliferative Activities

Oriuchi N, Tamura M, Shibazaki T, Ohye C, Watanabe N, Tateno M, Tomiyoshi K, Hirano T, Inoue T, Endo K (Gunma Univ, Japan)
J Nucl Med 34:2085–2089, 1993   124-95-2-4

Background.—The usefulness of thallium-201 for localization of brain tumors, differentiation of high-grade malignancy from benign or low-grade malignancy, and estimation of the degree of residual tumor or recurrence has previously been reported. The clinical effectiveness of thallium-201 brain SPECT images was determined in patients with supraten-

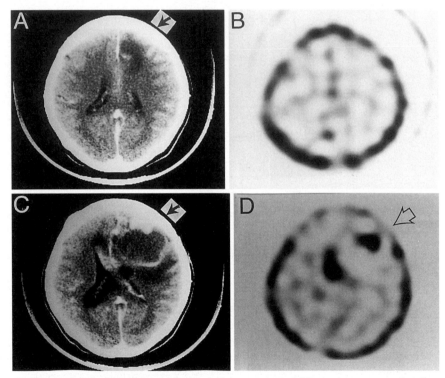

Fig 2–4.—Female, 40, with low-grade glioma. Contrast-enhanced CT scan demonstrates a low-density mass in the left frontal lobe (*arrow*) with enhancement in the medial portion (**A**). The SPECT image obtained 15 minutes after intravenous administration shows no accumulation in the lesion (**B**). Thallium-201 index, 101%; BUdR-LI, 0%. A contrast-enhanced CT scan (**C**) performed 19 months after the first CT scan demonstrates a ring-like enhanced mass in the left frontal lobe with a central low-density area (*arrow*). Marked edema and mass effect are shown. Thallium-201 brain SPECT performed the next day (**D**) demonstrates markedly increased accumulation in the medial and anterolateral margin of the lesion (*arrow*). Thallium-201 index, 157%, BUdR, 19%. Histologic diagnosis was glioblastoma. The patient died 31 months after the initial study. (Courtesy of Oriuchi N, Tamura M, Shibazaki T, et al: *J Nucl Med* 34:2085-2089, 1993.)

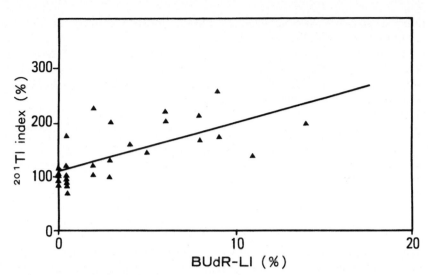

Fig 2–5.—Correlation between the thallium-201 index and the BUdR-LI in patients with glioma. Significant correlation was observed (n = 28; r = .67; P < .001). (Courtesy of Oriuchi N, Tamura M, Shibazaki T, et al: *J Nucl Med* 34:2085–2089, 1993.)

torial gliomas. In addition, the proliferative activities of neoplastic tissues were measured using bromodeoxyuridine (BUdR), a thymidine analogue.

Patients and Methods.—Twenty-eight patients with a mean age of 45.6 years were studied. All had supratentorial gliomas diagnosed that ranged in size from 3 to 9 cm. Thallium-201 SPECT studies were performed in all patients 1 to 37 days before surgical resection. In addition, 200 mg of IV BUdR per m² was administered 1 hour before surgery. An immunohistologic staining technique was used to detect BUdR-labeled cells from tumor specimens obtained at surgery. Follow-up continued for more than 25 months.

Results.—An association between the degree of thallium-201 uptake and histologic glioma grade was noted. In 12 of 14 patients with low-grade glioma, no accumulation of thallium-201 was observed at the tumor site. In addition, thallium-201 indexes, expressed as the count rate of the tumor site to the count rate over the contralateral normal region, were less than 113%. The BUdR-labeling index (LI) was also lower than 3% in all 14 patients with low-grade glioma (Fig 2–4). In 4 patients with grade III glioma, a definite accumulation of thallium-201 was noted at the lesion site, and indexes ranged from 122% to 162%; BUdR-LIs of 2% to 5% were also observed. Intense accumulation was found in the tumor sites of 10 patients with grade IV glioma. Thallium-201 indexes were more than 141% in these patients, with BUdR-LIs ranging from 2% to 14%. A significant association between the thallium-201 index and BUdR-LI was noted (Fig 2–5). In patients who died after surgery, the mean thallium-201 index and BUdR-LI were significantly higher than those in patients who survived 25 months postoperatively, at 173.2% compared with 122.4%, respectively.

Conclusion.—Supratentorial gliomas are effectively imaged with thallium-201 brain SPECT. In addition, the extent of the tumor can be fairly well predicted with this technique. Finally, the thallium-201 index reflects the proliferative activity of the tumor.

▶ This article confirms previous claims that malignant gliomas concentrate thallium better than more benign (low-grade) gliomas. A significant correlation was found between the thallium-201 index (tumor-to-contralateral site ratio) and tumor proliferative activity, as measured by a cell-labeling index after preoperative administration of bromodeoxyuridine. On inspection of Figure 2–5, however, the slope of the correlation is rather shallow, and the individual points are scattered. The standard error of the estimate was not given, but it is probably large. In an accompanying editorial (1), Tonami and Hisada point out that several factors influence the thallium index, including the size of the lesion, the amount of necrosis, the method of attenuation correction, and the spatial resolution (for smaller lesions). Will this thallium index ever be useful for patient management?—J.G. McAfee, M.D.

Reference

1. Tonami N, Hisada K: *J Nucl Med* 34:2089, 1993.

Thallium-201 Scanning for the Evaluation of Osteosarcoma and Soft-Tissue Sarcoma: A Study of the Evaluation and Predictability of the Histological Response to Chemotherapy
Menendez LR, Fideler BM, Mirra J (Univ of Southern California, Los Angeles)
J Bone Joint Surg (Am) 75A:526–531, 1993   124-95-2–5

Objective.—Different imaging techniques are used in the diagnosis, treatment planning, and follow-up of patients with osteosarcomas and soft tissue sarcomas. Thallium chloride is a readily available radionuclide that has rarely been studied in the evaluation of musculoskeletal tumors. The uptake of thallium by tumor cells is an active transport rather than a flow-dependent process; as a result, the scan can demonstrate the viability and metabolic activity of the pathologic cells. The use of thallium-201 (^{201}Tl) scanning was evaluated in patients with osteosarcoma and soft tissue sarcoma.

Methods.—Sequential thallium scans were performed before and after preoperative chemotherapy in 16 patients with high-grade sarcomas of the bone or soft tissue. Thallium uptake by the neoplasms was graded in a semiquantitative fashion by independent observers. Whether ^{201}Tl scanning could accurately determine the amount of viable tumor and predict the response to chemotherapy was investigated.

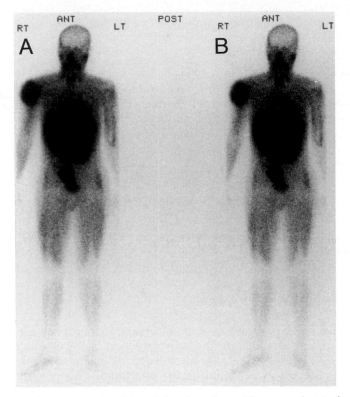

Fig 2–6.—Thallium scans made before and after chemotherapy. The scan on the **left** of each figure was made immediately after injection of thallium. Scan on **right** was made 90 minutes after injection. In **A,** a large lesion is demonstrated in the proximal aspect of the right humerus before chemotherapy. In **B,** there is dramatic improvement after chemotherapy. (Courtesy of Menendez LR, Fideler BM, Mirra J: J Bone Joint Surg [Am] 75A: 526–531, 1993.

Results.—Ten patients showed a reduced thallium uptake after chemotherapy (Fig 2–6). Nine of these patients also demonstrated a marked histologic response, with at least 95% tumor necrosis. The other 6 patients had no improvement on their postchemotherapy ^{201}Tl scans, and all had tumor necrosis of less than 95%. A marked response was noted in 5 of 8 patients with malignant fibrous histiocytoma and in 4 of 5 with Ewing's sarcoma.

Conclusion.—In patients with osteosarcomas and soft tissue sarcomas, thallium chloride scanning appears to provide a more accurate reflection of tumor viability and metabolic activity than studies that use flow-dependent scanning agents. It is believed that sequential thallium scintigraphy has a role along with other imaging modalities in the diagnosis, treatment planning, and follow-up evaluation of patients with such tumors. Scanning with ^{201}Tl can predict the histologic response of these tumors to preoperative chemotherapy.

▶ This article does not give any information on the histologic comparison of pre- and postchemotherapy biopsy specimens or the duration of the chemotherapy. However, a good correlation was found between the degree of postchemotherapy tumor necrosis histologically and the decrease in thallium uptake after chemotherapy compared with prechemotherapy images.

The authors emphasize that estimates of histologic viability are prone to tissue sampling errors, whereas macroscopic thallium images are not. Although this is an interesting pilot study, it is doubtful that this radionuclide protocol will influence patient management significantly.—J.G. McAfee, M.D.

A Complementary Role for Thallium-201 Scintigraphy With Mammography in the Diagnosis of Breast Cancer

Lee VW, Sax EJ, McAneny DB, Pollack S, Blanchard RA, Beazley RM, Kavanah MT, Ward RJ (Boston Univ)

J Nucl Med 34:2095–2100, 1993   124-95-2-6

Objective.—Physical examination and mammography are sensitive but not very specific methods for the early detection of breast cancer. Subsequent surgical biopsy is commonly needed to diagnose the lesion that has been detected as being malignant or benign. The potential role of

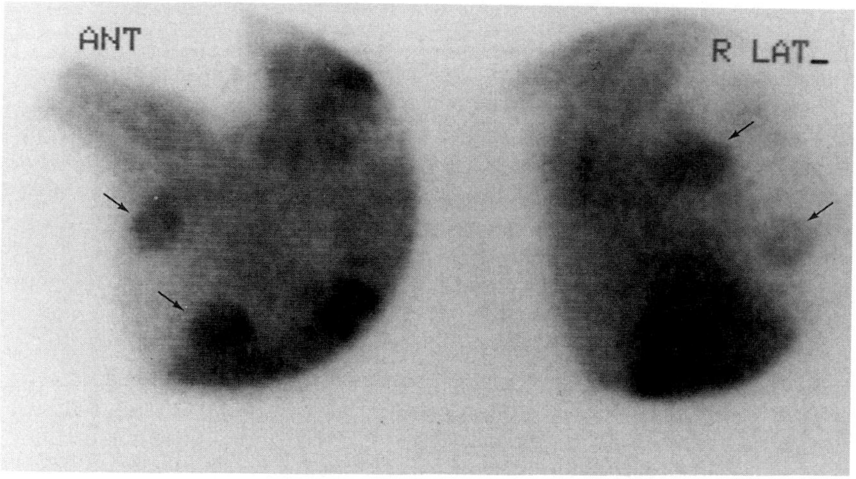

Fig 2–7.—Woman, 61, who had a large palpable mass at her right breast. Mammogram demonstrated a 6-cm lobulated mass without calcification in her right breast. Thallium scintigraphy detected large round areas of marked increased uptake at the right breast and axilla (*arrows*). The normal myocardium showed high uptake of thallium and should not be mistaken as abnormal uptake on the left side. (Courtesy of Lee VW, Sax EJ, McAneny DB, et al: *J Nucl Med* 34:2095–2100, 1993.)

thallium breast scanning as a complementary method for the diagnosis of breast cancer was examined.

Methods.—Forty patients with breast abnormalities that were discovered by mammography, physical examination, or a combination of the 2 were entered in the study; 2 of the patients were men. The patients were divided into 2 groups: group A, which included 30 patients with no previous history of breast cancer but who were scheduled for biopsy or surgery, and group B, which included patients with suspected local recurrence of breast cancer related to palpable nodules around the surgical sites. Thallium scintigraphy was performed in each patient, and the results were read in blinded fashion by independent reviewers. The sensitivity and specificity of thallium breast scanning were examined.

Results.—Thallium scans of 32 breasts in 30 patients were obtained before biopsy or surgery in group A. A pathologic diagnosis was obtained in 31 breasts in 29 patients. There were 7 true positive thallium scans and 22 true negative scans in this group, along with 2 false negative and 1 false positive scans. Of the 7 scans in group B patients, 5 were true positive and 1 each was true negative and false negative. The specificity of thallium scanning for cancer was 96%, and the sensitivity was 80% (Fig 2–7).

Conclusion.—Thallium scanning has a high specificity and moderately high sensitivity in the diagnosis of breast cancer. Further study will be needed to see whether the combination of mammographic and scintigraphic findings can reduce the number of breast biopsy procedures performed. Possible roles for scintigraphy could include scanning of the axilla for lymph node metastases, evaluation of the contralateral breast, and as a baseline for comparison with postoperative scans.

▶ As the authors point out, a much larger experience will be needed to assess the true value of thallium imaging of breast lesions, particularly in the differentiation of benign from malignant lesions.

If this procedure proves worthwhile, special small cameras, analogous to x-ray mammographic machines, may have to be developed for optimal breast and axillary imaging.—J.G. McAfee, M.D.

Utility of Thallium-201 and Iodine-123 Metaiodobenzylguanidine in the Scintigraphic Detection of Neuroendocrine Neoplasia
Montravers F, Coutris G, Sarda L, Mensch B, Talbot J-N (Faculté de Médecine Saint Antoine, Paris)
Eur J Nucl Med 20:1070–1077, 1993   124-95-2-7

Background.—Metaiodobenzylguanidine (MIBG) is an imaging marker that is specific for pheochromocytomas and neuroblastomas. It can also detect, with low sensitivity, other neuroendocrine tumors, including medullary thyroid carcinomas, paragangliomas, and carcinoid

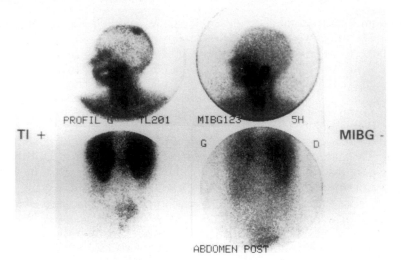

Fig 2–8.—Above, left lateral views of the skull. Skull metastasis of paraganglioma with uptake of thallium **(left)** and no uptake of MIBG **(right). Below,** posterior views of the abdomen. Sacrum metastasis of paraganglioma in another patient with uptake of thallium **(left)** and no uptake of MIBG **(right).** (Courtesy of Montravers F, Coutris G, Sarda L, et al: *Eur J Nucl Med* 20:1070–1077, 1993.)

tumors. Thallium-201 detects tumors with high sensitivity but low specificity. Using a combination of these 2 agents in scintigraphic studies may improve neuroendocrine tumor detection.

Methods.—In a 4-year study, 101 patients who were referred with suspected or confirmed neuroendocrine tumors underwent 137 scintigraphic examinations. Both MIBG and thallium were used. Scans were performed 20 minutes after the IV injection of 27 μCi (1 MBq per kg) of thallium per kg. The patient then received an IV injection of Iodine-123 MIBG, 110 μCi/kg (4 MBq/kg). Scans were performed 5 and 24 hours after the injection.

Results.—Neuroendocrine tumor was excluded in 43 patients. Dual-agent scintigraphy was negative in 40 of these patients; histologic data excluded neuroendocrine tumor in the other 3. Histologic data were used to diagnose neuroendocrine tumors in the remaining 58 patients. Eighteen patients had pheochromocytomas; 16 were detected by MIBG, 1 by both agents. Two patients had neuroblastoma; 1 was detected by MIBG, the other was not detected by either agent. Thallium was more sensitive in detecting medullary thyroid carcinoma; 23 of 30 localizations were detected by thallium alone, 1 by MIBG alone, and 2 by both agents. Dual-agent scintigraphy was most useful in detecting paragangliomas. Five of 12 paragangliomas were detected by MIBG, 5 more were detected by thallium (Fig 2–8).

Discussion.—In diagnosing neuroblastomas and pheochromocytomas, MIBG but not thallium is useful. Thallium but not MIBG is useful in diagnosing medullary thyroid carcinoma. However, 1 preoperative MIBG scan is recommended to detect an associated pheochromocytoma. Both agents should be used to diagnose paragangliomas, because different tumors within the same patient may take up different agents.

▶ This is an excellent comparison of the efficacy of the 2 different agents used in determining neuroendocrine tumors. However, this probably is not the final answer, with the advent of technetium-99m sestamibi as a tumor agent and with the recent Food and Drug Administration approval of the indium-111 octreotide analogue.—J.G. McAfee, M.D.

Iodine-131-Metaiodobenzylguanidine Scintigraphy in Preoperative and Postoperative Evaluation of Paragangliomas: Comparison With CT and MRI
Maurea S, Cuocolo A, Reynolds JC, Tumeh SS, Begley MG, Linehan WM, Norton JA, Walther MM, Keiser HR, Neumann RD (Warren G Magnuson Clinical Ctr; Natl Cancer Inst, Bethesda, Md; Natl Heart, Lung and Blood Inst, Bethesda, Md)
J Nucl Med 34:173–179, 1993   124-95-2–8

Background.—In patients who have functioning paragangliomas diagnosed, accurate localization of the disease is crucial for planning and assessment of treatment. Although CT and MRI play an important role in identifying these tumors before surgery, both procedures can fail to locate tumors in areas of previous surgery, and they may not detect extraadrenal or metastatic disease. Iodine-131 metaiodobenzylguanidine (MIBG) scintigraphy is another imaging technique that can effectively locate paragangliomas in areas that are distorted by tumor growth or previous surgery. Moreover, MIBG whole-body examinations are useful for detecting tumors stemming from unexpected locations. In preoperative and postoperative assessment of patients with paragangliomas, MIBG scanning was compared with CT and MRI.

Patients and Methods.—Thirty-six patients with a mean age of 37 ± 11 years were studied. They were divided into 2 groups according to surgical history. Group 1 had 21 patients with no previous surgery for paraganglioma. Group 2 had 15 patients who were evaluated after previous surgery for adrenal or extra-adrenal paragangliomas. Clinical diagnosis of functioning paragangliomas was based on typical signs and symptoms of disease or abnormal levels of urinary catecholamines or metabolites. All patients underwent evaluation with MIBG, CT, and MRI; sensitivity, specificity, and accuracy values were determined.

Results.—Benign adrenal disease was primarily noted in group 1 patients. In group 2 patients, malignant or extra-adrenal tumors were frequently observed. Transmission CT and MRI were found to be more sensitive than MIBG in group 1 patients, at 100%, 100%, and 82%, respectively. However, MIBG was the most specific at 100%. In group 2 patients, MIBG scintigraphy and MRI were more sensitive than CT, at 83%, 83%, and 75%, respectively. However, MIBG was again found to be the most specific at 100%. In patients with recurrent disease who were more likely to have malignant and extra-adrenal tumors, MIBG was the preferred initial modality. This was followed by MRI and CT images to provide better anatomical detail.

Conclusion.—The modalities of MIBG, CT, and MRI proved to be complementary for assessing patients with functioning paragangliomas. However, CT and MRI are the preferred procedures for patients with a clearly abnormal biochemical test when they are first seen. In these patients, tumors are frequently found in the adrenal, and CT and MRI sensitivity is high. However, when biochemical tests are not diagnostic, MIBG can effectively confirm or rule out pheochromocytoma.

▶ In a companion editorial to this paper (1), Dr. Jean-François Chatal suggests CT alone could be used for intra-adrenal pheochromocytomas, and iodine-131 MIBG could be used for finding extra-adrenal or recurrent tumors, in combination with the other 2 modalities (MRI for intra-abdominal tumors and continuous or spiral CT for thoracic lesions). He points out the persistent controversies regarding the terminology of pheochromocytomas and paragangliomas and the differences in preference for various biochemical tests.

Whenever the results of other types of images or biochemical tests are in doubt, the authors of this article contend that MIBG imaging can be helpful, because of its high specificity.—J.G. McAfee, M.D.

Reference

1. Chatal, J-F: *J Nucl Med* 34:180, 1993.

Treatment of Malignant Phaeochromocytoma, Paraganglioma and Carcinoid Tumours With ^{131}I-Metaiodobenzylguanidine
Bomanji J, Britton KE, Ur E, Hawkins L, Grossman AB, Besser GM (St Bartholomew's Hosp, London)
Nucl Med Commun 14:856–861, 1993   124-95-2–9

Introduction.—Radioiodinated metaiodobenzylguanidine (MIBG) concentrates in malignant pheochromocytoma, paraganglioma, and carcinoid tumors, and it has been used for treatment of tumors of neural crest origin.

Series.—Four patients with carcinoid tumors, 3 with paraganglioma, and 2 with malignant pheochromocytoma were treated with MIBG labeled with iodine-131 (^{131}I). In all patients, pretreatment scans made with ^{123}I-MIBG demonstrated metastases in soft tissue, and in 2 patients, in bone as well. The patients were followed for 8 months to 9 years after receiving ^{131}I-MIBG in cumulative doses of 4.8 to 40.1 GBq.

Results.—None of the patients had complete tumor regression response, but 3 had a partial tumor response lasting 40, 50, and 108 months, respectively, and thus have remained in remission; 3 patients had progressive disease. Forty-seven lesions were detected on baseline diagnostic and treatment images in the 9 patients, whereas only 20 were detected after treatment. Five of the 9 patients had a complete symptomatic response to treatment, and 3 others had a partial response. Six of the 9 patients had an objective normal response. The 1 serious adverse effect was mild liver failure in a patient with extensive hepatic metastases.

Conclusion.—Although treatment with ^{131}I-MIBG, is not curative, it does provide temporary palliation for some patients with metastatic pheochromocytoma, paraganglioma, and carcinoid tumors.

▶ These rather mixed therapeutic results are in keeping with those of other small series of patients previously reported. The mean therapeutic dose in this series was 170 mCi of ^{131}I-MIBG (range, 84 to 214 mCi). From 1 to 6 doses were given; as a result, the cumulative administered doses ranged from 129 to 1,085 mCi (mean, 495 mCi). The estimated cumulative absorbed dose varied from 100 to 10,000 rad.

The authors found that the response to this therapy was slow; even the symptomatic response took 3 to 6 months. Therefore, they recommended that the patient's life expectancy should be at least 1 year before undertaking this method of palliation.—J.G. McAfee, M.D.

Sinus Histiocytosis With Massive Lymphadenopathy: Skeletal Involvement

Lehnert M, Eisenschenk A, Dienemann D, Linnarz M (Free Univ, Berlin)
Arch Orthop Trauma Surg 113:53–56, 1993   124-95-2–10

Background.—Sinus histiocytosis with massive lymphadenopathy (SHML) is characterized by paleness, frequently swollen cervical lymph nodes, and subfebrile temperatures. Laboratory features can include accelerated blood sedimentation, hypergammaglobulinemia, and leukocytosis. Skeletal involvement is known to occur in approximately 5% to 10% of patients with this disorder. To date, the pathogenesis of SHML is unclear, although immune system dysfunction or a bacterial- or virus-associated infection may be involved. The clinical, radiographic, and pathologic manifestations of SHML were reviewed.

Case Report.—Woman, 64, had been seen 2.5 years previously for ear, nose, and throat (ENT) treatment of a therapy-resistant cold with constant secretion and increasing recurrent epistaxis. After 12 months of illness, she reported swelling and pain in various skeletal regions, including the right ankle joint, the left olecranon, and the cuboid bones of both feet. Multiple osseous lesions were revealed on scintigraphic, radiologic, and CT imaging (Figs 2–9 and 2–10). Subsequent biopsy specimens revealed the histomorphologic findings typical for SHML, including infiltration by large macrophages with massive hemophagocy-

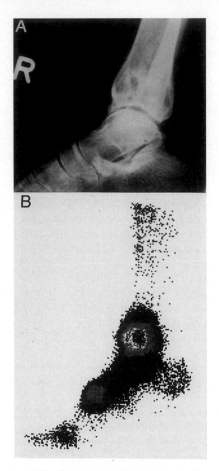

Fig 2–9.—A, cortical and medullary lytic lesions of the distal right tibia. **B,** technetium bone scan showing high uptake in the region of the right distal tibia and os cuboideum. (Courtesy of Lehnert M, Eisenschenk A, Dienemann D, et al: *Arch Orthop Trauma Surg* 113:53–56, 1993.)

tosis and a high plasma cell content associated with focal bone destruction. Operative resection of the left cuboid, which was reportedly the most painful region during walking, was performed. The defect was filled with an autologous bone transplant. The fixation material was removed 8 weeks postoperatively after good osseous consolidation of the implant. No radiologic signs of recurrence have been noted, and the patient remains symptom free. The other bone lesions have not been surgically treated, because the patient needed to first undergo ENT treatment. General medication therapy was not required.

Conclusion.—In patients with SHML, skeletal manifestations do not affect any specific bone regions or bones. Radiologic alterations can be nonspecific and may resemble osseous manifestations noted in histiocy-

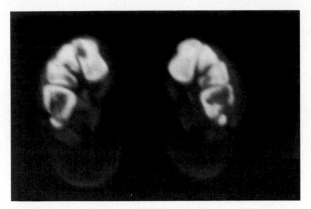

Fig 2–10.—Computed tomography scan showing expansile lesions of both ossa cuboidei. (Courtesy of Lehnert M, Eisenschenk A, Dienemann D, et al: *Arch Orthop Trauma Surg* 113:53–56, 1993.)

tosis X, metastasizing neuroblastoma, multifocal osteomyelitis, neurofibromatosis, or sarcoidosis.

▶ Although this condition is known as Rosai and Dorfman disease, it was actually described 8 years earlier by Lennert, but he did not get any of the credit. A registry of this disease in 1988 included 365 patients (1).

Microscopically numerous histiocytes are merely prominent distractors of secondary importance that are elicited in response to cytokine production of other cells in this condition, rather than a primary proliferation, as in malignant histiocytosis. It is a generally indolent condition, often with neutrophilic infiltration and microabscesses, as well as pale histocytes and plasma cells that distend the lymph node sinusoids (2).

Sinus histiocytosis can occur at any age, with the mean age being 20 years, but 62% of patients are younger than 10 years old. Cervical lymph nodes are involved in 97%, and 80% have involvement of other nodal areas at least microscopically (3). Extranodal disease occurs in about 30%, mostly in the head and neck. Any organ can be involved, especially the eyelids and the orbits, cutaneous and subcutaneous infiltrates.

Any bone can be involved, and the disphosphonate images have no characteristic features. However, gallium images are often positive, especially at the sites of nodal disease (3, 4).—J.G. McAfee, M.D.

References

1. Foucar E, et al: *Arch Dermatol* 124:1211, 1988.
2. Baden E, et al: *Oral Surg Oral Med Oral Pathol* 64:320, 1987.
3. McAlister WH, et al: *Pediatr Radiol* 20:425, 1990.
4. Pastakia B, Weiss SH: *Clin Nucl Med* 12:877, 1987.

Beguiled by the Gallium: Thymic Rebound in an Adult After Chemotherapy for Hodgkin's Disease

Burns DE, Schiffman FJ (Brown Univ, Providence, RI)
Chest 104:1916–1919, 1993   124-95-2–11

Background.—Gallium scanning has been found to be useful in diagnosis, staging, and differentiating between residual active disease or relapse and benign mediastinal enlargement after chemotherapy in patients with Hodgkin's and non-Hodgkin's lymphomas. However, in adult patients, gallium uptake in the mediastinum after chemotherapy may be indicative of benign thymic hyperplasia rather than tumor recurrence, as evidenced by a recent case report.

Case Report.—Woman, 18, reported general malaise, back pain, and a persistent cough of 6 weeks' duration after an upper respiratory tract infection. Cervical lymphadenopathy was found during physical examination, and a chest radiograph showed mediastinal enlargement. She was given a diagnosis of Hodgkin's disease that involved the mediastinal lymph nodes and lung parenchyma after a staging workup. A pretreatment gallium-67 scan revealed increased uptake in the mediastinum. Treatment consisted of 6 monthly cycles of chemotherapy. After treatment, the chest radiograph and chest CT showed resolution of disease, and a repeat gallium scan yielded normal results. A subsequent surveillance gallium scan that was performed 4 months later showed increased activity in the mediastinal and hilar regions. Corresponding chest CT and MRI revealed a retrosternal mass. Before initiating aggressive treatment for presumed disease recurrence, a biopsy of the mass was performed, which revealed normal thymus tissue. This mediastinal mass, which was now considered as thymus, remained evident on both MRI and chest CT. However, a gallium scan performed 10 weeks after the biopsy did not show abnormal radionuclide uptake in the mediastinum, despite the persistent mass. The patient has remained disease free for more than 3 years after initial treatment. The most recent radiographic examinations, including a normal gallium scan and stable CT and MRI, have verified the absence of disease recurrence.

Conclusion.—After chemotherapy, thymus enlargement can occur in adults with Hodgkin's disease. This may be considered when interpreting imaging studies, including gallium scans.

▶ This is a good, brief review of the problems in interpreting gallium images of the mediastinum, but it does not emphasize the superiority of SPECT over planar imaging.

After chemotherapy for mediastinal Hodgkin's disease, residual masses may be the result of persistent disease, relapse, or benign fibrosis. In such situations, gallium determines the presence of a viable tumor better than CT or MRI. However, in young adults, after chemotherapy for Hodgkin's disease, thymic enlargement (the result of thymic rebound or hyperplasia) can be seen by CT, MR, or gallium images. This is more common in children after chemotherapy for malignant neoplasms; the incidence may be as high as 40%.

The contours of the mediastinal enlargement tend to be more globular in neoplasms than in benign thymic enlargement. False negative gallium images, on the other hand, are likely to occur in the presence of a viable tumor if they are performed too soon after chemotherapy (within the first 6 weeks).—J.G. McAfee, M.D.

Gallium-67 Uptake in a Mass of Benign Transformation Mimicking Recurrence of Nodular Lymphocytic Predominance Hodgkin's Disease

Bar-Shalom R, Ben-Arie Y, Gaitini D, Epelbaum R, Parmett S, Israel O, Front D (Rambam Med Ctr, Haifa, Israel; Technion-Israel Inst of Technology, Haifa, Israel)
J Nucl Med 35:465–468, 1994   124-95-2-12

Background.—Gallium-67 is not tumor-specific, although it is used widely to manage patients with lymphoma. The reasons for its uptake in nonmalignant and premalignant lesions associated with lymphoma should be recognized.

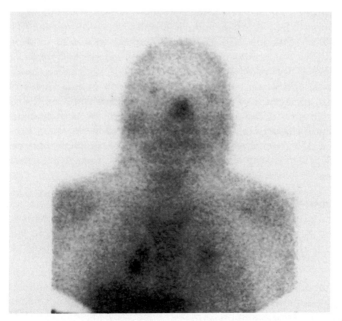

Fig 2–11.—Gallium-67 scintigraphy done 6 months later shows bilateral prominent parahilar pathologic uptake. (Courtesy of Bar-Shalom R, Ben-Arie Y, Gaitini D, et al: *J Nucl Med* 35:465–468, 1994.)

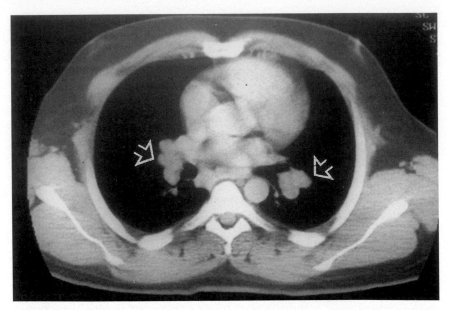

Fig 2–12.—Computed tomographic scan of the chest at the level of the hila shows bilateral lobular masses representing enlarged lymph nodes (*arrows*). After intravenous administration of contrast material, vascular enhancement is seen, whereas lymph nodes do not enhance. (Courtesy of Bar-Shalom R, Ben-Arie Y, Gaitini D, et al: *J Nucl Med* 35:465–468, 1994.)

Case Report.—Man, 31, with nodular lymphocytic-predominance Hodgkin's disease (HD) in remission, had a gallium-67 uptake in a mass of progressively transformed germinal centers and a sarcoid-like reaction that mimicked recurrence. Gallium-67 was taken up on 2 occasions, suggesting recurrence. The first time, abnormal uptake was observed in axillary lymph nodes. The second time, the abnormal uptake was in mediastinal and parahilar lymph nodes (Figs 2–11 and 2–12). On both occasions, the histology of the lesions demonstrated progressively transformed germinal centers and a sarcoid-like reaction but no signs of HD (Fig 2–13). After several months, the bilateral parahilar abnormal uptake disappeared spontaneously without treatment. The CT mass regressed but did not disappear.

Conclusion.—The appearance of a new mass taking up gallium-67 in lymphocytic-predominant HD during continuous clinical remission does not necessarily indicate a recurrence and need for therapy. In such cases a biopsy should be done to determine the nature of the lesion.

▶ Here is another danger in the interpretation of gallium scans for lymphomas. The authors point out that nodular lymphocytic predominant Hodgkin's disease is more common in males, especially those 30 to 40 years of age, with a high rate of relapse but with good response to therapy. However, there is no method, short of biopsy and careful histology, for distinguishing a

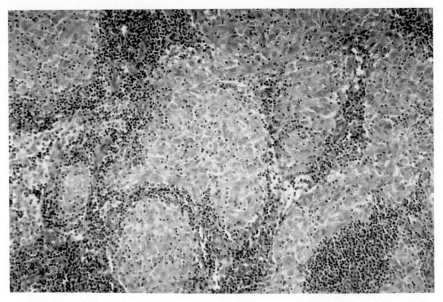

Fig 2–13.—Histology of the hilar lymph node (hematoxylin and eosin; original magnification, ×50). Most of the lymphatic normal tissue is replaced by many epitheloid cell granulomas in a sarcoid-like reaction. (Courtesy of Bar-Shalom R, Ben-Arie Y, Gaitini D, et al: *J Nucl Med* 35:465-468, 1994.)

recurrence from progressively transformed germinal centers in lymph nodes, a benign reaction that regresses spontaneously.—J.G. McAfee, M.D.

Thallium-201 Scintigraphy for Assessment of a Gallium-67-Avid Mediastinal Mass Following Therapy for Hodgkin's Disease

Harris EW, Rakow JI, Weiner M, Agress H Jr (Hackensack Med Ctr, NJ)
J Nucl Med 34:1326–1330, 1993   124-95-2–13

Introduction.—The usefulness of thallium-201 (^{201}Tl) imaging in distinguishing thymic rebound from recurrent tumor after chemotherapy for Hodgkin's disease in pediatric patients was illustrated.

Case Report.—Boy, 5 years, had a painless mass on the left side of his neck. A biopsy specimen revealed nodular sclerosing Hodgkin's disease. Initial and 4-month follow-up gallium-67 (^{67}Ga) scans and CT of the chest did not indicate any mediastinal abnormalities. The patient was treated with chemotherapy. After 8 months, at the completion of chemotherapy, the results of the patient's physical examination were normal. However, follow-up ^{67}Ga scans indicated increased mediastinal activity, and CT indicated an anterior mediastinal mass. Scintigraphy with ^{201}Tl demonstrated no significant mediastinal uptake. Follow-up ^{67}Ga and CT imaging demonstrated steady decrease in the mediastinal mass and activity.

Conclusion.—The addition of ²⁰¹Tl scans to CT and ⁶⁷Ga imaging is a noninvasive technique to differentiate thymic rebound from recurrent tumor in pediatric patients after chemotherapy for Hodgkin's disease.

▶ This is the third article on this subject! An interesting editorial (1) accompanying this article cautions that we do not have all the answers about ⁶⁷Ga and other approaches in distinguishing benign mediastinal uptake from lymphoma after treatment.

Illustrations show a child in whom thallium was taken up with much less intensity than gallium in lymphoma and a teenager who had increased thallium uptake in the thymus without mediastinal disease after chemotherapy. Benign bilateral gallium hilar uptake in adults that is sometimes unrelated to treatment is also mentioned.

More experience is probably needed regarding the evaluation of the efficacy of thallium for these mediastinal problems, let alone trials of the newer tumor agents, sestamibi and Octreoscan.—J.G. McAfee, M.D.

Reference

1. Israel O, Front D: *J Nucl Med* 34:1330, 1993.

Soft-Tissue Tumors: Diagnosis With Tc-99m (V) Dimercaptosuccinic Acid Scintigraphy
Kobayashi H, Sakahara H, Hosono M, Shirato M, Endo K, Kotoura Y, Yamamuro T, Konishi J (Kyoto Univ, Japan)
Radiology 190:277–280, 1994   124-95-2-14

Background.—Diagnosing malignancy in patients with soft tissue tumors is often difficult, especially when the patients have a low-grade malignancy. Because soft tissue sarcomas are not homogenous, histologic examination may only detect a portion of the tumors as malignant. Scintigraphy is often used to aid diagnosis. Both gallium-67 citrate and technetium-99m (⁹⁹ᵐTc) (V) dimercaptosuccinic acid (DMSA) have been used as tumor-seeking agents in radionuclide imaging to diagnose soft tissue tumors. Technetium-99m (V) DSMA was compared with gallium-67 citrate for sensitivity and specificity in patients with a variety of soft tissue tumors.

Methods.—Thirty-eight female and 38 male patients in whom there was histologic proof of soft tissue tumors or tumorous lesions that were 2 cm or greater in diameter underwent ⁹⁹ᵐTc (V) DSMA scintigraphy. Fifty-seven of these patients also underwent gallium-67 citrate scintigraphy within 2 weeks. The findings were compared (Fig 2–14).

Results.—Technetium-99m (V) DMSA uptake was clear in all malignant soft tissue tumors (primary sarcomas and metastatic carcinomas) and highly recurrent benign lesions (extra-abdominal desmoids and

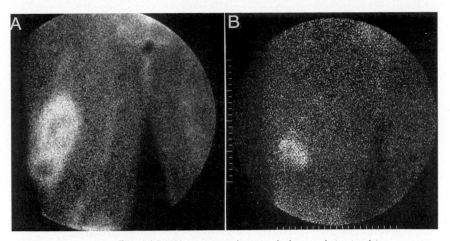

Fig 2–14.—Case 1. **A,** ⁹⁹ᵐTc (V) DMSA scintigram shows marked accumulation in a leiomyosarcoma of the right thigh. The lower part of the tumor shows a lack of radionuclide uptake. **B,** gallium-67 citrate scintigram of the tumor shows uptake at the site within the lesion where ⁹⁹ᵐTc (V) DMSA did not accumulate. (Courtesy of Kobayashi H, Sakahara H, Hosono M, et al: *Radiology* 190:277–280, 1994.)

tenosynovial giant-cell tumors) and almost all inflammatory tumorous lesions and angiomatous tumors (superficial and intramuscular hemangiomas). Sometimes, uptake did not occur in such benign soft tissue tumors as leiomyomas, neurinomas, lipomas, and myxomas. Gallium-67 citrate uptake was clear in all inflammatory lesions and soft tissue metastases of adenocarcinomas and in 57% (8 of 14) of soft tissue sarcomas, 20% (2 of 10) of highly recurrent benign tumors, and 11% (2 of 19) of benign soft tissue tumors. Gallium-67 uptake was not found to be specific for malignant soft tissue tumors.

Conclusion.—Technetium-99m (V) DMSA was clearly superior to gallium-67 citrate as an agent for diagnosing all malignant and highly recurrent benign soft tissue tumors. It showed a 100% sensitivity (all 19 tumors) for malignant tumors as opposed to 57% (8 of 14 tumors) for gallium-67 citrate. Lack of ⁹⁹ᵐTc (V) DMSA uptake could be an indication that a tumor is not malignant. Diagnosis of soft tissue tumors by ⁹⁹ᵐTc (V) DMSA scintigraphy has clinical advantages over other radiologic methods (e.g., MRI and angiography).

▶ This tumor-seeking agent has been around for more than a decade. Its name, ⁹⁹ᵐTc (V) DMSA, is really a misnomer, because it is not an acid. It is prepared at a pH of 8 or higher, with a minimal amount of stannous ion; therefore, it is really DMS-alkaline. It does not concentrate highly in the renal cortex, as regular ⁹⁹ᵐTc - DMSA does.

Most of the published images using this agent have been tumors of either the extremities or head and neck, rather than the solid malignancies of the torso that are more difficult to demonstrate. Unlike gallium, it is not tumor-specific and it shows inflammatory lesions such as synovitis or sarcoid granulomas.

The authors have not presented evidence that it has clinical advantages over other imaging modalities, such as MRI.—J.G. McAfee, M.D.

Intra-Arterial Infusion of Tc-99m MAA: A Case of Highly Selective Targeting of Liver Metastases and Shunting

Roos JC, Teule GJJ (Free Univ Hosp, Amsterdam)
Clin Nucl Med 19:219–220, 1994   124-95-2-15

Background.—Liver metastases may be treated by regionally administering chemotherapeutic agents. Technetium-99m macroaggregated albumin (^{99m}Tc-MAA) may be infused through the hepatic artery to determine proper catheter placement and tumor perfusion selectivity.

Case Report.—Man, 55, with hypertension and diabetes mellitus underwent a sigmoid resection of a primary malignant tumor. He was receiving angiotensin-converting enzyme inhibition for hypertension. Because of the presence of liver metastases, a catheter was placed in the hepatic artery for regional chemotherapeutic treatment. The patient was assessed after ^{99m}Tc-MAA was delivered through the hepatic artery (Figs 2–15 and 2–16). Despite systemic treatment with

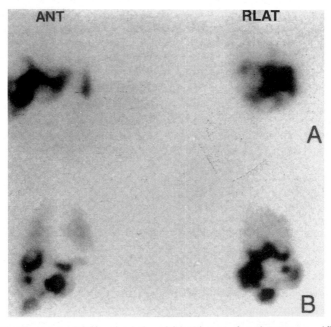

Fig 2–15.—The anterior (*ANT*) and right lateral (*RLAT*) views after administration of ^{99m}Tc colloid intravenously (**A**) and after ^{99m}Tc-MAA through the hepatic artery (**B**). (Courtesy of Roos JC, Teule GJJ: *Clin Nucl Med* 19:219-220, 1994.)

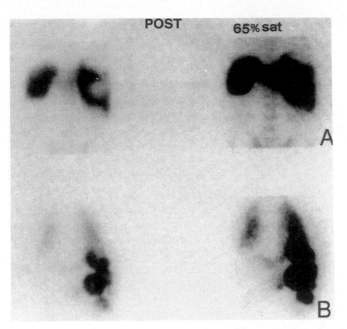

Fig 2-16.—The posterior (*POST*) views after administration of ^{99m}Tc colloid intravenously (**A**) and after ^{99m}Tc-MAA through the hepatic artery (**B**) without and with 65% saturation (65%sat). (Courtesy of Roos JC, Teule GJJ: *Clin Nucl Med* 19:219-220, 1994.)

a vasoactive drug that theoretically reduces flow to metastases, the scintigrams demonstrated a highly selective perfusion of the metastases and significant shunting.

Conclusion.—When regional perfusion studies and intra-arterial treatment are done, a possible effect of concomitant vasoactive medication on targeting and systemic side effects must be considered. In this patient, the catheter became infected and no more treatments could be given. The finding of increased toxicity associated with increased systemic shunting is not consistent in the literature, however.

▶ In the authors' references, there seems to be a correlation between the magnitude of the tumor-to-normal liver concentration ratio, systemic shunting as assessed by lung uptake of the ^{99m}Tc-MAA, and the degree of toxicity of chemotherapeutic agents. The degree of shunting varies widely in different individuals in the absence of any vasoactive agents. With increasing doses of vasoactive agents, the tumor-to-liver concentration ratio, lung uptake, and chemotherapy toxicity progressively increase.

As Kaplan and associates (1) note, vasoactive induction of shunting might occur in the tumor, in the normal liver, or disproportionately in both.—J.G. McAfee, M.D.

Reference

1. Kaplan WD, et al: *J Clin Oncol* 11:1266, 1984.

A Case of Metastatic Malignancy Masquerading as a Hepatic Hemangioma on Labeled Red Blood Cell Scintigraphy

Farlow DC, Little JM, Gruenewald SM, Antico VF, O'Neill P (Westmead Hosp, Sydney, Australia)
J Nucl Med 34:1172–1174, 1993
124-95-2-16

Background.—Technetium-99m red blood cell (RBC) scintigraphy can distinguish hemangiomas from other masses. As such, this procedure plays an important diagnostic role in patients with focal liver lesions, because a firm diagnosis of hemangioma frequently precludes the need for subsequent investigations and treatment. Although uncommon, false positive technetium-99m RBC findings can occur. Such a finding was de-

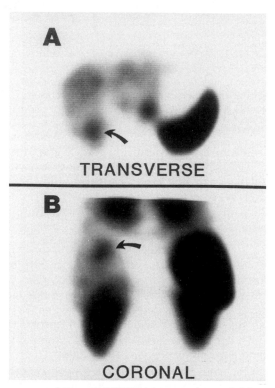

Fig 2–17.—A, transverse and **(B)** coronal SPECT images reveal a rounded focus of increased blood pooling in the posterior portion of the right lobe of the liver (*arrows*). (Courtesy of Farlow DC, Little JM, Gruenewald SM, et al: *J Nucl Med* 34:1172–1174, 1993.)

scribed in a patient with malignant neuroendocrine carcinoma of the stomach.

Case Report.—Woman, 36, with established metastatic gastric neuroendocrine carcinoma was evaluated for a 2-cm echogenic mass located in the right lobe of the liver, as demonstrated on ultrasound. Technetium-99m RBC scintigraphy was performed. A typical appearance of hepatic hemangioma was noted, including perfusion to blood-pool mismatch and an increase in blood-pool activity from early to delayed images. The site and degree of delayed blood pooling were further demonstrated on single-photon emission CT (SPECT) images (Fig 2–17). Because of these findings, the patient was managed conservatively, and biopsy was not performed. However, progressive lesion enlargement was noted on subsequent CT scanning, and smaller satellite foci were also apparent. Liver resection of the right lobe was performed, and several metastases up to 8 cm in diameter were found. They were histopathologically similar to the primary gastric neuroendocrine carcinoma. No evidence of hemangioma was noted.

Conclusion.—Few examples of false positive technetium-99m RBC scans have been reported. The findings in this patient underscore the need for cautious assessment of focal liver masses, even when scintigraphy reveals features typically associated with cavernous hemangioma.

▶ This hepatic malignancy perfectly mimicked a cavernous hemangioma by appearing on delay images without evidence in the perfusion or early images. The authors cite a handful of other reported malignancies, including hepatomas, that have produced false positive red cell images. However, they are unusual, considering the popularity of this study to avoid needle biopsies of hemangiomas. I think the quality of SPECT imaging with red cells labeled in vitro is superior to that of in vitro methods.—J.G. McAfee, M.D.

Radioimmunodetection of Solid Tumors: Future Horizons and Applications for Radioimmunotherapy

McKearn TJ (CYTO-GEN Corp, Princeton, NJ)
Cancer 71:4302–4313, 1993   124-95-2-17

Introduction.—Today, 17 years after the advent of hybridoma technology, radioimmunodetection of solid tumors by monoclonal antibody–based imaging techniques has a definitive clinical role. The initial immunoscintigraphic agents had definite limitations, notably suboptimal tumor-to-background radiolocalization ratio and immunogenic properties. Most clinical studies of radioimmunodetection methods for tumors have involved the use of intact murine antibodies as immunoscintigraphic-targeting vehicles.

Strategies for Improvement.—Attempts to make the antibodies used for immunodetection more human and, therefore, less immunogenic have involved construction of chimeric murine/human antibodies and transplantation of murine complementary–determining regions into the human immunoglobulin framework. An ultimate step would be production of human monoclonal antibodies. Lower doses of protein may well lessen the immunogenicity of murine-derived immunoscintigraphic agents. It should be possible, through selective enzymatic digestion of intact immunoglobulins or protein engineering techniques, to make smaller tumor-targeting vehicles. Improving the linkage between the tumor-targeting vehicle and radionuclide should make the delivery system more efficient. Another approach to improving radioimmunodetection entails modulating either tumor or host attributes. Limited success has been achieved in augmenting the delivery of radiolabeled antibody to tumor sites by increasing vascular permeability and tumor blood flow, either pharmacologically or by means such as hyperthermia and external beam radiation. Expression of some tumor antigens might be enhanced by administering recombinant human interferons. Use of a combination of radiolabeled antibodies directed against different tumor-associated antigens could make immunoscintigraphy more sensitive.

▶ Although progress in the development of radiolabeled monoclonal antibodies for imaging has been slow in the first 17 years since the advent of hybridoma technology, it is worthwhile to check on review articles such as this.

The author lists only 3 monoclonal antibodies that have undergone extensive clinical trials, and only 1 of these has been approved for marketing. Most of the review summarizes potential future biological and technical improvements, including protein engineering for smaller nonantigenic tumor targeting moieties. To date, monoclonal antibodies have been more successful in lymphomas than in the so-called solid tumors.—J.G. McAfee, M.D.

Immunodiagnosis of Tumours
von Kleist S, Bombardieri E, Buraggi G, Gion M, Hertel A, Hör G, Noujaim A, Schwartz M, Senekowitsch R, Wittekind C (Inst of Immunobiology, Freiburg, Germany; Natl Inst of Cancer Research, Milan, Italy; Regional Gen Hosp, Venice, Italy; et al)
Eur J Cancer 29:1622–1630, 1993   124-95-2–18

In Vitro Methods.—A number of tumor markers have been proposed for detecting breast carcinoma. The CA 15/3 assay appears to be more sensitive than carcinoembryonic antigen (CEA), and it correlates more closely with the extent of disease. The optimal marker for colorectal carcinoma is CEA. Neuron-specific enolase may be used to monitor the responsiveness of small-cell lung cancer to treatment and the progression of disease. A good marker for adenocarcinomas of the lung is CEA, whereas squamous cell carcinoma antigen is the optimal marker for squamous carcinomas. Pancreatic carcinomas are best evaluated using CA 19/9. The tumor markers used for gastric carcinoma include CEA,

CA 50, CA 19/9, and a new marker, TAG 72. Alpha fetoprotein (AFP) is a valuable tumor marker for hepatocellular carcinoma. Both AFP and human chorionic gonadotropin (HCG) serve as markers for non-seminomatous germ-cell tumors of the testis, whereas HCG alone is used for trophoblastic malignancies in females. Prostate-specific antigen is a tissue-specific marker for prostatic carcinoma. Ovarian cancers can be detected using CA 125. A large number of immune sera reactive with various intracellular structures are now available for distinguishing between malignant and normal cells.

In Vivo Methods.—Radioimmunodetection (RID) techniques based on murine monoclonal antibodies have been used in clinical oncology for more than a decade. Initial enthusiasm was dampened by the results of larger clinical trials. However, RID is a safe procedure. Antibody F(ab') fragments and short-lived radionuclides such as technetium-99m can be used. A truly tumor-specific antigen is not yet available.

▶ This is a summary of a consensus workshop of the European School of Oncology at Milan in October 1992. It reviews the progress in the development of tumor markers for in vitro tests and radioimmunoimaging.

Twenty clinically useful in vitro markers and 7 more new markers are listed and discussed. Most of these reliably correlate with tumor mass, and increased marker levels generally are not seen in the early tumor stages. The major drawback in tumor imaging has been that so few have had extensive clinical trials.—J.G. McAfee, M.D.

Satellite PET and Lung Cancer: A Prospective Study in Surgical Patients

Slosman DO, Spiliopoulos A, Couson F, Nicod L, Louis O, Lemoine R, Donath A, Junod AF (Geneva Univ Hosp)
Nucl Med Commun 14:955–961, 1993   124-95-2–19

Background.—Positron emission tomography appears to be a reliable, noninvasive technique for imaging the proliferative activity of malignant tissue, particularly with ^{18}F-labeled fluorodeoxyglucose (FDG). The potential role of PET scanning in a satellite center was evaluated prospectively as an adjunct to conventional methods for estimating the likelihood of pulmonary malignancy. The sensitivity of lung cancer detection was therefore determined by FDG-PET imaging before exploratory or therapeutic thoracotomy.

Patients and Methods.—Thirty-six patients who were referred for pulmonary PET scanning before surgery were studied. All had abnormal chest roentgenograms and suspected lung cancer. After PET scans, findings were assessed qualitatively and semiquantitatively.

Results.—Malignant pulmonary lesions were found in 31 of 36 patients. Of them, a focal increase in FDG pulmonary uptake was observed in 29 patients, similar to that seen in a female patient 65 years of age (Fig 2–18). Benign pulmonary lesions were demonstrated in 5 patients; negative PET scans were noted in 3 of these patients. As a result, the sensitivity of lung cancer detection by FDG-PET was 93.5%. After bayesian analysis, it was found that FDG-PET could best serve populations with a low prevalence of lung cancer.

Conclusion.—Adequate clinical information can be obtained in a satellite PET center using a simple FDG-PET scanning protocol. In addition, the information provided may aid in determining subsequent patient management.

▶ About half of all single pulmonary nodules by chest x-ray films and CT are malignant. No noninvasive method has been developed to avoid using thoracotomy for most benign nodules.

This clinical study of single nodules and suspected lung cancers was performed with ¹⁸F-FDG, because its high tumor-nontarget ratios are clearly su-

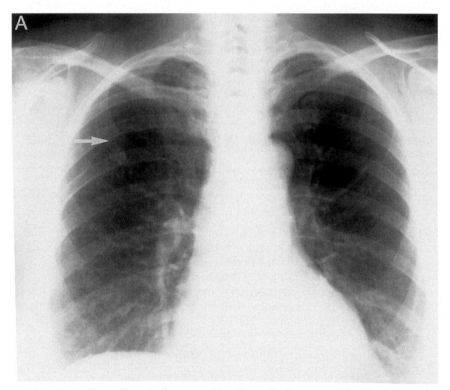

Fig 2–18.—A, chest radiograph of a woman, 65, with a small pulmonary nodule of the right superior lobe (*arrow*). **B,** CT scan of the nodule showing no calcification or spiculation. **C,** transverse sections of the PET examination showing the presence of a small, unique 9-mm-diameter hyperactive focal nod-

(continued)

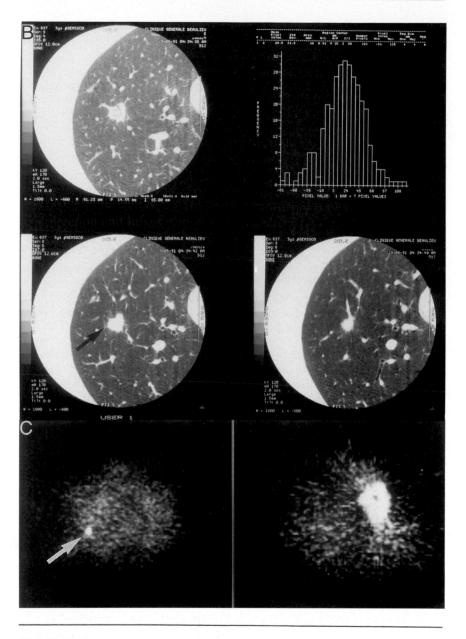

Fig 2–18 (cont).

ular abnormality with a tumor-to-normal tissue ratio of 2.7 (**left**) and normal myocardial FDG uptake (**right**). A segmentectomy was performed, and histologic examination revealed the presence of a small adenocarcinoma, 1.2 cm in diameter. (Courtesy of Slosman DO, Spiliopoulos A, Couson F, et al: *Nucl Med Commun* 14:955–961, 1993.)

perior to those of any other agent. The PET studies were simplified in a satellite PET facility, where the chest was scanned, for 20–30 minutes, 40–60 minutes after injection of commercial FDG.

The authors concluded that FDG-PET will still not avoid thoracotomy, despite its high sensitivity for malignancy (93.5%). The 2 false negatives occurred in unusual tumors, 1 in a fibrohyaline scar and the other a small polypoid tumor that infiltrated only the surface of the bronchial wall. The 2 false positives were inflammatory lesions—invasive aspergillosis and a plasmocytic granuloma.—J.G. McAfee, M.D.

Discordance Between F-18 Fluorodeoxyglucose Uptake and Contrast Enhancement in a Brain Abscess
Meyer MA, Frey KA, Schwaiger M (Univ of Michigan, Ann Arbor)
Clin Nucl Med 18:682–684, 1993   124-95-2-20

Introduction.—Infectious processes of the CNS may accumulate fluorodeoxyglucose (FDG) on positron emission tomographic imaging. Therefore, problems may occur when evaluating patients with a CNS mass. Because of the increase in AIDS in IV drug abusers, intracerebral abscess has been seen more frequently.

Case Report.—Woman, 29, an IV drug abuser who was also HIV-negative, had a fever of 104°F and left-sided hemiplegia. The fever had developed 5 days before admission and was accompanied by headache and vomiting. In addition to hemiplegia, her face was numb and her speech slurred. Intravenous heroin had been used until 2 months before admission. A homonymous left–visual-field defect was evident along with a left-sided sensory deficit and dense left hemiplegia that included the face. Janeway lesions on the feet, conjunctival hemorrhages, and oral thrush were noted. Blood cultures yielded coagulase-positive *Staphylococcus,* and the patient was given IV gentamicin and vancomycin. Transesophageal echocardiography revealed a shaggy 2-cm vegetation in the left atrium, part of which was mobile. Positron emission tomography with ^{18}F-FDG showed extensive hypometabolism throughout the right hemisphere and in the left cerebellum. A focus of intense uptake was seen between the right thalamus and caudate head, representing the center of the abscess. Mild uptake was noted in the superior aspect of the abscess wall. The patient improved during a 42-day course of antibiotic therapy but was left with a slight facial droop.

Discussion.—Only 1 other case of glucose consumption by a brain abscess has previously been reported. Positron emission tomography with FDG and contrast study may yield discordant findings in patients with CNS infection.

▶ This is another reminder that ^{18}F-FDG does not localize exclusively in neoplasms but in some inflammatory lesions with active metabolism as well. Perhaps thallium-201 SPECT can better distinguish inflammatory from neoplastic lesions. This is a common problem in patients with AIDS, in whom the incidence of intracranial lymphoma, toxoplasmosis, fungal infections, and abscesses is high.—J.G. McAfee, M.D.

Lymphoscintigraphy in High-Risk Melanoma of the Trunk: Predicting Draining Node Groups, Defining Lymphatic Channels and Locating the Sentinel Node
Uren RF, Howman-Giles RB, Shaw HM, Thompson JF, McCarthy WH (Royal Prince Alfred Hosp, Sydney, New South Wales, Australia)
J Nucl Med 34:1435–1440, 1993   124-95-2-21

Background.—Previous studies have shown that 37% of patients with melanomas thicker than 1.5 mm but clinically impalpable lymph nodes have micrometastases in nodes excised during elective lymph node dissection (ND). Wide local excision (WLE) with concurrent early ND improves the prognosis in these patients. The usefulness of cutaneous lymphoscintigraphy (LS) for identifying draining node groups in patients with high-risk melanoma of the trunk and its accuracy in locating the sentinel node or nodes in draining lymph node groups were determined.

Patients.—Cutaneous LS was performed in 159 men and 50 women with high-risk melanoma of the trunk but no palpable lymph nodes. The sentinel node was defined as the first node in a draining lymph node group to accept and retain the isotope tracer. The skin overlying the sentinel node was marked with an indelible pen. All excised lymph nodes were examined for the presence of metastatic melanoma by hematoxylin and eosin staining.

Results.—Cutaneous LS accurately identified drainage to 1 or more draining lymph node groups in 187 (89%) of the 209 patients. Lymphoscintigraphy had a sensitivity of 94% for detecting draining sites that contained metastases. It was possible to mark the major lymph node channels on the skin before dissection. Most patients had multiple draining lymph channels with widely varying patterns and numbers of draining lymph node channels. Lymphoscintigraphy allowed accurate localization of the sentinel node or nodes in each draining lymph node group.

Conclusion.—Lymphoscintigraphy provides important information on patients with melanoma of the trunk undergoing WLE who are being considered for concurrent elective ND.

▶ Lymphoscintigraphy was previously performed with technetium-99 antimony sulphur colloid, but attempts to obtain approval from the Food and Drug Administration were unsuccessful. The only approved commercial agent is technetium-99m albumin (Amersham), and this is satisfactory.

For lymphoscintigraphy imaging (1), the management of regional lymph node drainage of malignant melanoma remains highly controversial. Two prospective randomized trials (by the World Health Organization and Mayo

Clinic) and a more recent study (2) did not show any survival benefit from elective ND of nonpalpable nodes. Long-term survival is only effective in approximately 4% of all patients with elective dissections, but this effect is diluted by the lack of benefit in most patients in larger series (3).

On the other hand, therapeutic ND of palpable nodes is clearly beneficial, resulting in 20% to 30% long-term survivors (3). Scintigraphy is helpful in demonstrating unexpected drainage sites or ambiguous drainage into 2 or more nodal lesions (2).—J.G. McAfee, M.D.

References

1. Nawaz MK, et al: *Clin Nucl Med* 15:794, 1990.
2. Coit DG, Brennan MF: *Surgery* 113:128, 1993.
3. Singluff CL Jr, Stidham KR, Ricci WM, et al: *Ann Surg* 219:120, 1994.

Clinical Utility of Bone Scan Features of Pleural Effusion: Sensitivity and Specificity for Malignancy Based on Pleural Fluid Cytopathology

Sandler ED, Hattner RS, Parisi MT, Miller TR (Univ of California, San Francisco)

J Nucl Med 35:429–431, 1994   124-95-2-22

Background. —Although asymmetric chest activity with malignant and benign pleural effusions has been reported in bone scans, the clinical value of this finding is unclear. Specific scintigraphic criteria for malignant pleural effusion were developed and assessed retrospectively.

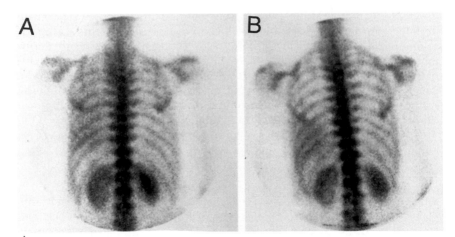

Fig 2–19.—Posterior thoracic bone scans. **A,** supine, and **(B)** erect of a man, 63, with renal cell carcinoma demonstrates layering of his malignant pleural effusion. (Courtesy of Sandler ED, Hattner RS, Parisi MT, et al: *J Nucl Med* 35:429-431, 1994.)

Methods.—Pleural fluid was obtained from 850 patients during 5 years. In 74 patients, bone scans were done within 2 months of thoracentesis. The scans and cytologic findings were evaluated by a consensus panel.

Findings.—The effusions were cytologically malignant in 34%, indeterminate in 12%, and benign in 54%. Based on cytopathology, bone scans detected malignant pleural effusions with a sensitivity of 34% to 50% and a specificity of 78% to 89%. True sensitivity and specificity averaged 42% and 84%, respectively (Fig 2–19).

Conclusion.—The bone scan is often the first examination to suggest pleural metastasis. When it is detected on a bone scan, it should be pursued beyond negative or indeterminate pleural fluid cytologic findings.

▶ This is a more detailed study of diphosphonate imaging in pleural effusions than has been reported previously. The presence of increased diffuse activity in a homithorax did not correlate well with positive cytology for malignant cells in the pleural fluid. Sixty-two of the 74 patients with pleural effusions had a primary malignancy, but only 25 had positive cytopathology (40%), and only 10 of these patients had a positive image. On the other hand, there were 5 patients with positive images and negative cytology and another 5 positives with indeterminate cytology.—J.G. McAfee, M.D.

3 Infection and Inflammation

Introduction

With so many antibiotics, radioisotopic approaches, and other imaging modalities available these days, how well do we now resolve the mysteries of fever of unknown origin (FUO)? In an older classic paper (1) that analyzed 100 cases of FUO, the criteria were illness of longer than 3 weeks; a temperature greater than 101°F (38.3°C) on several occasions; and a diagnosis that was uncertain after 1 week of study in the hospital.

At follow-up, the diagnosis in two thirds of these patients fell into 1 of 3 major categories—infections in 36 patients, neoplasms in 19, and collagen diseases (primarily rheumatic fever and disseminated lupus) in 13. No diagnosis could be made in only 7 patients. The common causes of infection (in descending order) were tuberculosis, liver and biliary infections, bacterial endocarditis, abdominal abscess, and pyelonephritis. The neoplasms included disseminated carcinomatosis, lymphomas, and leukemias.

These authors noted that the relative frequency of these entities varied from one era to another and also varied with different diagnostic criteria. In a later analysis of 128 cases seen before 1971 (2), the "big 3" remained almost unchanged—infection, 40% neoplasms (especially lymphomas), 20%, and collagen-vascular diseases, 15%. These authors believed that obscure fevers are most often caused by atypical manifestations of common diseases and that only about 25% were the result of less common diseases.

In a review of 67 patients with pyrexia of unknown origin who were imaged with gallium (3), a surprisingly large number (50) had positive images. Thirty-two had abdominal lesions, 12 had lesions of the chest, and 6 had lesions at other sites. Thirty-two had localized pyogenic infections, 3 had tuberculosis, 5 had neoplasms, and 6 had noninfectious lesions. Presumably, gallium would not be positive in most collagen diseases. Of 25 children with a fever of longer than 2 weeks but without localizing signs, gallium scans were positive in only one (4).

In a series of patients reported at a later time, who had FUO and were imaged with indium-111 leukocytes, the number was relatively small, and the proportion of patients with proven sepsis was relatively low. This change could be the result of improved detection of septic lesions by other newer modalities.

Moreover, many cases of FUO disappeared spontaneously without explanation. In one series of 32 patients (5), only 5 patients had positive indium-111 leukocyte images resulting from infection. Moreover, abnormal uptake occurred in non-Hodgkin's lymphoma lesions and intestinal uptake in a patient with Whipple's disease.

In another series of 28 patients (6), there were only 3 true positive leukocyte images from bacterial infections, 2 false positive images from swallowed pus from respiratory infections, and 2 others in collagen vascular diseases. Images were negative in tuberculosis and a fungal infection. In another study (7), it was concluded that indium-111 leukocyte imaging had a high sensitivity for detecting foci of infection in patients after surgery, but it was not very rewarding in spontaneous FUO.

The changing experience in the recent literature supports the impression that FUO caused by sepsis in patients without AIDS are becoming less frequent because of better diagnostic methods. Labeled leukoctyes appear to be effective in detecting pyogenic sepsis. However, gallium appears to be more versatile in detecting a variety of inflammatory lesions in FUO.

The first article (Abstract 124-95-3-1) describes the use of technetium-99m antigranulocyte monoclonal antibody in FUO.

John G. McAfee, M.D.

References

1. Petersdorf RG, Beeson PB: Fever of unexplained origin: Report of 100 cases. *Medicine* 40:1–30, 1961.
2. Jacoby GA, Swartz MN: Fever of undetermined origin. *N Engl J Med* 289:1407–1410, 1973.
3. Hilson AJW, Maisey MN: Gallium-67 scanning in pyrexia of unknown origin. *BMJ* 4:1330–1331, 1979.
4. Buonomo C, Treves ST: Gallium scanning in children with fever of unknown origin. *Pediatr Radiol* 23:307–310, 1993.
5. Schmidt KG, Rasmussen JM, Sorensen PJ, et al: Indium-111-granulocyte scintigraphy in the evaluation of patient with fever of undetermined origin. *Scand J Infect Dis* 19:339–345, 1987.
6. Davies SG, Garvie NW: The role of Indium-labeled leukocyte imaging in pyrexia of unknown origin. *Br J Radiol* 63:850–854, 1990.
7. MacSweeney JE, Peters AM, Lavender JP: Indium labelled leukocyte scanning in pyrexia of unknown origin. *Clin Radiol* 42:414–417, 1990.

Use of Immunoscintigraphy in the Diagnosis of Fever of Unknown Origin

Becker W, Dölkemeyer U, Gramatzki M, Schneider MU, Scheele J, Wolf F (Univ of Erlangen-Nuremberg, Erlangen, Germany)

Eur J Nucl Med 20:1078–1083, 1993   124-95-3–1

Introduction.—Thirty-four consecutive patients with a diagnosis of fever of unknown origin (FUO) were examined by immunoscintigraphy with technetium-99m (^{99m}Tc)–labeled antigranulocyte antibody anti-NCA-95. In such patients, the cause of fever cannot be determined despite intensive investigation. Although ^{99m}Tc-labeled antigranulocyte antibodies have been used successfully in the diagnosis of various localized infections, this was its first application with immunoscintigraphy to localize pathology in patients with FUO.

Patients and Methods.—Those in the patient group ranged in age from 25 to 85 years; 20 were men and 14 were women. Fever of unknown origin was defined as a rectal temperature of 38.3°C for at least 2 weeks and an inpatient status for longer than 1 week. No diagnosis had been established after full biochemical and hematologic studies and appropriate radiographic investigation. Scans were obtained at both 3–6 hours and 18–24 hours after injection of the antibody in 19 patients; in 15, the scans were obtained at 18–24 hours post injection. Three experienced nuclear physicians who did not have access to the results of other clinical investigations read the scans. All patients received antibiotics for more than 10 days before the scans.

Results.—In 8 patients, the site of infection was correctly diagnosed by immunoscintigraphy as the cause of FUO. Seven of 12 patients with a false negative scan had endocarditis, and immunoscintigraphy was unable to visualize the small moving focus of infection on the heart valve. The cause of FUO was not discovered in 4 patients during a follow-up of at least 3 months. Overall, 58.8% of patients had an infectious cause of FUO, and 30.2% had a benign or malignant hematologic disease, pancreatitis, or thyrotoxicosis.

Conclusion.—Immunoscintigraphy with ^{99m}Tc–anti–NCA-95 scanning localized infectious causes of FUO, with the exception of endocarditis. The overall diagnostic sensitivity of immunoscintigraphy for infection was low (40%), but its specificity was high (92%). The positive predictive value was calculated to be 88% and the negative predictive value was calculated to be 52%. In addition to endocarditis, pneumonia, and small brain abscesses (no more than .5 cm in diameter) were associated with false negative scans.

▶ The yield of positive images, which were found in 8 of 34 patients, is better than that in other series that describe the role of radionuclide imaging in patients with fever of unknown origin. Everyone has had little or no success in imaging subacute bacterial endocarditis. A major drawback with this agent is the in vivo elution of technetium-99m from the monoclonal antibody, resulting in urinary excretion. As a result, its value in urinary infections is limited, which is similar to the problem with ^{99m}Tc hexamethyleneamine-oxime–labeled leukocytes.—J.G. McAfee, M.D.

Nuclear Medicine and AIDS

O'Doherty MJ, Nunan TO (St Thomas Hosp, London)
Nucl Med Commun 14:830–848, 1993   124-95-3–2

Objective.—The prevalence of HIV infection is increasing steadily, and a proposed reclassification may increase the number of patients who are considered to have AIDS. The HIV-related challenges to the nuclear medicine clinician, including the infection risk to staff and patients, investigation of the diseases of immunocompromised patients, and the use of radiotracers to assess therapy were studied.

Infection Risk.—Needlestick injuries carry the risk of both hepatitis B and HIV infection. The risk of HIV infection from a needlestick injury is low, and it can be further minimized by not resheathing needles or by using a ready-made sheath holder. When needlestick injuries do occur, the injured individual should be offered zidovudine. Precautions are also needed for staff who perform in vitro blood labeling procedures and for avoiding droplet spread of other pathogens from patients with AIDS in the department.

Investigation of HIV-Infected Patients.—The spread of HIV infection also means that the nuclear medicine differential diagnosis must be expanded for high-risk patients. Consequently, more patients are coming to the nuclear medicine department with such previously rare diagnoses as *Pneumocystis carinii* pneumonia, Kaposi's sarcoma, and others. The broad range of opportunistic infections and unusual tumors must be considered in interpreting the nuclear medicine abnormalities of high-risk patients. The techniques for evaluating opportunistic infections in severely immunocompromised patients include lung technetium-99m DTPA aerosol clearance studies and donor leukocyte and gallium scanning. Nuclear medicine studies may be performed not only for respiratory infections such as *P. carinii* pneumonia, but also for gastrointestinal problems, abdominal infection and inflammation, neurologic problems, the musculoskeletal system, and other systems (Figs 3–1, 3–2, and 3–3).

Evaluation of Therapies.—Nuclear medicine techniques can also be used to monitor the effect of therapy against HIV itself or against opportunistic infections. Such techniques enable comparison of devices to ensure the delivery of effective drug dosages to the lungs or the response of tumors to therapy using metabolic markers.

Summary.—Some of the ramifications of the AIDS epidemic on the practice of nuclear medicine were outlined. As patients live longer and the pattern of the disease changes, it will be important to assess the effects and delivery of drugs, the development of suitable imaging for Kaposi's sarcoma to define the total body tumor load, and the use of positron emission tomographic imaging isotopes to assess the effects of antiviral drugs on brain metabolism.

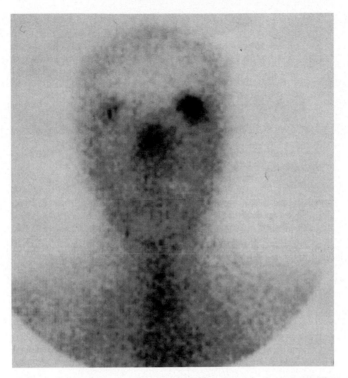

Fig 3–1.—Gallium-67 scan appearance in a patient with cytomegalovirus retinitis. The scan shows greater uptake in the right eye compared with the left. (Courtesy of O'Doherty MJ, Nunan TO: *Nucl Med Commun* 14:830–848, 1993.)

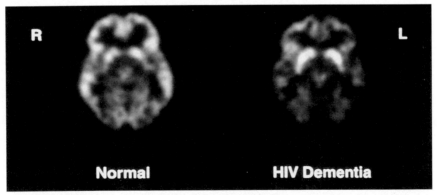

Fig 3–2.—^{18}F-fluorodeoxyglucose study in a patient with HIV encephalopathy and a normal patient. The scan of the patient with HIV shows the relative increased uptake in the basal ganglia caused by the diffuse, slightly patchy decreased uptake in the cortex. The patient was not taking medication at the time of the scan. (Courtesy of O'Doherty MJ, Nunan TO: *Nucl Med Commun* 14:830–848, 1993.)

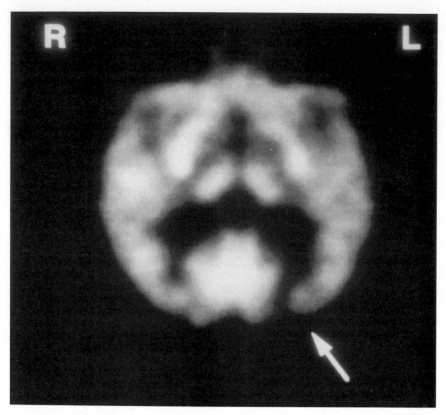

Fig 3–3.—^{18}F-fluorodeoxyglucose study in a patient with HIV who was seen with a quadrantanopia. The scan shows low uptake in a space-occupying lesion in the left occipital region (*arrow*). This is more likely to represent an infective process than cerebral lymphoma. (From O'Doherty MJ, Nunan TO: *Nucl Med Commun* 14:830–848, 1993. Courtesy of O'Doherty MJ, Lewis P, Nunan TO: *Lancet* i:242–243, 1993.)

▶ This excellent, detailed review is impossible to summarize adequately in an abstract. In the authors' experience, measurement of the lung clearance of technetium-99m DTPA is better than gallium-67 for detecting *Pneumocystis* pneumonia. They advocate donor-labeled leukocytes for suspected bacterial infections and gallium-67 for viral or mycobacterial infections and lymphomas.

Gastric uptake of gallium in patients with AIDS may be the result of gastritis or lymphoma. Increased bowel activity is not a totally reliable indication of bowel infections. A bacillary angiomatous skin lesion may simulate Kaposi's sarcoma, but it often involves bone at distant sites and can be treated with erythromycin. Previous excellent reviews of this subject can be found in the references below.—J.G. McAfee, M.D.

References

1. Vanarthos WJ: *RadioGraphics* 12:731, 1992.
2. Miller RF: *Eur J Nucl Med* 16:103, 1990.

Tc-99m DISIDA Hepatobiliary Scintigraphy in AIDS Cholangitis

Brunetti JC, Van Heertum RL, Kempf JS, Yudd AP, Farman J (St Vincent's Hosp and Med Ctr, New York; Columbia-Presbyterian Med Ctr, New York)
Clin Nucl Med 19:36–42, 1994   124-95-3-3

Background.—Cholangitis is a well-recognized complication of AIDS, often heralded by abnormally elevated liver function tests and liver enzymes. Endoscopic retrograde cholangiopancreatography (ECRP) is the method of choice for diagnosis, but it may be unsuccessful in patients with anatomical variations or stenosis of the ampulla of Vater. Hepatobiliary scintigraphy is definitely indicated in some cases of possible AIDS-related cholangitis.

Methods.—The technetium-99m DISIDA scans in 16 patients with documented AIDS cholangitis were reviewed with the goal of evaluating the spectrum of disease-related changes. There were 15 men and 1 woman (mean age, 36 years). The diagnosis was made by means of either ECRP with aspiration or biopsy or by the presence of characteristic sonographic or CT findings with positive stool culture and at least 6 months of follow-up. The investigators graded each scan for parenchymal function, gallbladder visualization, presence of ductal dilatation, and time of intestinal activity.

Findings.—Three different patterns were noted on hepatobiliary scans. Thirty-eight percent of the scans showed a cholangitis pattern, with focal ductal dilatation and focal narrowing and focal or diffuse parenchymal retention. Another 38% showed ductal dilatation without focal narrowing but with diffuse parenchymal retention (Fig 3–4). The remaining 25% of the scans displayed severe diffuse parenchymal retention with or without ductal abnormality. In 9 studies there was no visualization of the gallbladder, and in 2, gallbladder visualization was delayed.

Conclusion.—Although other findings may differ, patients studied had abnormal parenchymal retention usually with some degree of ductal abnormality.

▶ Patients with AIDS frequently are seen with right upper quadrant pain, and about 60% of them have cholangitis. This is another cause of nonvisualization of the gallbladder (9 of 16 patients in this series and delayed visualization in 2 patients). As in other reported series, the most common pathogens were *Cryptosporidium* and cytomegalovirus.—J.G. McAfee, M.D.

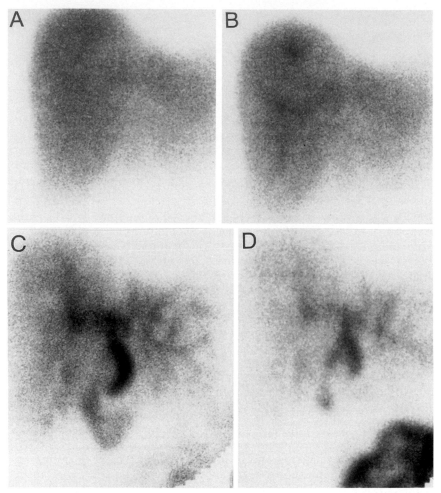

Fig 3–4.—Technetium-99m DISIDA bone scans obtained in a man, 40, with a history of intravenous drug abuse and cryptosporidial diarrhea. The patient had abdominal pain and abnormal liver function tests at presentation. Anterior images at (**A**) 1 minute, and (**B**) 5 minutes, show slightly heterogeneous uptake with early visualization of the dilated intrahepatic ducts at 5 minutes. **C,** anterior image at 1 hour shows diffuse dilatation of intra- and extrahepatic ducts. **D,** anterior image at 2 hours shows diffuse parenchymal retention, stasis in dilated ducts, and nonvisualization of the gallbladder. (Courtesy of Brunetti JC, Van Heertum RL, Kempf JS, et al: *Clin Nucl Med* 19:36–42, 1994.)

Infectious Diseases in Competitive Sports

Goodman RA, Thacker SB, Solomon SL, Osterholm MT, Hughes JM (Ctrs for Disease Control and Prevention, Atlanta, Ga; Minnesota Dept of Health, Minneapolis)
JAMA 271:862–867, 1994   124-95-3–4

Introduction.—More than 5 million high school and college students take part in organized, competitive sports. Although most of the literature on the health risks of sports has focused on injuries and noninfectious cutaneous and musculoskeletal problems, recent reports have raised concern about infectious disease outbreaks among athletes. A literature review was done to clarify the occurrence of infectious diseases among athletes or in sports settings.

Methods.—The review included a comprehensive search of the medical literature as well as 2 newspaper data bases. Articles describing cases or outbreaks of disease in which exposure to an infectious agent seemed likely to have occurred during sports training or competition were sought.

Findings.—Thirty-eight such reports from 1964 through 1993 were identified in a review of the medical literature. Most of the infectious agents were viruses, although fungi and gram-negative and -positive bacteria were also reported. Twenty-four reports involved person-to-person spread; half of them involved herpes simplex virus transmission among wrestlers. Other organisms that are spread in this way included *Staphylococcus aureus,* group A streptococci, hepatitis B virus, and several fungi; sports involved included wrestling, basketball, football, and rugby. There were 9 reports of a common-source spread of infectious agents, mainly involving enteroviruses. These cases commonly involved oral contamination of shared drinking water. The 5 reports of the spread of airborne measles included basketball games, wrestling matches, and gymnastic meets; potential exposure to spectators was entailed in several of these cases. Another 28 reports were identified from the newspaper databases, half of them involving basketball games.

Conclusion.—The risk of infectious disease in sports involves the athlete, the team, and spectators or others who may become exposed to infectious agents as a result of sports-related activities. Many of these outbreaks follow the seasonal patterns of disease transmission. Those responsible for the health of athletes must be aware of the infectious diseases the occur in sports and how to prevent them.

▶ Although this subject is only remotely related to nuclear medicine, it is an excellent survey for physicians who deal with patients with sports injuries and related problems. Skin infections from various organisms and viral infections of other organ systems predominate.

Herpes simplex in wrestlers is the most common single infection. Self-limited flulike illnesses in groups of athletes are common, and occasional outbreaks of measles and enterovirus infections occur. There have also been nasty outbreaks of echovirus infections with aseptic meningitis.

Although there are a few instances of direct transmission of hepatitis B, there are no known direct contact transmissions of HIV reported in athletic contact sports, despite all the hoopla in the sports media.—J.G. McAfee, M.D.

Usefulness of Gallium-67-Citrate Scans in Patients With Acute Disseminated Tuberculosis and Comparison With Chest X-Rays

Kao C-H, Wang S-J, Liao S-Q, Lin W-Y, Hsu C-Y (Taichung Veterans Gen Hosp, Taiwan, Republic of China)
J Nucl Med 34:1918–1921, 1993   124-95-3–5

Introduction.—In investigating the patient with possible acute disseminated tuberculosis (TB), the goal is to prove that the infection is TB as quickly as possible to allow prompt treatment. A positive gallium-67 (^{67}Ga) scan can increase the chances of detecting active TB. However, chest radiography is the best method for detecting miliary TB in the chest in acute disseminated disease. The value of ^{67}Ga scanning in patients with acute disseminated TB was evaluated by comparison of lung scintigraphy findings with those of chest radiography.

Methods.—The subjects were 16 patients who were admitted to a Taiwanese hospital with a diagnosis of acute disseminated TB. All had positive cultures of *Mycobacterium tuberculosis* from more than 1 source, a positive biopsy at necropsy, and/or a chest radiograph showing a miliary nodular pattern. Tuberculosis was localized using the chest radiographic and ^{67}Ga scanning findings.

Results.—Disseminated disease was not detected at chest radiography in 25% of patients. Although 11 of 12 patients had lesions in a miliary pattern, only 1 of them had focal changes (Fig 3–5). Gallium-67 scanning showed extrapulmonary disease in 50% of patients. Nineteen percent of lung scans were negative, 69% showed grade 1 or 2 disease, and only 12% showed grade 3 disease. A diffuse pattern was evident in 10 of 13 patients with positive scans. Underlying malignancy or immunocompromised disease was present in 56% of patients.

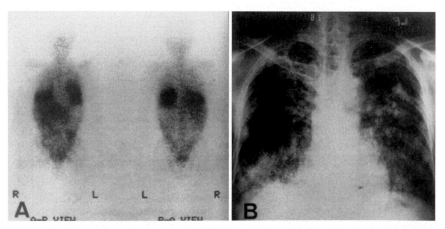

Fig 3–5.—Images obtained in a man, 56. **A,** ^{67}Ga lung scan reveals intensely localized uptake in the lower portions of both lungs, but the chest radiograph **(B)** shows a miliary pattern lesion. (Courtesy of Kao C-H, Wang S-J, Liao S-Q, et al: *J Nucl Med* 34:1918–1921, 1993.)

Conclusion.—These findings suggest that the combination of ⁶⁷Ga scanning and chest radiography is needed to avoid missing the diagnosis of acute disseminated tuberculosis. This is particularly so in high-risk patients. The ⁶⁷Ga scan findings may range from a negative picture to greater than liver uptake; whole body scans can clearly show the extrapulmonary TB focus.

▶ Unfortunately, tuberculous bugs are still alive and well, especially atypical organisms that are resistant to antibiotics in immunocompromised patients. These authors provide a strong argument that both chest x-ray films and ⁶⁷Ga imaging are needed in disseminated disease. In their patients, either modality alone would miss many lesions—19% false negative gallium chest images, with failure to detect disseminated disease in 25% by chest x-ray films alone.—J.G. McAfee, M.D.

Successful Gallium-67 Imaging of North American Pulmonary Blastomycosis

Dayanikli BF, Weissman AF, Wahl RL (Univ of Michigan, Ann Arbor)
J Nucl Med 34:958–960, 1993   124-95-3–6

Background.—Previously, South American blastomycosis has been imaged with gallium-67 (⁶⁷Ga) imaging. This imaging modality was successful in a case of North American pulmonary blastomycosis.

Case Report.—Man, 41, was previously healthy before he was seen with a 2-month history of febrile illness associated with a right lower lobe infiltrate and possible diagnosis of pulmonary blastomycosis. Computed tomography showed a masslike consolidation in the right lower lobe with a central area of reduced attenuation that was associated with a small right pleural effusion. A bone scan showed increased tracer uptake in the proximal upper extremity and lower extremity muscles and uptake in the ribs, concordant with intramuscular injections and history of trauma. A gallium scan, which was obtained using a medium-energy, parallel-hole collimator 24 hours after intravenous administration of 5 mCi of ⁶⁷Ga, showed increased uptake in the right lower lung field, corresponding to an area of infiltrate shown at CT. The pathologic diagnosis of pulmonary blastomycosis was confirmed.

Conclusion.—In this patient, North American pulmonary blastomycosis was imaged successfully with ⁶⁷Ga. Clinical, radiologic, and biopsy results were correlated.

▶ Add blastomycosis to your long list for the differential diagnosis of focal pulmonary uptake of ⁶⁷Ga.—J.G. McAfee, M.D.

Gallium-67 Scintigraphy in Borderline Lepromatous Leprosy

Mouratidis B, Lomas FE (Royal Canberra Hosp, Australia)
Australas Radiol 37:270–271, 1993   124-95-3-7

Introduction.—Leprosy is a chronic granulomatous infection that affects superficial tissues and appears in several forms. It is not usually included in the differential diagnosis of pyrexia of unknown origin (PUO). However, gallium-67 scintigraphy suggested the diagnosis of borderline lepromatous leprosy in a patient with PUO.

Case Report.—Woman, 38, had edema of her hands and feet, fever, weakness, lethargy, weight loss, and joint stiffness. Her skin had darkened, and she had a generalized erythematous rash. Her face and extremities had mild subcutaneous and neural thickening. The results of chest radiograph and bone marrow biopsy were nondiagnostic. Laboratory serum tests revealed elevations of γ-globulin, C-reactive protein, and angiotensin-converting enzyme. Gallium-67 scintigraphy showed increased uptake in the face (particularly the malar region) and thighs. A skin biopsy specimen taken from the thigh provided definitive diagnosis of borderline lepromatous leprosy.

Discussion.—The skin pigmentation changes, subcutaneous and neural thickening, and elevated angiotensin-converting enzyme were clinically consistent with the final diagnosis. Gallium-67 citrate visualizes areas of direct bacterial uptake and thereby localizes the focus of inflammatory lesions. In patients with PUO, this method allows the clinician to identify the area in which a biopsy should be performed, thereby yielding highly accurate diagnostic data.

▶ There are still 20 million people worldwide who have this disease.—J.G. McAfee, M.D.

The Detection of Ventricular Dysfunction and Carditis in Children With Kawasaki Disease Using Equilibrium Multigated Blood Pooling Ventriculography and ^{99}Tc^{m}-HMPAO-Labelled WBC Heart Scans

Kao CH, Hsieh KS, Wang YL, Wang SJ, Yeh SH (Taichung Veterans Gen Hosp, Taiwan, Republic of China)
Nucl Med Commun 14:539–543, 1993   124-95-3-8

Background.—Mucocutaneous lymph node syndrome, or Kawasaki disease, commonly affects infants and children younger than age 4 years. The etiology and pathogenesis of this acute febrile illness are unknown. Most patients have certain cardiovascular signs that are believed to result from coronary artery vasculitis with aneurysms, myocarditis, pericarditis, or endocarditis. The signs are gallop rhythm and distant heart sounds, pericardial effusion, and ECG abnormalities. Nearly all patients with Kawasaki disease are thought to have myocarditis.

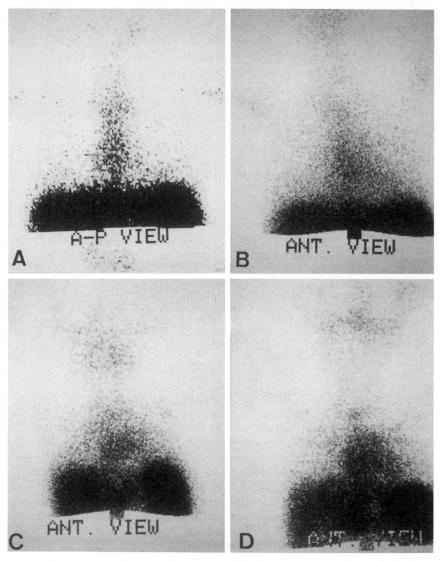

Fig 3–6.—A–D, the 24-hour anterior myocardial images after IV injection of technetium-99m HMPAO-labeled white blood cells. **A,** score 0. **B,** score 1. **C,** score 2. **D,** score 3. (Courtesy of Kao CH, Hsieh KS, Wang YL, et al: *Nucl Med Commun* 14:539–543, 1993.)

Objective.—Equilibrium multigated blood pooling ventriculography was used to evaluate biventricular function and technetium-99m hexamethylpropyleneamine oxime (HMPAO)–labeled white blood cell (WBC) heart scans were used to evaluate carditis in children with Kawasaki disease.

Methods.—Twenty-six boys and 11 girls with Kawasaki disease, aged 2.8 ± 2.2 years, were evaluated. Equilibrium multigated blood pooling ventriculography was performed with a digital gamma camera equipped to focus on the left ventricle and technetium-99m–labeled red blood cells. The cardiac image sequence generated high temporal resolution biventricular time-activity curves. Computer analysis of these curves calculated the left and right ventricular ejection fractions (LVEF and RVEF). After IV injection of technetium-99m HMPAO-labeled WBCs, a gamma camera was used to produce 24-hour myocardial imaging in left lateral, left anterior oblique, and anterior views. Two independent physicians interpreted and graded the scans. Scoring was done as follows: 0: < bone marrow uptake; 1: = marrow uptake; 2: > marrow uptake; 3: ≥ liver uptake (Fig 3–6).

Results.—Forty-three percent of the patients with Kawasaki disease who had severe carditis when evaluated by technetium-WBC also had the worst LVEFs and RVEFs when evaluated by equilibrium multigated blood pooling ventriculography. Twenty-four percent of the patients with mild carditis by technetium-WBC had the best LVEFs and RVEFs. The rest of the children (32%) were found to have both moderately severe carditis and biventricular function.

Conclusion.—The severity of carditis in children with Kawasaki disease is related to the degree of impairment in left and right ventricular function. Technetium-WBC imaging not only can determine the severity of carditis, but it also can predict ventricular functional impairment. Because it does both accurately, technetium-WBC should be used to evaluate children with Kawasaki disease.

▶ Kawasaki disease is much more common worldwide than was originally thought. It is now being encountered in older children as well and rarely in adults. Early diagnosis is of the utmost importance. It is easily confused with an acute infection, but antibiotics are not effective. The proper treatment, aspirin, and a single massive infusion of immune globulin (2 g/kg) given over 10 hours, markedly reduces the incidence of cardiac complications if it is given either as soon as possible or within the first week of symptoms; it also reduces the fever (1).

Echocardiography is widely used in the United States to assess the coronary arteries and ventricular contractability immediately and after about 6 weeks. If permanent cardiac damage occurs, it almost always is detectable in the first 40 days.

This article suggests that labeled leukocyte imaging can detect myocarditis without coronary artery involvement, but proper treatment should not be delayed to obtain images at 24 hours.—J.G. McAfee, M.D.

Reference

1. Newburger JW, et al: *N Engl J Med* 324:1633, 1991.

Technetium-99m Hexamethylpropylene Amine Oxime Labelled Leucocyte Scintigraphy in Ulcerative Colitis and Crohn's Disease

Papós M, Nagy F, Láng J, Csernay L (Albert Szent-Györgyi Med Univ, Szeged, Hungary; County Hosp, Szeged)
Eur J Nucl Med 20:766–769, 1993   124-95-3–9

Objective.—Adequate follow-up of patients with inflammatory bowel diseases requires a knowledge of current clinical activity and the extent of involved bowel segments. The value of technetium-99m hexamethylpropyleneamine oxime (^{99m}Tc-HMPAO)–labeled leukocyte scintigraphy (LS) in ulcerative colitis and Crohn's disease was examined.

Patients and Methods.—Thirty patients with ulcerative colitis underwent a total of 45 investigations. Those in the group had a mean age of 40.4 years and a mean duration of disease of 6.3 years. Fifty-three investigations were done in 34 patients with Crohn's disease. Their mean age

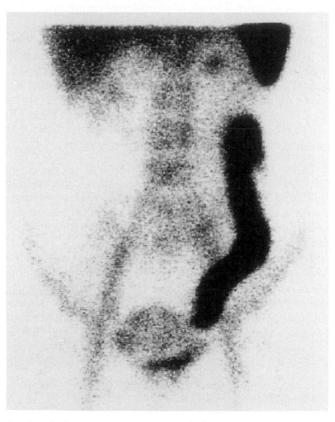

Fig 3–7.—Four-hour leukocyte scan in woman, 35, with ulcerative colitis. There is intense leukocyte accumulation in descending colon and rectosigmoid. (Courtesy of Papós M, Nagy F, Láng J, et al: *Eur J Nucl Med* 20:766–769, 1993.)

was 36.9 years, and their mean duration of disease was 7.2 years. All diagnoses were proved by histology or surgery. Anterior images were obtained 30 minutes and 2 and 4 hours (Fig 3–7) after reinjection of the labeled leukocytes. The segmental extent of the inflammation and the grade of leukocyte uptake were calculated and were then compared with laboratory and colonoscopy findings.

Results.—The average lipophilic complex yield of ^{99m}Tc-HMPAO was 93% and the mean labeling efficacy was 57%. The viability of the leukocytes averaged 98% and was not affected by the separation and labeling procedure. One hundred three of the 168 examined segments were found to be active on colonoscopy, biopsy, or x-ray investigation. Scintigraphy yielded false negative findings in 25 active segments (or an overall sensitivity of 76%) and false positive findings in 5 inactive segments. The sensitivity of leukocyte scintigraphy was higher in ulcerative colitis (87%) than in Crohn's disease (82% in the small intestine but only 53% in the large bowel). Correlations between scintigraphic activity values and the Best index and laboratory parameters of inflammation were significant in ulcerative colitis but not in Crohn's disease.

Conclusion.—The sensitivity of leukocyte scintigraphy was found to be higher in ulcerative colitis (87%) than in Crohn's disease (53% in the large bowel and 82% in the small intestine). The specificity was similar in the 2 diseases (93% in ulcerative colitis and 89% and 100% in Crohn's disease, corresponding to the large bowel and the small intestine). The discrepancies are probably the result of differences in cellular response—in Crohn's disease the infiltration is primarily lymphocytic, whereas in ulcerative colitis, granulocytes predominate.

▶ Labeled leukocyte studies in inflammatory bowel disease appear to be popular in Europe. However, in the United States, gastroenterologists tend to rely on clinical and other laboratory findings to assess the activity of the intrinsic bowel diseases and request imaging primarily for extrinsic abdominal inflammatory lesions (1).

The incidence of false positive results is surprisingly low in this study. Others (2) have experienced problems in distinguishing normal bowel activity from inflammatory disease—a difficulty not encountered with indium-111–labeled leukocytes. Some have quantitated the activity of intrinsic bowel inflammatory lesions after indium-111 leukocytes by counting stool collections, but nuclear technologists do not like to do this.—J.G. McAfee, M.D.

References

1. Best WR, et al: *Gastroenterology* 70:439, 1976.
2. Mountford PJ, et al: *J Nucl Med* 31:311, 1990.

Mesenteric Lymphadenitis Depicted by Indium 111-Labeled White Blood Cell Imaging

Achong DM, Oates E, Harris B (Tufts Univ, Boston; New England Med Ctr, Boston)

J Pediatr Surg 28:1550–1552, 1993   124-95-3-10

Introduction.—In an acutely ill child with abdominal pain and pharyngitis the diagnosis can be difficult. One possibility is mesenteric lymphadenitis, an ill-defined condition that is commonly associated with acute upper respiratory infection. A case in which indium-111–labeled white blood cell (^{111}In WBC) scintigraphy helped make the diagnosis of mesenteric lymphadenitis was examined.

Case Report.—Boy, 4 years, had a fever, leukocytosis, pharyngitis, and abdominal pain. A localized irritative process was suggested by the abdominal plain x-ray film finding of small air-fluid levels at the cecal tip. On abdominal CT, the retrocecal soft tissues were thickened. Indium-111 WBC scintigraphy demonstrated mild focal uptake in the right lower abdomen from 3 to 24 hours after injection. The nasopharynx and cervical lymph nodes also showed abnormal WBC localization (Figs 3–8, 3–9, and 3–10). Taken together, the abdominal and head and neck WBC activity and the physical findings suggested the diagnosis of mesenteric lymphadenitis/pharyngitis syndrome. The child's condition resolved gradually during 5 days; his Epstein-Barr viral titers were consistent with reactivated infection.

Discussion.—In children with abdominal pain and concomitant pharyngitis, the differential diagnosis should include mesenteric lymphadenitis associated with systemic infection. Persistent abdominal accumulation of labeled WBCs is an abnormal finding that on its own suggests an in-

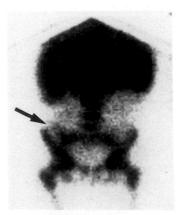

Fig 3–8.—Three-hour anterior abdominal image shows abnormal ^{111}In WBC localization in the right lower quadrant (*arrow*). (Courtesy of Achong DM, Oates E, Harris B: *J Pediatr Surg* 28:1550–1552, 1993).

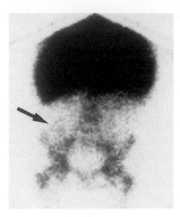

Fig 3–9.—Focal ¹¹¹In WBC activity persists in the right lower abdomen 24 hours post injection (*arrow*). As with Figure 3-8, the image is intentionally highly contrasted to emphasize the subtle abnormal abdominal WBC accumulation relative to the marked (but normal) liver and spleen uptake. (Courtesy of Achong DM, Oates E, Harris B: *J Pediatr Surg* 28:1550-1552, 1993.)

flammatory process (e.g., appendicitis). Mesenteric lymphadenitis is suspected when there are also other foci of uptake consistent with an upper respiratory infection.

▶ The challenge of right lower quadrant pain in children and young adults is to avoid surgery in acute mesenteric lymphadenitis but to avoid any undue delay in surgery for acute appendicitis. Early leukocyte imaging can be helpful with equivocal clinical findings.

As the authors point out, ¹¹¹In activity in the right lower abdomen may be the result of swallowed exudation from pharyngeal infections; therefore,

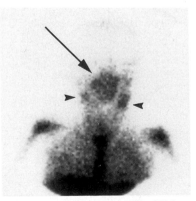

Fig 3–10.—Anterior head and neck view shows abnormal ¹¹¹In WBC accumulation in the nasopharynx (*arrow*) and cervical lymph nodes (*arrowheads*). (Courtesy of Achong DM, Oates E, Harris B: *J Pediatr Surg* 28:1550-1552, 1993.)

early images at 1 to 4 hours are important in patients with right lower quadrant pain.

The authors cite an older reference that is an excellent review (1). The organisms that cause this condition are still in question. Staphylococcal, beta-hemolytic streptococcal, and *Pasteurella* strains are sometimes recovered, but viruses are more commonly implicated, such as adenoviruses or Epstein-Barr virus, which causes infectious mononucleosis. Recent reports include infections from *Yersinia* organisms; typical or atypical mycobacterial infections, especially in children with AIDS; and cat-scratch bacilli. Children with acute appendicitis have lower serum levels of α-interferon than do those with right lower quadrant pain from other inflammatory causes.—J.G. McAfee, M.D.

Reference

1. Blattner RJ: *J Pediatr* 74:479, 1969.

Diagnosis of Infection in Ununited Fractures: Combined Imaging With Indium-111-Labeled Leukocytes and Technetium-99m Methylene Diphosphonate

Nepola JV, Seabold JE, Marsh JL, Kirchner PT, El-Khoury GY (Univ of Iowa, Iowa City)
J Bone Joint Surg (Am) 75A:1816–1822, 1993   124-95-3-11

Introduction.—Plain radiography often fails to reveal osteomyelitis in patients with ununited fractures. Combined scintigraphy with indium-111–labeled leukocytes and technetium-99m methylene diphosphonate was used to evaluate ununited fractures in patients with an increased likelihood of infection. This method of preoperative evaluation for osteomyelitis was compared with results of cultures of open bone.

Patients and Methods.—One hundred two sites of delayed union or nonunion in 96 patients were evaluated by combined scintigraphy. Tissue from the sites in question was obtained for culture at the time of operation. The patient group included 68 males and 28 females, ranging in age from 11 to 75 years. The tibia (55) and the femur (23) were the most commonly involved sites. Forty-seven patients had a history of drainage or wound infection, and 42 fractures had originally been open. A study was considered positive for osteomyelitis when uptake of the indium-111–labeled leukocytes at the involved site was greater than that in the adjacent or contralateral bone marrow and coincided with the site of concentration of technetium-99m methylene diphosphonate in bone.

Results.—Cultures of bone obtained intraoperatively were positive for 29% of sites and negative for 71%. When compared with these results, the combined imaging method yielded 25 true positive, 59 true negative, 11 false positive, 4 false negative, and 3 indeterminate interpretations. Therefore, in the diagnosis of osteomyelitis, combined scintigraphy had a sensitivity of 86%, a specificity of 84%, an accuracy of 82%, a positive predictive value of 69%, and a negative predictive value of 94%.

Conclusion.—Combined indium-111–labeled leukocytes and technetium-99m methylene diphosphonate scintigraphy is recommended for screening patients with nonunion or delayed union fractures or arthrodesis who are at risk for infection. Risk factors include a history of an open fracture, a wound complication, drainage, or radiologic findings suggestive of infection. Patients who have a closed fracture or uncomplicated internal fixation have a low rate of infection and should not require the combined imaging.

▶ This study indicates that the results of this combined imaging technique for detecting infection in nonunion or delayed union fractures are good, but leukocyte images may be false positive if the fractures involve a joint or adjacent metaphyseal regions. The methylene diphosphonate images, which are almost always positive in unhealed fractures, are useful only for localizing the foci of leukocyte accumulation in soft tissues or bones.

In some reported series of acute uncomplicated fractures, positive leukocyte images have been found, probably as a result of neutrophilic infiltration of the hematoma at the fracture site. The lesions at sites of nonunion or delayed union apparently are different. The relatively high sensitivity of detection of these old lesions contradicts the old adage that neutrophils do not migrate to old inflammatory lesions.—J.G. McAfee, M.D.

Preliminary Results on Scintigraphic Evaluation of Malignant External Otitis
Malamitsi J, Maragoudakis P, Papafragou K, Koukouliou V, Kalatzis Y, Adamopoulos G, Proukakis C (Univ of Athens, Greece; Hippocrateion Hosp, Athens, Greece)
Eur J Nucl Med 20:511–514, 1993   124-95-3–12

Introduction.—Malignant external otitis (MEO), a potentially fatal condition, occurs in diabetic and immunosuppressed patients. The infection may involve the temporal bone, mastoid process, and surrounding tissues. Bone sepsis at the base of the skull, resulting in massive thrombophlebitis of the brain, can cause death. *Pseudomonas aeruginosa* is usually isolated from cultures. Scintigraphic findings in 6 patients were reported.

Patients and Methods.—Four diabetic patients and 1 latent diabetic patient were given a clinical diagnosis of external otitis with suspected MEO. The sixth patient was presumed cured of MEO. All the patients underwent methylene diphosphonate (MDP), nanocolloid, and gallium SPECT imaging studies with quantitative analysis of regions of interest (ROI) and count profile curves. Studies that were considered to be positive had increased uptake on all the scintigraphic studies, and ROI quotients were much higher over the lesion than on the normal side.

Results.—Four patients, all with a difficult course of disease, had positive results on almost all scintigraphic studies for MEO. In one diabetic patient with negative results on all 3 studies, MEO was ruled out. This patient received a short course of antibiotics and was dismissed free of symptoms. The sixth patient, who was presumed cured of MEO, had scintigraphic findings suggestive of continuing low-grade bone infection. Prolonged treatment was recommended because of the likelihood of relapse.

Conclusion.—The classic Chandler's triad for MEO, consisting of diabetes, granuloma, and *P. aeruginosa*, is not always present. Therefore, a fourth criterion is proposed on the basis of these findings: scintigraphic demonstration of skull base infection. Gallium and nanocolloid, as markers of bone and soft tissue infection, gave increased uptake earlier than MDP. These studies are also useful in follow-up, because uptake is promptly reduced with decreasing inflammatory activity. The combination of all 3 modalities is recommended for evaluation of suspected MEO.

▶ As these authors indicate, demonstrating the presence or absence of osteomyelitis of the petrous temporal bone in otitis media is important. Unfortunately, judging by the lesion-to-normal side uptake ratios of the 3 agents provided in Table 1 in the original article, the calculated ratios were in error. The recalculated ratios were highest with MDP and lowest with gallium. However, in following the results of antibiotic therapy, gallium-67 should be the agent of choice, because MDP images tend to remain positive forever in adult inactive osteomyelitis.

Labeled leukocyte images in malignant otitis are sometimes unconvincing, because these immunocompromised patients apparently do not have normal neutrophilic migration to inflammatory stimuli.—J.G. McAfee, M.D.

Use of Bone Scan in Management of Patients With Peripheral Gangrene Due to Fulminant Meningococcemia

Hamdy RC, Babyn PS, Krajbich JI (Univ of Toronto)
J Pediatr Orthop 13:447–451, 1993 124-95-3-13

Objective.—Ten percent of patients with meningococcal disease will have the disastrous complication of fulminant meningococcemia, leading to ischemic lesions of any organ system, including the skeleton. In about 10% of patients with this complication, gangrene of the extremities will develop, probably as a result of disseminated intravascular coagulation and vasculitis. Such gangrene does not follow any uniform pattern, which may make it difficult to assess the proper level of amputation.

Technetium bone scintigraphy was performed in 4 children with fulminant meningococcemia and peripheral gangrene.

Patients.—The patients, drawn from a series of 53 patients with fulminant meningococcemia, all required amputation for extensive gangrene of the extremities. All showed a progressive, patchy, irregular gangrene within the first 2 hospital days. Over the next 3 weeks, the level of gangrene appeared to become demarcated in 12 limbs, but it could not be clinically determined in the remaining 4. All patients underwent bone scanning 2–5 weeks after the onset of illness. All scans were performed by the standard technique, with special attention to blood pool and flow phases.

Outcomes.—All extremities examined in each of the patients showed variable absent uptake in the distal portion of the limbs. All patients had delayed amputation of all 4 limbs. In 13 limbs, the level of amputation was based mainly on the bone scan level; 84% of these amputations were successful. The bone scan confirmed the clinical impression in 5 limbs with a clinically demarcated level of gangrene and revealed a more distal level than the clinical estimate in 5 other limbs. Bone scanning was useful in deciding on the level of amputation in 4 limbs with no clearly demarcated level of gangrene. Bone scan findings were ignored in 1 limb, in which revision amputation was later necessary to the level initially suggested by the bone scan.

Conclusion.—Bone scanning appears to be a useful adjunct in determining the appropriate level of amputation in patients with fulminant meningococcemia and extensive peripheral gangrene. It is most useful in patchy gangrenous areas in which there may be islands of viable tissue. Bone scanning should be done soon after the onset of gangrene to enable an early decision on the level of amputation and avoidance of unnecessary skin grafts.

▶ This is another example of an effective use of bone scanning not for diagnosis but as a demarcation guide for amputation, which is similar to its use in patients with severe frostbite in a previous report (1).

In the authors' review of the literature, they found 53 patients with gangrene from meningococcemia in 17 reports. In these previous reports, skeletal imaging was largely neglected.—J.G. McAfee, M.D.

Reference

1. Lisbona R, Rosenthall L: *J Trauma* 16:989, 1976.

Diagnostic Images: Gas-Forming Infections
Adamson DJA, Smith CC, Smith FW (Aberdeen Royal Infirmary, Scotland)
Postgrad Med J 69:581–582, 1993   1 2 4-95-3–1 4

Introduction.—Both clostridial and nonclostridial gas gangrene can appear without a history of trauma or surgery. Such a case was described in the leg of an elderly patient.

Case Report.—Woman, 89, experienced confusion and difficulty walking. Her left thigh was swollen and erythematous and had associated crepitus. A pelvic x-ray and a bone scan detected gas gangrene in the tissues of the left thigh. Surgery was not performed because the patient was a poor anesthetic risk. Instead, she was treated by antibiotics and the release of pus. Her recovery was slow but complete.

Conclusion.—A case of gas gangrene that was not associated with recent trauma or surgery was reported. Although the patient recovered with antibiotic therapy alone, the preferred treatment is surgical excision of necrotic tissue.

▶ This case report contrasts with the preceding paper, where vascular occlusion was a major contributing factor in the onset of gangrene that required amputation. The 89-year-old female described in this report may have been immunocompromised, but apparently she had no major vascular occlusion and recovered from the osteomyelitis and gangrene by antibiotic treatment and drainage without surgery.—J.G. McAfee, M.D.

Technetium-99m-HMPAO-Labeled Leukocytes and Technetium-99m-Labeled Human Polyclonal Immunoglobulin G in Diagnosis of Focal Purulent Disease
Hovi I, Taavitsainen M, Lantto T, Vorne M, Paul R, Remes K (Helsinki Univ Hosp; Päijät-Häme Central Hosp, Lahti, Finland; Turku Univ Central Hosp, Finland)
J Nucl Med 34:1428–1434, 1993   124-95-3–15

Introduction.—A number of radionuclear techniques have been introduced in recent years for the evaluation of infectious and inflammatory diseases. The relative clinical usefulness of these new methods has not been established. The usefulness of technetium-99m (^{99m}Tc) hexamethylpropyleneamine oxime (HMPAO)–labeled leukocytes was compared with that of ^{99m}Tc-labeled polyclonal human immunoglobulin G (Technescan HIG) for the detection of focal purulent disease or an inflammatory reaction specifically caused by microbiological agents and characterized by immigration of large numbers of leukocytes.

Patients and Methods.—Thirty patients with a mean age of 55 years and a known or strongly suspected focal infection were examined using the 2 imaging methods. Two of the patients were examined twice with labeled leukocytes, and 1 was examined twice with labeled HIG. The interval between leukocyte and immunoglobulin imaging was usually 48 to 96 hours. Two nuclear physicians who were blinded to the clinical in-

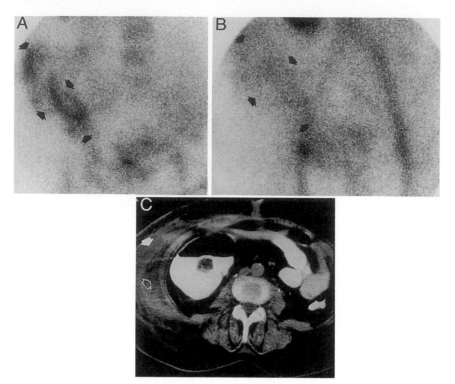

Fig 3–11.—Postoperative cellulitis and abscess. **A,** ^{99m}Tc-leukocyte scan at 4 hours showing stronger accumulation of tracer; lesion better delineated than in the ^{99m}Tc-HIG scan at 5 hours. **B,** *arrows* indicate corresponding areas. **C,** CT scan revealing edema *(filled arrow)* and small collection of fluid *(open arrow)* in the abdominal wall. (Courtesy of Hovi I, Taavitsainen M, Lantto T, et al: *J Nucl Med* 34:1428–1434, 1993.)

formation and 2 radiologists who were aware of the clinical history analyzed the scans.

Results.—Labeled HIG had a sensitivity of 58%, a specificity of 82%, an overall accuracy of 67%, a positive predictive value of 85%, and a negative predictive value of 53%; corresponding values for leukocyte imaging were 84%, 100%, 90%, 100%, and 79%. In no instance was the ^{99m}Tc-HIG imaging method better than the ^{99m}Tc-HMPAO leukocyte scan (Fig 3–11), and the overall accuracy of the leukocyte scan was significantly better than that of the HIG scan. Focal purulent disease was the final diagnosis in 19 patients.

Conclusion.—In cases of suspected focal infection, scintigraphy with ^{99m}Tc-labeled leukocytes is the preferable method. Directly labeled HIG is not recommended as the primary scintigraphic method in such cases, although it may be of value in the assessment of nonpurulent inflammations and reactive arthropathies.

► This seems to be a fair clinical comparison of the 2 agents. Sixteen of the 30 patients were first injected with ^{99m}Tc-HIG; in the other 14 patients, the ^{99m}Tc-labeled leukocytes were injected first. The mean injected activities were 7 mCi (260 MBq) of ^{99m}Tc for the labeled leukocytes and 8 mCi (300 MBq) of ^{99m}Tc-HIG.

If you were septic, would you like a diagnostic study with a sensitivity of detection of only 58% for ^{99m}Tc-HIG? Other workers have found too many false positives with labeled HIG as well.—J.G. McAfee, M.D.

Multidose Use of Exametazime for Leukocyte Labelling: A New Approach Using Tin Enhancement
Solanki C, Li DJ, Wong A, Miles KA, Sampson CB (Addenbrookes Hosp, Cambridge, England)
Nucl Med Commun 14:1035–1040, 1993   124-95-3–16

Background.—Technetium-99m (^{99m}Tc) exametazime–labeled leukocytes are widely used in many nuclear medicine applications. Because of the rapid oxidation of the small amount of stannous chloride in the available freeze-dried kit, reconstituted exametazime is inherently unstable. Whether the addition of stannous ion to previously reconstituted exametazime could maintain satisfactory levels of primary complex for cell labeling was confirmed, the volume of stannous fluoride solution needed for optimal levels of primary complex was determined, a protocol for cell labeling in which a vial of exametazime is used more efficiently was developed, and the suitability of tin-enhanced exametazime for clinical studies was investigated.

Methods and Findings.—Freshly prepared stannous solution, .1 mL, was mixed with .3 mL (25 µg) of exametazime solution and 400 to 500 MBq of pertechnetate. Mixed leukocytes from 50-mL blood samples from 114 patients were labeled. The ^{99m}Tc-exametazime used for labeling was prepared by tin enhancement. The exametazime had been reconstituted as long as 5 months earlier. The median labeling efficiency was 72%, ranging from 30% to 96%. Up to 15 doses of exametazime for leukocyte labeling could be prepared from 1 vial because of the small volumes used.

Conclusion.—The multidose use of reconstituted exametazime can be achieved by adding suitable amounts of tin to replace that lost through oxidation. A kit preparation permitted a fixed, reproducible amount of stannous ion to be added to reconstituted exametazime. With tin enhancement, satisfactory levels of radiochemical purity and labeling efficiency were obtained.

► Technetium-99m hexamethylpropyleneamine oxime (HMPAO) is still the best technetium radiopharmaceutical for labeling leukocytes in vitro for imaging foci of infection. This application of this agent appears to exceed its use for brain imaging. However, it is highly unstable and variable in clinical performance. Consequently, many modifications in its preparation have been proposed to prevent its rapid deterioration in vitro. This stannous ion addition method seems to work.

The authors demonstrated no change in labeling efficiency for leukocyte suspensions using HMPAO solutions up to 150 days old. Another method that appears to work is the addition of stable sodium iodide (1).—J.G. McAfee, M.D.

Reference

1. Millar AM: *Nucl Med Commun* 13:306, 1992.

Tc-99m Labeled Monoclonal Antibodies Against Granulocytes (BW 250/183) in the Detection of Appendicitis

Biersack HJ, Overbeck B, Ott G, Kania U, Briele B, Kropp J, Bockisch A, Grünwald F, Hotze AL, Hirner A, Shih WJ (Univ of Bonn, Germany; Waldkrankenhaus Bonn, Germany; Univ of Kentucky, Lexington)
Clin Nucl Med 18:371–376, 1993   124-95-3–17

Background.—Localizing focal sites of inflammation in the abdomen is important clinically, especially in cases of suspected appendicitis. The results of scintigraphy with technetium-99m (^{99m}Tc)–labeled monoclonal antibodies against granulocytes (BW 250/183) in such cases were reported.

Methods.—Thirty-two patients with suspected appendicitis underwent scintigraphy 2 hours after the tracer was injected. All patients also underwent surgery, with a histologic assessment of resected tissue.

Findings.—Seventeen patients had acute appendicitis, of whom 12 had right positive scans, for a sensitivity of 71%. Acute appendicitis could have been excluded in 15 cases. In 11 of these, the scan was true negative, for a specificity of 73%. Overall accuracy was 72%.

Conclusion.—The use of ^{99m}Tc antigranulocyte monoclonal antibodies may overcome the problems of the ^{99m}Tc hexamethylpropyleneamine oxime granulocyte and indium-111 oxine approaches, such as nonspecific intestinal activity and untimeliness. Technetium-99m–labeled antigranulocyte antibodies can be used in emergency procedures and may play a role in the management of patients with suspected appendicitis.

▶ These results do not look good enough. If one relied solely on this imaging procedure, would any surgeon be pleased with missing 3 of every 10 patients with acute or subacute appendicitis and 27% false positives? Results in the 18 female patients were worse than those in the males. There were only 3 true positive results in females, 5 false negatives, and 7 true negatives, but there were 3 false positives.

Unfortunately, in women 21 to 40 years old, the negative laparotomy rate for acute appendicitis is as high as 45%. In males, the imaging results were better (only one false positive and no false negatives). However, the negative laparotomy rate in males is much lower than that in females.—J.G. McAfee, M.D.

Comparison of ^{99}Tc^{m}Labelled Specific Murine Anti-CD4 Monoclonal Antibodies and Nonspecific Human Immunoglobulin for Imaging Inflamed Joints in Rheumatoid Arthritis
Kinne RW, Becker W, Schwab J, Horneff G, Schwarz A, Kalden JR, Emmrich F, Burmester GR, Wolf F (Univ of Erlangen-Nuremberg, Germany; Radiochemical Lab of the Behring Werke [Hoechst AG], Frankfurt, Germany)
Nucl Med Commun 14:667–675, 1993   124-95-3–18

Background.—Technetium-99m–labeled anti-CD4 monoclonal antibodies (MAbs) can be used to image inflamed joints in patients with rheumatoid arthritis (RA). The MAbs recognize the CD4 molecule expressed on T-helper cells and, with a lower density, on macrophages, both of which are found in abundance in RA inflammatory infiltrates. However, it is unclear whether the uptake of anti-CD4 MAbs is different from that of control immunoglobulins with irrelevant specificity.

Methods and Findings.—Eight patients with severe, active RA were assessed after IV injection of a technetium-99m–labeled murine antihuman CD4 MAb or polyclonal human immunoglobulin. Five patients received both the anti-CD4 MAb and human immunoglobulin. Anterior and posterior whole-body and joint scans were acquired 1, 4, and 24 hours after injection. As early as 4 hours after injection, the antihuman CD4 MAb demonstrated a greater target-to-background ratio by area-of-interest technique in arthritic knee and elbow joints compared with polyclonal human immunoglobulin used for conventional imaging.

Conclusion.—The anti-CD4 MAb permits more specific detection of inflammatory infiltrates that are rich in CD4-positive cells. Because anti-CD4 MAbs preferentially bind to mononuclear cells that infiltrate chronically inflamed joints but not to granulocytes characteristic of acute inflammation, they may also be used to differentiate chronic joint inflammation from other joint disorders.

▶ Although this is an elegant method of imaging inflamed rheumatoid joints, will it be important clinically? Many rheumatologists remain skeptical about the necessity of joint imaging with any radioactive agent, because the images correlate so closely with clinical findings. On the other hand, some like objective information about changes in uptake in response to therapy.—J.G. McAfee, M.D.

Technetium-99m-Labeled Hydrazino Nicotinamide Derivatized Chemotactic Peptide Analogs for Imaging Focal Sites of Bacterial Infection

Babich JW, Solomon H, Pike MC, Kroon D, Graham W, Abrams MJ, Tompkins RG, Rubin RH, Fischman AJ (Massachusetts Gen Hosp, Boston; Shriners Burns Inst, Boston; RW Johnson Pharmaceutical Research Inst, Raritan, NJ; et al)

J Nucl Med 34:1964–1974, 1993   124-95-3-19

Background.—Prompt identification, localization, and characterization of the focal sites of infection is a critical step in treating patients with fever, especially when localizing symptoms are not present. Recently, indium-111–labeled chemotactic peptides were found to be effective in the external imaging of focal infection sites in rats. Four hydrazino nicotinamide (HYNIC)–derivatized chemotactic peptide analogues were synthesized and assessed for both in vitro bioactivity and receptor binding.

Methods and Findings.—The peptides—For-NleLFK-HYNIC (HP1), For-MLFK-HYNIC (HP2), For-MLFNH(CH2)6NH-HYNIC (HP3), and For-MLF-(D)-K-HYNIC (HP4)—were radiolabeled with technetium-99m (^{99m}Tc) by a glucoheptonate cotranschelation. Their biodistribution in rats was determined at 5, 30, 60, and 120 minutes after injection. Peptide localization at sites of deep thigh *Escherichia coli* infection was determined by radioactivity measures in excised rat and rabbit tissues and through scintillation camera images obtained in rabbits. All peptides maintained biological activity and the ability to bind to the oligopeptide chemoattractant receptor on human polymorphonuclear leukocytes. Radiolabeled peptides were incubated with ^{99m}Tc-glucoheptonate and isolated by means of high-pressure liquid chromatography at specific activities of greater than 10,000 mCi/μM. Technetium-99m–labeled peptides retained receptor binding with EC_{50}s of less than 10 nM, and all 4 peptides were cleared rapidly from blood. Biodistributions of the individual peptides were similar. Accumulation levels in most normal tissues were low. All peptides concentrated at the infection sites in rats within 1 hour of injection. Images of the infection sites obtained in rabbits were outstanding, with target-to-background ratios of more than 20:1 at 15 hours after injection.

Conclusion.—Hydrazino nicotinamide–derivatized chemotactic peptide analogues retain receptor binding and biological activity. They are readily labeled with ^{99m}Tc at very high specific activities and are excellent radiopharmaceuticals for imaging focal infection sites. These molecules have many advantages over current radionuclide methods for localizing infection sites, and they merit further study.

▶ This article summarizes a great deal of experimental work in synthetic and analytical chemistry, radiochemistry, and biodistribution studies in rodents.

The authors have succeeded in achieving extremely high specific activities (about 10–100 pmol of ^{99m}Tc per mCi) to avoid the sudden marked neutropenia and other biological effects of microgram quantities of these peptides. The current preparation is painstaking, requiring fresh generator eluate and a terminal separation of the co-ligand glucoheptonate and other unbound ^{99m}Tc.

From the rodent biodistribution data presented, only about 10% of the injected radioactivity remains in the circulation by 5 minutes. By imaging, the radiolabeled activated cells sequestered chiefly in the lungs, liver, and spleen. In the rats with thigh infections, the infected-to-normal muscle concentration ratios at 2 hours were low (2 to 3), but they were high in the rabbit at 17 hours. However, at that time, most of the blood radioactivity was not cell bound.

The utility of the ^{99m}Tc chemotactic peptides for imaging infections will probably remain controversial for some time. More detailed studies are needed on the distribution of cell bound and plasma activity in the blood at various time intervals. Their evaluation compared with other available agents will require experiments in nonrodent species, because most of the circulating leukocytes in rodents are lymphocytes and not neutrophils.—J.G. McAfee, M.D.

Biodistribution and Imaging Studies of Technetium-99m-Labeled Liposomes in Rats With Focal Infection
Goins B, Klipper R, Rudolph AS, Cliff RO, Blumhardt R, Phillips WT (Univ of Texas Health Science Ctr, San Antonio; Naval Research Lab, Washington, DC)
J Nucl Med 34:2160–2168, 1993   124-95-3-20

Background.—Much research has been performed regarding the use of radiopharmaceutical agents for the noninvasive location of infection sites. Liposomes are spherical lipid bilayers that can carry a variety of drugs or radionuclides in their aqueous space and, therefore, have potential diagnostic imaging applications. A procedure was developed to label liposomes containing reduced glutathione (GSH) with technetium-99m (^{99m}Tc) using the lipophilic chelator hexamethylpropyleneamine oxime (HMPAO).

Methods.—The value of ^{99m}Tc liposomes in detecting focal infection sites in rats was evaluated. The rats were first infected in the thigh by intramuscular *Staphylococcus aureus* injection. Twenty-four hours later, ^{99m}Tc liposome, gallium-67 (^{67}Ga) citrate, or ^{99m}Tc human serum albumin (HSA) was injected intravenously. The rats were imaged using a gamma camera and killed at 4, 24, or 48 hours for tissue biodistribution studies.

Findings.—Abscesses were prominently localized within 2 hours in rats after ^{99m}Tc liposome injection and continued to increase in activity for up to 24 hours. This was not observed in rats that were given ^{67}Ga citrate or ^{99m}Tc-HSA. Mean abscess-to-muscle ratios determined from

24-hour biodistribution data obtained from tissue sampling were 35.3, 4.1, and 8 for [99mTc] liposomes, [67Ga] citrate, and [99mTc]-HSA, respectively.

Conclusion.—Technetium-99m liposomes labeled with this procedure were superior to the common radiopharmaceuticals used for infection imaging, and they may replace labeled leukocytes in localizing focal infection sites in some cases. The [99mTc] liposomes are easy to label, have a high labeling efficiency, and would be readily available in kit form.

▶ This is a novel [99mTc] radiopharmaceutical for imaging abscesses. The authors have succeeded in preparing liposomes much smaller than previous attempts by others, thereby slowing the plasma clearance by the reticuloendothelial organs. Their preparation is stable in vivo, unlike most [99mTc] albumin chelates, which are unstable after 2 or 3 hours.

The negligible liposomal activity in the gastrointestinal and urinary tracts is a significant advantage over other [99mTc] preparations. In the rat abscesses, the liposomal concentration was a little lower than that of gallium at 24 hours.

The abscess-to-muscle ratio was higher with the liposomes, because their muscle concentration was only one tenth that of gallium.

Is the mechanism of abscess localization of liposomes simply increased capillary permeability and faster plasma clearance? It would be interesting to compare the liposomes with indium-111–labeled leukocytes in a nonrodent species.—J.G. McAfee, M.D.

4 Musculoskeletal

Introduction

For decades, the interest in bone metabolism and disease has been dominated by studies of bone mineral and the biochemicals that control it, such as parathormone, calcitonin, and vitamin D. The mineral phase is easily imaged by several modalities. In nuclear medicine imaging, we have several agents for bone mineral and marrow but none for the organic phase. Clinicians have relied on serum alkaline phosphatase as an indicator of osteoblastic activity and hydroxyproline for bone loss. The biochemistry of bone matrix and the variety of cells in osseous tissue have been neglected in the past, but this has changed in recent years. The explosion of knowledge about these organic components of bone is beginning to have an impact on clinical practice.

Of 12 or 13 different collagens, at least 5 are in bone matrix, and type I is the major constituent (1). Many special bone proteins compose only 10% of the bone matrix, including osteocalcin, osteonectin, alkaline phosphatase, fibronectin, thrombospondin, proteoglycans, sialoproteins, bone acidic glycoprotein, and growth factors.

Osteocalcin, a small protein in osteoblasts, osteocytes, and matrix represents only 1% of noncollagen protein (2), but it leaks into plasma and urine and is a valuable indicator of osteoblastic activity. Osteocalcin radioimmunoassay urinary levels are high in hyperparathyroidism and Paget's disease and low in idiopathic or alcoholic osteoporosis and neoplastic hypercalcemia. The levels are high in the flare phenomenon of skeletal metastases usually from breast or prostate carcinoma, but they are not elevated with metastatic progression (3).

Bone has a great regenerating capacity for healing breaks and gaps by repeating the developmental process of embryonic skeletal formation. Various autologous cells that are transplanted into living connective tissue induce ectopic bone formation. Likewise, extracts of demineralized bone reduce ectopic bone by migrating mesenchymal cells, transforming first into chondrocytes and chondroblasts and later into osteoblasts and osteoclasts (4).

Purified bone extracts may contain as many as 7 osteogenic proteins, and at least 3 produce ectopic bone in experimental animals. Osteogenic protein is variously known as bone morphogenetic protein, osteogenin, and osteoinductive factor. Recombinant osteogenic protein-1 is available and has successfully filled in large segmental bone defects in animals (5).

Adult human bone cells were first cultured in 1979 for metabolic experiments. In 1992, cultured human osteoblasts successfully seeded demineralized human bank bone (6). It is likely that the combination of osteoconductive materials (inert titanium, calcium phosphate, ceramics, coral, and other graft substitutes), osteogenic proteins, and cultured autologous osteoblasts (osteoinductive) will be widely used in orthopedics to replace large segments of bone electively (7).

As the population ages, the prevalence of osteoporosis and secondary fractures undoubtedly will increase. Diphosphonate imaging probably will be used to assess the viability of these biogenic grafts in a manner similar to our current studies of autologous grafts.

John G. McAfee, M.D.

References

1. Robey PG: The biochemistry of bone. *Endocrinol Metab Clin North Am* 18:859–902, 1989.
2. Triffit JT: Editorial Review: The special proteins of bone tissue. *Clin Sci* 72:399–408, 1987.
3. Coleman RE, Mashiter G, Whitaker KB, et al: Bone scan flare predicts successful therapy for bone metastases. *J Nucl Med* 29:1354–1359, 1988.
4. Wozney JM, Rosen V, Celeste AJ, et al: Novel regulators of bone formation: Molecular clones and activities. *Science* 242:1528–1534, 1988.
5. Cook SD, Baffes GC, Wolfe MW, et al: The effect of recombinant human osteogenic protein-1 on healing of large segmental bone defects. *J Bone Joint Surg (Br)* 74-B:284–286, 1992.
6. Nolan PC, Nicholas RM, Mulholland BJ, et al: Culture of human osteoblasts on demineralized bone: a possible means of graft enhancement. *J Bone Joint Surg (Br)* 74-B:284–286, 1992.
7. Nolan PC, Hankey DP, Mollan RAB, et al: Large bony defects: Can bone cell culture fill the gap? *Cell Transplant* 3:351–353, 1994.

Osteomyelitis of the Pelvis

Rand N, Mosheiff R, Matan Y, Porat S, Shapiro M, Liebergall M (Hadassah-Hebrew Univ Med Centre, Jerusalem)
J Bone Joint Surg (Br) 75B:731–733, 1993   124-95-4-1

Background.—Osteomyelitis of the pelvis is rare and difficult to diagnose. Classification systems have been based on the anatomical location of the symptoms and physical signs: hip joint syndrome, abdominal syndrome, buttock syndrome, and sciatic or lumbar disk syndrome. The location of the symptoms and signs may depend on the direction in which pus drains from the infected bone.

Series.—All patients, 3 males and 1 female, aged 14 to 27 years, had delayed diagnosis. The symptoms in the 4 patients were low-grade fever and hip joint syndrome; intermittent fever with buttock and hip joint syndrome; high fever, right lower quadrant abdominal pain, and hip joint syndrome; and intermittent fever and buttock syndrome, respectively. White blood cell counts ranged from 7,000 to 15,000 per mm³, and the erythrocyte sedimentation rate ranged from 15 to 140 mm/hr. Three patients had technetium-99m bone scanning. In 2, the results were normal, and in 1, increased uptake was noted. A CT scan demonstrated a lytic lesion in all cases. In 1, collections were observed on both sides of the iliac crest, and in another, collections were seen in the hip and buttock. All patients recovered after extensive surgical drainage and antibiotic therapy.

Conclusion.—Pelvic osteomyelitis is a diagnostic challenge, because of its rarity and clinical signs that mimic other diseases. Its estimated incidence ranges from 2% to 11% among all patients with bone infections. The iliac bone is most commonly affected, perhaps because it is the largest pelvic bone with the richest blood supply. Possible causes include mild trauma and urinary tract infection; Crohn's disease is also associated with it. Bone scanning results can be false negative.

▶ These 4 patients were young, and in 3 the offending organisms were co-agulase-positive staphylococci. This article shows again that purely osteolytic lesions often are missed on planar bone scans. Perhaps a gallium or labeled leukocyte scan might have helped to make the diagnosis earlier, but they were not mentioned. The authors refer to a previous paper by Young (1) in which Young notes that "Trunkal osteomyelitis is always a clinical challenge. The pelvic and vertebral bones are deeply placed and their movements are minimal, so that the usual signs of bone infection (tenderness, limitation of motion) are missing."—J.G. McAfee, M.D.

Reference

1. Young F: *Surg Gynecol Obstet* 58:986, 1934.

Pubic Osteomyelitis Caused by *Staphylococcus simulans*
Sturgess I, Martin FC, Eykyn S (St Thomas' Hosp, London)
Postgrad Med J 69:927–929, 1993   124-95-4–2

Background.—Hospital-acquired infections with coagulase-negative staphylococci are becoming more common, especially with the use of intravenous devices. A case of *Staphylococcus simulans*, an unusual species, was examined.

Case Report.—Woman, 77, sought medical help for a profound right hemiparesis and dense dysphagia from a left cerebral infarction. Previously, she had been active and independent. Her history included noninsulin-dependent diabetes mellitus for 14 years, which was controlled by diet and tolbutamide. She also had had psoriasis since childhood. Six months after she was seen, she had pain in the right groin. No abnormalities were found on plain radiographs or isotope bone scan. A month later, her functional ability was found to be deteriorating. A tender pubic symphysis was found, and pubic osteomyelitis was diagnosed. Blood cultures grew *S. simulans* that were fully sensitive to all antistaphylococcal antibiotics. Initially, the pubic symphysis was normal radiologically but within a week rarefaction was detected. A diphosphonate bone scan then showed a localized hot spot. Antibiotic therapy was stopped after 25 days of treatment. However, her pain recurred 3 days later, and flucloxacillin and fusidic acid were administered for another 31 days.

Conclusion.—In this patient, positive blood cultures, an increased serum C-reactive protein, and the clinical picture were virtually diagnostic of pubic osteomyelitis. This condition has been reported in previously healthy children and intravenous drug abusers. In elderly individuals, it usually follows genitourinary procedures; gram-negative organisms predominate in such patients.

▶ This is another type of pelvic osteomyelitis. The infection usually spreads across the symphysis to the other side. Because the pubic bones are superficial, tenderness is usually elicited early on palpation and confirmed on bone scans and radiographs.—J.G. McAfee, M.D.

Histologically Proven Pressure Sore-Related Osteomyelitis in the Setting of Negative Technetium Bone Scans: Case Report
Burdge DR, Gribble MJ (Univ of British Columbia, Vancouver, Canada)
Am J Phys Med Rehabil 72:386–389, 1993   124-95-4–3

Background.—Pressure sores often develop in patients with spinal cord injury, stroke, or debilitating medical diseases. Contiguous osteomyelitis, a well-documented complication of pressure ulcers, is difficult to diagnose and treat. Technetium bone scanning has been found to be a very sensitive but nonspecific diagnostic test for osteomyelitis. Negative bone scans are believed to virtually exclude bone infection.

Series.—Three paraplegic men, aged 19 to 51 years, were evaluated for pressure ulcers. Technetium bone scanning showed no abnormality in all men; however, bone biopsy demonstrated the characteristic histopathologic changes of osteomyelitis. Pressure sore–related polymicrobial osteomyelitis was diagnosed.

Conclusion.—In patients with pressure ulcers for whom the level of clinical suspicion for osteomyelitis is high, a bone biopsy should be routine. Bone biopsy is the standard of reference for diagnosis of osteomyelitis, which can be present even when bone scanning results are normal.

▶ These authors review the varied results of bone scanning in pressure-sore osteomyelitis of the ischial tuberosities in paraplegic or bedridden patients. The sensitivity of detection is different from that of the common type of hematogenous osteomyelitis in viable bone.

In other reports that include less advanced lesions, bone scans are usually positive, although the specificity is poor. However, in the advanced lesions described in this study, the bone was exposed, necrotic, fragmented, and eroded. Such lesions that do not have a blood supply are better evaluated by radiography and CT. Even needle biopsy can miss the sites of osteomyelitis; sometimes, open surgical biopsy is required to make the diagnosis.—J.G. McAfee, M.D.

The Computer-Generated Bone Marrow Subtraction Image: A Valuable Adjunct to Combined In-111 WBC/Tc-99m in Sulfur Colloid Scintigraphy for Musculoskeletal Infection

Achong DM, Oates E (Tufts Univ, Boston)
Clin Nucl Med 19:188–193, 1994   124-95-4-4

Background. Osseous and soft tissue infection can be accurately diagnosed by indium-111–labeled white blood cell (WBC) scintigraphy. These images can be compared visually with concurrent technetium-99m sulfur colloid (SC) bone marrow (BM) images to distinguish physiologic BM variations in distribution from pathologic WBC accumulation in the assessment of the central, marrow-containing skeleton. The value of the computer-generated BM subtraction image in identifying and localizing infection was compared with that of standard visual evaluation of combined WBC/SC images.

Methods and Findings.—Thirty-one patients underwent combined WBC/SC with BM subtraction imaging. Infection was found in 21 of 36 possible sites. Two sites that were not noted on visual inspection were identified on BM subtraction images. Bone marrow subtraction had a

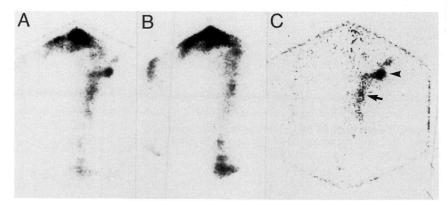

Fig 4–1.—A, interior WBC image demonstrates patchy uptake throughout the left femur with an intense focus of activity in the lateral thigh. **B,** modified sequential SC BM and (**C**) subtraction images identify both soft tissue sinus tract (*arrowhead*) and osseous (*arrow*) infections. Distal femoral WBC uptake corresponds to normal BM. (Courtesy of Achong DM, Oates E: *Clin Nucl Med* 19:188–193, 1994.)

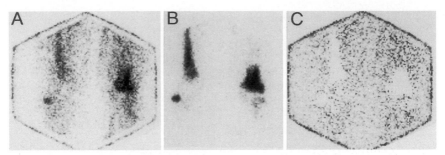

Fig 4–2.—A, anterior view of the knees demonstrates discrete, asymmetric WBC accumulation in the distal left femur. **B,** simple sequential BM image shows SC uptake in the same distribution as labeled WBCs. **C,** subtraction image confirms that WBC accumulation corresponds exactly to normal BM. (Courtesy of Achong DM, Oates E: *Clin Nucl Med* 19:188–193, 1994.)

sensitivity of 95%, a specificity of 93%, and an accuracy of 94%. For visual assessment of WBC and SC images, these values were 86%, 93%, and 89%, respectively (Figs 4–1 and 4–2).

Conclusion.—Computer-assisted BM subtraction imaging is a useful adjunct to combined WBC/SC scintigraphy, improving its overall sensitivity and accuracy. It increased the certainty of the diagnosis in this study.

▶ The use of marrow imaging that was complementary to labeled leukocyte imaging was first proposed by King and associates (1) and was confirmed by Palestro and colleagues for infected prostheses (2). The subtraction technique appears to be a worthwhile refinement for distinguishing osteomyelitis from irregularities in distribution of hematopoietic marrow. It can be particularly helpful when infection is suspected as a complication of preexisting abnormalities, such as osteoarthritis, compound fractures, postsurgical procedures, or prostheses.—J.G. McAfee, M.D.

References

1. King AD, et al: *Eur J Nucl Med* 17:148, 1990.
2. Palestro CJ, et al: *Radiology* 179:645, 1991.

Imaging Features of Musculoskeletal Brucellosis
Al-Shahed MS, Sharif HS, Haddad MC, Aabed MY, Sammak BM, Mutairi MA (Riyadh Armed Forces Hosp, Saudi Arabia)
RadioGraphics 14:333–348, 1994   124-95-4–5

Background.—Brucellosis, a zoonosis of worldwide distribution, is endemic in some areas. Its most common complication is musculoskeletal involvement; usually the spine is affected. The imaging features of musculoskeletal brucellosis were examined.

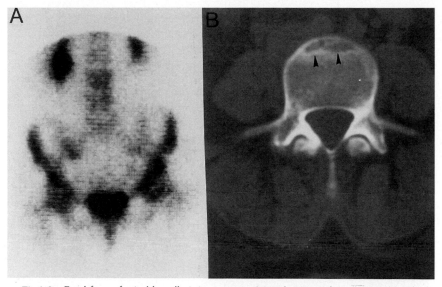

Fig 4–3.—Focal form of spinal brucellosis in a woman, 26, with systemic brucellosis and low back pain. **A,** scintigram shows focal increased uptake in the bodies of L3 and L4 and the right sacroiliac joint. This was seen only on the anterior view. The plain radiographic findings were normal. **B,** axial CT image obtained at the level of the superior end plate of L4 shows erosion (*arrowheads*) and normal paraspinal soft tissue. (Courtesy of Al-Shahed MS, Sharif HS, Haddad MC, et al: *Radiographics* 14:333–348, 1994.)

Methods and Findings.—Three hundred thirty-four patients with radiologically proved musculoskeletal brucellosis were seen between 1985 and 1993. Spinal involvement was focal or diffuse and had a predilection for the lumbar region. Hallmarks of the focal form included erosions and sclerosis in vertebral end-plates anteriorly, focal changes of inflammation by scintigraphy or MRI, and intact disks (Fig 4-3). Diffuse brucellar spondylitis was characterized by osteomyelitis of neighboring vertebrae, involvement of the intervening disk, and moderate epidural extension (Fig 4-4). Most joints with scintigraphic signs of disease were normal on radiography. The sacroiliac and knee joints are most often involved. Only a few patients had evidence of osteomyelitis, destructive arthritis (Fig 4-5), or myositis.

Conclusion.—Radiologic evidence of brucellosis can be seen in 68.8% of symptomatic sites. Bone scintigraphy is a sensitive screening method. Plain radiographs effectively demonstrate focal lesions, and MRI is best for assessment and follow-up of the diffuse form.

▶ In Saudi Arabia, brucellosis is common because the consumption of raw milk is popular. The disease also is common in South America, Spain, and Italy. This article describes the disease in detail and defines the relative roles of scintigraphy, CT, and MRI in musculoskeletal involvement.—J.G. McAfee, M.D.

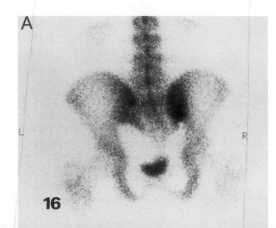

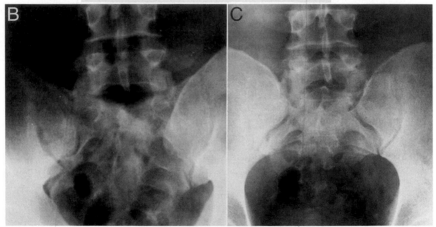

Fig 4–4.—Brucellar arthritis in a man, 25, with brucellosis and pain in the right sacroiliac joint. **A,** posterior scintigram shows increased uptake in the right sacroiliac joint. Increased uptake was also clearly seen on the anterior view (not shown). **B,** plain radiograph shows minimal widening of the sacroiliac joint with small erosions. **C,** radiograph obtained 6 months later shows narrowing of the right sacroiliac joint and minimal bone sclerosis. (Courtesy of Al-Shahed MS, Sharif HS, Haddad MC, et al: *Radiographics* 14:333–348, 1994.)

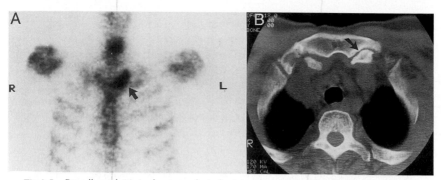

Fig 4–5.—Brucellar arthritis in the sternoclavicular joint in a man, 55, with systemic brucellosis and pain in that joint. **A,** scintigram shows a marked increased uptake in the lower cervical spine and the left sternoclavicular joint (*arrow*). **B,** axial CT image obtained at the level of the sternoclavicular joint shows marked cartilage loss and subarticular erosion in the joint (*arrow*). (Courtesy of Al-Shahed MS, Sharif HS, Haddad MC, et al: *Radiographics* 14:333–348, 1994.)

Multifocal Osteoarticular Tuberculosis: Report of Four Cases and Review of Management

Muradali D, Gold WL, Vellend H, Becker E (Toronto Hosp; Univ of Toronto)
Clin Infect Dis 17:204–209, 1993   124-95-4–6

Purpose.—In multifocal osteoarticular tuberculosis, there are at least 2 simultaneous, noncontiguous bone or joint lesions caused by *Mycobacterium tuberculosis.* This condition is often unrecognized in areas that are not endemic for tuberculosis, so diagnosis is delayed. Four cases of multifocal tuberculous osteomyelitis were reviewed.

Patients.—The patients were 3 women and 1 man, 16 to 38 years of age; all were immigrants to Canada, 2 from the Philippines and 2 from Africa. The patients were seen between 1985 and 1992. The condition involved local bone pain in all cases; 2 patients had a history of fever and 1 was seen with a draining sinus. The clinical and radiographic findings led to a presumptive diagnosis of malignancy in all cases (Fig 4–6). None of the patients showed any signs of pulmonary involvement. Histopathologic findings that were consistent with tuberculous osteomyelitis led to initiation of antituberculous chemotherapy in 2 patients; in the other 2, treatment did not begin until the culture results were obtained. Antibiotic therapy succeeded in 3 patients, and the fourth also required emergency anterior spinal decompression. Further skeletal lesions developed after the course of antibiotics in 2 patients.

Conclusion.—This experience illustrates the need to consider multifocal osteoarticular tuberculosis in patients from endemic areas who have multiple destructive osseous lesions. Pulmonary involvement need not be present, and involvement is not limited to the axial skeleton. The clinical

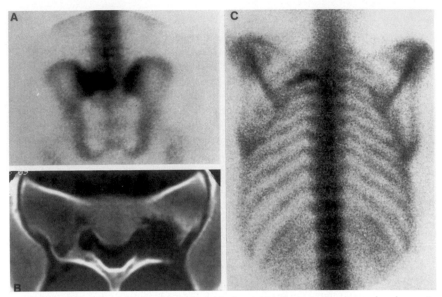

Fig 4–6.—Images obtained in a man, 26, who had an initial diagnosis of malignant lymphoma. **A,** bone scan of the pelvis shows increased activity in the area of the left sacroiliac joint. **B,** CT scan of the pelvis shows a destructive lesion of the left sacral ala. **C,** bone scan (posterior view) shows increased activity at the left third rib. (Courtesy of Muradali D, Gold WL, Vellend H, et al: *Clin Infect Dis* 17:204–209, 1993.)

and radiographic signs may be indistinguishable from those of malignancy.

▶ This article provides us with a stern reminder that tuberculosis and other granulomatous diseases can mimic multifocal malignancies on different imaging modalities, including bone scans. Missed diagnoses are serious, because most of the lesions respond to antituberculous antibiotics.—J.G. McAfee, M.D.

Multiple Atypical Bone Involvement in Sarcoidosis
Mañá J, Segarra MI, Casas R, Mairal L, Fernández-Nogués F (Univ of Barcelona)
J Rheumatol 20:394–396, 1993   124-95-4-7

Background.—Accurate differential diagnosis of atypical locations of bone sarcoidosis is required to distinguish neoplastic, infectious, metabolic, or granulomatous diseases. A case of sarcoidosis involved multiple osteolytic skull lesions and other atypical bone involvement.

Case Report.—Woman, 54, evaluated for nonspecific thoracic pain, was referred because a chest radiograph showed right paratracheal and left hilar lymph

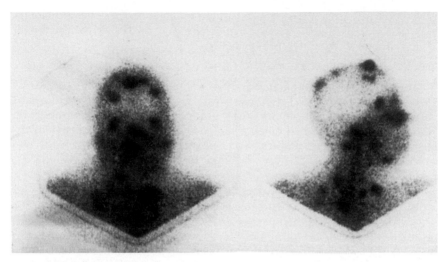

Fig 4–7.—Gallium scan showing multiple uptakes in skull, right mandibular bone, both parotid glands, and cervical and supraclavicular lymph nodes. (Courtesy of Maña J, Segarra MI, Casas R, et al: *J Rheumatol* 20:394–396, 1993.)

nodes. A gallium scan showed increased uptake at these locations and in the apex of the right lung. Thoracic CT revealed hilar and mediastinal lymph node enlargement. Results of the physical examination, tuberculin skin test, and respiratory function tests were normal. The serum level of angiotensin-converting enzyme was also normal. The lesions were not visible at a 5-month follow-up. Eight months after first seen, she returned with multiple nodules at the scalp and bilateral cervical and supraclavicular lymph nodes. A skull radiograph revealed multiple osteolytic lesions. A gallium scan showed multiple foci of increased uptake in the skull, the right side of the mandible, both parotid glands, and cervical and supraclavicular lymph nodes (Fig 4–7). A technetium-99m diphosphonate bone scan revealed hot spots in her skull, right mandibular bone, and right clavicle (Fig 4–8). Radiographs of the right clavicle and jaw confirmed the presence of osteolytic lesions. A CT scan demonstrated multiple skull lesions with normal brain parenchyma. The scalp nodules were contiguous with the skull lesions. Biopsies

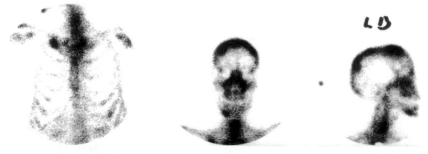

Fig 4–8.—Radionuclide bone scan revealing hot spots in skull, right mandibular bone, and right clavicle. (Courtesy of Maña J, Segarra MI, Casas R, et al: *J Rheumatol* 20:394–396, 1993.)

of the skull and cervical lymph node showed multiple noncaseating granulomas that stained and cultured negative for fungus and mycobacteria. The lymph nodes responded to prednisone, 40 mg/day, and maintenance doses of 20 mg/day were required for long-term control.

Discussion.—The frequency of bone involvement in sarcoidosis is probably underestimated, because most lesions are asymptomatic and most sarcoidosis patients do not undergo bone scintigraphy. The breadth of the differential diagnosis of osteolytic lesions mandates histologic confirmation of atypical bone involvement in patients with sarcoidosis.

▶ Radiologic evidence of bone involvement in sarcoidosis varies from 1% to 13% in different series. In the largest series of 425 cases in Spain (1), the incidence of bone involvement was 2%. Osteolysis of the fingers or toes is the most common manifestation. The lesions can be lytic or sclerotic, and they can be easily missed, because they usually are asymptomatic. Diphosphonate imaging demonstrates more lesions than either radiography or gallium imaging. Involvement of the skull and mandible is rare.—J.G. McAfee, M.D.

Reference

1. Badrinas F, et al: *Med Clin (Barc)* 93:81, 1989.

Sarcoidosis Involving Skeletal Muscle: Imaging Findings and Relative Value of Imaging Procedures
Otake S (Nagoya City Univ, Japan)
AJR 162:369–375, 1994   124-95-4-8

Introduction.—Muscular sarcoidosis is a rare condition that was first reported in 1908. Two clinical types of the disorder have been defined: nodular and myopathic. The imaging features of both types were presented, and the ability of various imaging procedures in assessment of muscular sarcoidosis was compared.

Patients and Methods.—Twenty-eight patients, including 20 with the nodular type of muscular sarcoidosis and 8 with the myopathic type, comprised the study group. All but 1 of the patients were women; their mean age was 56 years. The results of MRI were available in all cases. Also, 17 patients with the nodular type and 6 with the myopathic type underwent gallium-67 (^{67}Ga) scintigraphy. Sonography was performed in 6 patients with nodular muscular sarcoidosis; 2 in this group who were thought to have malignant tumors underwent angiography.

Results.—Patients with the nodular type of muscular sarcoidosis had lesions that were long and extended along muscle fibers (Fig 4-9). A star-shaped central structure of decreased signal intensity was demon-

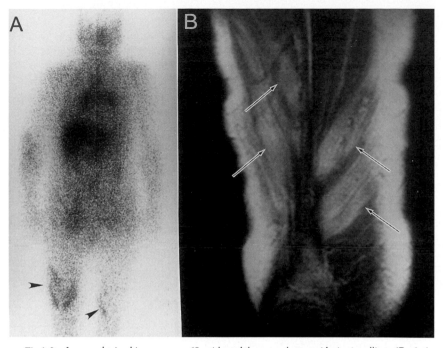

Fig 4–9.—Images obtained in a woman, 68, with nodular muscular sarcoidosis. **A,** gallium-67 scintigram shows multiple areas of increased uptake of radionuclide in both thighs (*arrowheads*) and in inguinal lymph nodes on both sides. **B,** proton density-weighted coronal MRI (repetition time, 1,800 ms; echo time, 50 ms) of the right thigh shows multiple nodules (*arrows*) corresponding to areas of increased radionuclide uptake seen on the ⁶⁷Ga scintigram. (Courtesy of Otake S: AJR 162:369-375, 1994.)

strated on axial MR images. Coronal and sagittal images revealed 3 stripes; the outer ones were of increased signal intensity, and an inner stripe had decreased signal intensity. Using gadopentetate dimeglumine, the peripheral area of the nodular lesions was enhanced. Sonograms demonstrated the central structure to be hyperechoic, whereas the peripheral area was hypoechoic relative to surrounding tissue. In patients with nodular involvement, CT and angiography were of less diagnostic value. Myopathic involvement was visualized only with ⁶⁷Ga scintigraphy (Fig 4-10); no abnormalities were apparent on MR images. The scintigrams showed diffuse increased uptake of radionuclide in 3 of 6 patients.

Conclusion.—Muscular sarcoidosis, like general sarcoidosis, affects women more often than men. Magnetic resonance imaging yields fairly specific findings in patients with the nodular type, and it is the preferred diagnostic method. Scintigraphy with ⁶⁷Ga is useful for screening the whole body and was the only imaging method that allowed identification

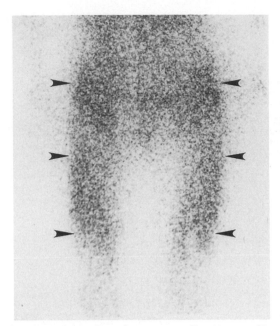

Fig 4–10.—Gallium-67 scintigram obtained in a woman, 53, with myopathic sarcoidosis. Diffuse increased uptake is seen in the thighs (*bottom 4 arrowheads*) and buttocks (*upper 2 arrowheads*). (Courtesy of Otake S: AJR 162:369-375, 1994.)

of myopathic sarcoidosis. Patients with myopathic sarcoidosis had no abnormalities on MRI.

▶ Involvement of skeletal muscle in sarcoidosis has been considered unusual, but it was present in 6% of patients in this series. Have we been missing this by neglecting to obtain gallium images of the buttocks and thighs in women, the most common sites of involvement?

In the nodular type, gallium images show increased uptake in stripes that correspond to the direction of muscle fibers; they are similar to the long nodules described on MR coronal images. The diffuse gallium activity seen in the myopathic type in 3 of 6 patients was not demonstrated by other imaging modalities.—J.G. McAfee, M.D.

Detection of Hypervascular Brown Tumors on Three-Phase Bone Scan

Jordan KG, Telepak RJ, Spaeth J (Univ of New Mexico, Albuquerque)
J Nucl Med 34:2188–2190, 1993   124-95-4–9

Background.—Although they are generally associated with primary hyperparathyroidism, brown tumors can occur with renal osteodystrophy. The manifestations of brown tumors vary on bone scans and plain radio-

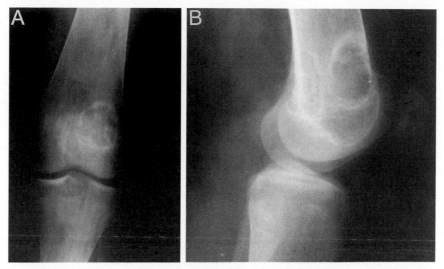

Fig 4–11.—Anteroposterior and lateral views of left knee. Lytic metaphyseal lesion with narrow zone of transition. (Courtesy of Jordan KG, Telepak RJ, Spaeth J: *J Nucl Med* 34:2188–2190, 1993.)

graphs. Detection of a hypervascular brown tumor on a 3-phase bone scan was reported.

Case Report.—Woman, 20, with a history of renal transplantation at age 11 years, underwent a 3-phase technetium-99m methyldiphosphonate (^{99m}Tc-MDP) bone scan after detection of several new lytic lesions in the left acetabulum and right femoral neck. She had a history of avascular necrosis of the left hip secondary to chronic steroid usage. Now, she was experiencing both chronic transplant rejection and hyperparathyroidism with a normal serum level of calcium and an elevated level of parathyroid hormone, 1,440 pg/mL. Plain pelvic, knee, and chest radiographs revealed multiple lucent lesions with sclerotic borders (Fig 4–11). The blood-pool phase of ^{99m}Tc-MDP imaging revealed a focal area of significantly increased activity in the distal left femur, consistent with the location of the lesion on the plain radiograph (Fig 4–12). The flow phase revealed increased activity with an intensity equal to that of the femoral artery. Immediate and delayed images revealed increased activity in the distal left femur and left acetabulum; delayed images also demonstrated increased activity in the right femoral neck, right scapula, and multiple ribs bilaterally. An open biopsy specimen of the left acetabular lesion revealed thinned cortex of the superior pubic ramus and ilium. A dark pink, slightly hemorrhagic tumor was resected. Microscopic examination revealed areas of fibroblasts and histiocytes with scattered clusters of giant cells that were consistent with brown tumor.

Conclusion.—This case demonstrates a significantly increased accumulation of ^{99m}Tc-MDP on all 3 bone scan phases in a biopsy-proved multiple brown tumor associated with secondary hyperparathyroidism. In the correct clinical setting, brown tumors should be included in the

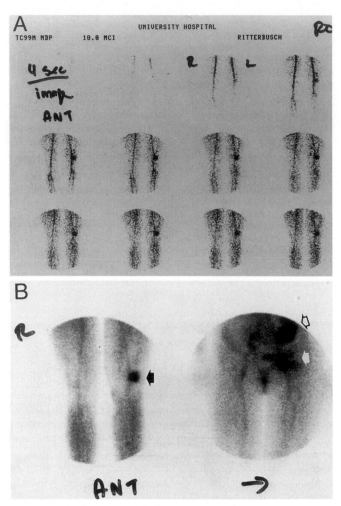

Fig 4–12.—A, ⁹⁹ᵐTc-MDP flow study of the lower extremities. Anterior images demonstrated markedly increased flow to distal left femoral lesion. **B,** ⁹⁹ᵐTc-MDP immediate-phase images. Increased activity in left femoral lesion (*black arrow*), left hip (*white arrow*), and left pelvic transplant (*arrowhead*). (Courtesy of Jordan KG, Telepak RJ, Spaeth J: *J Nucl Med* 34:2188–2190, 1993.)

differential diagnosis for focal accumulation of ⁹⁹ᵐTc-MDP on bone scans.

▶ Multiple brown tumors resulting from primary or secondary hyperparathyroidism are rarely seen these days, because the diagnosis is made biochemically at earlier stages of the disease, before more advanced skeletal lesions appear. However, multiple lesions can mimic skeletal metastases, a potentially serious mistake, because both conditions produce hypercalcemia.—J.G. McAfee, M.D.

Tibial Insufficiency Fractures in Adult Renal Transplant Recipients
Larcos G, Gruenewald SM (Westmead Hosp, NSW, Australia)
Clin Nucl Med 19:212–214, 1994   124-95-4-10

Background.—The skeletal complications of osteonecrosis and osteopenia can be seen in renal transplant recipients. Fractures often occur in such cases, usually in the femora, pelvis, or vertebrae. Two sedentary adult allograft recipients with leg pain had bone scintigraphy, serial radi-

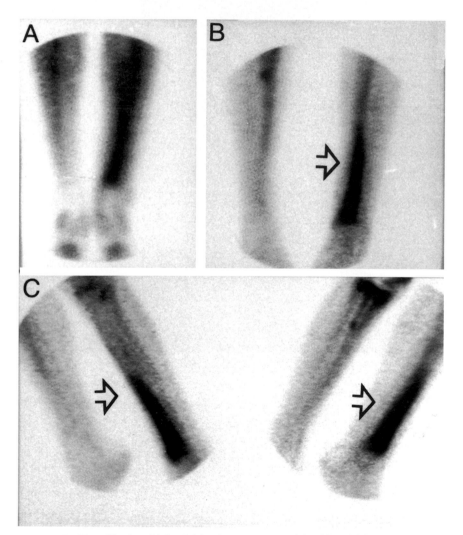

Fig 4–13.—Planar blood pool (**A**) and delayed static in anterior (**B**) and lateral (**C**) projections show an hyperemic longitudinal area of radiopharmaceutical uptake involving the anterior aspect of the tibial shaft (*arrow*). (Courtesy of Larcos G, Gruenewald SM: *Clin Nucl Med* 19:212-214, 1994.)

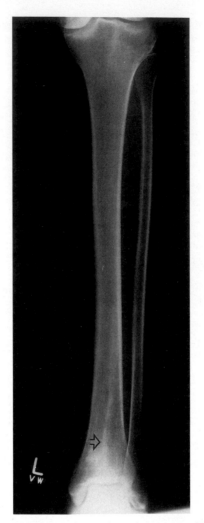

Fig 4–14.—Plain radiograph confirming fracture (*arrow*). (Courtesy of Larcos G, Gruenewald SM: *Clin Nucl Med* 19:212-214, 1994.)

ographs, and clinical findings that suggested insufficiency fractures of the tibiae.

Case Report.—Woman, 52, had discomfort over the anterior aspect of the left tibia 6 years after a second allograft kidney transplantation. She had experienced avascular necrosis of the medial plateau of the right tibia 5 years after the first allograft and underwent arthroplasty at that time. Bone scintigraphy revealed moderately increased radiopharmaceutical uptake of the anterior aspect of the left tibia longitudinally. This was associated with hyperemia on the blood pool images (Fig 4–13). Plain radiography revealed a linear area of sclerosis in the same place as the scintigraphic abnormality, which was consistent with a fracture (Fig 4–14).

Conclusion.—Adult renal transplant recipients may sustain insufficiency fractures in unusual locations. Although they are uncommon, these fractures should be considered in the differential diagnosis of renal allograft recipients with leg pain.

▶ Renal osteodystrophy, long-term dialysis, prolonged steroid therapy, and β_2-microglobulin–induced amyloidosis frequently result in the complications of osteonecrosis and/or fractures. As many as 44% of renal transplant patients have radiologic bone changes.

In 1 series of 225 transplant patients (1), aseptic necrosis involved the hips in 25%, the knees in 5%, the humeral heads in 3%, and other sites in 1%. Fractures may occur in as many as 26% of patients (2). The common sites are the ribs, ischiopubic rami, femoral neck, vertebrae metatarsals, and rarely in the tibiae.—J.G. McAfee, M.D.

References

1. Griffiths HJ, et al: *Radiology* 113:621, 1974.
2. Elmstedt E, Suahn T: *Acta Orthop Scand* 52:279, 1981.

Increased Skeletal Uptake of Tc-99m Methylene Diphosphonate in Milk-Alkali Syndrome

Campbell SB, MacFarlane DJ, Fleming SJ, Khafagi FA (Royal Brisbane Hosp, Australia)
Clin Nucl Med 19:207–211, 1994 124-95-4-11

Background.—Milk-alkali syndrome is characterized by hypercalcemia, alkalosis, and renal impairment associated with ingestion of large amounts of calcium and absorbable alkali by persons with dyspeptic symptoms. Currently, technetium-99m methylene diphosphonate (MDP) bone scanning is often used to assess hypercalcemia with a low parathyroid hormone (PTH) level, but the appearance of the technetium-99m MDP scan in patients with milk alkali syndrome has not been well described.

Case Report.—Man, 54, who was taking an over-the-counter antacid preparation for gastroesophageal reflux, sought medical attention for a 3-week history of back pain, increased thirst, polyuria, nausea, vomiting, and pruritis. A technetium-99m MDP bone scan, obtained in the initial assessment of the hypercalcemia, was markedly abnormal. The metabolic pattern of tracer uptake observed was similar to that seen in hyperparathyroidism and humoral hypercalcemia. However, the diffusely increased uptake involved the calvaria and long bones, whereas the axial skeletal appeared relatively normal. No focal lesions were present to suggest metastases, brown tumors, or Looser zones. About 5 months after the antacid and excessive calcium intake were stopped and the patient was well hydrated, the bone images appeared almost normal, and the biochemical markers were normal.

Conclusion.—The technetium-99m MDP bone scan done in the initial assessment of hypercalcemia revealed a "metabolic" pattern of tracer uptake similar to but not identical to that in patients with hyperparathyroidism and humoral hypercalcemia. The bone scan appearance returned to normal after the antacid and calcium were withdrawn.

▶ This syndrome will probably become rare, because a variety of drugs are so effective in managing peptic ulcer, including the H_2-receptor antagonists (e.g., cimetidine, famotidine, and ranitidine), the proton pump inhibitor omeprazole, sucralfate, nonabsorbable antacid bismuth subsalicylate (PeptoBismol), and antibacterials against *Helicobacter pylori*, such as metronidazole, tetracycline, or amoxicillin.

However, the syndrome tends to occur in self-medicating patients who take absorbable antacids and have a high-calcium diet. The parathormone levels may be high, as in hyperparathyroidism, or they may be low. A careful history should avoid confusion of the syndrome with hyperparathyroidism and other metabolic bone diseases.—J.G. McAfee, M.D.

Osteomalacia in a Patient With Anorexia Nervosa
Verbruggen LA, Bruyland M, Shahabpour M (Vrije Universiteit Brussel, Brussels, Belgium)
J Rheumatol 20:512–517, 1993   124-95-4–12

Objective.—Anorexia nervosa is a common condition in young women. It can result in amenorrhea. Osteoporosis is another well-recognized complication. A woman with anorexia nervosa and fractures had a combination of osteoporosis and osteomalacia.

Case Report.—Woman, 32, with a history of anorexia nervosa since adolescence, was hospitalized with progressive diffuse skeletal pain, weakness, and gait disturbance. She had denied any somatic illness previously and refused treatment; she had been amenorrheic for several years. Her bone pain had increased during the 2 previous winters. She reported a particular aversion to dairy products and dietary fat. She had a low normal serum calcium level and very low calciuria. The bone fraction of alkaline phosphatase was markedly elevated, and she had severely low vitamin D and B_{12} levels. She had recently sustained a spontaneous fracture of her right clavicle. Radiographs showed severe generalized osteopenia, and diphosphonate images showed bilateral juxta-articular increased uptake of many joints, sternum, multiple ribs, and symphysis pubis, as observed in osteomalacic metabolic bone disease. Increased foci were seen at the right clavicular fracture (Looser lines, etc.). Imaging studies showed Looser lines and

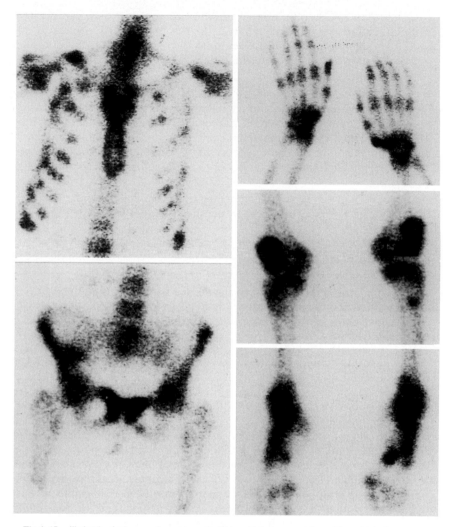

Fig 4–15.—Skeletal scintigrams show generally high radioisotope uptake, with multiple hyperactive regions in the ribs, the right clavicula, the wrists, several hand articulations, and the distal phalanx of the left thumb, the right iliac bone, bilaterally around the symphysis pubis, the knees, the proximal part of the left fibula, the ankles, and first metatarsal. (Courtesy of Verbruggen LA, Bruyland M, Shahabpour M: *J Rheumatol* 20:512-517, 1993.)

pseudofractures in a finger, fibula, and malleolus. Magnetic resonance imaging of the knee demonstrated evidence of a femoral pseudofracture, along with medullary changes (Fig 4-15). The lumbar bone mineral content was very low, and there were further signs of secondary hyperparathyroidism. The patient left the hospital before investigations were completed, refused therapy, and died at home the next year.

Conclusion.—Osteomalacia, in addition to osteoporosis, can occur as a complication of anorexia nervosa. In this patient, osteomalacia and secondary hypoparathyroidism seem to have resulted from complete avoidance of milk products, along with a low-fat and low-protein diet.

▶ The prevalence of anorexia nervosa is increasing, especially in young women from adolescence to approximately 25 years of age. Osteoporosis is a well-known complication, but superimposed osteomalacia is uncommon. The latter should be recognized biochemically and by multiple foci of increased uptake on bone scans, because osteoporosis does not ordinarily produce imaging abnormalities in the absence of fractures.—J.G. McAfee, M.D.

Intraosseous Fat Necrosis and Infarction Associated With Pancreatitis
Bayo F III, Massie JD, Sebes J (Univ of Tennessee, Memphis)
Clin Nucl Med 18:837–839, 1993   124-95-4–13

Introduction.—Pancreatitis can have serious sequelae, including lipase embolization and eventual multiple lytic bone lesions. Although this syndrome has been observed clinically, it is rare and therefore is often belatedly diagnosed.

Case Report.—Black man, 19, was hospitalized with progressive bilateral lytic cortical lesions of the fibula and tibia. Six months earlier, he had sustained an abdominal gunshot injury and pancreatitis. He was rehospitalized 1 month later with painful, swollen knees and ankles. Radiographs showed cortical lytic lesions of the tibia and fibula. A 3-phase technetium-99m methylene diphosphonate bone scan showed several pockets of increased activity distributed linearly and symmetrically along the tibias on both the arterial and blood pool images (Fig 4–16). The same distribution of linear uptake appeared on a gallium-67 citrate scan. The findings from ultrasound, CT, and an upper gastrointestinal series were consistent with pancreatitis. One month later, plain radiographs revealed that the lytic cortical lesions had progressed. After a nondiagnostic bone biopsy and a segmental osteotomy, bone infarction and fat necrosis of the tibia were the final pathologic diagnosis.

Discussion.—Intraosseous fat necrosis and infarction are relatively rare sequelae of both acute and chronic pancreatitis. Subcutaneous fat necrosis, arthritis, pleuritis, or pericarditis plus pancreatitis can indicate this syndrome. Clinically, the bone and joint symptoms dominate the lesser abdominal ones. Radiographs show lytic cortical lesions of the long bones, which appear similar to metastasis. Triple-phase bone scan findings indicate high bone turnover and periarticular activity consistent with periarticular fat necrosis and inflammatory changes in the bone. Clinical, radiographic, and bone scan findings must be correlated to make a definitive diagnosis.

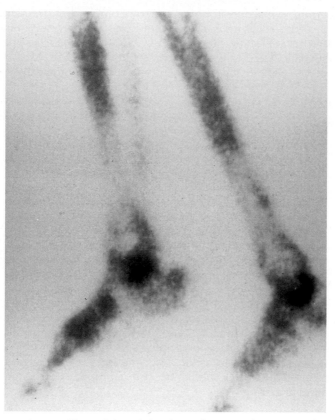

Fig 4–16.—Technetium-99m methylene diphosphonate bone scan showing multiple areas of increased activity in a linear and symmetric distribution along the tibia. Findings are consistent with an inflammatory process, trauma, and periostosis secondary to hypertrophic osteoarthropathy. (Courtesy of Bayo III F, Massie JD, Sebes J: *Clin Nucl Med* 18:837–839, 1993.)

▶ In the differential diagnosis of the scan findings, the authors mention an inflammatory process that includes osteomyelitis, traumatic periostitis, hypertrophic osteoarthropathy, and malignancy. Osteomyelitis and malignancy would be unusual for this bilateral, almost symmetrical process. The clinical and radiographic findings also favored a diffuse inflammatory process. Fortunately, this entity is rare.—J.G. McAfee, M.D.

How Does Iliac Crest Bone Marrow Biopsy Compare With Imaging in the Detection of Bone Metastases in Small Cell Lung Cancer?
Perrin-Resche I, Bizais Y, Buhe T, Fiche M (Centre Hospitalier Universitaire de Nantes, France)
Eur J Nucl Med 20:420–425, 1993   124-95-4-14

Background.—Iliac crest bone marrow biopsy has frequently been used as the gold standard for detecting bone marrow metastases in patients with small-cell lung cancer (SCLC). However, its false positive rate is probably high. The findings of bone scintigraphy (BS), MRI, and bone marrow biopsy were compared in patients with pathologically confirmed SCLC.

Methods.—Forty-eight consecutive patients were studied; 45 were assessable. The 3 tests were done within 1 week, during which no treatment was performed. Whole body scans and spot views in anterior and posterior projections were taken. The thoracolumbar spine, sternum, and pelvis were scanned with MRI spin-echo T1-weighted sequences. The acquisition time was less than 45 minutes.

Findings.—Only 5 bone marrow biopsy examinations were positive. Bone scintigraphy and MRI were also positive in these cases. Among the remaining 42, in which biopsy results were negative, both BS and MRI were positive in 10 cases and both were negative in 21 cases, MRI was positive and BS negative in 5 cases, and BS was positive and MRI negative in 6 cases. Follow-up scans confirmed the initial findings in most cases where either BS or MRI was positive.

Conclusion.—Bone marrow biopsy is more invasive and appears to be less sensitive than BS or MRI for detecting bone metastases. For detecting small spinal or pelvic metastases, MRI appears to be more sensitive than BS. Whole body bone scintigraphy is more sensitive in finding skull, costal, or peripheral disease. For detecting bone metastases in patients with SCLC, BS and MRI should be combined. This combination may replace bone marrow biopsy.

▶ The reputation of marrow biopsy, the gold standard for detecting metastases in small-cell carcinoma and other malignancies, has become tarnished in recent years. In another larger series of 112 patients with small-cell cancer (1), 8% had a positive biopsy and negative bone scan, but 22% had a positive bone scan and negative biopsy. Both studies were positive in only 9%. In that series, the correlation time between the 2 studies was poor.

In Europe, marrow imaging has become popular (2), particularly with particle nanocolloid (3) (Nanocoll, Solco Basel, Switzerland), because it achieves a high concentration in the marrow. However, it is not available in the United States.—J.G. McAfee, M.D.

References

1. Levitan N, et al: *Cancer* 56:652, 1985.
2. Reske SN: *Eur J Nucl Med* 18:203, 1991.
3. de Schrijver M, et al: *Nucl Med Commun* 8:895, 1987.

24 Hour/3 Hour Radio-Uptake Technique for Differentiating Degenerative and Malignant Bony Lesions in Bone Scanning

Kashyap R, Bhatnagar A, Mondal A, Sawroop K (Inst of Nuclear Medicine and Allied Sciences, Delhi, India)
Australas Radiol 37:198–200, 1993   1 2 4-95-4–1 5

Background.—The ability to differentiate bony metastases from degenerative lesions is very important. Although routine bone scanning with technetium-99m methylene diphosphonate is the method of choice for detecting bony lesions, it has a low specificity. An experience with 24-hour/3-hour radio-uptake ratio (24 hr/3 hr RUR) was described.

Methods.—Thirty patients with cancer (mean age, 52 years) were included. Seventeen had breast cancer; 8, prostate cancer; 2, lung cancer; and 1 each, renal cell carcinoma, thyroid cancer, and multiple myeloma. A 24 hr/3 hr RUR, the lesion-to-nonlesion ratio was used to differentiate metastatic from degenerative lesions, with the difference in radio-uptake behavior of the 2 lesions being used as the criterion.

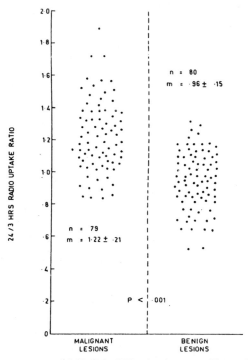

Fig 4–17.—Distribution pattern of 24 hr/3 hr RUR of malignant and benign bone lesions. Malignant lesions, $n = 79$; $m = 1.22 \pm .21$. Benign lesions, $n = 80$; $m = .96 \pm .15$. Difference significant at $P < .001$. (Courtesy of Kashyap R, Bhatnagar A, Mondal A, et al: *Australas Radiol* 37:198–200, 1993.)

Findings.—The RUR distribution curves of malignant and degenerative lesions differed significantly. The RUR of malignant lesions exceeded the critical point of 1.12, and the RUR of degenerative lesions was less than the critical point. The sensitivity was 68%; specificity, 80%; and accuracy, 74% (Fig 4–17).

Conclusion.—The 24 hr/3 hr RUR method appears to be a useful, cost-effective way to differentiate bony lesions. The RUR distribution curves of malignant and degenerative lesions were significantly different in the current series.

▶ This idea, which was originally proposed by Citrin and associates (1), seems to resurface every few years. However, the results of this study do not look promising—32% false negatives and 20% false positives for malignancies. Figure 4–17 shows a marked overlap in ratios between the benign and malignant lesions, despite the statistically valid difference between the mean ratios. As a result, this approach probably will not replace careful correlation of bone scans with other modalities, such as radiography, CT, and MRI.—J.G. McAfee, M.D.

Reference

1. Citrin DL, et al: *J Nucl Med* 16:886, 1975.

Diagnosis of Osteoid Osteoma in the Child
Kaweblum M, Lehman WB, Bash J, Grant AD, Strongwater A (Hosp for Joint Diseases Orthopaedic Inst, New York)
Orthop Rev 22:1305–1313, 1993   124-95-4-16

Background.—Diagnosing osteoid osteoma in young children is challenging because they cannot give an accurate history. New and previously reported cases of osteoid osteoma in children younger than 5 years of age were reviewed.

Patients and Findings.—Fifty-two cases from the literature and 7 new cases from the Hospital for Joint Diseases were analyzed. Osteoid osteoma occurred in the lower extremity in 73% of patients and in the upper extremity in 15% (Fig 4–18). Children who were just beginning to walk were especially difficult to diagnose. Although pain was the most common clinical manifestation, 12% of the children had no pain. The next most common findings were limp, tenderness, swelling, and atrophy (Fig 4–19). Technetium bone scans were very effective in identifying the tumor when standard radiographs were negative. Computed tomography enabled visualization and exact localization of the tumors in all the children studied. More than one fourth of the children had bone deformities and leg length discrepancies.

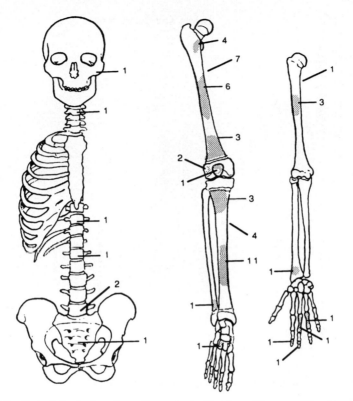

Fig 4–18.—Skeletal distribution of osteoid osteoma in 59 patients. (Courtesy of Kaweblum M, Lehman WB, Bash J, et al: *Orthop Rev* 22:1305–1313, 1993.)

Conclusion.—Diagnosis was very difficult in 30% of the cases reviewed, because the children's symptoms mimicked many other diseases. The recommended treatment is miniblock excision.

▶ This excellent review contains many details about this benign bone tumor. Twenty five of the 59 children were given an erroneous diagnosis before the osteoid osteoma was identified, and 9 of these were wrongly called osteomyelitis.

One patient had negative radiographs, and 2 had negative bone scans before a third scan with pinhole collimator showed the lesion in the distal femoral epiphysis adjacent to the growth plate. Another had negative radiographs and bone scan but had a positive scan 3 months later. In 3 cases, x-ray results were negative with positive bone scans. In lesions of the lumbar spine, there is usually scoliosis with convexity to the opposite side, because of muscle spasm on the side of the lesion.—J.G. McAfee, M.D.

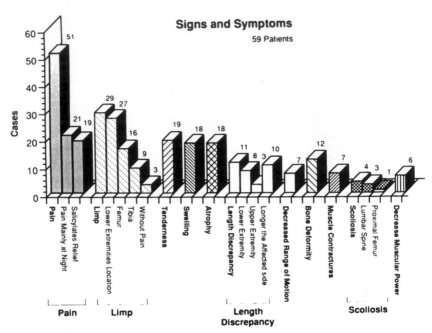

Fig 4-19.—Signs and symptoms of osteoid osteoma in 59 patients. (Courtesy of Kaweblum M, Lehman WB, Bash J, et al: *Orthop Rev* 22:1305–1313, 1993.)

Scintigraphy of Spinal Disorders in Adolescents
Mandell GA, Harcke HT (Alfred I duPont Inst, Wilmington, Del)
Skeletal Radiol 22:393–401, 1993   124-95-4-17

Inflammatory and Infectious Conditions.—Initial radiographs of the spine may be normal in both diskitis and vertebral osteomyelitis. However, bone scintigraphy can predate radiographic changes in both conditions by 3 to 6 weeks (Fig 4–20). Pin-hole collimation and SPECT helped to clarify the distribution of the increased tracer activity. A gallium-67 scan may aid in identifying the focus of infection when the bone scan is negative or equivocal.

Tumor and Tumor-Like Lesions.—The osteoid osteoma is the most common tumor involving the axial skeleton in adolescents. Because of their avidity for the bone-seeking radiopharmaceutical, the osteoid-forming nidus of the osteoid osteoma and the osteoblastoma (Fig 4–21) lend themselves to identification with bone scintigraphy.

Trauma.—With bone scintigraphy, the radiographic signs of occult fractures and stress fractures can be anticipated by weeks or months. In some cases, scintigraphy allows differentiation of occult fractures from developmental variations in the cervical spine.

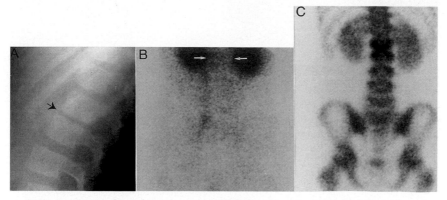

Fig 4–20.—Images obtained in a person with diskitis. **A,** lateral radiograph of the lumbar spine shows indistinctness of end plates and narrowing of the intervening disk space at L1-2 (*arrow*). **B,** posterior blood-pool planar bone scan of the abdomen demonstrates increased uptake at 2 vertebral levels between the lower poles of the kidneys (*arrows*). **C,** posterior delayed planar bone scan shows increased uptake involving L1 and L2 and the intervening disk space. (Courtesy of Mandell GA, Harcke HT: *Skeletal Radiol* 22:393-401, 1993.)

Spondylolysis and Pseudoarthrosis.—Both bone scintigraphy and plain radiographs may be normal; as a result, SPECT is now advocated to demonstrate the small foci of increased activity produced by many spondylolyses (Fig 4-22). This modality also increases the sensitivity of bone scanning for detection of the pseudoarthrosis by enhancing the area of subtly increased activity.

Conclusion.—Patterns of bone tracer uptake together with plain radiographic findings help to differentiate disease processes that affect the spine in adolescents. The accuracy of this imaging method is highly dependent on technique. Single-photon emission CT should now be rou-

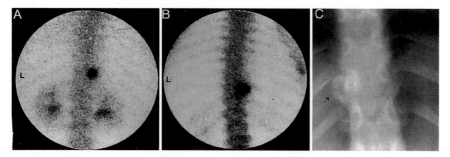

Fig 4–21.—Images obtained in a person with osteoblastoma. **A,** posterior blood-pool planar bone scan shows an intense ovoid area of increased uptake on the right side of the lower thoracic spine. **B,** posterior delayed planar bone scan shows intense focal radiotracer accumulation on the right side of T11. **C,** anteroposterior linear tomogram of the lower thoracic spine demonstrates a lytic lesion (*arrow*) in the overgrown transverse process on the right side of T11. (Courtesy of Mandell GA, Harcke HT: *Skeletal Radiol* 22:393-401, 1993.)

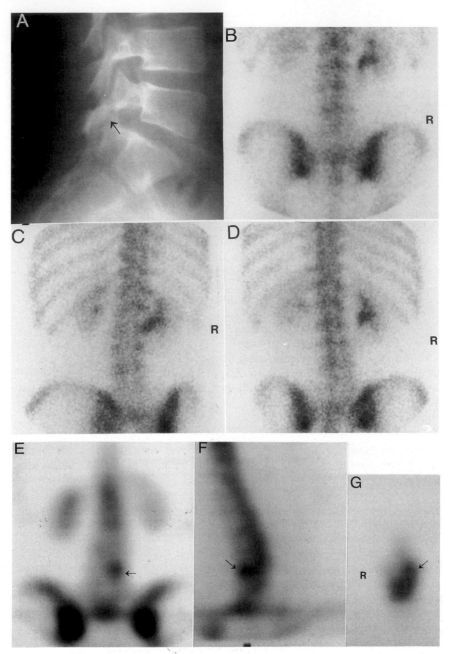

Fig 4–22.—Images obtained in a patient with suspected spondylolysis but without evidence on plain radiographs. **A,** lateral radiographic view of lumbosacral region, with a suspected area of sclerosis and/or lysis (*arrow*) indicated. **B–D,** bone scans. Posterior and both oblique delayed planar images of the lumbosacral spine have no evidence of increased uptake. **E–G,** coronal, sagittal, and transaxial SPECT projections demonstrate increased uptake (*arrow*) in the region of pars interarticularis on the left side of L4 (**bottom** of image in **G**). (Courtesy of Mandell GA, Harcke HT: *Skeletal Radiol* 22:393–401, 1993.)

tinely included for each study in cases of normal or equivocal planar images.

▶ This paper contains plenty of good, detailed information. In developmental spinal abnormalities, such as Scheuermann's disease, the anatomical changes are best demonstrated by radiographs, CT, and MRI.

Bone scans are usually positive in diskitis and osteomyelitis before they are in other imaging modalities; however, gallium images may not be positive in indolent diskitis.

Unlike osteoid osteomas of the pelvis or lower limbs, a spinal lesion may be purely lytic and hard to find on plain radiographs. The nidus may be only millimeters in diameter, whereas osteoblastomas usually produce larger lytic areas. Both lesions have intense uptake on bone scans. With portable probe detectors, intraoperative guidance can be provided for the location and extent of the lesions. Bone scans of the spine with central photopenia and a peripheral rim of increased activity (a doughnut appearance) may be the result of aneurysmal bone cysts, unicameral bone cysts, or giant-cell tumors. Eosinophilic granulomas of the spine are usually photopenic and may show vertebral collapse or deformity, but they are better demonstrated by other modalities.

In suspected trauma, the authors suggest waiting for 24 hours before performing the bone scan.—J.G. McAfee, M.D.

SPECT Evaluation of Unilateral Spondylolysis
Lusins JO, Elting JJ, Cicoria AD, Goldsmith SJ (AO Fox Mem Hosp, Oneonta, NY; Mt Sinai School of Medicine, New York)
Clin Nucl Med 19:1–5, 1994   124-95-4–18

Background.—Lumbar spondylolysis, which occurs in 6% of American adults, must be considered when assessing patients with low back complaints. Typically, spondylolysis occurs bilaterally, but 3 cases of unilateral spondylolysis were identified from a consecutive series of 65 patients with spondylolysis. Lumbar CT and SPECT were used in the assessment of all 3 patients.

Case Report.—Boy, 16 years, was referred for a neurologic assessment after 3 months of unsuccessful conservative treatment for back pain. He had sustained direct trauma to the low back while playing football. He reported that he had experienced back pain after exercise for 5 years. This pain usually decreased after restricted activity, but it did not remit. The neurologic assessment yielded no positive findings. Computed tomography showed spondylolysis on the left at L5. Degenerative changes in the opposite facet were observed on the right. A SPECT scan demonstrated increased activity in the right L5-S1 facet joint (Fig 4–23).

Conclusion.—All 3 patients with unilateral spondylolysis had positive scans. However, SPECT findings were definitive in each case, necessitat-

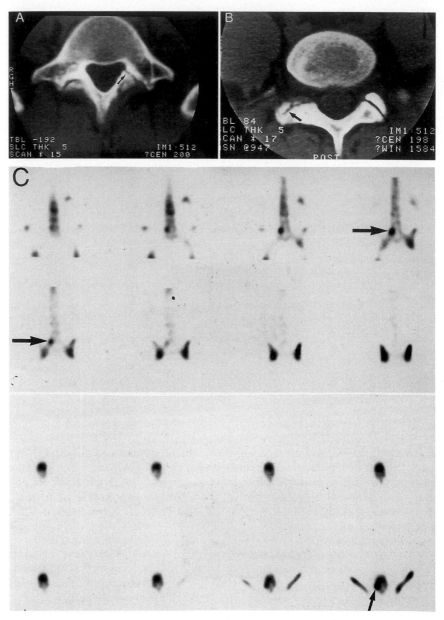

Fig 4–23.—Computed tomography through L5 of a boy, 16 years, with a back injury, shows (**A, far left**) unilateral spondylolysis on the left (*arrow*) with (**B, left**) degenerative changes in the facet on the opposite side (*arrow*). The SPECT scan at this level (**C, below**) shows increased activity at the site of the degenerated facet on the coronal and transaxial views (*arrows*). (Courtesy of Lusins JO, Elting JJ, Cicoria AD: *Clin Nucl Med* 19:1–5, 1994.)

ing consideration of the natural history of both unilateral and bilateral spondylolysis in the interpretation of SPECT activity.

▶ Good-quality SPECT images for low back pain are probably of the greatest help when planar images and CT studies are negative or equivocal. In a teaching session by Dr. Gary Gates some years ago, he observed that if you locate the intervertebral disk spaces on coronal or sagittal images, increased uptake encroaching on the disk space level is in an apophyseal joint, and pars activity is lower down. As in the authors' third patient, the increased uptake sometimes is in the vertebral bodies and not the posterior elements. I have seen bilaterally increased pars activity at L5 without visible CT defects (microfractures?).—J.G. McAfee, M.D.

Carpal Instability, the Missed Diagnosis in Patients With Clinically Suspected Scaphoid Fracture
Tiel-van Buul MMC, Bos KE, Dijkstra PF, van Beek EJR, Broekhuizen AH (Univ of Amsterdam)
Injury 24:257–262, 1993   124-95-4–19

Introduction.—Patients with scapholunate (S-L) dissociation, the most common cause of carpal instability, may lack radiologic signs in the presence of complete disruption of the S-L ligament. The mechanisms responsible for such an injury, as well as for scaphoid fractures, are hyperextension, ulnar deviation and intercarpal supination, which can occur during a fall on the outstretched hand. The incidence of carpal instability and its relationship to clinical and scintigraphic findings were determined in patients with suspected scaphoid fracture.

Methods.—The study group included a consecutive series of 160 patients who were treated for suspected scaphoid fracture after a fall on an outstretched hand. All were treated initially with immobilization in a below-elbow plaster. Patients whose initial radiographs were negative were referred for radionuclide bone scintigraphy. Immobilization was stopped if the bone scan was negative and continued if it was positive. Patients with a positive bone scan and persistently negative radiographs were treated as having a fractured scaphoid.

Results.—One hundred patients were followed for a mean of 26.8 months after injury. Twenty-two had clinical or radiologic signs of carpal instability (Fig 4–24). Compared with the 78 patients without evidence of carpal instability, those in this group had a significantly higher incidence of complaints (77% vs. 40%) and of a positive synovia test (64% vs. 21%). The 2 groups were similar in the percentage of patients with strength reduction and loss of wrist movement. Bone scans were not useful in detecting or excluding carpal instability (Fig 4–25). No additional information in the diagnosis of carpal instability was provided by the 3-phase bone scan.

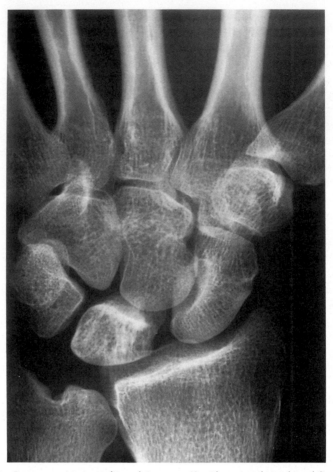

Fig 4–24.—Posteroanterior view radiograph in a man, 60, with suspected carpal instability (Watson's test positive); S-L distance greater than 3 mm. (Courtesy of Tiel-van Buul MMC, Bos KE, Dijkstra PF, et al: *Injury* 24:257–262, 1993.)

Conclusion.—Ligamentous disruption appears to be missed in a large number of patients with recent carpal injury. After a period of immobilization, the patient should undergo Watson's scaphoid test and the synovia stress test. Further radiodiagnostic tests should be ordered if radiographs are inconclusive. Persistent complaints suggest the presence of carpal instability or other complications.

▶ Scintigraphy is invaluable for detecting scaphoid injuries, but it does not tell the whole story. As a result, these authors also emphasize 4-view radiography, the synovia stress test, and Watson's test for carpal instability (see References 1 and 2).

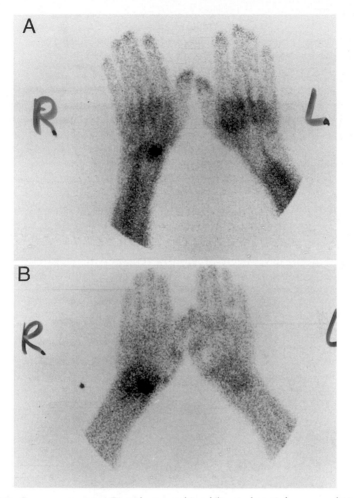

Fig 4–25.—Bone scan in a man, 71, without carpal instability. **A,** dynamic bone scan obtained 2–5 minutes after injection with hyperemia in the scaphoid region. **B,** static image with a hot spot in the same region, suggestive of scaphoid fracture. (Courtesy of Tiel-van Buul MMC, Bos KE, Dijkstra PF, et al: *Injury* 24:257–262, 1993.)

In a companion paper by the same authors (3), they conclude that patients with negative initial radiographs should still be treated in a below-elbow cast, including the whole thumb. Bone scanning should be done after 72 hours, and if it is positive, casting should be continued for 12 weeks. About two thirds with scaphoid hot spots on a bone scan had negative initial radiographs. After a minimum 1-year follow-up, 25% of the scaphoid hot spots could not be confirmed radiographically (were they healed fractures or over-diagnosis?).—J.G. McAfee, M.D.

References

1. Watson HK, et al: *J Bone Joint Surg (Am)* 68-A:345, 1986.
2. Watson HK, et al: *J Hand Surg (Am)* 13-A:657, 1988.
3. Tiel-van Buul MMC, et al: *J Bone Joint Surg (Br)* 75-B:61, 1993.

Fatigue Fractures of the Sacrum in Children: Two Case Reports and a Review of the Literature
Grier D, Wardell S, Sarwark J, Poznanski AK (Children's Mem Hosp, Chicago)
Skeletal Radiol 22:515–518, 1993   124-95-4-20

Introduction.—A fatigue fracture is one that typically occurs in young, active individuals. The lower extremities, particularly the tibia and metatarsals, are the most frequent sites for fatigue fractures in children and young adults. However, fatigue fractures of the sacrum are quite uncommon, and none have been previously reported in children. Two such cases were presented. However, the scintigraphic findings were similar in both cases.

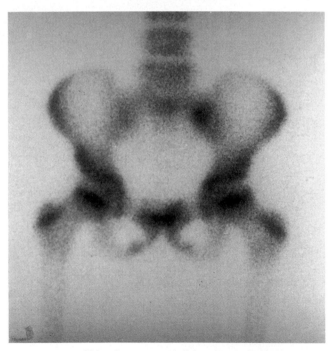

Fig 4–26.—Bone scintigram (delayed anterior view) of the pelvis shows focal increased activity in the left side of the sacrum. (Courtesy of Grier D, Wardell S, Sarwark J, et al: *Skeletal Radiol* 22:515–518, 1993.)

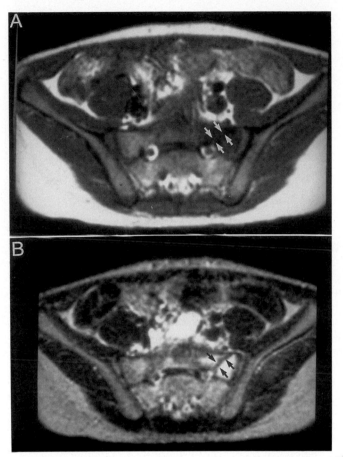

Fig 4–27.—Magnetic resonance images obtained through the sacral ala. **A,** axial T1-weighted image (repetition time, 483 ms; echo time, 11 ms) shows diffuse low marrow signal intensity with central linear signal void (*arrows*) in left sacral ala. **B,** axial T2-weighted image (repetition time, 2,500 ms; echo time, 80 ms) shows diffuse increased marrow signal intensity with central linear signal void (*arrows*) in the left sacral ala. (Courtesy of Grier D, Wardell S, Sarwark J, et al: *Skeletal Radiol* 22:515–518, 1993.)

Case Report.—Boy, 9 years, with no history of trauma, was seen with pain in the left superior sacral region. His symptoms had appeared gradually over a 4-week period. He had no history of fever, chills, or neurologic dysfunction. A physical examination revealed local tenderness over the left sacrum and posterior superior iliac spine. The FABER-Patrick and delayed Trendelenburg tests were positive on the left. An isotope bone scan showed a focal increase in activity in the left side of the sacrum (Fig 4–26). Both T1- and T2-weighted axial MRI showed a linear signal void in the left sacral ala that extended to an arcuate foramen (Fig 4–27). Computed tomography showed a linear band of medullary sclerosis at this site (Fig 4–28). The patient responded well to conservative treatment of the fatigue fracture of the left sacral ala.

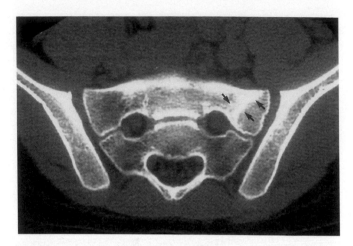

Fig 4–28.—Axial CT scan shows linear medullary sclerosis in left sacral ala extending to an arcuate foramen (*arrows*). (Courtesy of Grier D, Wardell S, Sarwark J, et al: *Skeletal Radiol* 22:515–518, 1993.)

Discussion.—Fatigue fractures in children may be difficult to diagnose if they occur at an unusual site or without a typical history. Sacral fatigue fractures have been reported in young adults who were involved in serious athletic training, but these fractures have not been described in children. Bone scintigraphy typically shows a focus of increased activity in the lateral part of the sacrum. Plain radiography was noncontributory to the diagnosis in the 2 cases reported here. Symptoms include low back pain of gradual onset that occasionally radiates to the hip or groin. Sacral fatigue fractures are treated conservatively with a period of non–weight-bearing and analgesics. Knowledge of typical MRI findings will enable the clinician to diagnose fatigue fractures of the sacrum in children and distinguish them from infection or malignancy.

▶ This is a good review of stress fractures. The authors make a clear distinction between fatigue fractures that result from abnormal or repetitive loading of normal bone (as seen in children and normal adults) and insufficiency fractures in abnormal bone, with reduced resistance to deformation resulting from osteoporosis, previous radiation, or other intrinsic bone lesions.

Sacral fractures are common in adults usually after falls on the buttocks. Because they often produce a horizontal band of increased uptake in the sacrum on diphosphonate images, they may be missed radiographically. On the other hand, these uncommon fatigue fractures in children usually cause a unilateral increase in the ala of the sacrum.—J.G. McAfee, M.D.

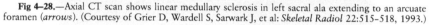

Tibiofibular Synostosis in Professional Basketball Players
Henry JH, Andersen AJ, Cothren CC (Orthopaedic Surgery and Athletic Med-

icine, PA, San Antonio, Tex; San Antonio Spurs Basketball Team)
Am J Sports Med 21:619–622, 1993   124-95-4-21

Objective.—Two cases of stress fracture of the tibia in professional basketball players that resulted in callus formation of the interosseous space were reviewed. A tibiofibular synostosis can cause shin splintlike pain as well as ankle pain.

Case 1.—Man 22, was originally seen for an injury to his calf. Despite treatment, he continued to complain of pain in the anterior compartment during play. A radiograph revealed an old stress fracture of the tibia and synostosis between the tibia and fibula. Anti-inflammatory medication and physical therapy provided little symptomatic relief. The patient had no problems during the off-season, yet his bone scan was positive at the next preseason physical examination. Computed tomography at this time revealed a tibiofibular synostosis. The player was later able to return to professional basketball.

Case 2.—Male professional basketball player, 28, also experienced pain re lated to a synostosis between the tibia and fibula. He was later traded, casted for 2 months, and eventually cut from the team. He is no longer playing basketball.

Discussion.—Both of these players had primarily anterior compartment–type pain that occurred only when running, cutting, and jumping. Rest and reduction of activity decreased their symptoms. Excision of their synostoses may be necessary in the future, but surgery has not yet been required for pain relief or resumption of activity.

▶ Congenital proximal tibiofibular synostosis is rare, but acquired synostosis in athletes is more common, usually at the junction of the middle and lower thirds of the tibia and fibula. Surgical excision has been beneficial to some patients. These lesions could easily be confused with fractures or stress fractures on diphosphonate images, but they are diagnosed definitively by radiography.—J.G. McAfee, M.D.

Overuse Ballet Injury of the Base of the Second Metatarsal: A Diagnostic Problem
Harrington T, Crichton KJ, Anderson IF (Royal North Shore Hosp, St Leonards, Australia; North Sydney Orthopaedic & Sports Medicine Centre, Crows Nest, Australia; Sports X-Ray Orthopaedic & Sports Medicine Radiology, Crows Nest, Sydney, Australia)
Am J Sports Med 21:591–598, 1993   124-95-4-22

Background.—Pain over the second metatarsal joint in ballerinas may be an indication of traumatic synovitis of the second tarsometatarsal joint or a stress fracture at the base of the second metatarsal. A prompt diagnosis is important, because each condition requires a different

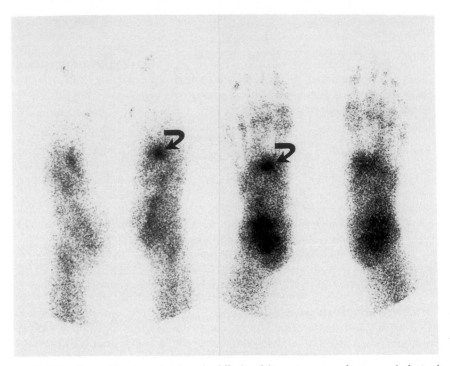

Fig 4–29.—Scans of 2 patients that show the difficulty of diagnosing a stress fracture on the basis of bone scan findings alone. The image on the **left** is from a patient with traumatic synovitis; that on the **right** is from a patient with a bone stress reaction. The symptomatic areas of isotope accumulation are indicated by *curved arrows*. Other areas of increased activity show that multiple sites of joint injury occur in ballerinas. (Courtesy of Harrington T, Crichton KJ, Anderson IF: *Am J Sports Med* 21:591-598, 1993.)

course of treatment. The case histories of 8 ballerinas treated for pain over the second metatarsal joint were reviewed.

Patients.—Eight ballerinas between 15 and 24 years of age complained of pain in the midfoot region that was worse en pointe and with jumps. Each dancer had a clinical examination, plain radiography, bone scanning, and MRI. All problems were unilateral.

Results.—Clinical examination, radiography, and scintigraphy did not differentiate bone stress from traumatic synovitis (Fig 4–29). A bone stress reaction at the base of the second metatarsal was demonstrated on MRI scans of 6 dancers (Fig 4–30) and a fracture line could be identified on 4 examinations. The other 2 dancers had normal MRI scans, and a diagnosis of traumatic synovitis was made by exclusion. Dancers with stress reactions were advised to rest and gradually return to dancing. Three ballerinas followed this advice and were symptom-free after 6 to 8 weeks of rest, and 3 dancers continued to dance against advice. The 2 dancers with traumatic synovitis were treated with nonsteroidal anti-in-

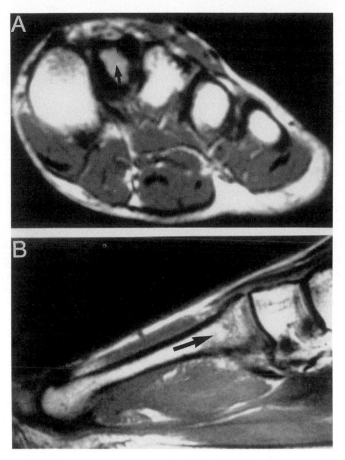

Fig 4–30.—Axial (**A**) and tilted sagittal T1-weighted (**B**) MR images of a patient with marked decrease in bone marrow signal in the base of the second metatarsal (*arrows*), but with no visible fracture line. This area normally has identical marrow signal intensity to that in the adjacent metatarsals. The findings here are believed to represent bone stress or trabecular microfracture. (Courtesy of Harrington T, Crichton KJ, Anderson IF: *Am J Sports Med* 21:591-598, 1993.)

flammatory drugs and passive mobilization and were allowed to continue dancing; both became symptom-free within 6 weeks.

Conclusion.—The prompt differential diagnosis of pain and tenderness over the second metatarsal joint in ballet dancers shortens the course of treatment.

▶ Apparently, these are common injuries in female ballet dancers (but in not males), but accounts of them are rarely found in the literature. Bone scans provide objective evidence of injury, but they cannot distinguish synovitis from stress fracture of the second metatarsal. Six of the 8 female dancers had a short first metatarsal (Morton's foot). When the fracture line of this stress fracture is visible, it involves the medial corner of the second metatarsal bone.—J.G. McAfee, M.D.

Vocal Cords Dysfunction Results From Heterotopic Ossification in a Patient With Burns
Lippin Y, Shvoron A, Faibel M, Tsur H (Chaim Sheba Med Ctr, Tel Hashomer, Israel; Tel Aviv Univ, Israel)
J Burn Care Rehabil 15:169–173, 1994   124-95-4-23

Introduction.—A man 38 years of age had limited movement of the vocal cords because of heterotopic ossification. This appears to be the first such case recorded.

Case Report.—Man, 38, had burns over 45% of his body and smoke inhalation injury. The initial treatment was fluid and plasma replacement, mechanical ventilation through a soft-cuffed endotrachial tube, and topical wound care. After 8 weeks, his general condition improved, but extubation failed because of ventilatory insufficiency. An uneventful permanent tracheostomy was performed. Pain and limited motion were detected in his ankles, although this area had not been burned. Radiographs indicated extra-articular ossification around both ankles. Laryngoscopy demonstrated very limited mobility of both vocal cords. Radiographs revealed fluffy calcified shadows in the neck. A technetium-99m scan revealed increased uptake in this region and around the ankles. Treatment was initiated with diphosphonate, but the patient was lost to follow-up after 6 months.

Conclusion.—The first reported case of vocal cord dysfunction resulting from heterotopic ossification around the cricoarytenoid joint was described.

▶ This is another unusual cause of extraosseous deposition of technetium-99m diphosphonates.—J.G. McAfee, M.D.

Extraskeletal Localization of MDP in Soft Tissue Secondary to Methotrexate Infiltration
Brown CV, Miller JH (Dept of Veterans Affairs Med Ctr, West Los Angeles; Childrens Hosp, Los Angeles)
Clin Nucl Med 19:357–358, 1994   124-95-4-24

Case Report.—Boy, 15 years, with non-Hodgkin's lymphoma had infiltration of a methotrexate infusion from a right forearm IV catheter that resulted in soft tissue erythema and swelling of the right arm. Six days later, a bone scan was done to assess the sudden onset of nontraumatic thoracic spine pain. Spine activity was normal, but uptake of technetium-99m methylene diphosphonate in the soft tissues of the right arm was greatly increased because of myonecrosis

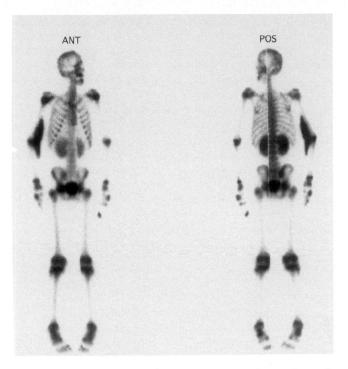

Fig 4–31.—Delayed anterior and posterior whole-body bone scintiphotographs reveal marked accumulation of methylene diphosphonate in the right medial humeral areas. Bone scintigraphy was performed 6 days after infiltration of methotrexate into the soft tissue of the right upper extremity. Accentuated renal uptake of tracer is present in these scintiphotographs secondary to antecedent cancer chemotherapy. (Courtesy of Brown CV, Miller JH: *Clin Nucl Med* 19:357–358, 1994.)

and soft tissue microcalcification (Fig 4–31). This is the first reported case of soft tissue uptake of skeletal tracers from chemotherapy extravasation.

▶ The high-intensity interstitial infiltration simulates a direct interstitial injection of the radioactive dose on interstitial infiltration of calcium infusions. Infiltration of any cytotoxic agent is not recommended.—J.G. McAfee, M.D.

5 Endocrine

Introduction

Perhaps clinical nuclear medicine began with the development of the thyroid uptake measurement and thyroid imaging, which for many years were the primary tests in the field. I still recall that one of the concerns expressed by the Chairman of Medicine at the Albert Einstein College of Medicine when I joined the faculty as Director of Nuclear Medicine was that my background was not in endocrinology, which was the most important aspect of nuclear medicine. Therefore, it is very gratifying to see that work in endocrinology and nuclear medicine is enjoying a bit of a resurgence after having decreased in importance in the field over the last 10 to 15 years.

The approval by the Food and Drug Administration of the use of somatostatin introduces us to an agent for endocrine tumors that has great promise. The improvements in parathyroid localization, especially with the introduction of sestamibi, have given us something to offer the clinician in that area. The treatment of thyroid disease with radionuclides remains the single greatest success story in the application of radioactive materials to therapy in both benign and malignant disease. We appear to be entering a time of revitalization of the field of "nuclear endocrinology."

M. Donald Blaufox, M.D., Ph.D.

Parathyroid Localization Prior to Primary Exploration
Shaha AR, LaRosa CA, Jaffe BM (State Univ of New York, Brooklyn)
Am J Surg 166:289–293, 1993   1 2 4-95-5–1

Background.—There is controversy regarding the use of parathyroid localization studies before primary exploration. If the preoperative diagnosis of primary hyperparathyroidism is correct, the success of primary surgical exploration exceeds 90% to 95%, precluding the need for preoperative localization. Recent experience suggests that parathyroid localization studies before primary exploration may be of great value under certain specific conditions.

Patients.—Within the past 8 years, 80 parathyroid explorations were performed for primary hyperparathyroidism. In the first 5 years, localization tests included sonography, thallium-technetium scanning, and CT.

Comparison of Various Noninvasive Studies in Parathyroid Localization Before Primary Exploration

	Ultrasound	Thallium-Technetium Scanning	Computed Tomography	Magnetic Resonance Imaging
Sensitivity	55%–88%	59%–96%	68%–95%	57%–82%
Specificity	95%–98%	90%–98%	89%	94%–97%

(Courtesy of Shaha AR, LaRosa CA, Jaffe BM: *Am J Surg* 166:289–293, 1993.)

In the latter 3 years, thallium-technetium scanning was used for specific indications before primary exploration.

Findings.—The enlarged thyroid gland was localized in 24 of 30 patients who underwent thallium-technetium scanning before primary exploration. The specific indications were diagnostic dilemmas, technical problems, and high-risk patient factors. In patients with mild asymptomatic hypercalcemia, preoperative localization confirmed the presence of a parathyroid adenoma and indicated whether surgery would be successful. Patient factors included those at high risk because of associated medical problems, including hypertension, congestive heart failure, and other cardiac problems. In those patients, preoperative localization ensured shorter operative times and less tedious dissections.

Discussion.—The use of parathyroid localization before primary exploration in selected patients helps achieve the very best results. The 4 currently used noninvasive localization studies—ultrasonography, technetium-thallium subtraction scanning, CT, and MRI—have almost identical success rates (table). Each of these studies has its own advantages and disadvantages, but the technetium-thallium scan is recommended because it is readily available, is easy to perform, and allows for easy interpretation as well as localization of ectopic parathyroid glands. The success rates of parathyroid localization using thallium-technetium scanning range from 75% to 80%, with sensitivity and specificity that exceed 90%.

▶ Shaha et al. report remarkably good sensitivity and specificity for parathyroid localization using thallium-technetium scanning. These impressive results probably are obtained because of the investigators' careful criteria for localization studies.

It is becoming increasingly apparent that the role of imaging is relatively limited in patients with suspected hyperplasia and secondary hyperparathyroidism and in those who are undergoing a first-time surgery. However, in patients in whom reexploration is necessary, the test becomes increasingly valuable. The substitution of technetium sestamibi for thallium also tends to make the test easier to perform and may improve the results.—M.D. Blaufox, M.D., Ph.D.

A Comparison of 10 MHz Ultrasound and 201-Thallium/99m-Technetium Subtraction Scanning in Primary Hyperparathyroidism

Gallacher SJ, Kelly P, Shand J, Logue FC, Cooke T, Boyle IT, McKillop JH (Glasgow Royal Infirmary, Scotland; Stobhill Hosp, Glasgow, Scotland)
Postgrad Med J 69:376–380, 1993   124-95-5-2

Background.—Debate continues regarding the routine preoperative localization of parathyroid adenomas and/or hyperplasia. Methods available include thallium-technetium subtraction scanning, high-resolution ultrasound, CT, and MRI.

Methods.—The 2 most commonly available techniques, 10-MHz ultrasound and thallium-201/technetium-99m subtraction scanning (Tl-Tc), were compared in 25 patients with primary hyperparathyroidism. Imaging findings were compared with surgical findings at neck exploration.

Results.—The Tl-Tc scanning had a sensitivity of 42% and a specificity of 97% compared with a sensitivity of 38% and specificity of 89% for ultrasound. Of the 9 cases in which both techniques were positive, they correctly localized the parathyroid adenoma in 8. Together, both methods were unable to localize abnormal parathyroid tissue in 44% of cases. The median gland size when both scans were negative was 170 mg compared with 750 mg when Tl-Tc scanning was correct, 960 mg when ultrasound was correct, and 980 mg when both techniques were correct.

Conclusion.—In the preoperative evaluation of patients with primary hyperparathyroidism, neither Tl-Tc scanning nor ultrasound appears to be sufficiently sensitive or specific for routine use. Perhaps further study can identify a role for use of both studies together.

Magnetic Resonance Imaging in Preoperative Localization of Diseased Parathyroid Glands: A Comparison With Isotope Scanning and Ultrasonography

Yao M, Jamieson C, Blend R (Wellesley Hosp, Toronto; Princess Margaret Hosp, Toronto)
Can J Surg 36:241–244, 1993   124-95-5-3

Background.—Surgical excision of diseased parathyroid glands is the definitive treatment for hyperparathyroidism; however, the procedure can damage recurrent laryngeal nerves and cause hypoparathyroidism postoperatively. Noninvasive techniques to localize the glands can be used preoperatively to minimize the risks by defining the area of disease for the surgeon.

Objective.—Because ultrasonography and thallium-technetium subtraction scintigraphy (TTSS) are the most widely used localizing techniques, the usefulness of MRI compared with that of ultrasonography and TTSS in localizing glands was evaluated.

Sensitivity of TTSS, Ultrasonography (US), and MRI in Detecting a Parathyroid Adenoma and Correctly Predicting the Side and Quadrant

Modality	Patients, no.	Detection of adenoma, %	Correct prediction of	
			Side, %	Quadrant, %
TTSS	27	67	48	7
US	27	44	33	26
MRI	11	36	36	9

(Courtesy of Yao M, Jamieson C, Blend R: *Can J Surg* 36:241-244, 1993.)

Methods.—Between July 1987 and April 1990, 1 or more of these localization studies were administered to 27 women and 10 men with primary hyperparathyroidism. Subsequently, all patients underwent surgical excision of their diseased glands by the same surgeon. Surgery confirmed the presence of parathyroid lesions. All but 1 patient had normal calcium levels after surgery, and they were deemed cured.

Operative results were compared with preoperative localization test findings. The sensitivity of each test was determined by analyzing how well the test detected the lesion, predicted the correct side where the lesion was located, and localized the specific quadrant of the lesion. Other factors were examined (e.g., lesion size, thyroid abnormalities, and the preoperative levels of calcium and parathormone) to determine any correlation with sensitivity.

Results.—The table shows the results of the sensitivity determinations for each test. The sensitivity of TTSS in detecting parathyroid adenoma was 67%, ultrasonography was 44%, and MRI was 36%. The sensitivity of TTSS in predicting the correct side was 48%, ultrasonography was 33%, and MRI was 36%. None of the differences were significant.

Once each test had detected a lesion, its probability of predicting the correct side was 73% for TTSS, 75% for ultrasonography, and 100% for MRI. Once the test had predicted the correct laterality, its probability of predicting the correct quadrant was 15% for TTSS, 78% for ultrasonography, and 25% for MRI.

Conclusion.—Magnetic resonance imaging was not superior to ultrasonography or TTSS in detecting parathyroid adenomas. No correlation was found between the sensitivity of a given test and the size of the lesion, the presence of thyroid abnormalities, or the calcium or parathormone levels seen before operation. Considering the high cost and limited sensitivity of all 3 tests, they are unnecessary for uncomplicated parathyroid disease.

▶ These articles (Abstracts 124-95-5–2 and 124-95-5–3) lend further support to the view that routine parathyroid imaging in uncomplicated patients is of dubious value. Furthermore, it provides data that none of the competing modalities—MRI, TTSS, or ultrasound—offers any significant advantage over radionuclide scanning.

It is interesting to note the wide range in reported sensitivities for all the tests used in the detection of parathyroid disease. Perhaps this is a reflection of considerable variation in patient populations and methodology. It will be interesting to see how these numbers change as more data are accumulated on the use of technetium-99m–sestamibi in parathyroid disease, which appears to be an easier technique both to perform and to interpret.—M.D. Blaufox, M.D., Ph.D.

Prospective Comparison of Technetium-99m-Sestamibi/Iodine-123 Radionuclide Scan Versus High-Resolution Ultrasonography for the Preoperative Localization of Abnormal Parathyroid Glands in Patients With Previously Unoperated Primary Hyperparathyroidism
Casas AT, Burke GJ, Sathyanarayana, Mansberger AR Jr, Wei JP (Med College of Georgia, Augusta)
Am J Surg 166:369–373, 1993   124-95-5–4

Objective.—Two methods of localizing abnormal parathyroid glands preoperatively—high-resolution ultrasonography and radionuclide subtraction imaging with iodine-123 (^{123}I) and technetium-99m (^{99m}Tc) sestamibi—were compared in a prospective series of 22 patients with a recent diagnosis of primary hyperparathyroidism. Sixteen patients had a solitary adenoma confirmed pathologically, 1 had 2 adenomas, and 5 had findings of diffuse parathyroid hyperplasia.

Methods.—Ultrasound studies were done using a real-time scanner and a 7.5-MHz linear-array probe. The thyroid was imaged with radioiodine, and, 4 hours later, technetium-labeled sestamibi was administered and the neck and upper thorax were imaged with a wide-field-of-view

Prospective Value of High-Resolution Ultrasonography Versus ^{99m}Tc-Sestamibi/^{123}I Scan		
	Ultrasound (%)	Sestamibi (%)
Adenoma		
Sensitivity	69	88
Specificity	100	100
Positive-predictive value	85	100
Hyperplasia		
Sensitivity	33	100
Specificity	100	88
Positive-predictive value	100	75

(Courtesy of Casas AT, Burke GJ, Sathyanarayana, et al: *Am J Surg* 166:369–373, 1993.)

gamma camera and parallel collimator. Digitalized images were analyzed by computer before generating the final subtraction images.

Results.—Nuclide scanning identified 14 of the 16 solitary adenomas preoperatively; both the sensitivity and specificity were 88%. Retrospectively, all these adenomas were identified. All 5 patients with diffuse parathyroid hyperplasia had scan findings consistent with hyperplasia, but individual glands were not differentiated. Ultrasonography was only 69% sensitive in identifying adenomas (table). Scanning with ^{99m}Tc-sestamibi was significantly more effective in localizing adenomas and identified smaller lesions than ultrasonography.

Conclusion.—Radionuclide imaging is perferable to high-resolution ultrasonography for localizing abnormal parathyroid glands in patients with primary hyperparathyroidism before initial neck dissection.

▶ This is another potential improvement in our ability to participate in the diagnosis of hyperparathyroidism. It is not yet clear whether ^{99m}Tc-sestamibi is going to greatly improve the technique or just simplify it. However, this article, which combines sestamibi with ^{123}I subtraction, presents very optimistic findings indeed. A word of caution: Do not assign too much value to the retrospective data. The real question is how well can we do before surgery.—M.D. Blaufox, M.D., Ph.D.

Dual Photon Absorptiometry for Bone Mineral Measurements Using a Gamma Camera
Valkema R, Prpic H, Blokland JAK, Camps JAJ, Papapoulos SE, Bijvoet OLM, Pauwels EKJ (Univ Hosp, Leiden, The Netherlands)
Acta Radiol 35:45–52, 1994   124-95-5-5

Objective.—With a gamma camera, dual-photon absorptiometry (DPA) can offer certain advantages, including low cost and a reduced radiation dose. The development and evaluation of a gamma camera that was modified for DPA by the addition of a commercially available collimator-source assembly were reported.

Methods.—In DPA with a gamma camera, each pixel in the image is regarded as a counting result of an independent detector. For each pixel, bone mineral content (BMC) is calculated using the attenuation of photons in both channels. A standard general-purpose gamma camera fitted with a commercial converging collimator assembly that was especially designed for DPA was used. Flood field studies, phantom measurements, and measurements in healthy volunteers were performed. Comparisons with a rectilinear DPA and a dual-energy x-ray (DEXA) system were also performed.

Results.—In the phantom studies, the 3 systems had a linear response in measurements of 4 vials, each containing a different amount of hydroxyapatite. Precision using the gamma camera system was 1.6% to

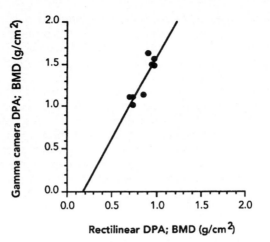

Fig 5–1.—Bone mineral density in vivo of the gamma camera densitometer compared with that for the rectilinear densitometer ($y = .35 + 1.94x$, $R^2 - .78$, P less than .01). (Courtesy of Valkema R, Prpic H, Blokland JAK, et al: *Acta Radiol* 35:45–52, 1994.)

2.8%. In the in vivo studies, there was good correlation between the results obtained with the rectilinear DPA and gamma camera systems. Directing the photon beam from posterior to anterior allowed for easy separation of the vertebrae using the gamma camera system.

Conclusion.—The validity and feasibility of bone mineral density measurements performed using a gamma camera were confirmed, with accuracy and linearity that were comparable to those of existing DPA systems (Fig 5–1). For purposes of clinical application, normal population values should be established. The divergent photon beam precludes accurate calculation of BMC or use of fixed regions of interest in follow-up measurements. Because DEXA remains more precise, gamma camera DPA cannot be recommended for individual patient follow-up.

▶ This report suggests an effort to create a more practical and perhaps useful approach to bone mineral measurements. I remember the Society of Nuclear Medicine meeting in 1981 when Lester Levy from Long Island Jewish Hospital first suggested using gamma camera measurements for BMD. Certainly, the ability to use the ubiquitous gamma camera for these measurements would enhance the appeal of using a nuclear medicine technique rather than the x-ray absorptiometry that is currently popular.

When we first introduced DPA bone mineral measurements at Montefiore Medical Center, a large number of physicians thought it was quite important to their patients' care, but when it became apparent that Medicare was not going to reimburse for this procedure, many of the physicians had to abandon its use because of their patients' inability to pay.

This is yet another example of the great disadvantage nuclear medicine as a relatively small discipline has in dealing with the government. The negative impact of the federal health care system on nuclear medicine through its ability to refuse payment has been a major contributor to problems of manpower and progress in the field. It is incredible that the federal regulators cannot understand the great value and cost-efficacy of nuclear medicine, and they do not have any sense of the incredible harm they are doing to the field through the difficulties they raise for reimbursement of common nuclear medicine procedures. The pay scales are arbitrary and capricious, and valuable procedures like DPA have suffered greatly from the federal agencies' unwillingness to accept the evidence of their usefulness. I cannot understand how a physician can be expected to treat a patient with agents whose success has been clearly shown to be unpredictable and some of which have been shown to be potentially dangerous and yet have no objective measure of the effect he/she is having on the patient's disease.—M.D. Blaufox, M.D., Ph.D.

Somatostatin Analogs for the Localization and Preoperative Treatment of an Adrenocorticotropin-Secreting Bronchial Carcinoid Tumor
Phlipponneau M, Nocaudie M, Epelbaum J, De Keyzer Y, Lalau JD, Marchandise X, Bertagna X (Centre Hospitalier Régional Universitaire, Amiens, France; Centre Hospitalier Régional Universitaire, Lille, France; INSERM U-159, Paris)
J Clin Endocrinol Metab 78:20–24, 1994   124-95-5–6

Introduction.—A bronchial carcinoid tumor may be difficult to detect by CT or MRI. Because neuroendocrine cells frequently express somatostatin receptors, the somatostatin analogue octreotide might prove helpful in locating a nonpituitary tumor in patients who are seen with ectopic adrenocorticotropic hormone (ACTH) syndrome.

Case Report.—Woman, 45, was seen with symptomatic hypokalemia of 3.1 mmol/L and hypercortisolism. Her appearance was typical for moderate Cushing's syndrome. Bone mineral density in the spine was markedly reduced. The serum cortisol level was 1,448 nmol/L and the plasma ACTH was 21.4 pmol/L. Urinary free cortisol excretion was unchanged during a high-dose dexamethasone suppression test, and the plasma ACTH did not respond to stimulation with ovine corticotropin-releasing factor. Abdominal CT showed moderate enlargement of the adrenal glands and the head of the pancreas. Thoracic CT revealed a possible 7-mm nodule in the left upper lobe. A 3-day course of octreotide led to marked clinical improvement and a substantial decline in plasma and urinary cortisol levels. Scintigraphy with ^{111}In-pentetreotide (Octreoscan) revealed a focus of abnormal uptake in the upper left lung at the exact site of the suspected nodule. Exploration, which was done after a month of octreotide therapy, revealed a small tumor at the expected site that was associated with a plasma ACTH gradient. The lesion proved to be a carcinoid tumor that contained immunoreactive ACTH in a concentration of 198 pmol/mg wet tissue weight.

Conclusion.—Radioanalogue scintigraphy with somatostatin is an accurate and noninvasive means of localizing occult neuroendocrine tumors. It may provide an alternative to inferior petrosal sinus sampling in patients who are suspected of having ectopic ACTH secretion whose pituitary is normal on MRI.

▶ This case report nicely illustrates a potential use for somatostatin imaging in a patient with an adrenocorticotropin-secreting bronchial carcinoid tumor. Now that somatostatin has been approved by the Food and Drug Administration, its use throughout the United States should greatly increase. Although the agent has been available in Europe for some time, its use has been relatively limited. I expect that in the next issue of the YEAR BOOK OF NUCLEAR MEDICINE we will be able to review considerably more publications concerning the application of somatostatin imaging of neuroendocrine tumors.—M.D. Blaufox, M.D., Ph.D.

Thyroid Hormones in Differentiated Thyroid Cancer
Samuel AM, Mehta MN, Desai KB (Bhabha Atomic Research Centre, Tata Mem Centre Annexe, Parel, Bombay, India)
Clin Nucl Med 19:49–53, 1994   124-95-5-7

Background.—Thyroglobulin (Tg) is present in most thyroid cancers and metastatic tissues; elevated Tg is a marker for thyroid cancer metastases. Thyroid cancers and their metastases concentrate iodine and are regulated by circulating thyroid-stimulating hormone (TSH). Six-week discontinuation of thyroxine (T_4) therapy leaves many patients euthyroid or grossly hypothyroid. The ability of metastases to synthesize triiodothyronine (T_3) and T_4 was evaluated.

Methods.—Serum levels of T_3, T_4, TSH, and Tg were estimated by routine radioimmunoassay methods in 136 differentiated thyroid cancer patients who were referred for radioiodine therapy. The patients had all discontinued T_4 at least 6 weeks earlier.

Results.—Among 83 patients with metastatic disease, 15 had functioning metastases with normal hormone production; all functioning metastases were follicular carcinomas of skeletal origin. Fifty-one patients with metastatic disease had elevated Tg; patients with skeletal metastases had the highest values. Levels of Tg were low in patients with residual thyroid disease. Radioiodine concentrated in the metastatic lesions. The metastatic lesion response to radioiodine was poor in patients with normal hormone levels; the response was better in patients with elevated Tg levels and low T_3/T_4 values whose metastatic sites were primarily in nodes or lungs. Residual thyroid tissue and nodal metastasis responded even better when Tg and thyroid hormone levels were low.

Conclusion.—A significant number of patients with metastatic thyroid cancer, particularly those with skeletal metastases of follicular carcinoma, synthesize thyroid hormone. These patients generally have significant Tg serum elevations and respond poorly to radioiodine. Prolonged observation is needed to differentiate the biological behavior of hormone-synthesizing tumors from that of those that do not synthesize hormones.

▶ Samuel et al. suggest that in their patient population, individuals with tumors, metastatic thyroid disease, and evidence of high thyroglobulin with normal hormone levels responded more poorly to treatment than patients with high thyroglobulin and low hormone levels. They indicated these patients had no remaining functioning normal thyroid tissue but do not offer much detail about this. Of course, the presence of thyroid tissue would be a major confounding factor. It is difficult to understand why increased production of thyroid hormone would be associated with decreased response, unless it results in a shorter residence time of the radioactive iodine in the tumor. If the authors' observations can be confirmed, this would suggest the need to develop a different treatment strategy for patients with skeletal metastases.—M.D. Blaufox, M.D., Ph.D.

Chromatographic Identification in Serum of Endogenously Radioiodinated Thyroid Hormones After Iodine-131 Whole-Body Scintigraphy in the Follow-Up of Patients With Differentiated Thyroid Carcinoma
Bianchi R, Iervasi G, Matteucci F, Turchi S, Cazzuola F, Bellina CR, Boni G, Molea N, Ferdeghini M, Toni MG, Mariani G (Univ of Pisa, Italy)
J Nucl Med 34:2032–2037, 1993   124-95-5–8

Introduction.—Serial iodine-131 (^{131}I) whole body scintigraphy (WBS) and serum thyroglobulin (hTg) assay are the conventional forms of follow-up for patients with differentiated thyroid cancer (DTC). The 2 techniques are not entirely sensitive, with a 15% to 20% incidence of discordant results. It may be possible to assay ^{131}I uptake in serum as thyroid products endogenously labeled with ^{131}I, even if the uptake is too low to be detected by WBS. This assumption was tested in a study using chromatography.

Methods.—The study sample comprised 125 patients who were undergoing routine monitoring after complete primary treatment for DTC, i.e., surgery and ^{131}I ablation. Eighty-four were women and 41 were men, with a mean age of 41 years. The chromatographic procedure was performed using a plasma sample taken 72 hours after administration of radioiodine for WBS. This specimen was fractionated on a Sephadex-G25 superfine column by first eluting all radioactive species except for the thyroid hormones then the radioiodothyronines. A combination of at least 3 confirmatory tests (e.g., standard radiographs, thallium-201 scan, positive uptake of therapeutic ^{131}I, and MRI) was the gold standard against which WBS, hTg, and chromatography were compared.

Diagnostic Performance Values (Bayesian Approach) of the 3 Tests Considered Either Singly or in Various Combinations (Values Given as Percentages)

	Sensitivity	Specificity	Accuracy	Positive predictive value	Negative predictive value
[131]I WBS	90.6	95.1	92.8	95.1	90.6
Serum hTg	60.9	100.0	80.0	100.0	70.9
Chromatography	98.4	100.0	99.2	100.0	98.4
[131]I WBS + Serum hTg	92.2	95.1	93.6	95.2	92.1
[131]I WBS + Chromatography	98.4	95.1	96.8	95.5	98.3
Chromatography + Serum hTg	100.0	100.0	100.0	100.0	100.0
[131]I WBS + Serum hTg + Chromatography	100.0	95.1	97.6	95.5	100.0

(Courtesy of Bianchi R, Iervasi G, Matteucci F, et al: *J Nucl Med* 34:2032–2037, 1993.)

Results.—Forty-nine percent of the patients were free of residual functioning thyroid tissue. Most of the remaining patients had benign thyroid tissue and were positive on chromatography; recurrent tumor was excluded by other means. Sensitivity in detecting functioning thyroid tissue was 98.4% for chromatography vs. 90.6% for WBS. Specificity was 100% and 95.1%, respectively, and accuracy was 99.2% vs. 92.8%. For hTg, sensitivity was 60.9%, specificity was 100%, and accuracy was 80%. With the combination of chromatography and hTg, sensitivity, specificity, and accuracy were all 100% (table).

Conclusion.—Chromatography for identification of endogenously radioiodinated thyroid hormones after ^{131}I WBS is a valuable addition to conventional procedures for the follow-up of patients with DTC. It is a very sensitive test for assessing the results of ^{131}I ablation of postsurgical residual thyroid tissue. The chromatographic method yielded no false positive results in this cohort.

▶ Bianchi et al. describe a relatively simple technique for determining the presence of endogenously radioiodinated thyroid hormones in the plasma after WBS of patients whose thyroid tissue has been ablated.

If the significance of circulating thyroid hormone in relation to therapy, as discussed in the preceding article (Abstract 124-95-5–7) can be confirmed, this technique could have a very important place. It also raises some serious questions. Samuel and associates tell us that there was no evidence of residual thyroid tissue in their patients, but this article suggests that it may be possible to detect radioiodinated thyroid hormone in patients in whom whole body imaging does not reveal any evidence of residual functioning tissue. On the other hand, it may be possible that the iodinated hormone they measured was coming from undetected metastases.

These 2 articles raise some interesting questions that may exert some influence on our procedures for the follow-up and evaluation of patients with thyroid cancer.—M.D. Blaufox, M.D., Ph.D.

Serum Thyroglobulin and Iodine-131 Whole-Body Scan in the Diagnosis and Assessment of Treatment for Metastatic Differentiated Thyroid Carcinoma
Lubin E, Mechlis-Frish S, Zatz S, Shimoni A, Segal K, Avraham A, Levy R, Feinmesser R (Beilinson Med Ctr, Petah Tiqva, Israel; Tel Aviv Univ, Israel)
J Nucl Med 35:257–262, 1994   124-95-5–9

Background.—For decades, patients who had undergone thyroidectomy for differentiated thyroid carcinoma (DTC) underwent periodic iodine-131 (^{131}I) whole body scanning. This approach has numerous disadvantages, including the need to suspend therapy for 6 weeks, question-

---

Results of ^{131}I Whole Body Scan

261 Ablated Patients

WBS	Metastasis Present		Absent
Positive	32		0
Negative	26		203
Sensitivity		55%	
Specificity		100%	
Accuracy		90%	

(Courtesy of Lubin E, Mechlis-Frish S, Zatz S, et al: *J Nucl Med* 35:257–262, 1994.)

able sensitivity, and low yield in detecting metastases. Experience with serum thyroglobulin (TG) in a series of 261 consecutive patients with DTC who had undergone total thyroidectomy and ablation was reported.

Methods.—The patients included 178 females and 83 males with histologically confirmed DTC. The mean follow-up was 8 years. Treatment was with near-total thyroidectomy and ablation with ^{131}I, on the basis of the postoperative evaluation. The serum TG was periodically measured using a noncompetitive immunoradiometric assay with no reduction in replacement therapy. Iodine-131 whole body scanning was performed after replacement therapy was suspended for 6 weeks or when thyroid-stimulating hormone (TSH) increased higher than 50 μU/mL. When radiologic procedures were performed with iodinated contrast media, patients waited 10 or more weeks before undergoing ^{131}I whole body scanning.

Results.—Of the 208 patients with serum TG consistently less than 10 ng/mL, 201 had no signs of metastases and were considered to be true negatives. Fifty-eight patients with proven metastases were followed for a mean of 7 years. Eighty-eight percent of them had high serum TG assays while they were receiving full replacement therapy. Iodine-131 whole body scanning localization was clear in 55% of these patients (table). In no instance did a patient with a positive whole body scan have a negative serum TG determination.

Conclusion.—Serum TG had a sensitivity of 88%, a specificity of 99%, and an accuracy of 97% in the recognition of metastases among DTC-ablated patients. The recommended protocol for evaluation of patients with DTC after surgery and ablation was clinical examination every 6 months for the first 3 years and yearly thereafter. In addition, serum TSH and TG measurements were taken at each visit, ultrasound of the neck was done yearly for the first 3 years and every 2 years thereafter, and chest radiography was done every 2 years. When any of these procedures raised the suspicion of active disease, ^{131}I whole body scanning was indicated.

▶ Lubin et al. describe a detailed, extensive experience with a more conventional and accepted means of assessing the diagnosis and treatment of metastatic DTC. Certainly, serial measurements of TG are much simpler than the methodology suggested in the preceding articles (Abstracts 124-95-5–7 and 124-95-5–8) and may be used as an indication for whole body scintigraphy.

Although TG measurements are highly specific, their sensitivity is only 88%. Some patients with metastases clearly are missed if TG is used as the sole marker. The supplementary techniques the authors recommend are ultrasound and chest radiography. Some consideration should also apparently be given to the measurement of thyroid hormone after whole body scintigraphy in an effort to bring the sensitivity closer to 100%.—M.D. Blaufox, M.D., Ph.D.

False-Positive Thyroid Cancer Metastasis on Whole-Body Radioiodine Scanning Due to Retained Radioactivity in the Oesophagus

Bakheet S, Hammami MM (King Faisal Specialist Hosp and Research Centre, Riyadh, Saudi Arabia)

Eur J Nucl Med 20:415–419, 1993   124-95-5–10

Introduction.—Most often the appearance of radioiodine uptake in the mediastinum in a patient with differentiated thyroid cancer signifies metastatic disease. Fifteen recent whole body radioiodine scans demonstrated a total of 19 mediastinal artifacts that resembled nodal or spinal metastases, but the artifacts resolved on delayed images that were acquired after eating and drinking or when the study was repeated within 1 week.

Methods.—Whole body radioiodine scans are made with 5 mCi of iodine-123, 4–6 weeks after withdrawing thyroxine. Six spot images are acquired within 10 minutes, starting 24 hours after nuclide ingestion in the form of a single capsule.

Findings.—The areas of radioiodine activity resembled metastases in the lymph nodes or spine (Fig 5–2). Seventeen foci of activity disap-

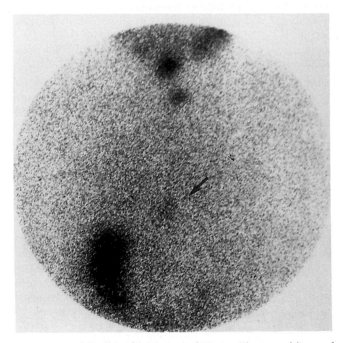

Fig 5–2.—Posterior view of the chest of a woman, aged 70 years. The *arrow* delineates focal activity in the lower mediastinum mimicking spinal metastasis. (Courtesy of Bakheet S, Hammami MM: *Eur J Nucl Med* 20:415–419, 1993.)

peared completely after the patient ate and drank, and 2 were absent when the study was repeated within 1 week of initial imaging.

Implications.—A falsely positive appearance of mediastinal radioiodine uptake is fairly frequent in patients with thyroid cancer and probably represents transient radioactivity in a normal esophagus. Further images acquired after drinking and eating should clarify the picture.

▶ The problems of artifacts in all the scanning procedures that we do are serious and numerous. Although it would seem improbable that the experienced observer would be misled by activity in the gastrointestinal system, it certainly is not out of the realm of possibility. These cases underscore an important point: Failure to recognize this possibility could certainly result in inappropriate treatment, especially in a busy nuclear medicine department if an inadequate number of views are obtained. Once again, this emphasizes that the technologist must perform the scan with close interaction with the nuclear medicine physician to carry out whatever additional maneuvers are necessary to clarify the findings.—M.D. Blaufox, M.D., Ph.D.

Diagnostic Use of Recombinant Human Thyrotropin in Patients With Thyroid Carcinoma (Phase I/II Study)
Meier CA, Braverman LE, Ebner SA, Veronikis I, Daniels GH, Ross DS, Deraska DJ, Davies TF, Valentine M, DeGroot LJ, Curran P, McEllin K, Reynolds J, Robbins J, Weintraub BD (NIH, Bethesda, Md; Univ of Massachusetts, Worcester; Massachusetts Gen Hosp, Boston; et al)
J Clin Endocrinol Metab 78:188–196, 1994   124-95-5-11

Background.—Radioiodine uptake and serum thyroglobulin (Tg) levels are the studies currently used to detect residual or metastatic thyroid tissue in patients with differentiated thyroid carcinoma. Both of these studies require that the patient be sufficiently hypothyroid for adequate endogenous thyroid-stimulating hormone (TSH) stimulation; nearly all

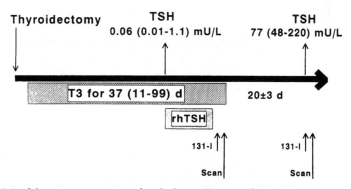

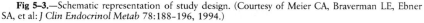
Fig 5–3.—Schematic representation of study design. (Courtesy of Meier CA, Braverman LE, Ebner SA, et al: *J Clin Endocrinol Metab* 78:188–196, 1994.)

patients have clinical hypothyroid symptoms during this period. With the use of recombinant human TSH (rhTSH), iodine-131 (^{131}I) uptake and Tg release can be stimulated from residual thyroid tissue in patients who are euthyroid.

Methods.—The safety, dosage, and efficacy of rhTSH in 19 patients with differentiated thyroid carcinoma were examined. The patients had recently undergone thyroidectomy and were receiving suppressive doses of triiodothyronine (T_3). They received 10–40-unit doses of rhTSH for 1–3 days. The day after the last dose, they were given 1–2 mCi of ^{131}I, followed 48 hours later by a neck and whole body scan. Triiodothyronine was discontinued for a median of 19 days, resulting in marked elevation of endogenous serum TSH levels. A second dose of ^{131}I was then given, followed 48 hours later by a repeat whole body scan (Fig 5–3).

Results.—There were no major adverse effects of rhTSH, although 16% of the patients who received the higher doses reported nausea. Psychometric measures of quality of life were much better during rhTSH treatment than after T_3 withdrawal. Serum TSH peaked 2–8 hours after rhTSH injection, to 127 mU/L with the 10-unit dose, 309 mU/L with the 20-unit dose, and 510 mU/L with the 30-unit dose. Twenty-four hours after injection, TSH levels decreased to 83, 173, and 463 mU/L, respectively.

In 63% of the patients, both thyroid scans were of similar quality and showed a similar number of abnormal ^{131}I uptake sites. Sixteen percent of the patients had additional uptake sites in the chest and thyroid bed on the rhTSH scan that were not visible on the hypothyroid scan. Another 16% had additional lesions shown only after T_3 withdrawal. One patient had an uptake focus that was better demonstrated after rhTSH than after withdrawal. The scan made after rhTSH showed a lower amount of radioiodine uptake in the thyroid bed in 68% of the patients. However, after correction for the increased whole body retention of ^{131}I during hypothyroidism, uptake was comparable to that after T_3 withdrawal. Nearly three fourths of the patients had at least twice the serum Tg levels in response to rhTSH; the same patients had a similar Tg response to T_3 withdrawal. In all but 1 of these, the increase was quantitatively lower after rhTSH.

Conclusion.—Preliminary data suggest that rhTSH is a safe and effective method of stimulating ^{131}I uptake and Tg secretion without causing symptoms of hypothyroidism. The optimal dose regimen of rhTSH would appear to be 10–20 units/day given during 1 or more days before radioiodine administration. Proof of the efficacy of rhTSH awaits a phase III trial.

▶ In patients with thyroid disease, TSH has always been a potentially useful modality that is fraught with many difficulties. Now we have the era of recombinant gene technology and a new source of human thyrotropin. Meier et al. presented a promising use of rhTSH in patients with thyroid carcinoma.

It is particularly noteworthy that in their experience, this drug appeared to be safe and was effective in stimulating ^{131}I uptake and Tg secretion without the need for or disadvantage of inducing hypothyroidism.—M.D. Blaufox, M.D., Ph.D.

Assessment of the Efficacy of Iodine-131 for Thyroid Ablation
Comtois R, Thériault C, Del Vecchio P (Univ of Montreal)
J Nucl Med 34:1927–1930, 1993   124-95-5–12

Purpose.—Iodine-131 ablation of residual thyroid tissue is customary in patients who have undergone near-total thyroidectomy for thyroid carcinoma. However, opinions differ as to which patients should receive iodine-131 and at what doses; the trend has been toward lower doses. The effectiveness of thyroid ablation using 1,110 MBq of iodine-131 was evaluated.

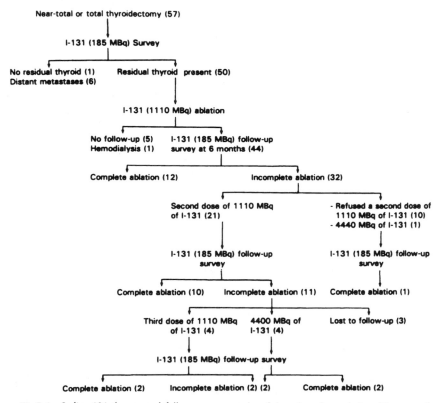

Fig 5–4.—Iodine-131 therapy and follow-up scan results of the selected population. (Courtesy of Comtois R, Thériault C, Del Vecchio P: *J Nucl Med* 34:1927–1930, 1993.)

Methods.—The study included 57 patients who underwent near-total thyroidectomy for papillary, mixed, or follicular thyroid carcinoma. Four months later, after 5–6 weeks of withdrawal of L-thyroxine, the patients underwent whole body scanning with 185 MBq of iodine-131, with planimetry of the thyroid scan used to measure residual thyroid area. Ablation therapy using a 1,110-MBq dose of iodine-131 was performed within 5 days in all patients except 6 who had distant metastases and 1 with no residual thyroid tissue. All but 6 of these patients were followed up 6 months later with repeat iodine-131 scanning (Fig 5–4).

Results.—Ablation was successful in 27% of the patients. The total body area was smaller in patients with total thyroid ablation, 1.63 vs. 1.83 m², as was residual thyroid tissue, 1.4 vs. 2 cm². Patients with successful ablation were also somewhat less likely to have associated goiter, 11% vs. 40%. The total thyroid ablation was achieved in 53% of the patients with 1 or more of the following characteristics: total body area less than 1.9 m², residual thyroid tissue less than 2.1 cm², and no associated previous diffuse or multinodular goiter. By contrast, ablation was successful in only 11% of the patients without these characteristics.

Conclusion.—A single, 1,110-MBq dose of iodine-131 is sufficient to achieve ablation of a functioning thyroid remnant in more than one fourth of the patients after near-total thyroidectomy. Total ablation is more likely in patients with a lower total body area, smaller residual thyroid tissue, and no associated previous diffuse or multinodular goiter. Other patients may need higher iodine-131 doses to achieve total ablation.

▶ Given a patient with thyroid cancer, how much thyroid should be removed? Should the remaining tissue be ablated with radioiodine therapy? How much radioiodine therapy should the patient be given? These questions have almost an infinite number of answers. The rationale (or lack of rationale) of dealing with residual thyroid tissue has been a problem almost since radioiodine was first introduced to treat thyroid cancer.

These authors report their experience using an ablative dose that is at the low end for post-thyroidectomy remnant ablation. Only 27% of the patients were ablated successfully, which does not attest very well to the use of this low dose, which we abandoned at Montefiore many years ago. However, the authors describe some of the characteristics that increase the likelihood of successful ablation with a low dose, which might be worth considering in some circumstances.—M.D. Blaufox, M.D., Ph.D.

Peripheral Facial Nerve Palsy After High-Dose Radioiodine Therapy in Patients With Papillary Thyroid Carcinoma

Levenson D, Gulec S, Sonenberg M, Lai E, Goldsmith SJ, Larson SM (Mem

Sloan-Kettering Cancer Ctr, New York)
Ann Intern Med 120:576–578, 1994   124-95-5-13

Introduction.—Sialoadenitis is a common complication of radioiodine therapy, but an extensive MEDLINE search failed to reveal any association between such treatment and facial nerve palsy. Two patients had parotitis and facial palsy develop after receiving radioiodine.

Case 1.—Man, 51, with locally invasive papillary thyroid carcinoma had a recurrence 19 years after thyroidectomy. After his second operation, he received 29 mCi of iodine-131 (^{131}I). His parotid glands became markedly engorged and tender within 24 hours. He lost his taste sensation, and, after 9 days, a partial right peripheral facial palsy developed. Prednisone was given for 5 days, and facial nerve function was nearly normal at 3 months although xerostomia persisted.

Case 2.—Man, 60, who had locally invasive papillary cancer of the thyroid, received an estimated radiation dose to the thyroid cancer of 13,400 rad and a blood dose of 200 rad from ^{131}I. Mild parotid tenderness developed, as well as a right peripheral facial palsy, which almost completely resolved within the ensuing months.

Discussion.—Inflammation of the facial nerve might have led to peripheral facial paralysis in these patients. An alternative cause is direct radiation injury of the facial nerve.

▶ Many of us tend to regard radioiodine therapy as an extremely well tolerated procedure with remarkably few adverse effects. Certainly, we do not often think of the development of facial nerve palsy after radioiodine therapy. It is a disturbing complication, but, fortunately, the patients appear to have regained most of their neurologic function. Although it is possible that the development of Bell's palsy was coincidental and not directly related to the radiation, these cases reports should remind us that we should not take the safety of the use of radioactive materials for granted. Although remarkably well tolerated and certainly preferable to many alternative procedures, the administration of high doses of radioactivity has risks.—M.D. Blaufox, M.D. Ph.D.

Intraoperative Detection of Pheochromocytoma With Iodine-125 Labelled *Meta*-Iodobenzylguanidine: A Feasibility Study

Ricard M, Tenenbaum F, Schlumberger M, Travagli J-P, Lumbroso J, Revillon Y, Parmentier C (Institut Gustave-Roussy, Villejuif, France; Hôpital Necker, Paris)
Eur J Nucl Med 20:426–430, 1993   124-95-5-14

Background.—Surgical removal of neoplastic tissue is the most effective treatment for pheochromocytoma. Radiolabeled preoperative probes are useful for localizing osteoid osteoma, thyroid carcinoma, and neuroendocrine tumors, particularly in patients with ectopic or unusual localization. Radiolabeled *meta*-iodobenzylguanidine (mIBG) and surgical treatment for pheochromocytoma in 6 patients with significant mIBG tumor uptake were described.

Clinical Procedure.—Before surgery, tumor foci were localized scintigraphically using mIBG labeled with iodine-123. Single-photon emission CT was performed when required for precise localization; data were superimposed on CT scans. Precise uptake sites were noted using skin marks or internal structures such as bones. Forty-eight hours before surgery, Lugol's solution was administered to suppress thyroid iodine uptake; then, mIBG labeled with iodine-125 was injected. Iodine-125 doses ranged from 740 kBq to 37 MBq, based on probe sensitivity. Tumor counting rates were noted before and after surgical excision. The reference activity level was measured in blood from large vessels. Urinary metanephrine excretion was measured before and 90 days after surgery.

Results.—Tumor foci were found in all cases. Count rates, obtained with the CdTe detector, were 10–50 counts s^{-1} for blood background; ∼40 to more than 1,000 counts s^{-1} before excision; 5–100 counts s^{-1} after excision. The before-after counting rate ratio was ∼4 to more than 25.

Conclusion.—The hypothesis that all tumor foci concentrate the tracer was supported. The use of mIBG labeled with iodine-125 and a miniaturized CdTe probe is a feasible reoperation procedure in pheochromocytoma.

▶ Although the decision to use radioactive materials in the operating suite is not simple, there are many potential advantages. Iodine-125 is relatively safe because of the low energy of its emission, and when it is used with a miniaturized CdTe probe, it may have a role in the localization of certain tumors that are difficult to locate during surgery. Certainly, it may help reduce the operating time and the associated surgical morbidity. In this situation, labeling MIBG with ^{125}I proved to be useful in the localization of pheochromocytoma intraoperatively. Other intraoperative procedures, including localization of melanoma of the eye, have used radionuclides, and, more recently, radiolabeled antibodies were used to localize tumors that show antibody uptake.

Although preoperative localization is surely highly preferred, there certainly are and will continue to be situations where techniques such as this may play an important role in leading the surgeon toward a successful removal of some type of space-occupying lesion that is difficult to find through simple palpation.—M.D. Blaufox, M.D., Ph.D.

Intraperitoneal Distribution Imaging Prior to Chromic Phosphate (P-32) Therapy in Ovarian Cancer Patients
Tulchinsky M, Eggli DF (Milton S Hershey Med Ctr/Penn State Univ Hosp,

Hershey, Pa)
Clin Nucl Med 19:43–48, 1994   124-95-5–15

Background.—Intraperitoneal distribution imaging (IDI) with technetium-labeled sulfur colloid has been used in patients with malignant ascites at the time that phosphate-32–labeled chromic phosphate is instilled. About 1 L of ascitic fluid is left in place, but it appears that intraperitoneal loculation of the nuclide may be associated with significant side effects. There is increasing evidence that chromic phosphate is an effective measure in some patients with localized ovarian cancer.

Literature Search.—A MEDLINE search revealed only 11 articles that dealt with the technical aspects of IDI. No consistency was observed in the techniques used among the various groups of investigators.

Personal Experience.—Eight patients with ovarian cancer had 1 L of normal saline and 1 mCi of technetium-labeled sulfur colloid infused intraperitoneally for IDI. All completed the standard IDI protocol, and none had complaints during or after the procedure. All patients had free peritoneal distribution of radionuclide. Loculation was noted in 1 patient who had had only 250 mL of saline infused, but free intraperitoneal distribution was observed when the study was repeated using the standard high-volume approach.

Technical Aspects.—Effective intraperitoneal chemotherapy requires that the entire peritoneal surface be exposed to the therapeutic agent. Consistent results can be obtained with IDI when a total of 1 L of fluid is instilled and when 500 mL of normal saline is administered before infusion of the radionuclide.

▶ As often happens with procedures that appear to be very simple and straightforward, there is very little in the literature concerning them. This of course is related to the medical profession's fascination with zebras, whereas large herds of cows and obvious but extremely important problems receive relatively little attention.

The authors have nicely formalized IDI by reviewing the methodology and some of the important problems that can be associated with it. In particular, they point out the potential for mistakenly diagnosing a loculation if an insufficient amount of saline is used for the technetium sulfur colloid distribution study. Such an error could have important therapeutic implications.—M.D. Blaufox, M.D., Ph.D.

Positron Emission Tomography of Thyroid Masses

Adler LP, Bloom AD (Univ Hosps of Cleveland, Ohio)
Thyroid 3:195–200, 1993   124-95-5–16

Background.—Improvements in diagnostic techniques have reduced the number of patients with thyroid nodules who undergo surgical excision. Malignancy rates in recently reported surgical series have improved from 20% to 45%. The value of PET using [^{18}F]2-deoxy-2-fluoro-D-glucose (FDG) for the differential diagnosis of thyroid nodules was examined.

Methods.—The study sample included 9 patients, 7 with solitary thyroid nodules and 2 with dominant nodules in multinodular goiters. Surgical resection was planned in all patients because of the suspicion of carcinoma. The patients underwent PET after administration of FDG. The reconstructed images were subjected to both subjective and quantitative analysis.

Results.—Four of the lesions were follicular adenomas, 3 were papillary carcinomas, and 2 were multinodular goiters. Two of the cancers were seen as areas of intensely increased FDG accumulation; the third was very small, resulting in reduced apparent uptake. Four of the 6 benign lesions also appeared as areas of increased FDG uptake. Visual analysis alone did not distinguish the malignant from the benign lesions. The mean dose uptake ratio (DUR)—calculated by adjusting the FDG uptake for the patient's weight and net dose administered—was higher in the malignant lesions: The DUR was more than 8.5 in all 3 cancers and less than 6.5 in all 6 benign lesions. The 2 categories of benign lesions showed no difference in DUR.

Conclusion.—This preliminary study yielded promising results with PET for the differential diagnosis of thyroid nodules. If PET could be offered selectively to patients with suspicious cytologic findings, it could avoid surgery in some of those with benign disease and facilitate definitive surgery in those with malignancies. Further research is needed to confirm the ability of FDG PET to discriminate between benign and malignant follicular neoplasms.

▶ The use of PET to differentiate thyroid cancer from benign disease would seem at first to be a little like using an elephant to kill an ant. However, the authors suggest that the technique has some promise, and, on second thought, it may have real clinical potential.

To consider its value, you must compare the cost of PET with the cost of thyroid surgery. Once surgery becomes involved, patient management gets considerably more expensive. If a significant number of patients could be spared surgery by having PET instead, it would more than justify itself in terms of cost. Unfortunately, the world tends to look only at the price of the procedure and not at the price of alternative procedures; this is another example. Positron emission tomography has the potential to be a highly cost-effective procedure.—M.D. Blaufox, M.D., Ph.D.

The Effect of Fine-Needle Aspiration Biopsy on the Thyroid Scan
Gordon DL, Wagner R, Dillehay GL, Khedkar N, Martinez CJ, Bayer W, Brooks MH (Loyola Univ of Chicago, Maywood, Ill; Lutheran Gen Hosp, Park

Ridge, III)
Clin Nucl Med 18:495–497, 1993   124-95-5–17

Introduction.—Fine-needle aspiration biopsy (FNAB) is currently used for preoperative distinction between benign and malignant thyroid disease. Although it is assumed that FNAB will not alter the isotope uptake pattern on a thyroid scan, the effect of the biopsy procedure on the scan pattern has not been evaluated. Thyroid scans were performed on 11 patients before and after FNAB and were compared to determine whether a change in the scan pattern occurred.

Methods.—After a thyroid scan with either technetium-99m or iodine-123 isotopes, FNAB was performed on 11 patients with nodular thyroid disease. The biopsy was directed at the area that on scan revealed increased isotope uptake (e.g., a hot or warm nodule or an enlarged lobe with an increased isotope uptake). After the FNAB, the thyroid scan was repeated within 7 weeks (mean, 10 days) using the same isotope; the patterns of isotope distribution on the scans taken before and after FNAB were compared.

Results.—In 9 patients, post-FNAB thyroid scans did not reveal a change in the pattern of isotope uptake compared with initial thyroid scans. However, changes were seen in the post-FNAB thyroid scans of 2 patients. One patient, who had a cytologic diagnosis of colloid goiter, had a decrease in isotope uptake in 2 areas of the thyroid scan that had contained 2 warm nodules (Fig 5–5); 1 needle aspiration had been performed on each of these nodules. In the second patient, a nodule that had been aspirated 3 times showed a decrease in isotope uptake.

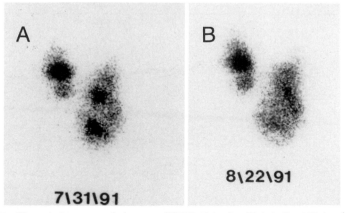

Fig 5–5.—Change in isotope uptake because of FNAB of the thyroid. **A,** iodine-123 thyroid scan of a colloid goiter before FNAB showing a nodule in the right lobe and 2 nodules in the left lobe that concentrate isotope more densely than the remainder of the gland. **B,** 1 day after FNAB of the thyroid, the 2 nodules in the left lobe fail to demonstrate increased radioiodine concentration. (Courtesy of Gordon DL, Wagner R, Dillehay GL, et al: *Clin Nucl Med* 18:495–497, 1993.)

Conclusion.—Fine-needle aspiration biopsy altered the isotope uptake on a thyroid scan in 2 of 11 patients studied. The change in isotope uptake after FNAB might have affected the management of these patients if the nodules had represented only the uptake in a follicular neoplasm rather than in colloid goiters. Hemorrhage, necrosis, and infarction are possible effects of FNAB, any of which can alter the scan pattern of a thyroid nodule. To avoid possible changes in the isotope uptake of thyroid nodules, radionuclide scanning should be performed before FNAB.

▶ I included this article because the point it makes seems so obvious that it could be the subject of an article. I would think that under most circumstances no one would attempt a thyroid scan in a patient who has recently had a needle inserted into that thyroid. The physician would have anticipated that the insertion of the needle, with its associated bleeding and inflammatory response, no matter how minimal, could have an effect on the reliability of the scan.

The authors have proven that this common-sense assumption is indeed correct. It would seem to me that it should be a given in nuclear medicine that any type of intervention in a patient before radionuclide imaging may have an adverse effect on the accuracy of our procedures.—M.D. Blaufox, M.D., Ph.D.

Call Mosby Document Express at **1 (800) 55-MOSBY** to obtain copies of the original source documents of articles featured or referenced in the YEAR BOOK series.

6 Renal

Introduction

Progress in nuclear medicine appears to be moving in leaps and bounds rather than in steady increments. During the last several years, we have seen major innovations in the nephrologic applications of radionuclides. Now, we appear to have entered a phase of consolidation, and the advances are somewhat less dramatic.

There still is a major lack of material in the area of urinary tract infection. I am convinced this is an extremely important application of radionuclide methodology that has been sadly neglected.

Another area where there is need for continuing study and innovation is diuretic renography. As with most areas in nephrology, we associate the work in the field with only a few names. More investigators need to become interested in this area and to take advantage of its unrealized potential.

M. Donald Blaufox, M.D., Ph.D.

First Experience in Healthy Volunteers With Technetium-99m L,L-Ethylenedicysteine, a New Renal Imaging Agent
Van Nerom CG, Bormans GM, De Roo MJ, Verbruggen AM (U Z Gasthuisberg, Leuven, Belgium)
Eur J Nucl Med 20:738–746, 1993   124-95-6–1

Introduction.—Studies in animals suggest that technetium-99m L,L-ethylenedicysteine (^{99m}Tc-L,L-EC) is a potentially useful radioactive tracer for renal function studies. It is easily prepared, has a long shelf life, and shows negligible uptake by surrounding tissues. The initial results with ^{99m}Tc-L,L-EC in humans were described.

Methods.—Six healthy men were used to compare ^{99m}Tc-L,L-EC and ^{99m}Tc mercaptoacetyltriglycine (MAG$_3$). Dynamic kidney and bladder images were obtained for up to 30 minutes after IV injection of either tracer, 18.5 MBq, with 1.85 MBq of iodine-131 O-iodohippurate in 2 mL of saline as an internal biological standard. Regions of interest in the kidneys and background activity were compared, and plasma radioactivity was measured with both radiotracers at intervals ranging from 2 to 60 minutes.

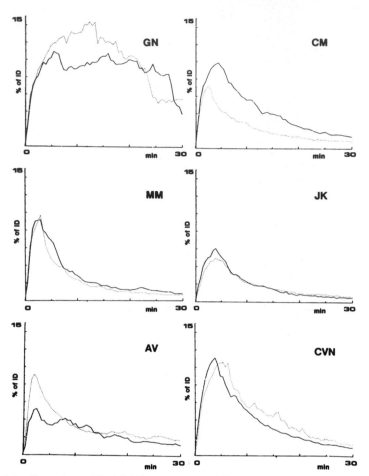

Fig 6–1.—Comparison of the left kidney renograms of ^{99m}Tc-MAG$_3$ (*solid line*) and ^{99m}Tc–L,L-EC (*dotted line*) in the 6 volunteers. (Courtesy of Van Nerom CG, Bormans GM, De Roo MJ, et al: *Eur J Nucl Med* 20:738–746, 1993.)

Results.—Analogue images taken with the 2 tracers were of equal diagnostic values, and the renograms were similar in all men (Fig 6–1). The mean plasma clearance was 382.9 mL/min/1.73 m² with ^{99m}Tc-MAG$_3$ vs. 460.2 mL/min/1.73 m² with ^{99m}Tc–L,L-EC. Urinary excretion values were 69.4% vs. 66.5% of the injected dose at 30 minutes and 83.1% vs. 79.8% at 60 minutes, respectively. Plasma protein binding of ^{99m}Tc-L,L-EC was 31% vs. 88% for ^{99m}Tc-MAG$_3$. In addition, the volume of distribution was greater with ^{99m}Tc–L,L-EC.

Conclusion.—The ^{99m}Tc–L,L-EC combination is a very promising new radiotracer for functional kidney evaluation. The exact mechanism of its high plasma clearance is unknown, but further studies in patients are warranted.

▶ Ethylenedicysteine made its appearance around 1992. Since that time, it has moved rapidly from the laboratory to trials in humans. Its physiologic action appears to be quite interesting, and it compares favorably with ^{99m}Tc-MAG$_3$. However, MAG$_3$ has the advantages of being the first approved technetium-labeled tubular agent in the United States and extensive distribution throughout Europe. For ethylenedicysteine to establish a place in the evaluation of renal disease with radionuclides, it will be necessary for the investigators either to demonstrate its superiority in some application or its economic advantage. We await further clarification of these issues.—M.D. Blaufox, M.D., Ph.D.

The Variability of Processing of Technetium-99m DTPA Renography: Role of Interpolative Background Subtraction
Hurwitz GA, Champagne CL, Gravelle DR, Smith FJ, Powe JE (Univ of Western Ontario, London, Canada; Victoria Hosp, London, Ont, Canada)
Clin Nucl Med 18:273–277, 1993   124-95-6–2

Introduction.—The performance of quantitative renography could potentially be improved by the application of interpolative background subtraction (IBS). The potential benefits of IBS as applied to technetium-99m (^{99m}Tc) DTPA renography were assessed.

Methods.—Seventy-six patients with hypertension underwent ^{99m}Tc scintigraphy for evaluation of possible renal arterial stenosis. After rapid bolus injections of 300–700 MBq of ^{99m}Tc-DTPA, differential renal uptake was measured by considering the integrated counts during the 1–3 minute interval after injection. Using a routine method for differential function, the counts in each kidney were corrected for background subtraction using an operator-selected crescentic region lateral to each kidney. A 1–3-minute integrated image and commercial software for the

Differential Renal Function With DTPA: Normal Values in 24
Patients With Hypertension in Series A

Technique	Mean (% left)	Normal Range (% left)	Replication* (r value)
Routine BGS	52	46–58	0.89
No BGS	51	44–57	0.95
Interpolative BGS	51	43–59	0.98
Early (1–2 min)	52	44–61	0.79

Abbreviation: BGS, background subtraction.
* Each value was performed twice and averaged.
(Courtesy of Hurwitz GA, Champagne CL, Gravelle DR, et al: *Clin Nucl Med* 18:273–277, 1993.)

quantitation of myocardial images with thallium-201 were used to apply the IBS technique separately to each kidney. The same renal outlines as were used for the routine analysis were used to calculate differential uptake without background subtraction. The software program also simultaneously calculated background-subtracted uptake on the integrated 1–2-minute data. A renographic 3-sample slope/intercept technique was used for simultaneous determination of the glomerular filtration rate.

Results.—In a series of patients with normal renal anatomy, each method yielded a mean value for left renal function that was slightly greater than 50% of the total (table). Use of IBS or omission of background subtraction yielded a slightly narrower range of normal. Although correlation between the sets of repeated measures was reasonable with all techniques, the use of IBS more closely replicated the values. Replicability was lessened by use of only the 1–2-minute data.

In another test set, the use of IBS reduced the standard deviation by 51% in the patients with normal renal arteries, by 26% in those with unilateral stenosis, and by 58% in those with bilateral stenoses. Correlations between the mean values obtained by the routine technique vs. any other were very good although omission of background subtraction during the 1–3-minute uptake phase resulted in a slope of the line that was significantly lower than 1. In the same set of patients, the IBS and routine techniques were closely correlated.

Conclusion.—Use of the IBS technique could reduce the variability of measurements made in ^{99m}Tc-DTPA renography. The IBS method preserves the depiction of renal asymmetry and performs better in the case of reduced renal function. The technique could be highly valuable in assessing the effects of drug treatment, angioplasty, or surgical revascularization, especially in patients with overall impairment of renal function.

▶ To subtract or not to subtract, that is the question. Whether it be nobler to suffer the slings and arrows of no background subtraction and so on, and so on, and so on. Hurwitz et al. advocate an interpolative method for background subtraction. However, I am not convinced that the background subtraction problem has indeed been solved. Until someone can demonstrate a really significant difference in diagnostic capability through background subtraction and that the background being subtracted improves results and corresponds to the real background, it remains a method for massaging the data. Although improved precision of any technique is certainly highly desirable, the goal we all seek is improved accuracy.—M.D. Blaufox, M.D., Ph.D.

Measurement of Normal Renal Artery Blood Flow: Cine Phase-Contrast MR Imaging vs Clearance of *p*-Aminohippurate
Wolf RL, King BF, Torres VE, Wilson DM, Ehman RL (Mayo Clinic and Found, Rochester, Minn)
AJR 161:995–1002, 1993   124-95-6–3

Background.—One disadvantage of determining renal blood flow measurements based on renal clearance of *p*-aminohippurate is that the kidneys are not studied separately. In addition, temporal resolution is poor, and normal renal function is required. A reliable quantitative, noninvasive technique for assessing renal hemodynamics would be useful for investigating renal vascular diseases and the effects of treatment. Cine phase-contrast MRI was compared with renal clearance of *p*-aminohippurate, which is currently defined as the gold standard test for measurement of normal renal blood flow.

Participants and Methods.—Ten healthy volunteers were included in the study. Bilateral oblique and sagittal cine phase-contrast MRIs were simultaneously acquired. Imaging planes were oriented perpendicular to the left and right renal arteries to measure through-plane flow. Velocity encoding was 150 cm/sec in 7 of the 10 and 100 cm/sec in 8 of the 10 participants. The selection of MRI parameters for flow measurements was based on studies that showed appropriate spatial resolution and imaging plane perpendicular to the flow axis are the most critical controllable elements for reducing errors. In 6 participants, axial cine phase-contrast images of the abdominal aorta above and below the origin of the renal arteries were obtained. In these instances, renal blood flow was evaluated by measuring the difference between suprarenal and infrarenal aortic flow. Immediately after MRI measurements, renal clearance of *p*-aminohippurate was determined in all participants.

Results.—Renal blood flow measurements obtained with cine phase-contrast MRI closely paralleled those obtained using clearance of *p*-aminohippurate (Fig 6–2). The mean difference at a velocity encoding of 150 cm/sec was 69 mL/min. At a velocity encoding of 100 cm/sec, the mean difference was 39 mL/min. Aortic flow measurements with cine phase-contrast MRI were less reliable for assessing renal blood flow than measurements in the individual renal arteries. Compared with renal blood flow determined using clearance of *p*-aminohippurate, a mean difference of −75 mL/min was noted.

Conclusion.—Cine phase-contrast MRI for noninvasive measurement of renal blood flow is a promising technique. Results closely paralleled those obtained using clearance of *p*-aminohippurate. Moreover, the MRI procedure is quicker, can be used to determine unilateral or bilateral renal blood flow, and does not rely on renal function.

▶ Although Wolf et al. clearly know better, they use the term renal blood flow and *p*-aminohippurate (PAH) clearance interchangeably. The clearance of PAH is limited by renal blood flow, but it may be very different from the actual renal blood flow, depending on the extraction fraction of the kidney. Because extraction fraction varies, even in normal individuals, considerable error can occur when renal blood flow is estimated using PAH clearance. The use of PAH clearance to validate a technique for renal blood flow may make this problem even worse, because apples and oranges are being compared.

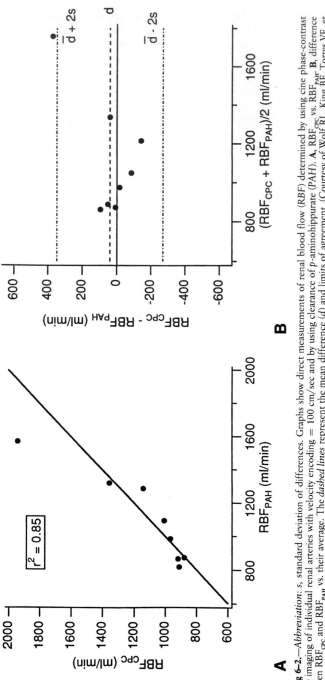

Fig 6-2.—*Abbreviation: s,* standard deviation of differences. Graphs show direct measurements of renal blood flow (RBF) determined by using cine phase-contrast (CPC) imaging of individual renal arteries with velocity encoding = 100 cm/sec and by using clearance of *p*-aminohippurate (PAH). **A,** RBF$_{CPC}$ vs. RBF$_{PAH}$. **B,** difference between RBF$_{CPC}$ and RBF$_{PAH}$ vs. their average. The *dashed lines* represent the mean difference (*d*) and limits of agreement. (Courtesy of Wolf RL, King BF, Torres VE, et al: AJR 161:995–1002, 1993.)

However, this interesting study demonstrates some progress in application of phase-contrast MRI for the measurement of blood flow through the renal arteries. Although the authors correct for the extraction ratio, they make the assumption that it is the same in all individuals. They rightfully correct for the hematocrit, but again, it is the arterial hematocrit that must be corrected and not the venous hematocrit. It is not clear from their article which correction they used, but presumably it was the venous hematocrit.—M.D. Blaufox, M.D., Ph.D.

Improved Formulas for the Estimation of Renal Depth in Adults
Taylor A, Lewis C, Giacometti A, Hall EC, Barefield KP (Emory Univ, Atlanta, Ga)
J Nucl Med 34:1766–1769, 1993   124-95-6–4

Background.—An effective renal plasma flow or the glomerular filtration rate can be calculated by techniques based on the percentage injected dose of technetium-99m DTPA in the kidney 1–2 or 2–3 minutes after injection. These algorithms incorporate the Tonnesen formulas for estimating renal depth, which were derived from ultrasound measurements obtained at an oblique angle in patients who were seated. However, radionuclide renographic studies are generally done with the patient in the supine position.

Methods.—Renal depths calculated by the Tonnesen equations were compared with actual depths measured by CT in 126 patients. Those with obvious abdominal or renal disease were excluded. Renal depth was measured as the distance from the skin to the anterior and posterior surfaces of the kidney at the renal hilum. A set of regressive equations for estimating kidney depth was derived based on age, height, and weight; then the equations were applied prospectively to a new set of 75 patients.

Results.—The calculated renal depth by the Tonnesen formulas tended to underestimate the actual renal depth. Age, height, and weight were the important predictive variables; sex was not predictive. The equations derived from pooling of both data sets were: right renal depth (mm) = 151.3 weight (kg)/height (cm) + .22 age − .77 and left renal depth (mm) = 161.7 weight (kg)/height (cm) + .27 age − 9.4. Correlation coefficients were .81 for the right and .83 for the left kidney; corresponding standard errors of the estimate were 10.1 and 10.2 mm (Fig 6–3).

Conclusion.—New equations, based on CT measurements in supine patients were provided for the estimation of renal depth in adults. These equations give a much better estimate than the widely used Tonnesen equations. A relative uptake measurement outside the 56/44 range is un-

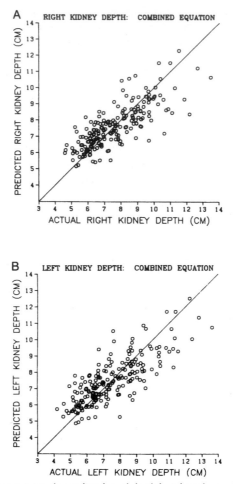

Fig 6–3.—*Solid line* represents the predicted renal depth based on the combined equations for the right (**A**) and left (**B**) kidneys. The *circles* represent the CT-determined depths. (Courtesy of Taylor A, Lewis C, Giacometti A, et al: *J Nucl Med* 34:1766–1769, 1993.)

likely to reflect differences in tissue attenuation caused by differences in renal depth.

▶ Tip Taylor's contributions to the field of renal nuclear medicine have been outstanding. However, in this particular issue, I must disagree with him. Although I believe that the formulas he presents for measurement of renal depth are an improvement over what has been available, they remain an inaccurate way of correcting this problem.

The renal depth will tend to vary from population to population, because there are undoubtedly differences based on race and sex. The actual difference accounted for by these equations is extremely small. Renal depth becomes a real problem in those patients with a significant disparity between the 2 sides. There is no way of predicting which patients these will be, and the formula cannot adequately correct for them. Therefore, it seems to me that there is very little to be gained by correcting for renal depth using a formula, if the goal is to prevent erroneous measurements in patients in whom a significant difference in renal depth exists.—M.D. Blaufox, M.D., Ph.D.

In Vivo Determination of Radiation Dose in Kidneys and Bladder During Renogram: A New Approach

Nikiforidis G, Karatrandou A, Vassilakos P (Univ of Patras, Rio-Patras, Greece)
Nucl Med Commun 14:611–617, 1993   124-95-6-5

Background.—Medical Internal Radiation Dose (MIRD) Committee equations and a reference man are typically used to calculate the radiation dose absorbed by a patient from a radiopharmaceutical. However, these estimations assume that the patient is normal and has the characteristics of the reference man, whereas certain pathologic conditions can present large deviations from normal. A study was conducted using real data to determine the radiation dose in the kidneys and bladder during renography.

Methods and Results.—In the study protocol, processing of frames obtained in the various stages of the renogram permitted measurement of the kidney and bladder mass and the time distribution of radioactivity in these organs (Fig 6–4). The mean dosimetric results for normal renograms agreed with the MIRD estimates of kidney-absorbed dose. However, dose estimation for individuals was very approximate. For some pathologic conditions, including hydronephrosis and bilateral acute tu-

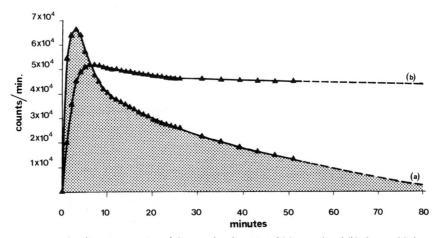

Fig 6–4.—Graphic representation of the cumulated activity of (*a*) normal and (*b*) abnormal kidney during renogram. (Courtesy of Nikiforidis G, Karatrandou A, Vassilakos P: *Nucl Med Commun* 14:611–617, 1993.)

bular necrosis with normal uptake, estimated values were 5–40 times higher than the normative data. The large intrinsic variability in renal function and mass associated with these diseases was confirmed by the high value of the standard deviation for dose absorbed by the kidneys.

Conclusion.—This approach to in vivo determination of the radiation dose to the kidneys and bladder during renography yields estimates similar to the MIRD values for normal individuals, but it produces very significant deviations in pathologic ones. The mass of the kidney is reduced or its clearance is retarded in certain pathologic conditions, affecting the mass of the "source" and "target" organs and the biodistribution of the radiopharmaceuticals. The new approach could be modified for separate determination of the appropriate dose of pelvis and parenchyma through selection of their regions of interest and identification of the respective activity curves.

▶ The nuclear medicine community has become relatively blasé about radiation dose in recent years. One of our earliest attractions was that the radiation dose incurred in most radionuclide procedures was far lower than that in a comparable radiographic procedure. In recent years, this is no longer true, as larger and larger doses of radioactivity are used to achieve better and better count statistics.

It is important that we continue to pay some attention to radiation dosimetry, and as this article points out, assumptions made for reference man (or woman) may not be accurate in certain pathologic conditions, and we may be seriously underestimating the amount of radiation we are giving to patients in some situations. Although the presence of disease may justify using a somewhat higher radiation dose than in a normal patient, it does not justify a cavalier attitude.—M.D. Blaufox, M.D., Ph.D.

Does Early Pyeloplasty Really Avert Loss of Renal Function? A Retrospective Review

MacNeily AE, Maizels M, Kaplan WE, Firlit CF, Conway JJ (Children's Mem Hosp, Chicago; Northwestern Univ, Chicago)
J Urol 150:769–773, 1993   124-95-6–6

Objective.—The optimal timing for repair of congenital obstruction of the ureteropelvic junction is controversial. Advocates of early repair maintain that it can avert future loss of renal function, whereas others suggest that surgery should be reserved for children who have symptoms or whose renal function declines. Diuresis radionuclide renograms were reviewed to determine the best way of assessing relative renal function in children with unilateral ureteropelvic junction obstruction.

Methods.—One hundred sixty-seven diuretic radionuclide renograms—half preoperative, half postoperative—performed in 75 patients within an 8-year period were reviewed. The most common abnormalities were antenatal hydronephrosis in 35% of patients and urinary tract infection or sepsis in 24%; the median age at first renography was 36 weeks. All patients had renography done before surgery, a normal contralateral kidney, and no other abnormalities that might have affected renal function. One- and 3-minute scintillation count data were used to compute the differential function of the affected kidney. The differential function is the area under the renogram curve between 1 and 3 minutes after injection.

Results.—There was no age- or presentation-related decline in the percentage of differential function on the initial renogram. The average between the 1- and 3-minute values on any given examination was only half the standard deviation of any calculated percentage of differential function. Change in the postoperative percentage of differential function was also unaffected by age at presentation, type of presentation, postoperative complications, or surgeon.

Conclusion.—Early pyeloplasty does not prevent loss of renal function in children with congenital ureteropelvic junction obstruction. The effects of surgical timing on relevant clinical factors and renal physiologic functions remain to be determined.

▶ This study nicely demonstrates the application of nuclear medicine methodology in urologic disease. Although the findings are going to cause some controversy, it remains an approach to a very important problem, the resolution of which would be almost impossible to attempt without the availability of radionuclide renography.—M.D. Blaufox, M.D., Ph.D.

Correlation of Ultrasound and Renal Scintigraphy in Children With Unilateral Hydronephrosis in Primary Workup
Nitzsche EU, Zimmerhackl LB, Hawkins RA, Stöver B, Frankenschmidt A, Sigmund G, Choi Y, Hoh CK, Moser EA (Univ of California, Los Angeles; Albert-Ludwigs-Univ, Freiburg, Germany)
Pediatr Nephrol 7:138–142, 1993   1 2 4-95-6–7

Introduction.—Ureteropelvic junction narrowing, usually seen as hydronephrosis, is the most common congenital abnormality of the urinary tract. Hydronephrosis can be accurately detected in infants and children by the use of ultrasound. Renal scintigraphy with various radiopharmaceuticals provides information on renal function and is routinely correlated with ultrasound when patients are imaged. The relationship between ultrasound morphologic findings and relative renal function, quantified with dynamic technetium-99m mercaptotriacetylglycine imaging, was retrospectively studied.

Patients and Methods.—The study group included 142 children, ranging in age from newborn to adolescent, with unilateral hydronephrosis. The condition was detected by ultrasound screening in 71 patients and

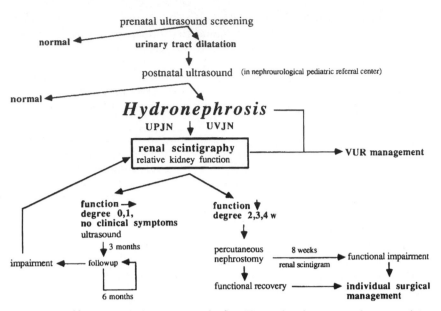

Fig 6–5.—*Abbreviations:* VUR, vesicoureteral reflux; W, complete diagnostic workup required. Diagnostic algorithm for hydronephrosis. (Courtesy of Nitzsche EU, Zimmerhackl LB, Hawkins RA, et al: *Pediatr Nephrol* 7:138–142, 1993.)

diagnosed after urinary tract infection or symptoms in the remaining 71 patients. Renal scintigraphy and ultrasound were performed in the same week. Three blinded readers defined the degree of hydronephrosis observed at ultrasound on a scale from 0 (normal) to 4 (severe dilatation of renal pelvis and calices and minimal residual parenchyma evident). Relative renal function based on scintigraphic findings was graded as 0 (normal) to 4 (essentially nonfunctional, 0% to 9% relative renal function).

Results.—Of the 142 abnormal kidneys, 81 were hydronephrotic secondary to ureteropelvic junction narrowing and 21 were hydronephrotic because of ureterovesical junction narrowing. Twenty-four kidney-ureteral units were refluxive, and 16 appeared to be hydronephrotic secondary to various pathologies. Observer agreement for ultrasound hydronephrosis grading was 72%. An inverse relationship existed between ultrasound morphology and scintigraphically quantified relative kidney function, indicating that ultrasound fails to estimate the potential reduction of relative kidney function in patients with more severe hydronephrosis.

Conclusion.—Because hydronephrosis does not always affect renal function, the functional status of hydronephrotic kidneys must be assessed by renal scintigraphy. A diagnostic algorithm for hydronephrosis is provided (Fig 6–5). By combining the morphologic findings of ultrasound and the functional data obtained with renal scintigraphy, patients who need surgical intervention can be distinguished from those for whom conservative management is appropriate.

▶ This article explores and provides a very reasonable algorithm for the relative roles of ultrasound and renal scintigraphy in pediatric patients with hydronephrosis. The point is made once again that routine radiographic procedures are primarily morphologic and cannot be relied on for functional information. This is the dominant role of nuclear medicine and renal scintigraphy. I certainly agree that in most situations, the initial test for examining the urinary tract should be a noninvasive, nonradiation test such as ultrasound. Once an abnormality is established, the role of the nuclear medicine procedures takes on great importance.—M.D. Blaufox, M.D., Ph.D.

Scintigraphic Evaluation of the Short- and Long-Term Renal Effects of Oral Felodipine Using Technetium-99m-Mercaptoacetyl Triglycine
Özdemir O, Erbas B, Ugur Ö, Varoglu E, Erbengi G, Bekdik C, Oram E (Hacettepe Univ, Ankara, Turkey)
Am J Nephrol 13:249–254, 1993   124-95-6–8

Purpose.—The dihydropyridine calcium antagonist felodipine effectively reduces arterial blood pressure, with its selective primary action on the smooth muscle of the arterial resistance vessel. It also has a wide range of renal effects, such as reducing increased renal vascular resistance. Technetium-99m mercaptoacetyl triglycine (^{99m}Tc-MAG$_3$) was used to investigate the short- and long-term effects of felodipine on renal perfusion and tubular function.

Methods.—Twelve patients with essential hypertension (mean age, 49 years) were studied by renal scintigraphy using ^{99m}Tc-MAG$_3$. Scans were performed at baseline, 2 hours after oral administration of 5 mg of felodipine, and 4 weeks later while patients were receiving 5 to 10 mg of felodipine per day.

Results.—Felodipine therapy significantly reduced the systolic and diastolic blood pressures, from 159/105 to 141/87 mm Hg. No significant change in heart rate was noted. The perfusion index initially decreased from 246 to 194, suggesting an increase in renal blood flow; however, no change occurred during chronic administration, when the perfusion index was 230. The initial dose of felodipine resulted in a nonsignificant decrease in the total clearance of ^{99m}Tc-MAG$_3$, from 361 to 351 mL/min; however, long-term therapy yielded no change in renal perfusion or tubular function.

Conclusion.—Oral felodipine initially produces a significant increase in renal blood flow, possibly as a result of selective vasodilation. In the acute phase, a minimal decrease in tubular secretion occurs, possibly because of an inhibitor effect on tubular function. However, long-term felodipine therapy appears to have no effect on renal perfusion and tubular secretion function.

▶ It is particularly gratifying to see that this article on the use of radionuclide technology for evaluating the kidney was published in the *American Journal of Nephrology*. Despite the versatility of the many procedures available for evaluating the kidney with radiopharmaceuticals, nephrologists have been slow to fully understand the implications and importance of these techniques.

This study once again demonstrates the type of data that can be obtained relatively inexpensively and noninvasively and that is critical to the nephrologist's understanding of the management of patients with hypertension and renal disease.—M.D. Blaufox, M.D., Ph.D.

Differential Kidney Scans in Preoperative Evaluation of Kidney Donors

Shokeir AA, Gad HM, Shaaban AA, El-Kenawy MR, El-Sherif A, Shamaa MA, Bakr MA, Ghoneim MA (Urology and Nephrology Ctr, Mansoura, Egypt)
Transplant Proc 25:2327–2329, 1993   124-95-6–9

Introduction.—Living-related donors are still the main source of transplanted kidneys in many countries. Preoperative assessment of donor ensures that the kidneys are functioning well and equally. In the past, the choice to take the right or left kidney for transplantation has been based on the findings of morphologic studies. A radioisotopic method for selective determination of the glomerular filtration rate (GFR) to guide the choice of which kidney to use was described.

Methods.—Two hundred seventy-five live-donor nephrectomies were performed within a 5-year period. After preliminary medical evaluation, histocompatibility testing, and radiologic imaging, selective determination of the function of both kidneys was made using radioisotope renography. Technetium-99m DTPA was used, and a dynamic study was obtained at 1-minute intervals for 20 minutes with a scintillation camera. The glomerular clearance for each kidney was calculated by the equation $(dr/dt)/P$. The mean follow-up for the kidney recipients was 32 months.

Results.—No significant difference was noted between the mean combined renographic clearance and the mean 24-hour creatinine clearance: 113 vs. 115 mL/min, respectively. The average disparity in kidney clearance was 11 mL/min, with an expected 30% of kidney pairs showing a disparity in renographic clearance of more than 15 mL/min. When the clearance values were comparable, the choice of which kidney to harvest was made on an anatomical basis. When a significant difference was found, the selected side was usually determined on a functional basis, regardless of anatomical findings.

Conclusion.—Radioisotopic renography is recommended for differential evaluation of renal function as part of the preoperative evaluation of live kidney donors.

▶ Although I am a strong advocate of the extensive use of radionuclides in nephrology, I am not really sure I agree with the authors' recommendations. Given a normal patient with normal renal function and no evidence of kidney disease, it should not really matter which kidney is chosen for transplantation, because renal function should be reasonably similar. Therefore, the major determinant of which kidney to use for transplantation should be anatomy. In patients in whom there is some suspicion of a difference between the 2 kidneys, radioisotope studies clearly would be indicated. However, in general, it would appear that ultrasound should be sufficient. I would be concerned that the differences in function in some of the patients that the authors cite might be related more to methodologic issues than to a meaningful difference between the 2 sides. That the authors noted no difference in graft survival regardless of the baseline renal function lends further support to this assumption.—M.D. Blaufox, M.D., Ph. D.

Captopril Renoscintigraphy With Tc-99m DTPA in Patients With Suspected Renovascular Hypertension: Prospective and Retrospective Evaluation
Itoh K, Tsukamoto E, Nagao K, Nakada K, Kanegae K, Furudate M (Hokkaido Univ, Sapporo, Japan)
Clin Nucl Med 18:463–471, 1993   124-95-6–10

Objective.—Reliable and accurate noninvasive techniques are needed for the detection of renovascular hypertension (RVH). In captopril-augmented renoscintigraphy (CRS), the glomerular filtration rate declines in response to captopril challenge in the presence of renal artery stenosis. The diagnostic accuracy and limitations of CRS were clarified in a prospective study.

Patients.—Captopril-augmented renoscintigraphy was performed in 41 patients with suspected RVH during a 3½-year period. Sixteen patients proved to have RVH, 8 with bilateral renal artery stenosis, 6 with unilateral stenosis, and 2 with coarctation of the thoracic aorta. All but 2 of these patients received percutaneous transluminal angioplasty or surgical revascularization. The remaining 25 patients were excluded from having RVH by angiography and further studies.

Methods.—All of the patients underwent CRS. Captopril was given by mouth 1 hour before scintigraphy, with the latter patients in the series receiving a 50-mg dose. The scintigraphy was performed using technetium-99m DTPA with doses ranging from 185 MBq for children to 370 MBq for adults. After the dose was counted and administered by IV bolus injection, serial 3-second interval blood perfusion images and 2-minute interval sequential images were recorded. Absolute renal uptake of

Sensitivity and Specificity of Precaptopril and Postcaptopril Renoscintigraphy

	RVH Group			Non-RVH Group	Sensitivity	Specificity
	Total	Unilateral	Bilateral			
Prospective						
Baseline Study	(n = 16)	(n = 6)	(n = 10)	(n = 19)		
1. SRF ≤ 42%	10	5	5	7	63%	63%
Captopril	(n = 18)	(n = 7)	(n = 11)	(n = 25)		
1. CRR ≤ −20%	10	4	6	6	56%	76%
2. RNG (+)	8	4	4	1	44%	96%
3. CRR ≤ −20% or RNG (+)	12	4	8	6	67%	76%
4. CRR ≤ −20% and RNG (+)	8	4	4	1	44%	96%

Retrospective

Baseline Study	(n = 16)	(n = 6)	(n = 10)	(n = 19)		
1. SRF ≤ 45%	14	6	8	10	88%	47%
2. SRF ≤ 40%	10	5	5	6	63%	68%
Captopril	(n = 18)	(n = 7)	(n = 11)	(n = 25)		
1. CRR ≤ −25%	9	4	5	1	50%	96%
2. CRR ≤ −25% or RNG (+)	11	4	7	1	61%	96%
3. CRR ≤ −25% and RNG (+)	(n = 17) 8	(n = 7) 4	(n = 10) 4	(n = 25) 0	44%	100%
4. SRF ≤ 40%	10	6	4	3	59%	88%

Abbreviations: SRF, split renal function; CRR, captopril-induced reduction rate of renal function; RNG (+), change of the renogram to any of the high-graded types.
Note: The parenthesis indicates the number of studies.
(Courtesy of Itoh K, Tsukamoto E, Nagao K, et al: Clin Nucl Med 18:463–471, 1993.)

the individual kidney was calculated by a count-based gamma camera method, from which the glomerular filtration rate of each kidney was estimated. A relative split renal function of less than 42% of the total renal uptake was considered positive for unilateral renal artery involvement. Captopril-augmented renoscintigraphy was considered positive when there was more than a 20% decline in the captopril-induced reduction rate (CRR) or conversion to a higher-grade renographic pattern.

Results.—Based on split renal function analysis, the sensitivity and specificity of the baseline study were both 63%. The sensitivity of CRS was 67%, with a specificity of 76%. When the criterion for a positive study was changed to a 25% decline in CRR, the specificity of CRS improved to 96%, and the sensitivity declined to 61%. The captopril-induced changes in the configuration of the renogram were highly specific but not very sensitive (table). Patients who met both the renographic and CRR criteria were the most likely to have RVH. These criteria were frequently diagnostic in patients with bilateral stenosis and a variable scintigraphic response to captopril.

Conclusion.—Captopril renoscintigraphy is a very specific study for the evaluation of RVH. It is also useful in detecting functional renin dependency in the affected kidney before and after intervention and in deciding whether angiotensin-converting enzyme inhibitor treatment is indicated. However, its value is limited in certain situations (e.g., poorly preserved kidney function, long-term captopril therapy, previous surgical manipulation of the stenotic artery, and chronic renal parenchymal damage).

▶ This article from Japan adds a little more information to our knowledge of captopril renography, which has occupied an important place in the differential diagnosis of renovascular hypertension during the past several years. Although the authors' reported specificities are quite high, they provide somewhat less optimistic estimates of the sensitivity of the test. A table in the original article provides some detail about their sources of false positive and false negative studies, information that is useful in helping refine our understanding of the procedure.—M.D. Blaufox, M.D., Ph.D.

Aspirin Renography to Detect Unilateral Renovascular Hypertension
Imanishi M, Yano M, Hayashida K, Ishida Y, Takamiya M, Kimura G, Kojima S, Kawano Y, Matsushima Y, Matsuoka H, Omae T (Natl Cardiovascular Ctr, Osaka, Japan)
Kidney Int 45:1170–1176, 1994   124-95-6–11

Background.—Radionuclide renograms are widely used in screening for renovascular hypertension, but their sensitivity and specificity are low. The tracer iodine-123 orthoiodohippurate ([^{123}I]OIH) is commonly used for initial renographic examinations, because it is excreted from the

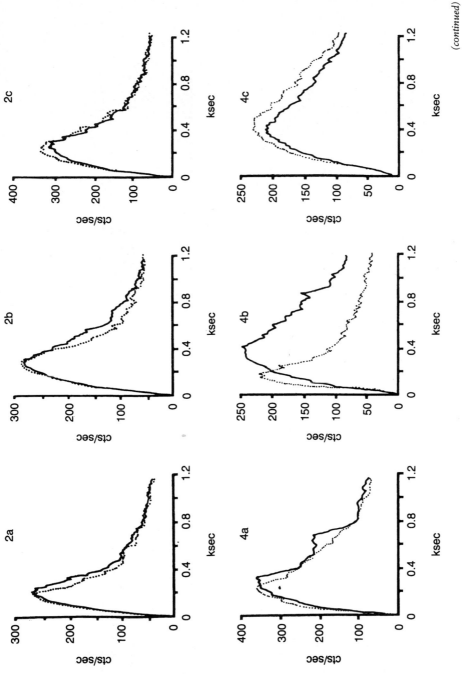

(continued)

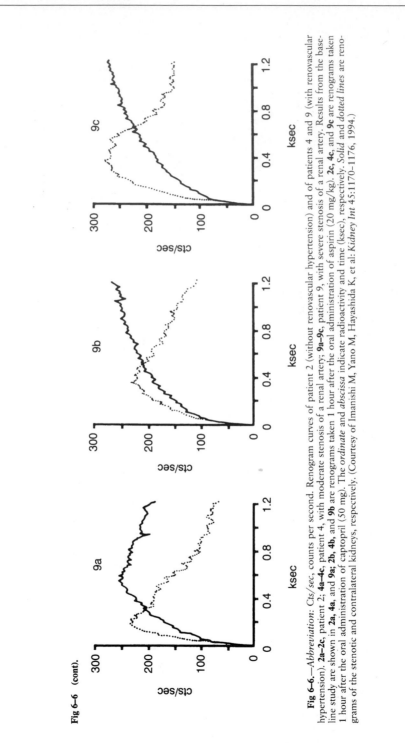

Fig 6-6 (cont).

Fig 6-6.—*Abbreviation:* Cts/sec, counts per second. Renogram curves of patient 2 (without renovascular hypertension) and of patients 4 and 9 (with renovascular hypertension). **2a–2c**, patient 2; **4a–4c**, patient 4, with moderate stenosis of a renal artery; **9a–9c**, patient 9, with severe stenosis of a renal artery. Results from the baseline study are shown in **2a, 4a**, and **9a; 2b, 4b**, and **9b** are renograms taken 1 hour after the oral administration of aspirin (20 mg/kg). **2c, 4c**, and **9c** are renograms taken 1 hour after the oral administration of captopril (50 mg). The *ordinate* and *abscissa* indicate radioactivity and time (ksec), respectively. *Solid* and *dotted lines* are renograms of the stenotic and contralateral kidneys, respectively. (Courtesy of Imanishi M, Yano M, Hayashida K, et al: *Kidney Int* 45:1170–1176, 1994.)

kidneys quickly and yields information about the overall renal function. Detection of renal arterial stenosis that causes hypertension might be increased in [^{123}I]OIH renography through inhibition of renal prostaglandin synthesis. Renography in combination with aspirin administration was used to examine patients with unilateral renal arterial stenosis.

Methods.—Eight patients with 45% to more than 90% stenosis were studied, along with 1 patient without stenoses. Most patients underwent radionuclide renography 3 times: once at baseline; again after the oral administration of aspirin, 20 mg/kg, an inhibitor of prostaglandin synthesis; and finally after the oral administration of captopril, 50 mg. A significant decrease in renal blood flow was defined as at least a 5-minute time to the peak in the renogram. A 2-minute difference in the peak times of the 2 kidneys was considered significant.

Results.—The time to the peak of the stenotic kidney was significantly delayed in both kidneys by both aspirin and captopril, but it was delayed to a greater extent in the stenotic kidney. Sensitivity in the detection of unilateral renovascular hypertension increased from 43% at the baseline study to 100% with aspirin. The control patient had no difference between the kidneys in the 3 renograms, whereas a patient with moderate stenosis had a significant difference only with aspirin renography. In a patient with severe stenosis, aspirin and captopril both increased the differences between the baseline renogram curves (Fig 6–6).

Conclusion.—The use of [^{123}I]OIH renography after aspirin administration may represent a new, noninvasive, sensitive method of detecting renovascular hypertension. Aspirin works by inhibiting prostaglandin synthesis, decreasing blood flow and the glomerular filtration rate, and thereby reducing urine flow rate in the stenotic kidney. At the dose used here, the inhibitory effects seem to be reversible and to cause little damage to the kidneys.

▶ This small study provides an interesting modification to captropril renography. It certainly is a simple and reasonably safe procedure and merits further study.

The authors' suggestion that they increased the sensitivity of the test from 43% to 100% using aspirin is of particular interest in view of the preceding article by Itoh and colleagues (Abstract 124-95-6-10), which also reported a relatively low sensitivity in a Japanese patient population. Although the low sensitivity noted with ordinary captopril renography in these studies may be related to the population study, other reports have had relatively disappointing sensitivities, so anything that would improve this safely is worth considering.—M.D. Blaufox, M.D., Ph.D.

Captopril Renal Scintigraphy in Patients With Hypertension and Chronic Renal Failure

Datseris IE, Bomanji JB, Brown EA, Nijran KS, Padhy AK, Siraj QH, Britton KE
(St Bartholomew's Hosp, London; Charing Cross Hosp, London)
J Nucl Med 35:251–254, 1994   124-95-6-12

Rationale.—Angiotensin-converting enzyme (ACE) inhibitors now are widely used to treat patients with hypertension and renal failure in the hope of conserving renal function. However, where the renin-angiotensin-aldosterone system is active, as in renal artery stenosis (RAS), ACE inhibitors can have adverse effects on renal function. A noninvasive method of detecting functionally significant RAS and predicting the effect of an ACE inhibitor on the kidneys would have considerable value.

Patients.—Captopril renal scintigraphy was evaluated in 41 patients who were hypertensive and in chronic renal failure. About half the patients had severe, uncontrolled hypertension; 14 had diabetic nephropathy; and 6 had intrinsic renal parenchymal disease, usually glomerulonephritis. Seven patients were in heart failure at the time they were seen. In all patients, the glomerular filtration rate was 50% of predicted normal or less.

Methods.—The ACE inhibitors were withdrawn a week before scintigraphy, which used a large-field-of-view gamma camera, a parallel-hole, low-energy collimator, and an on-line computer. Data were acquired immediately after the bolus injection of 80 MBq of technetium-99m mercaptoacetyltriglycine. Scintigraphy was repeated within a week, using oral captopril, 25 mg, 1 hour before the test.

Results.—No patient had side effects from orally administered captopril. The maximum decline in diastolic blood pressure was 25 mm Hg. Renal artery stenosis was confirmed in 5 of 7 patients who were thought to have a high probability of being so affected. Two of these patients had lower blood pressure and improved renal function after angioplasty. Fifteen patients had a low probability of RAS, and 19 had an indeterminate probability of RAS. The ACE treatment was continued or initiated in 14 patients with a low probability of RAS and in 9 with an indeterminate probability. In these patients, the mean parenchymal transit time was significantly reduced on the postcaptopril scintigram. Renal function remained stable or improved 6 months after scintigraphy. Of 11 patients without a reduced mean parenchymal transit time, 3 were placed on dialysis and the other 8 had no significant change in renal function.

Conclusion.—Captopril renal scintigraphy is a useful study in high-risk patients with hypertension and chronic renal failure. Abnormal findings are consistent with angiotensin II–dependent renovascular dysfunction. Patients with normal findings may benefit from treatment with an ACE inhibitor.

▶ This is a very useful study in a group of patients in whom it is particularly important to understand the role of captopril renography, because of problems with potential false positive and false negative studies.

The authors' suggestion that captopril renography may be useful in deciding whether to treat patients having chronic renal failure with ACE inhibitors is provocative.

I highly recommend this article as well as the editorial concerning it, which I wrote, which appears on page 254 of the same issue of the *Journal of Nuclear Medicine.*—M.D. Blaufox, M.D., Ph.D.

Quantitative Analysis of the Technetium-99m-DTPA Captopril Renogram: Contribution of Washout Parameters to the Diagnosis of Renal Artery Stenosis

Dey HM, Hoffer PB, Lerner E, Zubal IG, Setaro JF, Black HR (Yale Univ, New Haven, Conn; Veterans Affairs Med Ctr, West Haven, Conn)
J Nucl Med 34:1416–1419, 1993   1-24-95-6-13

Introduction.—There is great variation among reports of the sensitivity and specificity of captopril renography for the diagnosis of renal artery stenosis (RAS). Previously, encouraging results were reported with the criteria of a time to peak renal activity of 11 minutes or greater on the pre- or postcaptopril scan and/or a glomerular filtration rate (GFR) ratio between the kidneys of greater than 1.5 on the postcaptopril study. However, better results using diagnostic criteria based on the residual cortical activity of ^{131}I-hippuran have also been reported. The efficacy of DTPA washout parameters was compared with that of quantitative uptake criteria for the detection of RAS.

Methods.—The retrospective analysis included pre- and postcaptopril DTPA renograms from 88 patients with hypertension. Angiography demonstrated RAS in 45 patients and normal renal arteries in 43. Time-activity curves from the patients with essential hypertension were used to develop diagnostic washout criteria for a positive DTPA renogram. The

---

Sensitivity, Specificity, and Predictive Values

Diagnostic criterion	Sensitivity	Specificity	Positive predictive value	Negative predictive value
Original*	0.89	0.84	0.85	0.88
Washout†	0.67	0.79	0.77	0.69

* Original diagnostic criteria = time to peak and GFR ratio.
† Washout criteria = 20 and 30 min/peak ratios.
(Courtesy of Dey HM, Hoffer PB, Lerner E, et al: *J Nucl Med* 34: 1416–1419, 1993.)

criteria were based on the 20- and 30-min/peak activity ratios in each kidney.

Results.—On retrospective application of the washout criteria to the original patient date, RAS had a sensitivity of 67% and a specificity of 79%. Application of the previously reported criteria based on time to peak activity in each kidney and the GFR ratio between kidneys improved sensitivity to 89% and specificity to 84% (table).

Conclusion.—Quantitative analysis of the DTPA renogram using the time to peak and the GFR ratio is sensitive and specific for RAS. Accuracy is not improved by measurement of 20- and 30-min/peak renal activity ratios. Mean washout ratios are greater after captopril administration for kidneys with and without RAS.

▶ The contributions of this group to our use and understanding of captopril renography have been outstanding. However, our experience with captopril renography is at variance with theirs. We find the 20- or 30-minute/peak activity criterion ratio to be very useful and have had rather disappointing results with the 11-minute time to peak activity criterion. On the other hand, I believe that the single most useful measurement in a great many studies has been the GFR ratio of greater than 1.5 on the postcaptopril study. It may be the most useful parameter for centers that are using technetium DTPA as the diagnostic agent.—M.D. Blaufox, M.D., Ph.D.

Acute Transplant Artery Thrombosis Induced by Angiotensin-Converting Inhibitor in a Patient With Renovascular Hypertension
Dussol B, Nicolino F, Brunet P, Leonetti F, Siles S, Berland Y (Hôpital Sainte-Marguerite, Marseille, France; Hôpital de la Timone, Marseille, France)
Nephron 66:102–104, 1994   1 24-95-6–1 4

Background.—Many cases of acute renal failure are related to angiotensin-converting enzyme inhibitors. Most of these patients have renovascular disease and a marked decrease in renal perfusion pressure. A patient with acute thrombosis of a renal transplant artery after angiotensin-converting enzyme inhibitor treatment was described.

Case Report.—Man, 43, underwent renal transplantation because of end-stage renal failure resulting from chronic glomerulonephritis. The transplant artery anastomosed to the recipient's hypogastric artery. The patient's artery was larger than the transplant artery. Postoperatively, the patient had worsening hypertension, which was managed with verapamil, labetolol, and furosemide.

Two years later, the patient still had severe hypertension, 160/110 mm Hg. Digitalized angiography showed a 50% postanastomotic stenosis of the transplant artery. The patient was given captopril, 50 mg/day, which resulted in a dramatic decline in blood pressure and a deterioration of renal function. Captopril treatment was stopped; radiologists and vascular surgeons declined to perform a revascularization revision of the graft. After captopril was given for before-and-after renal scintigraphy, the graft was not visualized, and the creatinine clearance declined to 0. His blood pressure dropped dramatically, and the patient was admitted with anuric acute renal failure. Complete thrombosis developed in the transplant artery at arteriography; complete removal of the graft was necessary because of total necrosis. The patient was restarted on chronic hemodialysis.

Discussion.—In all such cases, occlusion is preceded by a dramatic decline in arterial pressure. The nonspecific mechanism of this thrombosis might be an abrupt decrease in renal perfusion pressure across the stenosis, with a resultant reduction in renal plasma flow.

▶ It is becoming increasingly clear that long-term angiotensin-converting enzyme inhibitor (ACEI) treatment has certain risks in patients with renovascular disease. However, it is important to note that no serious side effects have been reported in patients after a single dose of ACEI, and the captopril renogram remains a very safe test for enhancement of the differential diagnosis of renovascular hypertension. The administration of a single dose of captopril should not be regarded as dangerous. The major acute side effect is hypotension, which can be easily treated by placing the patient supine and administering saline if necessary. In patients in whom a significant risk is suspected, a smaller dose of captopril should be considered.—M.D. Blaufox, M.D., Ph.D.

Measurement of Tc-99m DTPA Serum Clearance for Estimating Glomerular Filtration Rate in Children With Cancer
Rodman JH, Maneval DC, Magill HL, Sunderland M (St Jude Children's Research Hosp, Memphis, Tenn)
Pharmacotherapy 13:10–16, 1993   124-95-6-15

Background.—The estimated technetium-99m (^{99m}Tc) DTPA clearance from blood samples with no urine collection serves as a reliable indicator of the glomerular filtration rate (GFR) in adults. However, its application to children has not been well studied.

Methods.—In 17 children with cancer, the disposition of ^{99m}Tc-DTPA, including the effects of binding and study design on serum clearance estimates, was investigated. Nine blood samples were obtained within 6 hours in each patient, and the total and free ^{99m}Tc in serum was measured. The free ^{99m}Tc-DTPA determinations were made by ultrafiltration. All 9 measured concentrations were used to create a 2-compartment model for ultrafiltrable ^{99m}Tc-DTPA, from which clearance estimates were derived. The results provided a reference value for the GFR in each patient.

Results.—The 2-compartment model provided the best description of total ^{99m}Tc-DTPA concentrations (Fig 6–7). However, the median total clearance of 35 mL/min was significantly lower than the ultrafiltrate clearance of 58 mL/min. Clearance estimates based on a 3-point subset

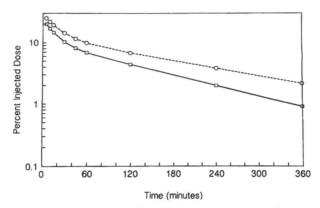

Fig 6–7.—Computer simulations illustrate the time course of total (*upper line*) and ultrafiltrable (*lower line*) ⁹⁹ᵐTc-DTPA after an IV bolus dose, using median estimates of pharmacokinetic parameters from all 17 children. (Courtesy of Rodman JH, Maneval DC, Magill HL, et al: *Pharmacotherapy* 13:10–16, 1993.)

of the ultrafiltrable data were used to examine the effects of a simplified sampling schedule. The median clearance was 69 mL/min, significantly higher than the reference GFR. There was good prediction of the reference estimates for the GFR after application of a correction factor to compensate for the limited sampling schedule.

Conclusion.—Consistent and practical estimates of the GFR in children can be obtained by the use of ultrafiltrable ⁹⁹ᵐTc-DTPA serum clearance and a limited sampling schedule. However, serum binding and study design are still potentially important confounding factors.

▶ The debate on how to measure renal function using radionuclide techniques continues. This reported method has many problems, especially because the reference method is in itself debatable, and the authors' final recommendation uses a correction factor. Our experience with using ultrafiltrates to estimate the GFR has been uniformly poor.

The problem of establishing an accepted technique for measuring renal function using radionuclides has been approached by the American College of Nuclear Physicians through its Quality Assurance Workshop and also by the Radionuclides in Nephrourology group, which is attempting to develop a consensus document. Hopefully, within a short time after this YEAR BOOK is published, general guidelines will be available for the measurement of GFR and other aspects of renal function using radionuclides. If we could all adopt a single, reliable method, it would take us a long way toward obtaining general acceptance of these techniques.—M.D. Blaufox, M.D., Ph.D.

A Simplified Technique for Radionuclide Hysterosalpingography

Jacobson A, Uszler JM (Santa Monica Hosp Med Ctr, Calif)
J Assist Reprod Genet 10:4–10, 1993   124-95-6–16

Background.—The fallopian tubes function in sperm and egg transport. However, there has been no physiologic test for competency in this function. The radionuclide hysterosalpingogram (RNHSG) attempts

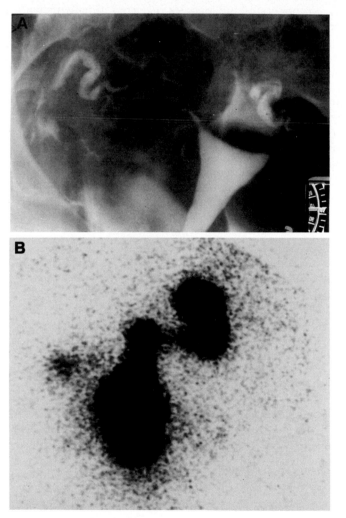

Fig 6–8.—A, bilateral patency on the HSG. **B,** RNHSG with good function on the left, but the right tube has decreased activity with slow transport. (Courtesy of Jacobson A, Uszler JM: *J Assist Reprod Genet* 10:4-10, 1993.)

to provide a physiologic functional assay of transport. A simpler, faster RNHSG method was described.

Methods.—Forty-four patients were recruited from an infertility clinic. A tuberculin syringe and a Tomcat catheter were used to deposit .1 mL of tracer medium in the uterus. Imaging was begun before tracer deposition.

Results.—Among those with patent tubes but no transport function by RNHSG, most had had pelvic inflammatory disease or endometriosis (Fig 6–8). No unassisted pregnancies occurred in patients who had nonfunctional tubes by RNHSG.

Conclusion.—Using the faster and simpler RNHSG technique described, the test takes less than 1 hour and requires no more than 100 μci of tracer. Positive results are usually obtained within 20 minutes. Intrauterine deposition of tracer with RNHSG imaging can provide a physiologic measurement of tubal transport function.

▶ We continue to see sporadic reports of the use of radionuclides for the evaluation of impedance and penile dysfunction and also for the performance of radionuclide hysterosalpingography. I have always thought that both of these techniques have very great potential.—M.D. Blaufox, M.D., Ph.D.

7 Gastrointestinal

Introduction

As has been true in previous years, most of this year's selections are about hepatobiliary imaging. They include fewer red blood cell studies than we have seen before and a few more studies using labeled white blood cells related to the gastrointestinal tract. A modest revival of interest in Meckel's scan may be starting as well.

Alexander Gottschalk, M.D.

The Hot Spot Hepatobiliary Scan in Focal Nodular Hyperplasia
Boulahdour H, Cherqui D, Charlotte F, Rahmouni A, Dhumeaux D, Zafrani ES, Meignan M (Univ Paris XII-Val de Marne, Créteil, France)
J Nucl Med 34:2105–2110, 1993   124-95-7–1

Purpose.—Some nuclear medicine tracers have been proposed as an aid to the diagnosis of focal nodular hyperplasia (FNH), a benign liver tumor with an innocuous natural history. A characteristic triad of findings in FNH has been reported: associated hypervascularization, normal uptake of colloids, and accumulation of hepatobiliary tracer. However, studies of FNH using colloid or hepatobiliary tracers have used different technical conditions and yielded inconsistent results. Both kinds of tracers were used under standardized technical conditions in a homogenous series of 14 patients with 25 pathologically proven FNH tumors.

Methods.—The patients were all women who had used oral contraceptives; 9 were asymptomatic. All of the tumors were diagnosed as FNH on pathologic examination of resected specimens or surgical biopsy specimens. All patients underwent 2 radionuclide scans within a 48-hour interval: a hepatobiliary scan using technetium-99m (^{99m}TC)-labeled trimethyl bromo-iminodiacetic acid (TBIDA) and a second scan using ^{99m}Tc-labeled rhenium colloid.

Results.—The hepatobiliary scans showed relatively normal TBIDA uptake in the region of the tumor. However, 92% of the lesions showed a hot spot of radioactivity during the clearance phase of the scan (Fig 7–1). This finding could appear early or late, depending on the relative contrast between the tumor and normal liver tissue, but it was always seen at 1 hour (table). A "doughnut" pattern within the hot spot, the result of a central defect, was seen in 3 tumors. During the perfusion

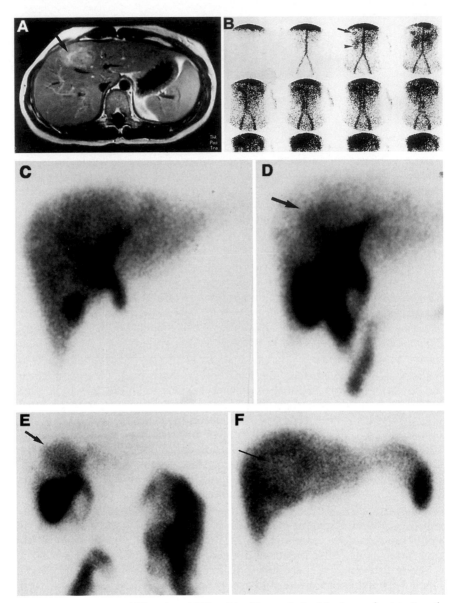

Fig 7–1.—Patient 2. **A,** MRI study; axial T1-weighted image obtained 4 minutes after injection of paramagnetic contrast agent: a 5-cm mass is visible in the right lobe of the liver with a hyperintense central scar (*arrow*). **B,** ^{99m}Tc-labeled TBIDA angiography; 1-second images. An early vascular activity (*arrow*) is demonstrated in the right lobe of the liver over the renal vascular activity area (*arrowhead*). **C,** TBIDA scan at 10 minutes. The uptake is rather homogenous throughout the liver. **D,** TBIDA scan at 35 minutes. A hot spot of hyperactivity appeared in the right lobe over the gallbladder (*arrow*). **E,** overexposed TBIDA scan at 60 minutes where the hot spot is obvious (*arrow*) but the normal liver has already cleared the tracer. **F,** colloid liver scan. A defect is seen in the quadrate lobe (*arrow*). In the inferior part of the liver's right lobe, a region of the gallbladder corresponds to a discrete hypoactivity area. (Courtesy of Boulahdour H, Cherqui D, Charlotte F, et al: *J Nucl Med* 34:2105–2110, 1993.)

Size, Location, and Imaging Characteristics of FNH Tumors

Patient no.	Tumor size (cm) and location*	TBIDA scan Hypervascularity	Time of detectability (min)	Colloid scan (activity)	US†	CT‡	MRI‡	Discrete sinusoidal dilatation**
1	(10) III	present	22	Hypo	Iso	+	+	absent
2	(5) IV	present	27	Hypo	Iso	–	+	present
3	(4.5) VII	present	35	Iso	Hyper	+	+	present
	(1.5) III	absent	18	Iso	nd	nd	nd	present
4	(8) VI, VII, VIII	present	30-D	Hypo	Hypo	+	+	B
5	(4) III	present	30	Hypo	Iso	+	+	present
	(1) IV	absent	nd	Iso	Iso	+	+	B
6	(5) I, VIII	present	50	Hypo	Iso	+	+	B
7	(5) VII	absent	30-D	Iso-D	Hyper	+	+	B
	(3) V	absent	25	Iso	nd	–	+	present
	(10) LL	present	20	Iso	Iso	+	+	present
8	(8) VII	present	38	Iso	Hyper	–	–	B
	(4) IV	absent	38	Iso	nd	–	+	E
	(1) VIII	absent	40	Iso	nd	nd	nd	B
	(10) I	present	38	Iso	Hyper	+	–	B

(continued)

Table (*continued*)

9	(5) IV	present	33	Iso	Iso	−	+	B
	(2) V	present	nd	Iso	nd	nd	nd	E
10	(5) III	present	35	Hypo	Hypo	+	+	absent
11	(7) III	present	28	Iso	Iso	+	−	absent
12	(3) VIII	present	33	Hypo	Hypo	+	+	B
	(1.5) VII	absent	60	Iso	Iso	−	+	present
	(5) II	present	27	Hypo	Hypo	+	+	present
	(3) III	present	27	Iso	nd	nd	nd	present
13	(8) III	present	30-D	Iso-D	Iso	+	+	absent
14	(4) IV	present	30	Hypo	Hypo	+	+	B

* Hepatic segments involved by the tumor; *nd*, not detected; *LL*, left lobe.
† Ultrasound: echogenicity.
‡ CT and MRI: (+) criteria for focal nodular hyperplasia are present; (−) 1 or more criteria are missing.
** At the vicinity of the tumor; *E*, tumors enucleated without normal liver parenchyma; *D*, doughnut pattern observed; *B*, FNH diagnosis performed only on surgical biopsy specimens.

(Courtesy of Boulahdour H, Cherqui D, Charlotte F, et al: *J Nucl Med* 34:2105–2110, 1993.)

phase, 76% of the tumor sites demonstrated hypervascularization. On the colloid scan, 64% showed normal colloid uptake. Computed tomography or MRI detected FNH in 84% of the cases, whereas 36% showed a focal defect. Tumor detectability was enhanced by late images, overexposed x-ray films, multiple views, and gallbladder excretion stimulation.

Conclusion.—Hepatobiliary scanning can be useful in the diagnosis of FNH. The high prevalence of hot spots noted may be the result of the careful and standardized technique used; the 50–60-minute views are important. The hot spot sign described may result from the unusual pathologic characteristics of FNH, including fibrosis, hyperplastic hepatocytes, and cholangiolar proliferation. They probably represent poor clearance of tracer from the region of FNH, with image contrast provided because the normal hepatocytes clear the tracer promptly.

▶ Although this is a small series, I like that all these patients had histologic proof. The authors go on to correctly state that there is no way to assess specificity without a large, prospective trial.

I think it is important to point out that these lesions almost certainly show up as hot spots on the delayed images because the FNH does not clear the tracer well, although the hepatocytes within it clearly function effectively. Remember that these authors are using the brominated variety of iminodiacetic acid (IDA), which clears extremely rapidly. If you use the diisopropyl variety, and the possibility of FNH crosses your mind, you might be well advised to get an ultradelayed image (e.g., 1½ to 2 hours). The combination of a normal colloid scan with a hot spot on the IDA study should be a dynamite diagnostic duo for FNH.—A. Gottschalk, M.D.

Cholescintigraphy in the Diagnosis of Acute Cholecystitis: Morphine Augmentation Is Superior to Delayed Imaging
Kim CK, Tse KMK, Juweid M, Mozley DP, Woda A, Alavi A (Hosp of the Univ of Pennsylvania, Philadelphia)
J Nucl Med 34:1866–1870, 1993   124-95-7-2

Introduction.—Previous research has suggested that morphine-augmented radionuclide hepatobiliary imaging is as useful as or more useful than delayed imaging for the diagnosis of acute cholecystitis. However, there have been few systematic comparisons of the efficacy of the 2 techniques. The scans of 306 consecutive patients were reviewed, focusing particularly on the negative predictive value (NPV) and positive predictive value (PPV) of morphine-augmented imaging.

Methods.—Approximately 185 MBq of technetium-99m diisopropyl-iminodiacetic acid (^{99m}Tc-DISIDA) was administered IV to each patient. In those cases where the gallbladder was not visualized within 1 hour despite the presence of radioactive bile in the common bile duct and the small bowel, .04 mg of morphine sulphate per kg was injected IV over 3 minutes. This was followed immediately by an additional 74 MBq of ^{99m}Tc-DISIDA. Planar images were then acquired for another 30 minutes. Findings were interpreted as being most consistent with acute cholecystitis if the gallbladder could still not be visualized.

Results.—The gallbladder was visualized within the first hour of study in 215 patients, 5 of whom were subsequently confirmed to have acute cholecystitis by postsurgical histopathology. As a result, the NPV of early gallbladder visualization was 98% in this group. Delayed images were obtained in 46 of the remaining 91 patients. Findings proved to be true positive in 17 cases, true negative in 10, and false positive in 19; none were false negative. Morphine-augmented studies yielded 24 true positive results, 15 true negative, 4 false positive, and 2 false negative. When the cases with gallbladder visualization within 1 hour were excluded, the PPV for acute cholecystitis was significantly lower with delayed imaging (47%) than with morphine augmentation (85%). Results were similar (PPV 59% vs. 86%) when analysis was confined to patients who underwent surgery. The techniques did not differ significantly in NPV (100% vs. 88%).

Conclusion.—Delayed imaging can be inconvenient and potentially disadvantageous to the patient. Delayed imaging also has a significantly lower specificity and PPV for acute cholecystitis than morphine-augmentation imaging. Sensitivity and NPV are slightly higher, although the difference is statistically insignificant for delayed imaging.

▶ What these authors don't tell us is how patients are assigned to each of the 2 imaging groups. For example, if the patients who got morphine were very ill and were expected to go to surgery stat, whereas those who got delayed imaging studies were not so ill, a severe patient selection bias could exist. Furthermore, each patient who got morphine got an extra 2 mCi of IDA at 1 hour. We don't know whether the delayed imaging patients did or not—another possible variable about which to worry.

Despite these objections, these data further confirm the efficacy of using morphine. Interested readers may want to look at this article in its entirety, because it contains a relevant literature review of both techniques.—A. Gottschalk, M.O.

Abnormal Gallbladder Nuclear Ejection Fraction Predicts Success of Cholecystectomy in Patients With Biliary Dyskinesia
Sorenson MK, Fancher S, Lang NP, Eidt JF, Broadwater JR (Univ of Arkansas, Little Rock)
Am J Surg 166:672–674, 1993   124-95-7–3

Introduction.—A small subset of patients with classic biliary colic who do not have documented gallstones by ultrasound or oral cholecystography may have biliary dyskinesia. The value of quantitative cholecystokinin

Quantitative Cholecystokinin Cholescintigraphy in
Patients With Upper Abdominal Pain

	Group 1* (%)	Group 2† (%)
No. of patients	11	6
Classic biliary colic	11 (100)	1 (17)
Mean gallbladder ejection fraction (range)	20.3 (7–33)	42 (38–45)
Cholecystectomy	11	0
Symptoms relieved	11 (100)	5‡ (83)

* GBEF was ≤ 35%.
† GBEF was > 35%.
‡ Five patients had esophagogastroduodenoscopy, which demonstrated gastritis/duodenitis, and symptom relief with H_2 blockers.
(Courtesy of Sorenson MK, Fancher S, Lang NP, et al: *Am J Surg* 166:672–674, 1993.)

cholescintigraphy was evaluated in identifying patients with abnormal gallbladder emptying who might benefit from cholecystectomy.

Patients and Methods.—A retrospective review was conducted of 18 patients who had gallbladder ejection fractions (GBEF) measured by cholecystokinin cholescintigraphy after ultrasound revealed no evidence of gallstones or biliary ductal dilatation. A GBEF less than or equal to 35% in response to cholecystokinin was considered abnormal. The 12 men and 6 women all had symptoms consistent with biliary tract disease.

Results.—Six of the patients had normal scans; the mean GBEF in this group was 42%. Eleven patients had abnormal scans with an ejection fraction of less than or equal to 35%; the mean GBEF in this group was 20.3%. One patient was excluded from analysis because the scan was indeterminate. All 11 patients with abnormal scans underwent cholecystectomy and experienced full resolution of their symptoms during a mean follow-up of 10 months; chronic cholecystitis was the pathologic diagnosis in all cases. Upper endoscopy led to a diagnosis of gastritis/duodenitis in 6 patients with normal scans. Five obtained relief of symptoms with H_2 blockers; the sixth patient, the only one of this group with classic biliary colic, was not helped by H_2 blockade (table).

Conclusion.—A GBEF of less than or equal to 35% can identify patients with biliary dyskinesia who will benefit from cholecystectomy. Patients with normal scans need further diagnostic testing to identify the source of their abdominal symptoms.

▶ I trust these data do not come as a surprise to you. I am delighted to see this in the surgical literature and hope that you will see more of these patients in your practice as a result.—A. Gottschalk, M.D.

The Diagnostic Value of Grading Hyperperfusion and the Rim Sign in Cholescintigraphy

Bohdiewicz PJ (William Beaumont Hosp, Royal Oak, Mich)
Clin Nucl Med 18:867–871, 1993   124-95-7–4

Objective.—The frequency of the rim sign and hyperperfusion in patients with acute cholecystitis (AC) was determined. Also tested was the hypothesis that a greater degree of hyperperfusion or rim sign is associated with greater severity of gallbladder disease in AC.

Methods.—Biliary scans of 84 hospitalized patients who were considered likely to have AC were retrospectively evaluated. Included among these scans were 55 that had a radionuclide angiography phase. The time to visualization of the gallbladder and small bowel was recorded as normal, delayed, or nonvisualized. Hyperperfusion and the rim sign were graded as mild or marked (Fig 7-2). The percentages of patients with various degrees of marked rim signs and hyperperfusion were calculated for each degree of cholecystitis, and vice versa.

Results.—Fifty-three of the 65 patients who had biliary scans with surgical and pathologic correlation had a final diagnosis of AC. Most (70%) of them were classified as "complicated" AC, defined by the presence of gangrene, perforation, empyema, necrosis, ulceration, or fibrous exudation. The rim sign was present in 47% of all patients with AC; 53% had hyperperfusion to the region of the gallbladder fossa. No patient with noncomplicated AC had a marked rim sign or marked hyperperfusion. Subdivision of the rim sign and hyperperfusion into a "marked" category substantially improved the specificity, positive predictive value, and likelihood ratio for the diagnosis of AC, particularly for the complicated subgroup when marked hyperperfusion or marked rim sign was the criterion used for a positive study.

Results.—There is an obvious association between a marked rim sign, marked hyperfusion, or both, and more severe acute cholecystitis. However, a mild rim sign is also clinically significant. Most of the patients with a mild rim sign or mild hyperperfusion had complicated AC.

▶ I suspect that you will not see anywhere near as many rim signs in your series as this author did, but I agree that when you see it, it is bad news. You had best phone the attending physician right away to let him/her know that you are sorely troubled.—A. Gottschalk, M.D.

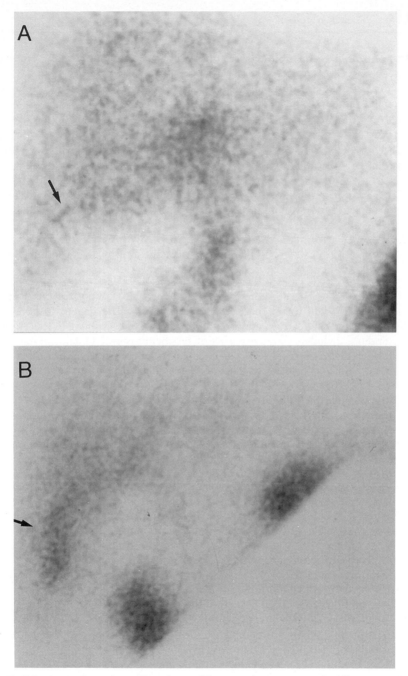

Fig 7–2.—A, anterior analogue image from a biliary scan demonstrating a "mild" rim sign of increased pericholecystic hepatic activity (*arrow*). **B,** anterior analogue image from a biliary scan demonstrating a "marked" rim sign of increased pericholecyst hepatic activity (*arrow*). (Courtesy of Bohdiewicz PJ: *Clin Nucl Med* 18:867–871, 1993.)

Radionuclide Hepatobiliary Scanning in Patients With AIDS-Related Sclerosing Cholangitis

Quinn D, Pocock N, Freund J, Kelleher A, Penny R, Brew B (St Vincent's Hosp, Darlinghurst, Australia)

Clin Nucl Med 18:417–422, 1993   124-95-7–5

Introduction.—Biliary disease, which is usually secondary to cryptosporidial or cytomegalovirus infection, is a common cause of abdominal pain in patients with AIDS. With accurate assessment and specific treatment, symptomatic improvement is possible. Ultrasound and endoscopic retrograde cholangiopancreatography (ERCP) have been the primary means of investigating suspected hepatobiliary diseases in AIDS. Data on the use of technetium-99m diisopropylphenylcarbamoylmethyl iminodiacetic acid (^{99m}Tc-DISIDA) cholescintigraphy in 3 patients with AIDS-related hepatobiliary disease confirmed by ERCP were reviewed.

Case Report.—Man, 49, homosexual, known to be HIV-positive for 5 years, was seen with right upper-quadrant abdominal pain. The patient had recently had cryptosporidial diarrhea but no other previous AIDS-defining illness. Abnormal findings included elevated results of biochemical liver function tests and a markedly reduced absolute CD4 cell count. Abdominal ultrasound revealed dilatation of both intrahepatic and extrahepatic ducts. These findings were confirmed on ERCP and revealed mucosal irregularity consistent with HIV-related sclerosing cholangitis. Further evidence of the diagnosis was provided by ^{99m}Tc-DISIDA cholescintigraphy. Treatment with diclazuril brought about some relief of symptoms. A repeat ^{99m}Tc-DISIDA scan showed a slight improvement in the percentage of tracer clearance from the hepatobiliary system in 40 minutes, from 3.6% at the initial study to 8.2% at follow-up.

Discussion.—Another patient who underwent radionuclide hepatobiliary scanning also showed focal duct dilatation with strictures in the biliary tree. A third demonstrated diffuse hepatic parenchymal retention, with marked delay in tracer washout. Identification of sclerosing cholangitis or papillary stenosis in HIV-positive patients is important because these conditions may respond to specific treatment. Radionuclide cholescintigraphy with ^{99m}Tc-DISIDA is widely available, is easy to perform, carries virtually no risk of adverse effects, and enables a quantitative estimation of biliary dysfunction. Radionuclide biliary scanning is useful in the evaluation of patients with AIDS who have right upper-quadrant pain, especially when ultrasound is inconclusive or the response to treatment must be monitored quantitatively.

▶ This is a nice discussion of AIDS-related sclerosing cholangitis. The iminodiacetic acid pattern clearly depends on which ducts are involved. If there is diffuse small-duct disease, none of the tracer gets cleared and you have a hepatitis type of picture. If some of the larger ducts are involved but some are not, you get regional increased activity with a delay in clearance. If more distal ducts are involved, you might get a pattern of generalized partial obstruction with diffuse duct dilatation and retention. If your images are very good, you will be fortunate enough to see that the dilatation of the biliary tree is not homogenous but has areas within it that are more dilatated than others, but you may not be so lucky.—A. Gottschalk, M.D.

Bile Duct Leakage After Laparoscopic Cholecystectomy Diagnosed by Radioisotopic Scanning
Politoske EJ (Univ of Southern California, Corona)
Clin Nucl Med 18:318–320, 1993   124-95-7–6

Background.—Laparoscopic cholecystectomy is quickly becoming the technique of choice for gallbladder removal. Compared with traditional cholecystectomy, it is associated with shorter hospital stays, less postoperative pain, and reduced costs. When performed by experienced surgeons, laparoscopic cholecystectomy is a safe procedure. However, there is a higher incidence of injury to the bile duct. Nuclear scintigraphy is a noninvasive method for diagnosing traumatic injury to the bile duct.

Case Report.—Woman, 37, had a major bile duct leak after undergoing an apparently successful laparoscopic cholecystectomy. After surgery, she reported generalized abdominal pain, nausea, and vomiting. Subsequently, jaundice and fever developed. Three days after surgery, 4 mCi of technetium-labeled meclofenamate (Meclomen) was injected IV, and the possibility of bile leakage or bile duct obstruction secondary to retained gallstones was investigated. Prompt visualization of the liver and biliary tree was achieved at 5 minutes. On sequential scans, a collection of radioactivity in the gallbladder fossa and right lobe of the liver was seen. The activity persisted in the gallbladder bed on delayed x-ray films and apparently increased in intensity and extended along the inferolateral margin of the right upper quadrant. The common bile duct was patent, with radioactivity extending into the small-bowel loops. A laparotomy was performed, and a significant bile leakage from the cystic duct stump was found. The patient's postoperative course was uneventful.

Conclusion.—In this patient, the complication of laparoscopic cholecystectomy was diagnosed promptly using nuclear scintigraphy. Use of radioisotopic scanning should be considered in patients with abdominal pain after laparoscopic cholecystectomy.

▶ This case highlights a diagnostic observation that I have found to be highly reliable over the years. When the iminodiacetic tracer outlines the contour of the liver, it is because it has leaked from the hepatocytes into the surrounding hepatic capsule. You then see it on the edges in the best tangential projection.

This case also illustrates that persistent pain after laparoscopic cholecystectomy is a good indication for cholescintigraphy. I had a similar case recently and made the diagnosis of subcapsular bile leak. In my case, drainage was satisfactorily performed by percutaneous-guided CT.—A. Gottschalk, M.D.

Prompt Visualization of the Gallbladder With a Rim Sign—Acute or Subacute Cholecystitis?

Morrison JC, Ramos-Gabatin A, Gelormini RG, Brown JW, Pitts NL (Wilford Hall USAF Med Ctr, Lackland AFB, Tex)
J Nucl Med 34:1169–1171, 1993   124-95-7-7

Background.—Photointense pericholecystic hepatic activity next to the gallbladder fossa—the PCHA or rim sign—correlates well with the presence of acute cholecystitis on iminodiacetic acid (IDA) scans. The positive predictive value of a rim sign for acute complicated cholecystitis is 94% when it is associated with nonvisualization of the gallbladder at 1 hour. In 1 patient who was immunosuppressed, a rim sign was observed on a technetium-99m diisopropylimidoacetic (DISIDA) scan, with prompt gallbladder visualization after bone marrow transplantation.

Case Report.—Man, 42, had signs and symptoms of acute cholecystitis. He had had autologous bone marrow transplantation for progressive multiple myeloma. Findings on gallbladder ultrasound suggested acute cholecystitis. A DISIDA scan demonstrated a rim sign, but there was normal gallbladder visual-

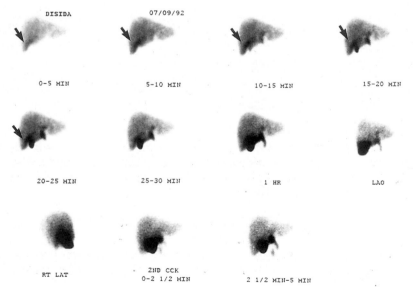

Fig 7–3.—Rim sign (*arrows*) seen in early hepatic phase and persisting throughout the study. (Courtesy of Wilford Hall Medical Center, San Antonio, Texas; and Morrison JC, Ramos-Gabatin A, Gelormini RG, et al: *J Nucl Med* 34:1169–1171, 1993.)

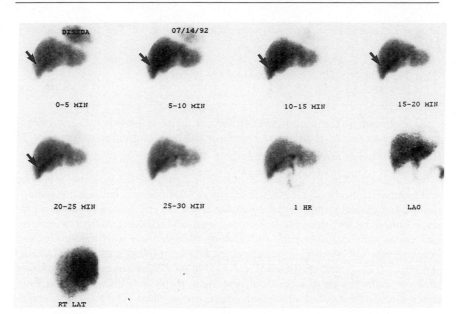

Fig 7–4.—Persistent rim sign (*arrows*) but no gallbladder visualization at 1 hour. (Courtesy of Wilford Hall Medical Center, San Antonio, Texas; and Morrison JC, Ramos-Gabatin A, Gelormini RG, et al: *J Nucl Med* 34:1169–1171, 1993.)

ization (Fig 7–3). Seventy-two hours later, when the patient's white blood cell (WBC) count was recovered, a repeat DISIDA scan showed a persistent rim sign but no gallbladder visualization at 1 hour (Fig 7–4). This pattern strongly predicted acute complicated cholecystitis. Biliary drainage with percutaneous cholecystotomy resulted in clinical improvement. Semielective cholecystectomy 8 weeks later confirmed the acute and chronic cholecystitis.

Conclusion.—Patients who are both immunocompromised and neutropenic may not have sufficient WBCs and secondary inflammatory cytokines to cause cystic duct obstruction. Whenever a rim sign is observed, with or without gallbladder visualization, acute or subacute cholecystitis should be suspected.

▶ These authors present an interesting case with an interesting hypothesis to explain it. I continue to believe that if you see a rim sign on a hepatobiliary study, it usually means trouble, so you need to give the attending surgeon a call and worry aloud to him/her. The unusual "variant" does nothing to change my mind.—A. Gottschalk, M.D.

Modern Concepts in Nonsurgical Management of Traumatic Biliary Fistulas

Horattas MC, Lewis RD, Fenton AH, Awender HM (Akron Gen Med Ctr, Ohio; Northeastern Ohio Univs College of Medicine)
J Trauma 36:186–189, 1994   124-95-7–8

Background.—Significant morbidity can arise if post-traumatic biliary tree injury or biliary fistulas are overlooked. Nonsurgical management of traumatic biliary fistulas was described.

Case Report.—Man, 27, who had been in an automobile accident, was alert and hemodynamically stable with multiple skeletal injuries, left-sided pneumothorax, and central intrahepatic hematoma (Fig 7–5). A CT scan revealed no intraperitoneal hemorrhage; the hematoma gradually resolved. After 2 weeks, he had upper right quadrant pain and abdominal distention with mildly elevated liver enzymes and bilirubin. A hepato-iminodiacetic (HIDA) scan revealed extensive biliary leakage into the pelvis (Fig 7–6). Under CT guidance, a percutaneous drainage catheter was placed along the right flank; 500 mL of bilious fluid drained immediately, and significant drainage continued. The next day, endoscopic retrograde cholangiopancreatography revealed single biliary fistulas in the left and right hepatic ducts. Transampullary stenting was accomplished. A HIDA scan 48 hours later revealed radionuclide flow into the duodenum with minimal extravasation, which correlated with minimal percutaneous catheter drainage.

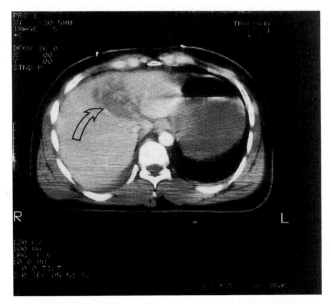

Fig 7–5.—Admission abdominal CT scan. (Courtesy of Horattas MC, Lewis RD, Fenton AH, et al: J Trauma 36:186–189, 1994.)

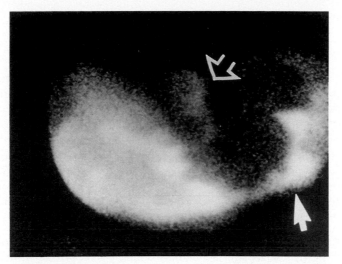

Fig 7–6.—HIDA scan demonstrating extravasation of bile outlining loops of small bowel (*lower arrow*) and minimal drainage into the duodenum (*upper arrow*). (Courtesy of Horattas MC, Lewis RD, Fenton AH, et al: *J Trauma* 36:186–189, 1994.)

Recovery was uneventful. The stent was removed after 6 weeks; a follow-up cholangiogram showed complete healing and no stenosis.

Discussion.—Diagnosis, drainage, and decompression are the keys to managing biliary fistulas. Radionuclide hepatobiliary scintigraphy is highly sensitive for identifying biliary leaks and fistulas, but it is less specific than cholangiography for delineating fistula location and anatomy. Persistent or excessive drainage may benefit from decreasing biliary tree pressure. Preferential bile drainage will continue in the biliary fistulas until the fistula tract resistance exceeds the resistance through the sphincter of Oddi. Normal biliary pressures are 300 mm H_2O or greater. Biliary tree decompression dramatically reduces fistular flow and leakage, allowing for rapid fistular maturation and closure.

▶ Figure 7–6 shows an even better example of the subcapsular bile leak outlining the contour of the liver. Note that the authors don't comment on this; they are only interested in the small-bowel visualization, but it is usually best to set the maximum diagnostic yield from the nuclear medicine studies used. In this case, the findings are best explained as showing both a subcapsular and intraperitoneal bile leak. The diagnosis of biliary fistula is then strongly suggested. As the authors point out, the 3 major components of the management of biliary fistulas are diagnosis, drainage, and decompression.

Another discussion of traumatic fistula describes the use of multiple imaging studies in a patient with "early profound jaundice following blunt hepatic trauma: resolution after lobectomy" (1).—A. Gottschalk, M.D.

Reference

1. Visner SL, et al: *J Trauma* 36:576, 1994.

Hepatobiliary Excretion of MAG3: Simulation of a Urinary Leak
Dogan AS, Kirchner PT (Univ of Iowa, Iowa City)
Clin Nucl Med 18:746–750, 1993   124-95-7–9

Introduction.—A case report illustrated the potential for an erroneous diagnosis of urinary leak in patients undergoing technetium-99m mercaptoacetyltriglycine (^{99m}Tc-MAG$_3$) scintigraphy for the evaluation of renal insufficiency. Biliary excretion of the tracer can be prominent in some cases, suggesting urinary extravasation.

Case Report.—Man, 50, was readmitted with acute renal failure (serum creatinine, 8.9 mg/dL) 3 days after undergoing double J-stent placement for bilateral hydronephrosis and obstruction of both ureters at the ureteropelvic junctions. A renal scintigram was performed to evaluate the possibility of acute urinary tract obstruction. The ^{99m}Tc-MAG$_3$ study revealed findings typical of renal insufficiency and suggested the presence of lower tract obstruction. Delayed images in the posterior and posterior oblique projections revealed significant tracer accumulation lateral to the right kidney (Fig 7–7), consistent with a urinary leak. Additional views subsequently showed this extrarenal activity to be tracer in the bowel and biliary system. There was a lack of discernible tracer activity in the urinary bladder during 6 hours, despite the appearance of tracer activity in both

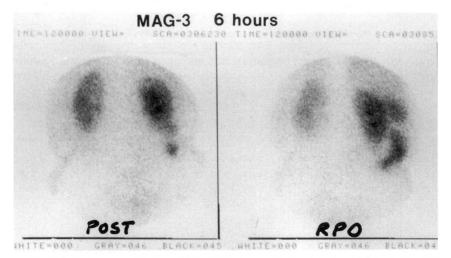

Fig 7–7.—Six hours post injection of ^{99m}Tc-MAG$_3$, tracer collection lateral and inferior to the right kidney is consistent with a urinary leak. Collecting system activity is now well defined on the **right**, but bladder activity still is not evident. (Courtesy of Dogan AS, Kirchner PT: *Clin Nucl Med* 18:746–750, 1993.)

collecting systems by 40 minutes. As a result, the patient was determined to have bilateral obstruction of the stented ureters, and he received percutaneous nephrostomy tubes. His symptoms improved rapidly, and he was discharged a week after admission with a serum creatinine level of 1.3 mg/dL.

Discussion.—A small amount of ^{99m}Tc-MAG$_3$ is excreted by the biliary system in normal patients; the amount can increase as much as 10-fold in patients with renal insufficiency. This case shows that any unusual or unexpected collections of tracer must be carefully investigated. Obstruction is unlikely, although it is not excluded, if neither the bladder nor the collecting system and ureter accumulate discernible tracer activity within several hours. Obstruction is almost certain if tracer is demonstrated in the upper tract and fails to reach the bladder or the Foley drainage bag in 10–30 minutes.

▶ Okay, we've been warned. Let's put the information these folks provide to good use. As the authors go on to illustrate in this article, if you simply remember to turn the patient over and take an anterior image if you are at all suspicious, the correct diagnosis is likely to become obvious.—A. Gottschalk, M.D.

Hepatic Hemangioma in Cirrhotics With Portal Hypertension: Evaluation With Tc-99m Red Blood Cell SPECT

Achong DM, Oates E (Tufts Univ, Boston)
Radiology 191:115–117, 1994   124-95-7-10

Introduction.—Portal hypertension results in extensive shunting of normal liver blood flow away from the liver. The effect of such abnor-

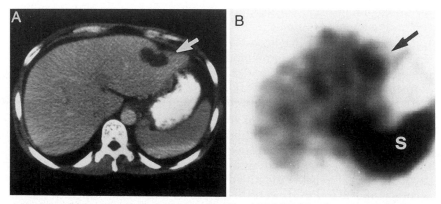

Fig 7–8.—*Abbreviation:* S, spleen. True positive CT and RBC SPECT studies. **A,** transaxial CT scan demonstrates a bi-lobed 4-cm × 2-cm lesion of low attenuation (*arrow*) in the left lobe of the liver. **B,** comparable transverse RBC SPECT scan shows focal RBC accumulation (*arrow*), characteristic of HH. The lesion has remained stable on serial CT scans for 3 years. (Courtesy of Achong DM, Oates, E: *Radiology* 191:115–117, 1994.)

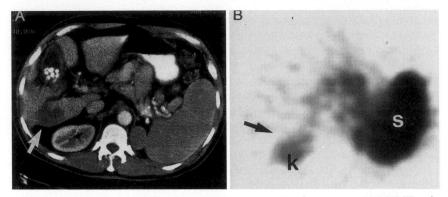

Fig 7–9.—*Abbreviations:* S, spleen; K, kidney. False positive CT and true negative RBC SPECT studies. **A,** transaxial CT scan demonstrates a 4.5-cm × 2-cm, ill-defined lesion of low attenuation (*arrow*) in an enlarged cuadate lobe. **B,** comparable transverse RBC SPECT scan shows no focal RBC accumulation (*arrow*). Thin-needle biopsy specimen revealed cirrhosis and fatty change. (Courtesy of Achong DM, Oates E: *Radiology* 191:115–117, 1994.)

mal liver blood flow dynamics on the diagnostic accuracy of technetium-99m–labeled red blood cell (RBC) SPECT was determined in patients with cirrhosis who were undergoing evaluation for hepatic hemangioma (HH).

Patients and Methods.—Fifteen individuals with cirrhosis and portal hypertension were identified from a retrospective review of 85 patients who underwent RBC SPECT for possible HH. These patients had a mean age of 53 years; 14 were men. Chronic alcohol abuse was the cause of liver disease in 8 patients. Nineteen lesions with a mean diameter of 3.5 cm were considered possible HHs on the basis of CT and/or ultrasound, and they were studied with RBC SPECT. Diagnosis of HH was based on the finding of focally increased activity greater than that of the surrounding liver, corresponding in location to the CT- or ultrasound-documented lesion.

Results.—The final diagnoses—determined by histopathologic analysis, lesion stability during a minimum of 1 year of follow-up, or hepatic angiography—were 6 HHs and 13 non-HHs. Red blood cell SPECT correctly identified 4 of the 6 HHs (Fig 7–8) and all 13 non-HHs (Fig 7–9). Both the HHs missed were small (1 and 1.4 cm in diameter).

Conclusion.—The premise of this study was that the substantial decrease in total flow and blood pool activity that occurs in portal hypertension could lead to false negative scintigraphic results for HH. Despite the presence of portal hypertension in this series of patients with cirrhosis, RBC SPECT reliably identified HH. The sensitivity, specificity, and accuracy of RBC SPECT were 67%, 100%, and 89%, respectively. For lesions greater than 1.4 cm in diameter, sensitivity increased to 100%.

▶ We would have been shocked had these data turned out otherwise. Remember, HHs are visualized as hot spots because they have a high blood volume (i.e., many venous lakes within the lesion). The rate at which these venous lakes fill is irrelevant. The fact that in cirrhosis much of the hepatic blood flows away from the liver only means you must wait long enough for the venous lakes to fill up with radiotracer and become visible. Fortunately, these authors have demonstrated that the pathology of the lesion is much more important to its visualization than the rate of blood flow.—A. Gottschalk, M.D.

The Accuracy of Technetium-99m-Labeled Red Cell Scintigraphy in Localizing Gastrointestinal Bleeding

Dusold R, Burke K, Carpentier W, Dyck WP (Texas A&M Univ Health Science Ctr, Temple)
Am J Gastroenterol 89:345–348, 1994   124-95-7-11

Introduction.—Previous studies have reported disparate results regarding the accuracy of technetium-99m–labeled red blood cell scintigraphy in localizing the site of gastrointestinal bleeding. In a retrospective review of 153 patients evaluated between 1981 and 1991, clinical and technical factors that contribute to scan accuracy were identified.

Patients and Methods.—The mean age of the patients was 66 years. Approximately half had at least 1 previous episode of gastrointestinal bleeding. A total of 174 tagged red blood scans were performed, using 3 different methods during the 10-year study. Patients were followed up by chart review for a mean of 698 days.

Results.—Ninety (59%) of the patients had 102 positive, tagged red blood cell scans and 63 (41%) had negative scans. The average transfusion requirement for the bleeding event leading to the scan did not differ significantly for patients with positive (6.3 units) and negative (5.9 units) scans. Other factors that had no influence on the incidence of

TABLE 1.—Positive-Scan Patients With Bleeding Localized by an Additional Procedure or Surgery

	Scan Localization			
	Left colon	Right colon	Other	Total
Localized				
Yes	6	17	10	33
No	0	5	6	11
Total	6	22	16	44
	100% (6/6)	77% (17/22)	62% (10/16)	75% (33/44)

(Courtesy of Dusold R, Burke K, Carpentier W, et al: *Am J Gastroenterol* 89:345-348, 1994.)

TABLE 2.—Influence of Timing on Scan Accuracy as Determined by an Additional Diagnostic Procedure or Surgery

	Time at Which Scan Proved Positive		
	<2 h	≥2 h	Total
Accurately localized bleeding site			
Yes	19	14	33
No	0	7	7
Total	19	21	40
	100% (19/19)	67% (14/21)	$p < 0.01$

Note: Excludes patients with an upper gastrointestinal bleeding source.
(Courtesy of Dusold R, Burke K, Carpentier W, et al: *Am J Gastroenterol* 89:345-348, 1994.)

scan positivity or accuracy of localization were patient age and sex and subjective description of the type of blood loss. Of the 90 patients with positive scans, 44 had a surgical procedure or additional diagnostic studies that localized the site of bleeding. Red blood scanning correctly identified 33 of these 44 sites, including all 6 left colon bleeding sites (Table 1). Twenty-two scans in the 44 patients were positive within 2 hours. Accuracy was 86% overall in these early positive scans, and it was 100% when the 3 patients with upper gastrointestinal bleeding were excluded (Table 2). Scans that were positive in 2 hours or more were less likely to be accurate.

Conclusion.—The technetium-labeled red blood cell scan is especially useful in localizing lower gastrointestinal bleeding, particularly in the left colon. Positivity within 2 hours was the most important factor that influenced scan reliability. Red blood cell scintigraphy is least reliable in the upper gastrointestinal tract; therefore, an upper gastrointestinal source of bleeding should be excluded before the scan.

▶ These results are not surprising. The authors point out that they imaged these patients under the camera for 2 hours. They do not make it clear whether they imaged continually for 2 hours or simply took serial pictures from time to time over the 2-hour period. At any rate, they go on to image at whatever interval seems prudent after 2 hours.

I have long believed that pee, pus, blood, and water run downhill. Add to this the ability of the colon to propel blood along very rapidly, and you are left with a situation that suggests you have very little chance to figure out where the blood came from if you are not imaging continually. Therefore, it makes sense that when there is very little colon left for the blood to move to (i.e., the left colon), the accuracy should be the highest. It also makes sense that when the patient is imaged at intervals (i.e., after 2 hours), the accuracy should be lousy. Therefore, these data fit my long-held view that once you stop continually imaging the patient, your ability to tell where a gastrointestinal bleed comes from probably depends more on your luck than your skill.—A. Gottschalk, M.D.

Prospective Comparative Study of Technetium-99m-WBCs and Indium-111-Granulocytes for the Examination of Patients With Inflammatory Bowel Disease

Arndt J-W, van der Sluys Veer A, Blok D, Griffioen G, Verspaget HW, Lamers CBHW, Pauwels EKJ (Univ Hosp, Leiden, The Netherlands)
J Nucl Med 34:1052–1057, 1993   124-95-7-12

Introduction.—A number of radiopharmaceuticals have been used to examine patients with inflammatory bowel disease (IBD). However, many, including indium-111 (^{111}In) granulocytes, have been time-consuming and difficult to prepare. The abilities of technetium-99m white blood cell (^{99m}Tc-WBC) scintigraphy and ^{111}In-granulocyte scintigraphy were compared in assessing the presence and location of active IBD.

Patients and Methods.—Fourteen patients, 7 men and 7 women with a mean age of 39 years, were investigated with the 2 examinations. Scintigraphically abnormal or discordant segments were evaluated by radiologic or endoscopic examination within 14 days of ^{99m}Tc-WBC scintigraphy. Twelve of the patients had Crohn's disease, and 2 had ulcerative colitis. To score the scintigrams for the presence or absence of pathologic activity, the bowel was divided into 9 segments; 111 segments were available for scoring.

Results.—A comparison of ^{99m}Tc-WBC images obtained 1 hour after injection and 3-hour ^{111}In-granulocyte images showed concordance for 102 of 111 (91.8%) bowel segments. Five segments appeared pathologic only on the ^{99m}Tc-WBC images and 4 were pathologic only on ^{111}In images. For 28 small-bowel segments, there were 3 positive concordant and 3 discordant segments, all ^{99m}Tc-WBC–positive (Fig 7–10). Two of 4 segments positive only on ^{111}In-granulocyte scintigrams were true positive at endoscopy, and 2 contained hardly any inflammatory lesions.

Conclusion.—Early imaging with ^{99m}Tc-WBCs is superior to imaging with ^{111}In-granulocytes for the evaluation of active IBD. Because of the higher dose and better imaging characteristics of the former method, images are acquired faster, can be obtained from different views, and have a higher spatial resolution. In addition, the radiation dose to the patient is lower with ^{99m}Tc-WBCs, and cell separation is simpler and less time-consuming.

▶ Nothing here is a surprise, but it is nice to have the data.—A. Gottschalk, M.D.

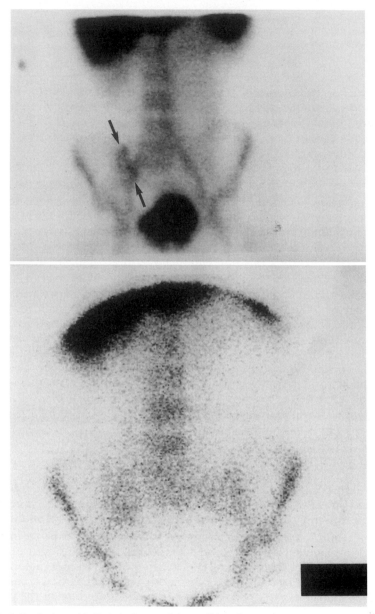

Fig 7–10.—Patient with Crohn's disease of the small bowel. Discordant images. Clear pathologic activity in the terminal ileum (*between the arrows*) on the 99mTc-WBC image (**top**). Normal 111In-granulocyte scintigram (**bottom**). (Courtesy of Arndt J-W, van der Sluys Veer A, Blok D, et al: *J Nucl Med* 34:1052–1057, 1993.)

Indium-111-White Blood Cell Scintigraphy in Crohn's Patients With Fistulae and Sinus Tracts

Even-Sapir E, Barnes DC, Martin RH, LeBrun GP (Victoria Gen Hosp, Halifax, NS, Canada)
J Nucl Med 35:245–250, 1994   124-95-7-13

Background.—Indium-111 white blood cell (^{111}In-WBC) scintigraphy can indicate the activity and extent of Crohn's disease, but its correlation with fistulization in Crohn's disease has not been established. The clinical usefulness of ^{111}In-WBC scintigraphy in patients with Crohn's disease who have fistulas and sinus tracts was evaluated.

Methods.—Indium-111 WBC images of 17 patients with Crohn's disease who had fistulas and sinus tracts were compared with radiographic results and surgical findings. Scintigraphic findings of this cohort and 50 consecutive abnormal ^{111}In-WBC studies from patients with Crohn's disease who had suspected active bowel disease but no known fistulas or sinus tracts were also compared.

Results.—The presence of concomitant intestinal and extraintestinal lesions on scintigraphy and the absence of distal luminal activity in patients without colostomy or bowel obstruction suggested the presence of fistulas. Indium-111–WBC imaging detected the drainage site of fistulas or accompanying deep abscesses. The scintigraphically determined extent of active bowel disease agreed completely with surgical findings in 14 of 17 patients; surgical and radiographic findings agreed in only 9 of 15 patients. All surgically proven abscesses were detected scintigraphically. Early images from 1 patient with a large ileosigmoid fistula detected a sigmoid abnormality that appeared normal at surgery (Fig 7–11).

Conclusion.—Indium-111–WBC scintigraphy is a useful adjunct to radiographic study, providing information essential to the appropriate

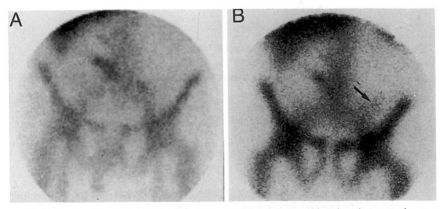

Fig 7–11.—Ileosigmoid fistula. **A,** early image. **B,** delayed image. Although early images detect a proximal intestinal lesion, there is no luminal activity distal to it. Note the activity in the sigmoid (*arrow*). (Courtesy of Even-Sapir E, Banes DC, Martin RH, et al: *J Nucl Med* 35:245–250, 1994.)

management of patients with Crohn's disease who have fistulas and sinus tracts.

▶ Some of the images shown in this article have subtle abnormalities. The use of technetium-99m–labeled white cells with their increased photon flux could be a major improvement if you are trying to make this diagnosis.—A. Gottschalk, M.D.

Indium Scanning in Assessment of Acute Crohn's Disease: A Prospective Study of Sensitivity and Correlation With Severity of Mucosal Damage

Heresbach D, Bretagne J-F, Raoul J-L, Moisan A, Siproudhis L, Devillers A, Gosselin M (Univ Hosp Pontchaillou, Rennes, France)
Dig Dis Sci 38:1601–1607, 1993   124-95-7-14

Background.—Indium-111 (^{111}In)–labeled granulocyte scanning has lower diagnostic sensitivity for the extent of Crohn's disease than for ulcerative colitis. The sensitivity of ^{111}In scanning may correlate with the severity of mucosal damage. The Crohn's disease endoscopic index of severity (CDEIS) is a new, reproducible, and valid assessment of mucosal

Comparison of Detailed Endoscopic Findings Between True Positive and False Negative Intestinal Segments at Scintigraphy

| | ^{111}In granulocyte scan at 3 hr | | |
	True positive (N = 51)	False negative (N = 19)	P
Percentage of the segmental surface involved by the disease (mean ± SD)	45 ± 38	25 ± 25	<0.01
Percentage of the segmental surface involved by ulcerations (mean ± SD)	26 ± 25	10 ± 9	<0.001
Presence of superficial ulceration			
Yes (%)	51 (100)	16 (84)	NS*
No (%)	0 (0)	3 (16)	
Presence of deep ulceration			
Yes (%)	20 (39)	0 (0)	NS
No (%)	31 (61)	19 (100)	

*NS, not significant.
(Courtesy of Heresbach D, Bretagne J-F, Raoul J-L: *Dig Dis Sci* 38:1601–1607, 1993.)

damage. The sensitivity of ^{111}In scanning for the extent and activity of Crohn's disease was reevaluated using the CDEIS.

Methods.—Colonoscopic and ^{111}In scintigraphic findings for 19 patients with active colonic or ileocolonic Crohn's disease were compared.

Results.—Active mucosal lesions were visible in 70 of 86 intestinal segments. Third-hour scintiscans revealed at least 1 positive intestinal segment in all patients. Among the 86 initial endoscopic segments, ^{111}In scanning suggested that 52 were positive and 34 were negative. Subsequent endoscopy confirmed 51 positive and 15 negative scintigraphies; thus, ^{111}In scanning had a 98% positive predictive value and a 44% negative predictive value. The sensitivity diagnosis of acute extent was 73% for ^{111}In scanning, although complete scintigraphy-endoscopy agreement occurred in only 32% of patients. The percentages of segmental surfaces involved in the disease and in ulceration only were significantly higher in true positive segments than in false negative segments (table). Thirty-nine percent of true positive segments and none of the false negative segments had deep ulcerations, but the difference was not significant.

Conclusion.—Indium-111–labeled granulocyte scanning results correlate well with endoscopic mucosal lesion severity in Crohn's disease. Nevertheless, scintigraphy may miss minor mucosal lesions.

▶ I am intrigued by the authors' suggestion that the lesions detected are those which require treatment and that those which are not detected by scintigraphy have no clinical significance. A prospective trial that proves this could cut down on the use of endoscopy and potentially decrease the cost of managing these patients.—A. Gottschalk, M.D.

Remnants of Normal Tissue in Polycystic Disease of the Liver: A Cause for Difficulty in the Interpretation of Indium-111 White Blood Cell Study
Even-Sapir E, Barnes DC, Iles SE (Victoria Gen Hosp, Halifax, NS, Canada)
Clin Nucl Med 18:967–969, 1993   124-95-7–15

Background.—Indium-111–labeled white blood cell (^{111}In-WBC) scanning identifies the infection site in patients with fever. Activity in areas other than the normal biodistribution of labeled WBC suggests infection. A case of diffuse hepatic disease, in which markedly altered radiopharmaceutical biodistribution confounded ^{111}In-WBC interpretation, was presented.

Case Report.—Man, 49, was febrile and had chronic hepatic and renal failure caused by polycystic disease. Anterior ^{111}In-WBC scintigraphy revealed uptake in the mid-abdomen (Fig 7–12); posteriorly, uptake was noted to the right of the spine. Scintigraphy did not differentiate normal liver tissue or infection site as the cause of abdominal ^{111}In-WBC uptake. Two days later, technetium-99m SC scintigraphy revealed the absence of functional tissue in the right lobe and multi-

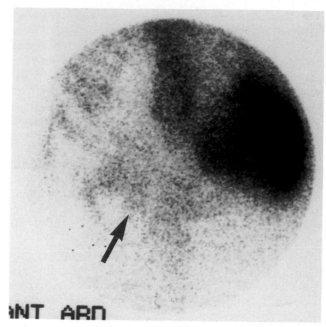

Fig 7–12.—Indium-111 WBC study. Diffuse uptake in the expected location of the liver is absent. Uptake is demonstrated in the mid-abdomen anteriorly (*arrow*). (Courtesy of Even-Sapir E, Barnes DC, Iles SE: *Clin Nucl Med* 18:967–969, 1993.)

ple photon-deficient areas in the remainder of the liver; remnants of functioning liver parenchyma corresponded to the abdominal site of ^{111}In-WBC uptake (Fig 7–13). During subsequent hepatectomy and nephrectomy and combined hepato-renal transplantation, no abdominal or hepatic abscesses were found. Pathologic examination of the specimen revealed diffuse replacement of normal liver tissue by cysts; only the caudate lobe was preserved.

Discussion.—Normal radiopharmaceutical uptake in the liver and spleen commonly obscures hepatic and splenic abscesses, infected cysts, and subphrenic and perihepatic abscesses. Correlation of a photon-deficient area on a technetium-99m SC image with normal ^{111}In-WBC images may reveal an infectious process in the liver or spleen. In this patient, the correlation indicated that remnants of liver tissue, rather than abscesses, caused the scintigraphic abnormality.

Conclusion.—Sulfur colloid imaging is useful in documenting a defect in a liver that appears normal on ^{111}In-WBC scintigraphy and in mapping remaining normal tissue in diffuse hepatic disease.

▶ This is a nice case, but it really represents déjà vu all over again. In general, any time you do "hot spot" imaging, warm (i.e., isoactive) lesions will be missed if you don't have a template to tell you where they should be. Examples include the use of a colloid liver scan to help detect a faintly active hem-

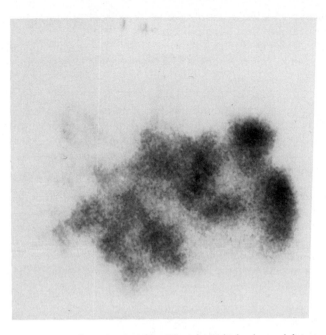

Fig 7–13.—Anterior view of a technetium-99m SC study. Multiple photon-deficient areas are detected in the liver with remnants of functioning parenchyma, which correspond to the foci of uptake on ¹¹¹In-WBC study. (Courtesy of Even-Sapir E, Barnes DC, Iles SE: *Clin Nucl Med* 18:967–969, 1993.)

angioma in the liver with labeled red blood cells, the use of a colloid liver scan to find a faintly active abscess in the liver with gallium, and the use of technetium bone scanning to find an area of incongruous uptake with gallium scanning to detect chronic osteomyelitis. Clearly, with the activity going to the liver in the usual white cell scan, a template colloid liver scan to show functional hepatic activity would seem mandatory to avoid a diagnostic disaster.

Other unusual cases that I have come across include "Image distortion due to massive ascites during Tc-99m RBC scanning for intestinal bleeding" (1) and "Grossly abnormal liver-spleen scan in a patient with veno-aclusive disease of the liver that normalized completely on follow-up" (2).—A. Gottschalk, M.D.

References

1. Conway SK, Briggs RC: *Clin Nucl Med* 18:520, 1993.
2. Joshi MJ, et al: *Clin Nucl Med* 18:590, 1993.

False-Positive Meckel's Imaging and True-Positive Imaging of a Gastrointestinal Bleed and Surgical Lesion

Spieth ME, Seder JS, Yuja RE, Kimura RL, Schroeder EV, Silvestri JH (LAC+King Med Ctr, Los Angeles; Community Mem Hosp, Ventura, Calif)
Clin Nucl Med 19:298–301, 1994   124-95-7-16

Introduction.—Pertechnetate has facilitated the diagnosis of Meckel's diverticulum, a lesion that is difficult to detect with conventional radiographic studies. In an unusual case of a false positive Meckel's scan, pathologic examination confirmed that the lesion removed at surgery was an unsuspected carcinoid tumor.

Case Report.—White woman, 76, was seen because of maroon-colored stools and lightheadedness. A colonoscopy did not reveal a discrete lesion. Iron tablets were prescribed, and she was discharged. Meckel's scan was performed several months later when the gastroenterologist suspected Meckel's diverticulum. Immediately after IV injection of 7.5 mCi of technetium-99m pertechnetate, physiologic activity was noted in the stomach blood pool and lateral to the stomach in

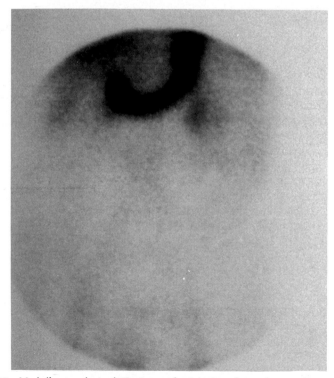

Fig 7–14.—Meckel's scan obtained 10 minutes after injection of pertechnetate. (Courtesy of Spieth ME, Seder JS, Yuja RE, et al: *Clin Nucl Med* 19:298–301, 1994.)

the left upper quadrant. The nuclear physician thought that the focus of activity was not in the usual position for a Meckel's diverticulum (Fig 7–14). Two weeks later when the patient underwent surgery, the appearance of the 1-cm ulcerated ileal lesion suggested a carcinoid. A short-bowel and single mesenteric node resection was performed followed by primary ileal anastomosis. Histopathologic examination demonstrated a classic carcinoid.

Discussion.—This is the third published case of a carcinoid tumor discovered by a false positive Meckel's scan. A negative scan does not exclude the presence of a Meckel's diverticulum, and there are numerous potential causes of false positive scans, the most common being gut activity visualized by secreted pertechnetate from the stomach and pertechnetate in the renal pelvis or ureter. Inflammatory and vascular lesions are uncommon causes of false positive Meckel's imaging.

▶ This is a rare but good thing to know. I cannot help but wonder whether the visualization resulted from the carcinoid tumor or the ulceration within it. Remember, right after injection, about 85% of the pertechnetate is still bound to plasma proteins and therefore could easily leak into the gut, just as colloid does. Finally, I also wonder what a loop of ileum was doing in the left upper quadrant.—A. Gottschalk, M.D.

Repeated Technetium-99m Pertechnetate Scanning for Children With Obscure Gastrointestinal Bleeding
Kong M-S, Huang S-C, Tzen K-Y, Lin J-N (Chang Gung Children's Hosp, Taipei, Taiwan, Republic of China)
J Pediatr Gastroenterol Nutr 18:284–287, 1994   124-95-7–17

Background.—Seven instances were reported in which children with massive gastrointestinal bleeding from ectopic gastric mucosae had false negative results from technetium-99m (^{99m}Tc) abdominal scans. Other

---

Summary of Patients With Obscure Gastrointestinal (GI) Bleeding From Ectopic
Gastric Mucosa

Case no.	Age at Dx	Sex	Duration of GI bleeding	Tc-99m scan –	Tc-99m scan +	Cause of – scan	Pathology
1	50 mo	m	8 mo	1	1	Bleed	Meckel
2	27 mo	m	21 mo	2	1	?	Duplication
3	27 mo	m	1.5 mo	1	1	Bleed	Meckel
4	7 mo	m	1 mo	1	1	?	Meckel
5	19 mo	m	2.5 mo	2	1	?	Duplication
6	19 mo	m	12 mo	1	1	No CE	Meckel
7	15 mo	m	7 mo	1	1	?	Meckel

Abbreviations: Dx, diagnosis; *Bleed,* bleeding; *CE,* cimetidine enhancement; *?,* unknown.
(Courtesy of Kong M-S, Huang S-C, Tzen K-Y, et al: *J Pediatr Gastroenterol Nutr* 18:284–287, 1994.)

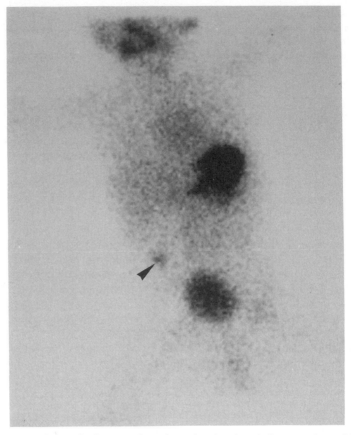

Fig 7–15.—Focal area of radioactivity (*arrow*) was found at the right lower quadrant of the abdomen of the patient with hemophilia. (Courtesy of Kong M-S, Huang S-C, Tzen K-Y, et al: *J Pediatr Gastroenterol Nutr* 18:284–287, 1994.)

examinations had failed to locate the source of the bleeding, and positive results were obtained only after repeated [99mTc] abdominal scans.

Patients and Methods.—The 7 children ranged in age from 7 to 50 months at diagnosis. The duration of gastrointestinal bleeding ranged from 1 month to 21 months. All had undergone various studies, including endoscopy, gastrointestinal series, angiography, and [99mTc]-labeled red blood cell scans, to search for the source of bleeding. These studies and the initial [99mTc] abdominal scans were negative in all cases. Two of the patients required a third scan before positive results were obtained. Surgical specimens confirmed the source of bleeding to be ectopic gastric tissue in 5 patients with Meckel's diverticulum and in 2 patients with enteric duplication (table).

Discussion.—The failure of a [99mTc] scan to detect ectopic gastric tissue in children with gastrointestinal hemorrhage does not exclude the diagnosis. Potential causes of false negative studies include an insufficient mass of gastric tissue, impaired blood supply, downstream washout of pertechnetate, excessive secretions, or suboptimal technique. In 1 child, a hemophiliac with active bleeding, the continued bleeding may have caused a washout of isotope, which produced negative results. The second scan, obtained after the bleeding diminished, was positive (Fig 7–15). As many as 3 ^{99m}Tc scans may be required in children with negative scans but a high level of suspicion for ectopic gastric mucosa.

▶ Good point.—A. Gottschalk, M.D.

Cholescintigraphic Study of Effect of Somatostatin Analog, Octreotide, on Bile Secretion and Gallbladder Emptying in Normal Subjects
Grimaldi C, Darcourt J, Harris AG, Lebot E, Lapalus F, Delmont J (Cabinet d'Hépato-Gastro-Entérologie, Nice, France; Nice Univ Hosp, France; Cedars Sinai Med Ctr, Los Angeles)
Dig Dis Sci 38:1718–1721, 1993   124-95-7–18

Introduction.—Octreotide is a long-acting somatostatin analogue that is used to control acromegaly and various gastrointestinal and pancreatic endocrine tumors. Gallstones are an expected side effect of long-term treatment. Native somatostatin inhibits emptying of the gallbladder, and reduces bile flow, and may increase bile cholesterol saturation.

Objective and Methods.—The effects of octreotide on hepatic bile secretion and gallbladder function were studied in 12 healthy individuals of both sexes whose median age was 46 years. Quantitative scintigraphy was performed using technetium-99m (^{99m}Tc)-labeled parabutyl iminodiacetic acid (PBIDA) and a wide-field-of-view gamma camera equipped with a computerized scintigraphic data analyzer. Dynamic imaging was continued for 90 minutes after injection of the radiopharmaceutical. The participants received either 100 μg of octreotide or a placebo in a double-blind manner 10 minutes before the radionuclide, and a fatty meal was served 1 hour later.

Results.—Peak hepatic radioactivity was insignificantly higher in octreotide-treated individuals, and the relative decrease in activity was significantly less in these individuals. The peak gallbladder activity after the fatty meal was achieved significantly later in the individuals who were given octreotide, and the ratio of tracer activity at 60 and 90 minutes was significantly higher when octreotide was given.

Conclusion.—Octreotide slows the hepatic release of ^{99m}Tc-labeled PBIDA, presumably because of reduced secretion of bile. It also inhibits postprandial contraction of the gallbladder.

▶ The good news is that the radioactive octreotide tracer that many of you will begin to use as a diagnostic agent to find endocrine and other type tumors (a new drug application was just granted last June) uses only about 10 µg of octreotides; in other words, about one tenth the dose given in this study. Consequently, you can probably forget the effect the tracer will have on gallbladder physiology.

The bad news is that as octreotide becomes a therapeutic option for patients with endocrine tumors, they may get gallstones. Therefore, you will have to know what octreotide does to gallbladder physiology to properly interpret your iminodiacetic acid scans.—A. Gottschalk, M.D.

Influence of the Menstrual Cycle and of Menopause on the Gastric Emptying Rate of Solids in Female Volunteers

Monés J, Carrió I, Calabuig R, Estorch M, Sainz S, Berná L, Vilardell F (Universitat Autònoma de Barcelona)
Eur J Nucl Med 20:600–602, 1993   124-95-7–19

Background.—Gastric emptying of both solids and liquids takes longer in women than in men. It is possible that the difference reflects an influence of estrogens and/or progesterone on gastric emptying. Studies have indicated that changes between phases of the menstrual cycle are minimal, although emptying becomes somewhat faster after menopause.

Objective.—The rate of gastric emptying of solids was estimated at various phases of the menstrual cycle in 15 premenopausal women, 22 to 35 years of age, who were not using oral contraception and in 10 postmenopausal women, 47 to 66 years of age, who had been menopausal for a year or longer. All were generally in good health.

Method.—Patients took a 96-MJ test meal, consisting of a sandwich, omelette, and orange juice, after fasting for 8 hours. Technetium-labeled human serum albumin was added to the egg of the omelette, and gastric radioactivity was monitored at 15-minute intervals, during which patients remained seated or walked around.

Findings.—Similar gastric emptying rates were recorded in the follicular and luteal phases of the cycle in premenopausal women and also in the premenopausal and postmenopausal women. From 41% to 52% of the labeled meal remained in the stomach after 90 minutes. The mean emptying half-times were in the range of 75–78 minutes in all groups.

Conclusion.—Neither gender nor menopausal status is an important factor when measuring gastric emptying in patients with disorders such as anorexia nervosa, bulimia, or nonulcerogenic dyspepsia.

▶ Viva la no difference.—A. Gottschalk, M.D.

Radioisotope Determination of Regional Colonic Transit in Severe Constipation: Comparison With Radio Opaque Markers

van der Sijp JRM, Kamm MA, Nightingale JMD, Britton KE, Mather SJ, Morris GP, Akkermans LMA, Lennard-Jones JE (St Mark's Hosp, London; St Bartholomew's Hosp, London; Univ Hosp, Utrecht, The Netherlands)
Gut 34:402–408, 1993   1 24-95-7-20

Background.—Radiopaque markers are widely used to measure whole-gut transit times in identifying patients with slowed intestinal transit. However, in patients who are constipated, altered colonic motility may lead to an erroneous designation of the site of colonic delay if radiopaque markers are used and radiographs are made infrequently.

Objective.—To accurately estimate regional colonic transit, the transit of an isotopically labeled test meal was determined in patients who simultaneously ingested radiopaque markers.

Methods.—Studies were done in 12 women, 24 to 55 years of age who, for unknown reasons, had bowel movements less often than once a week with a colon of normal diameter on barium enema examination. All of them described bloating and abdominal pain. Twelve men and women of similar age who denied gastrointestinal symptoms were also evaluated. After an overnight fast, the participants took a 630-kcal pancake containing indium-111 bound to microspheres of Amerlite resin. At the same time, the participants swallowed a first set of 20 barium-impregnated polyvinylchloride markers, and further sets were ingested 24 and 48 hours after the test meal. Scintigraphy began 6 hours after the meal and continued for 1 week or until all activity was absent from the colon.

Results.—All the constipated patients retained more than 20% of the ingested radiopaque markers at 96 hours. Four of them had no bowel action during the 1-week study, whereas the others averaged fewer than 2 bowel actions during this time. Constipated patients consistently had colonic transit values outside the normal range, reflecting delayed transit. Similar results were obtained using the isotopic and marker methods.

Conclusion.—Radioisotopic estimates of colonic transit provide accurate data on transit through individual regions of the colon. Radiopaque markers can be used to screen for delayed colonic transit.

▶ The authors go on to say that they believe the isotope technique is more accurate than the "well-established" radioopaque marker technique. Consequently, the isotope method may be the best to use to determine the effectiveness of therapy, particularly if therapy is directed at a localized region of the colon or rectum, for example, segmental surgical resection.—A. Gottschalk, M.D.

Physiopathological Significance of Thallium-201 Per Rectum Scintigraphy in Liver Cirrhosis

Urbain D, Muls V, Dupont M, Jeghers O, Thys O, Ham HR (Free Univ, Brussels, Belgium)

J Nucl Med 34:1642–1645, 1993   124-95-7-21

Background.—The physiopathologic significance of thallium-201 (^{201}Tl) per-rectum scintigraphy has not been established. The results of this method were compared with results obtained from direct measurement of inferior mesenteric shunting, portal pressure, liver cellular function, as evaluated by the Aminopyrine Breath Test, and the size of esophagogastric varices and spleen, which indirectly represented azygos and splenic shunts, respectively.

Methods and Findings.—The measures of portal systemic shunt estimated by the per-rectal method and those obtained by direct administration of the tracer in the inferior mesenteric artery were highly correlated. However, there was no correlation between ^{201}Tl per-rectal results and portal presssure or with azygos and splenic shunting. The correlation with the Aminopyrine Breath Test was fair. These findings may result from a change in both methods in patients with advanced liver disease.

Conclusion.—The ^{201}Tl per-rectal scintigraphy explores the portal systemic shunt, which depends almost solely on the inferior mesenteric territory. Although the limited territory explored by this method is probably a restrictive factor in the detection and quantitation of the total portal-systemic shunt, the specific information provided by the test may be helpful in defining clinical and biological profiles of patients with cirrhosis and inferior mesenteric shunting.

▶ I always try to have the tail end of this section represented by a tail-end study. In this case, the test is not very hard to perform, and you may wish to keep it in mind when machines like the Doppler unit in your place break down or some other instrumentation catastrophe occurs. It is good to remember that many tracers can be administered effectively per rectum. For example, Paul Harper (1) found out years ago that pertechnetate is effectively absorbed from the rectum. This type of information may be useful when you come across an obese veinless patient. It is always good to have a trump card to play (at least I did not say ace in the hole).—A. Gottschalk, M.D.

Reference

1. Harper PV, et al: Pharmacodynamics of some technetium-99m preparations, in *Radioactive Pharmaceuticals* proc. ORAU symposium, Nov, 1965.

8 Vascular

Introduction

The introduction of the Anger camera into nuclear medicine was associated with considerable enthusiasm about the possibility of examining perfusion and blood flow with radionuclide techniques. Early studies using bolus injections of technetium reviewed relative carotid blood flow, blood flow to the renal arteries, studies of aortic aneurysm, and many other vascular abnormalities. However, the introduction of Doppler techniques, improved arteriography, MRI, and plethysmography have largely eclipsed the role of radionuclides in the evaluation of diseases of the vascular system. Although the number of recent articles on this subject in nuclear medicine is relatively small, it is encouraging to know that some effort is still being made in this area. With the great versatility of radionuclide techniques, it is not unreasonable to anticipate some significant developments during the next several years as our technology improves.

M. Donald Blaufox, M.D., Ph.D.

Regional Distribution of ^{201}Tl During One-Leg Exercise: Comparison With Leg Blood Flow by Plethysmography
Seto H, Kageyama M, Futatsuya R, Shimizu M, Watanabe N, Wu Y, Kakishita M (Toyama Med and Pharmaceutical Univ, Japan)
Nucl Med Commun 14:810–813, 1993   124-95-8–1

Background.—Although many techniques are available for quantifying the arterial circulation in the legs at rest, there are no adequate methods for measuring regional blood flow during exercise in clinical settings. The validity of thallium-201 (^{201}Tl) distribution as an estimate of regional blood flow in the legs was assessed.

Methods.—Eleven men, mean age 61 years, without peripheral vascular disease were studied. Thallium-201 leg uptake was compared using whole body scintigraphy and simultaneously measured leg blood flow with plethysmography during 1-leg exercise. In addition, the ^{201}Tl leg uptake ratio and leg blood flow ratio were compared to exclude the effect of cardiac output variation in each man.

Findings.—The correlation between leg blood flow and ^{201}Tl leg uptake was good and highly linear. However, the ^{201}Tl leg uptake ratio

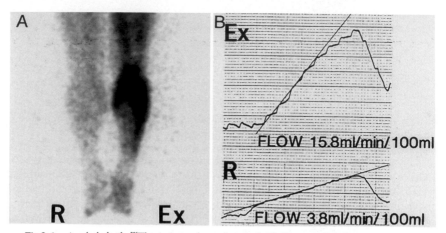

Fig 8–1.—A, whole body ^{201}Tl scintigram (posterior view). Thallium-201 uptake ratio (Ex/R) in the calf region is 3.94. **B,** plethysmographic data during 1-leg exercise. Leg blood flow ratio (Ex/R) is 4.16. (Courtesy of Seto H, Kageyama M, Futatsuya R, et al: *Nucl Med Commun* 14:810–813, 1993.)

somewhat underestimated the leg blood flow ratio as exercise became strenuous (Fig 8–1).

Conclusion.—Thallium-201 leg uptake and its ratio based on whole body scintigraphy were correlated closely with leg blood flow and its ratio by plethysmography during 1-leg exercise. As a result, the regional distribution of ^{201}Tl by whole body scintigraphy reflects regional blood flow in the legs during exercise.

▶ In view of the very high association between peripheral vascular disease and coronary artery disease, it is surprising that so little attention has been directed at adding an evaluation of peripheral blood flow to the thallium stress test. The authors provide another look at this technique, along with further justification for adding it to the evaluation of selected patients who are undergoing thallium stress tests.—M.D. Blaufox, M.D., Ph.D.

Radionuclide Limb Blood Flow Measurements to Resolve Diagnostic Problems in Vascular Surgery
Parkin A, Maughan J, Robinson PJ, Wilkinson D, Kerin MJ, Kester RC (St James's Univ NHS Hosp Trust, Leeds, England)
Nucl Med Commun 15:148–151, 1994   124-95-8–2

Introduction.—Although the most common cause of exercise-induced leg pain is peripheral vascular disease (PVD), diagnosis can be difficult. The usefulness of radionuclide extremity blood flow measurements was examined in 60 patients with an atypical appearance of intermittent claudication.

Methods.—All patients had below-knee blood flow measurements in both legs. For this technique, the patient is supine with the legs and feet over the gamma camera field. A blood pressure cuff placed just below the knee is inflated, and the tracer is injected. After 3 minutes for equilibration, the cuff is released and the rate of increase of activity within the extremity is recorded by the gamma camera every second for 100 seconds.

Results.—The normal range of below-knee extremity blood flow in healthy nonsmoking volunteers was 10–22 mL/100 mL of tissue/min. Thirty-two of the 60 patients included in this study had blood flow that was below the normal level in at least 1 leg. Significant vascular disease was proven in 31 patients; 1 refused to undergo further evaluation. Orthopedic disease was identified in 23 patients. In the 5 remaining patients, the symptoms resolved spontaneously.

Conclusion.—Radionuclide extremity blood flow evaluation is reliable and superior to assessment of peripheral pulses and measurement of the ankle to brachial pressure index for the diagnosis of PVD in patients with exercise-induced leg pain.

▶ This article presents a more quantitative approach to the measurement of peripheral blood flow than the preceding one (Abstract 124-95-8-1). Although a qualitative assessment may be adequate in most patients, in some, especially in those in whom some intervention is going to be carried out that must be evaluated, more objective numbers are probably required. However, it may be that the evaluation of blood flow after exercise has significant advantages, even though it is only a qualitative technique over a quantitative technique that can only be done at rest. Perhaps some combination of the 2 techniques would be optimal.—M.D. Blaufox, M.D., Ph.D.

A Comparative Study of Radionuclide Venography and Contrast Venography in the Diagnosis of Deep Venous Thrombosis

Kilpatrick TK, Gibson RN, Lichtenstein M, Neerhut P, Andrews J, Hopper J (Royal Melbourne Hosp, Victoria, Australia; Univ of Melbourne, Victoria, Australia)
Aust N Z J Med 23:641–645, 1993   124-95-8-3

Background.—The value of the radionuclide blood pool venogram in identifying deep venous thrombosis (DVT) has not been researched sufficiently, even though it has a lower complication rate than the gold standard of contrast x-ray venography. The relative accuracy and interobserver variability of radionuclide blood pool and x-ray contrast venography were compared.

Methods.—Radionuclide and contrast venography were compared prospectively in 39 patients. A meta-analysis was also performed on previously published studies.

Studies Comparing Accuracy of Technetium-99m–Labeled Erythrocyte Radionuclide Venography and Contrast Venography in the Diagnosis of DVT in the Proximal and Distal Leg

Study	Year	Patient no.	DVT site		Proximal		Distal	
			Proximal	Distal	Sens	Spec	Sens	Spec
Beswick[8]	1979	30	19	2	19/19 (100%)	8/9 (89%)	2/2 (100%)	8/9 (89%)
Kempi[9]	1981	27	10	6	8/10 (80%)	11/11 (100%)	4/6 (67%)	10/11 (91%)
Lisbona[10]	1982	35	17	4	17/17 (100%)	12/14 (86%)	3/4 (75%)	13/14 (93%)
Singer[11]	1984	21	9	2	8/9 (89%)	10/10 (100%)	2/2 (100%)	8/10 (80%)
Kilpatrick	1993	39	10	5	9/10 (90%)	22/24 (92%)	3/5 (60%)	22/24 (92%)
Mean value					94%	93%	74%	90%
Confidence intervals					85-98%	84-97%	50-89%	80-95%

(Courtesy of Kilpatrick TK, Gibson RN, Lichtenstein M, et al: *Aust N Z J Med* 23:641–645, 1993.)

Findings.—Interobserver variation was significant in radionuclide and contrast venograms, with values of 37% and 22%, respectively. Using consensus studies, the sensitivity and specificity of radionuclide venography were 87% and 83%, respectively, compared with those for contrast venography. In the proximal veins, the sensitivity and specificity were 90% and 92%, respectively, compared with 74% and 90% in the distal veins (table).

Conclusion.—The best diagnostic test for establishing or refuting the presence of DVT may vary with the nature of the clinical presentation. No 1 test is entirely accurate in diagnosing acute DVT; clinical data are mandatory for facilitating an accurate diagnosis and appropriate treatment. Although radionuclide venography is useful in excluding DVT and diagnosing proximal but not distal DVT, further research is needed to confirm the diagnostic accuracy of this method.

▶ Another old nuclear medicine technique is revisited and compared with the accepted gold standard. The comparative sensitivities and specificites of radionuclide and contrast venograms are surprisingly similar, and, not surprisingly, the interobserver variation for both techniques is quite large. This is another neglected technique that maybe we should be using more often in some clinical settings.—M.D. Blaufox, M.D., Ph.D.

Role of Radionuclide Venography in the Detection of Proximal Deep Vein Thrombosis: A Prospective Comparative Study

Mohamadiyeh MK, Shaban AA, El-Desouki M, Malabarey T, Ell PJ (King Khaled Univ Hosp, Riyadh, Saudi Arabia; Inst of Nucl Medicine, UCMSM, London)

Nucl Med Commun 14:1014–1022, 1993   124-95-8–4

Background.—Current diagnostic techniques fail to detect nearly half the cases of deep vein thrombosis (DVT), which can result in pulmonary embolism (PE). Radionuclide venography (RNV) is nonspecific for thrombosis, and some investigators have suggested that it be replaced with blood pool venography. However, RNV may be more helpful and convenient in the screening of DVT above the knee, especially in patients with signs or symptoms of PE.

Methods.—The role of radionuclide imaging techniques in the evaluation of thromboembolic disease was prospectively reevaluated. Forty-eight patients with suspected PE or DVT underwent RNV and ventilation-perfusion lung scintigraphy. Both studies were done using technetium-99m (^{99m}Tc)-labeled macroaggregated albumin. In addition, contrast venography and peripheral ^{99m}Tc-labeled red blood cell scintigraphy were performed in 32 patients.

Results.—The overall agreement rates were 89% for RNV and 88% for radionuclide blood pool venography. Disagreement rates increased at distal sites. Sensitivities were 90% and 88%, respectively, with specificities of 73% and 82%. Blood pool venography was no better than RNV in detecting DVT or confirming PE. Radionuclide venography detected the possible source of PE in 72% of the cases.

Conclusion.—Radionuclide venography remains a valid noninvasive technique for the detection of proximal DVT. It is especially helpful in improving the diagnostic accuracy of thromboembolism by demonstrated DVT in patients with a low or intermediate probability of PE. The clinical role of blood pool venography remains to be established.

▶ A significant advantage in doing RNV is the ability to combine it with a lung scan, thereby minimizing the cost of the procedure and providing a considerable amount of additional useful information in selected patients. If the use of blood pool RNV improved the sensitivity and specificity of the technique, this justification would be considerably weakened.

It is interesting that the authors report that blood pool venography does not appear to be a significantly better technique. Because the ultimate concern is the development of PE, and because the use of macroaggregated albumin for renography appears to yield comparable results to blood pool venography using stannous fluoride, it would be preferable to use the macroaggregated albumin and take advantage of the ability to perform a subsequent lung scan.—M.D. Blaufox, M.D., Ph.D.

Thrombus Imaging With Technetium-99m Synthetic Peptides Based Upon the Binding Domain of a Monoclonal Antibody to Activated Platelets

Knight LC, Radcliffe R, Maurer AH, Rodwell JD, Alvarez VL (Temple Univ, Philadelphia; Cytogen Corp, Princeton, NJ)
J Nucl Med 35:282–288, 1994   124-95-8-5

Background.—Monoclonal antibodies (Mabs) for fibrin or platelets have enabled vascular thrombus imaging; however, slow blood disappearance of even small antibody fragments impedes diagnosis. Synthetic oligopeptides that mimic active binding Mab regions or native glycoproteins may carry radiotracer and permit earlier thrombus imaging because they clear the blood more rapidly. Seven technetium-99m–labeled peptides were evaluated.

Methods.—The peptides were synthesized with amino acid sequences based on the primary binding region of platelet glycoprotein IIb/IIIa-directed Mab PAC1. Thirty minutes after creation of a fresh thrombus in the left jugular vein of rabbits, radiotracers were infused in a marginal ear vein on the contralateral side. To assess peptide behavior in mature lesions, thrombi were induced in the femoral veins of 7 dogs 24 hours before radiotracer administration.

Results.—In rabbits and dogs, peptide radioactivity left the blood pool quickly, appearing in the kidneys within 10 minutes. The percentage of the administered dose in the blood decreased to about 2% to 3% by 4 hours. In rabbits, clots were visible within 1 hour and focally positive by 2 hours. The area of uptake often extended into the jaw and ear, possibly related to clot progression in the vein. Clot-to-blood ratios were low for fibrinogen because of its slow blood disappearance. For rapidly clearing peptides, clot-to-blood ratios were less than 2:1. Glucoheptonate, a negative control, had significantly higher clot-to-blood and clot-to-muscle ratios than many of the peptides in rabbits. Of 2 peptides tested in dogs, only 1 produced a thrombus image. Technetium-99m glucoheptonate exhibited only diffuse uptake in the thrombus area. Thrombus-to-muscle ratios and peak thrombus uptake of the effective peptide were significantly lower than fibrinogen values.

Conclusion.—Labeled synthetic peptides are technically feasible, but absolute thrombus binding with these peptides is still insufficient to provide reliable imaging of preexisting thrombi.

Detection of Deep Venous Thrombi and Pulmonary Embolus With Technetium-99m-DD-3B6/22 Anti-Fibrin Monoclonal Antibody Fab' Fragment

Bautovich G, Angelides S, Lee F-T, Greenough R, Bundesen P, Murray P, Schmidt P, Waugh R, Harris J, Cameron K, Lambrecht RM, Basten A (Royal Prince Alfred Hosp, Sydney, Australia; Biomedicine and Health Program, Ansto, Menai, Australia; AGEN Biomedical Ltd, Brisbane, Australia; et al)
J Nucl Med 35:195–202, 1994   124-95-8-6

Introduction.—There is a great need for a noninvasive method that can provide reliable detection of deep venous thrombosis (DVT) and pulmonary embolism. Venous and arterial thrombi are largely composed of cross-linked fibrin. Initial research has shown that the antifibrin

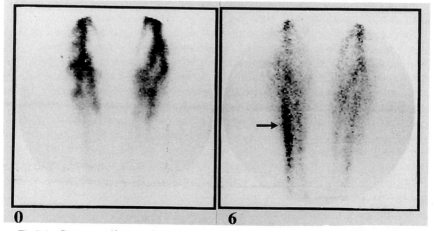

Fig 8–2.—Posterior calf views obtained at 0 and 6 hours after the injection of ^{99m}Tc-3B6. Tracer accumulation is increased in the peroneal vein region of the left calf (*arrow*). (Courtesy of Bautovich G, Angelides S, Lee F-T, et al: *J Nucl Med* 35:195–202, 1994.)

monoclonal antibody DD-3B6/22 has a high affinity for the DD domain of cross-linked fibrin, without cross-reaction with fibrinogen, fibrinogen degradation products, or fibrin monomer. The use of technetium-99m (^{99m}Tc)–labeled antifibrin DD-3B6/22 Fab' monoclonal antibody fragments for the detection of DVT and pulmonary embolism was evaluated.

Methods.—Participants were 20 patients with DVT, which was confirmed by contrast venography or venous duplex scanning. All were studied after injection of a 600-MBq dose of ^{99m}Tc-DD-3B6/22 Fab'. Planar images of the lower limbs were obtained at 0, 2, 6, and 24 hours and chest scintigrams at 6 and 24 hours. Nineteen patients were receiving heparin.

Results.—Imaging with the radioimmunoconjugate demonstrated all venographically documented calf (popliteal and femoral) thrombus sites. In the patients whose thrombi were confirmed by venous duplex scanning, imaging detected all but 2 calf thrombi in 2 patients with bilateral disease and other positive sites. Bilateral DVT with multiple sites was visualized in the popliteal and femoral regions of the calf in 5 patients. There was also 1 confirmed case of pulmonary embolus. Thrombus sites were documented at both 2 and 6 hours after injection (Fig 8–2). There were no adverse reactions, although there may have been 1 low-titer human anti-mouse antibody response.

Conclusion.—Results were promising with ^{99m}Tc-DD-3B6/22 Fab' for the noninvasive detection of DVT and pulmonary embolism. No allergic or toxic reactions have occurred so far. This radioimmunoconjugate may also hold potential for the gamma camera detection of the pathologic cross-linked fibrin associated with certain tumors.

▶ The search continues for a radionuclide marker of venous thrombosis. Numerous techniques have been introduced over the years, but none has met with adequate success.

As our techniques for identifying receptor ligands and antibodies continues, it should be possible to develop a radionuclide-labeled agent that binds specifically to a clot with a high affinity. The venography techniques suffer from our being required to look for a cold spot in a sea of activity, which is quite difficult, particularly in the distal veins. A hot spot induced by an agent that clears rapidly from the blood would be much easier to detect and could potentially be evaluated using a portable camera at the bedside in patients who could not be moved. The development of such a test should be possible with the skills we have today. The most surprising thing is that we do not have such a test yet. Knight and associates and Bautovitch and colleagues (Abstracts 124-95-8–5 and 124-95-8–6) appear to be pointing us in the right direction.—M.D. Blaufox, M.D., Ph.D.

Lymphoscintigraphy: A Reliable Test for the Diagnosis of Lymphedema

Ter S-E, Alavi A, Kim CK, Merli G (Hosp of the Univ of Pennsylvania, Philadel-

phia; Thomas Jefferson Univ Hosp, Philadelphia)
Clin Nucl Med 18:646–654, 1993   124-95-8-7

Objective.—The diagnostic value of lymphoscintigraphy using technetium-99m–labeled antimony trisulfide colloid was examined in 17 patients who were suspected of having lymphedema in 20 upper or lower extremities.

Methods.—A total dose of 1 mCi of radiopharmaceutical in a 1-mL volume was injected subcutaneously in 4 equal portions in the first and second interdigital spaces of the lower extremities bilaterally or in the second and third interdigital spaces of the upper extremities bilaterally. Static anterior images were recorded within the first hour and after 3–5 hours in most instances. Two experienced nuclear medicine physicians independently interpreted the images without knowledge of the patient's history or the results of other imaging studies. The time of appearance of activity in the inguinal or axillary lymph nodes showed whether lymph transport was delayed.

Findings.—Lymphoscintigraphy demonstrated an abnormal pattern in 8 of 11 extremities with primary or secondary lymphedema, for a sensitivity of 73%. Dermal backflow was the most common abnormality. Three extremities were mistakenly not imaged within the first hour after nuclide injection, and their delayed static images appeared normal. The image pattern was normal in all 9 extremities that were edematous for other reasons, making the study 100% specific.

Conclusion.—Lymphoscintigraphy done using technetium-99m–labeled antimony trisulfide colloid is a reliable noninvasive means of confirming the presence of lymphedema and can be conveniently used for repeated follow-up evaluation.

▶ This technique may be of some value in a limited number of patients. Unfortunately, technetium-99m antimony trisulfide is still an investigational new drug, and the supplier of the agent has ceased its production in the United States. Further investigation in this area should involve the identification of an alternate radiopharmaceutical and/or sufficient clinical justification to induce a manufacturer to supply the drug.—M.D. Blaufox, M.D., Ph.D.

Phantom Infection in Asymptomatic Vessels
Tsapakos MJ, Line BR (Albany Med Ctr, NY)
Clin Nucl Med 18:1101–1102, 1993   124-95-8-8

Background.—Technetium-99m autologous-labeled leukocyte scintigraphy is commonly used to locate abscess and infection sites. Two cases of phantom infection in asymptomatic vessels were reported.

Patients.—Two men, 69 and 70, had persistent tracer uptake in patent, uninfected, asymptomatic vessels. In 1 patient, who was being

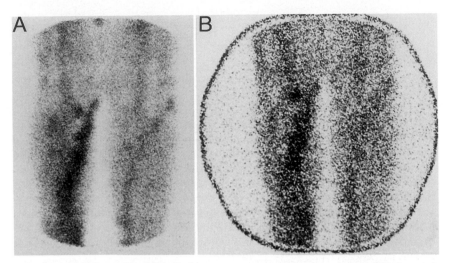

Fig 8–3.—Technetium-99m-labeled leukocytes were prepared using the procedure of Danpure et al. Technetium-99m white blood cell (WBC) images of the calf region at 2 hours (**A**) and 24 hours (**B**) in a man, 69 years of age. He reported an 8-month history of left ankle pain after removal of internal fixation pins. Technetium-99m WBC scintigraphy was requested to exclude osteomyelitis. Although the left ankle was unremarkable, there was increased tracer uptake along the contralateral anteromedial calf at both 2 and 24 hours. The uptake in the vessel relative to background is greater at 24 hours, a finding suggestive of infection. Prominent uptake at 2 and 24 hours has previously been described as indicative of infection with technetium-99m WBC and indium-111 WBC. (Courtesy of Tsapakos MJ, Line BR: *Clin Nucl Med* 18:1101–1102, 1993.)

screened for inflammatory disease of the ankle, tracer uptake was noted in a varicosity of the opposite lower extremity (Fig 8–3). In the other patient, uptake was seen in a prosthetic aorta-to-right common femoral artery bypass graft. An intraoperative swab biopsy specimen was uninfected.

Conclusion.—This is the first report of persistent tracer uptake in patent, uninfected vessels. The persistent margination of radiolabeled white blood cells results from unknown causes. A noninfectious etiology for white cell localization in varicosities and bypass grafts should be considered.

▶ One of the biggest problems that confronts nuclear medicine is that many of our procedures are very sensitive, but they tend to be highly nonspecific. Because of this lack of specificity, it is particularly important that the nuclear medicine physician be aware of the source of false positive studies.

Although this report concerns only 2 patients, it again makes apparent the need for the nuclear medicine practitioner to be thoroughly familiar with the patient's history and to examine the patient as part of the overall nuclear medicine examination.—M.D. Blaufox, M.D., Ph.D.

Adenomyosis as Seen on Blood Flow and Blood Pool Imaging During Bone Scintigraphy

Moreno AJ, Pacheco EJ, Carpenter AL, Rodriguez AA, Turnbull GL (William Beaumont Army Med Ctr, El Paso, Tex)

Clin Nucl Med 19:204–206, 1994   124-95-8-9

Introduction.—Bone scintigraphy can often be the source of extraskeletal information, particularly the blood flow and/or blood pool phases of the study. The importance of the blood flow and blood pool components of the bone scan was demonstrated in a patient with adenomyosis.

Case Report.—Woman, 42, complained of intermittent low-back and left lower-extremity pain for 5 months. Reflex sympathetic dystrophy of the left lower-extremity was considered a diagnostic possibility. The patient underwent a 3-phase bone scintigraphic study. On the blood flow and blood pool images, there was a large focus of increased activity in the right lower abdomen (Fig 8–4). Pelvic CT showed enlargement of the uterus, with apparent displacement to the right. Uterine involvement with diffuse adenomyosis was found at exploratory laparotomy.

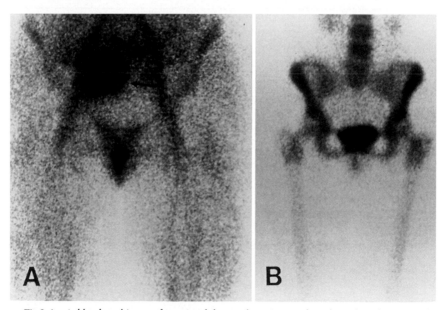

Fig 8–4.—A, blood pool image of anterior abdomen shows increased uptake in the right upper pelvic region (*arrow*). **B,** delayed static image of the anterior abdomen obtained 4 hours after injection of the radiopharmaceutical shows normal uptake in the skeleton and soft tissues. The abnormal activity was not seen in the delayed images. (Courtesy of Moreno AJ, Pacheco EJ, Carpenter AL, et al: *Clin Nucl Med* 19:204–206, 1994.)

Discussion.—Three-phase bone scanning may give important initial clues that a patient's symptoms are extraskeletal in origin. In this case, delayed bone scintigraphy would not have demonstrated the abnormality. The use of 3-phase bone scintigraphy, which consists of blood flow and blood pool images over the anterior pelvis, is recommended in the evaluation of women with lower-back or pelvic pain.

▶ Perhaps no examination in nuclear medicine provides as much information of general diagnostic importance as the bone scan. This case report, once again, attests to it and provides some support for the use of the 3-phase bone scintigraphic study in patients with unidentified low-back or pelvic pain.—M.D. Blaufox, M.D., Ph.D.

Call Mosby Document Express at **1 (800) 55-MOSBY** to obtain copies of the original source documents of articles featured or referenced in the YEAR BOOK series.

---

9 Central Nervous System

Introduction

This year's selections were drawn from a wide variety of publications in the United States and abroad. In the past, we have had several annual papers on the seizure patient, but there were none this year. New areas such as observer variability and standardization are emerging as important topics.

Alexander Gottschalk, M.D.

Regional Cerebral Blood Flow Improves With Treatment in Chronic Cocaine Polydrug Users

Holman BL, Mendelson J, Garada B, Teoh SK, Hallgring E, Johnson KA, Mello NK (Harvard Med School, Boston; McLean Hosp, Belmont, Mass)
J Nucl Med 34:723–727, 1993
124-95-9-1

Purpose.—Abnormal brain perfusion patterns, which are often indistinguishable from those of early AIDS dementia, have been reported in chronic cocaine users. High-resolution technetium-99m hexmethyl-propyleneamine-oxine SPECT was used to determine whether these perfusion defects are reversible.

Methods.—Ten cocaine-dependent polydrug users were admitted to an inpatient treatment facility. Regional cerebral blood flow (rCBF) was studied by SPECT 2 or 3 days after admission, as well as 7–8 days and 17–29 days after abstinence from drugs. Treatment included the opioid mixed agonist-antagonist buprenorphine, beginning 10 days after admission. Activity ratios for cortical regions relative to cerebellar activity were calculated, and regions were classified as initially abnormal, with an activity ratio less than .6; borderline, .6–.72; and normal, greater than .72.

Findings.—Regional CBF in abnormal zones increased by a mean of 11% by the second SPECT examination and by 23.8% at the third. For borderline cortical regions, the increase was 4.8% at 7–8 days and 11.1% at 17–29 days. Normal regions showed a 2.9% decrease at the second examination and a 2.7% increase at the third. Location of the cortical region did not affect the rCBF increase.

Conclusion.—Within the first month of inpatient treatment, chronic cocaine users have partial reversal of their brain perfusion defects. Blood flow may be increased by 45% in 3 or 4 weeks, although rCBF may not completely return to normal in all patients.

▶ Good stuff. The "before" and "after" pictures in the original article were a technical triumph to relate to each other because the interval between imaging was a matter of days. The authors normalized each SPECT scan location against a co-registered MRI study. The co-registration was done using each study to define surface contours of the brain, which were then correlated; in short, a master imaging tour de force. However, look at what has been accomplished. Not only are the data interesting in their own right, but if various treatment protocols ultimately must be compared, this group is in a perfect position to do so.—A. Gottschalk, M.D.

Comparative SPECT Study of Stroke Using Tc-99m ECD, I-123 IMP, and Tc-99m HMPAO
Matsuda H, Li YM, Higashi S, Sumiya H, Tsuji S, Kinuya K, Hisada K, Yamashita J (Kanazawa Univ Hosp, Japan)
Clin Nucl Med 18:754–758, 1993   1 24-95-9-2

Background.—Technetium-99m ethyl cysteinate dimer (^{99m}Tc-ECD), a new brain perfusion imaging agent, displays selective brain retention and rapid renal excretion. Although previous studies have documented the in vivo kinetics and dosimetry of this agent, there is little information on how it compares with other commercially available brain perfusion agents—iodine-123 iodoamphetamine (^{123}I-IMP) and ^{99m}Tc-hexamethyl-propyleneamine-oxime (HMPAO)—in the same patient.

Regional Sensitivity of Lesion Detection in Patients With Stroke in 3 Types of SPECT Scans

	SPECT Scan		
Brain Region	Tc-99m ECD	I-123 IMP	Tc-99m HMPAO
Cerebral cortex*	51% (61/120)	70% (84/120)	45% (37/80)
Cerebellum	58% (7/12)	67% (8/12)	63% (5/8)
Striatum	58% (7/12)	58% (7/12)	38% (3/8)
Thalamus	58% (7/12)	58% (7/12)	25% (2/8)
White matter	42% (5/12)	50% (6/12)	38% (3/8)

Note: Values in parentheses are number of regions of interest (ROI) pairs with abnormal asymmetric index values/total number of ROI pairs.
*P <.001 contingency table analysis.
(Courtesy of Matsuda H, Li YM, Higashi S, et al: *Clin Nucl Med* 18:754–758, 1993.)

Methods.—Twelve patients with chronic cerebrovascular disease underwent brain perfusion SPECT imaging using ^{99m}Tc-ECD. In addition, 8 patients underwent ^{123}I-IMP and ^{99m}Tc-HMPAO. The remaining 4 had ^{99m}Tc-ECD and ^{123}I-IMP scans.

Findings.—Iodine-123 IMP had a higher lesion sensitivity than ^{99m}Tc-ECD and ^{99m}Tc-HMPAO in the cerebral cortex, cerebellum, and white matter. Technetium-99m-ECD and ^{123}I-IMP had greater lesion sensitivity than ^{99m}Tc-HMPAO in the striatum and thalamus. Iodine-123 IMP had the highest lesion contrast in the cerebral cortex and cerebellum, and ^{99m}Tc-ECD had the highest contrast in the thalamus and striatum. Lesion contrast in all regions was greater with ^{99m}Tc-ECD than with ^{99m}Tc-HMPAO (table).

Conclusion.—There appears to be regional variation in the sensitivity of lesion detection and lesion contrast with ^{99m}Tc-ECD compared with ^{123}I-IMP. Technetium-99m ECD seems to be superior to ^{99m}Tc-HMPAO.

▶ Interesting data. We hope that by the time this YEAR BOOK comes out, ECD will be available to those who want to make this type of comparison.—A. Gottschalk, M.D.

Regional Cerebral Blood Flow Measured With *N*-Isopropyl-*p*-[^{123}I]Iodoamphetamine and Its Redistribution in Ischemic Cerebrovascular Disease
Odano I, Tsuchiya T, Nishihara M, Sakai K, Abe H, Tanaka R (Niigata Univ, Japan)
Stroke 24:1167–1172, 1993   124-95-9–3

Background.—When a low-perfusion region is seen as an area of reduced activity of radiotracer on an early image, the activity increases gradually, and the low perfusion disappears on a delayed image acquired 3–5 hours after iodine-123 iodoamphetamine (^{123}I-IMP) injection. This redistribution phenomenon is believed to reflect metabolic activity in viable cerebral tissue and to indicate a good clinical outcome in patients with cerebrovascular disease. However, the clinical and pathophysiologic significance of this phenomenon is debated.

Methods.—Sixteen patients with chronic infarction and 10 age-matched healthy controls underwent SPECT with N-isopropyl-*p*-[^{123}I]-iodoamphetamine. Participants ranged in age from 26 to 77 years. Regional cerebral blood flow was measured quantitatively by a microsphere model. The redistribution on delayed images was analyzed in ischemic lesions.

Findings.—The supratentorial mean cerebral blood flow as 52.7 mL/100 g/min, and the ratio of gray matter to white matter in controls was 2.34 mL/100 g/min. Low-activity regions of ischemic lesions on early images, which were classified into 2 abnormal zones—an infarct

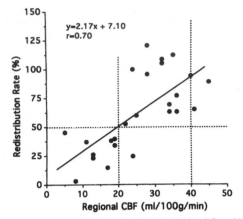

Fig 9-1.—Plot showing correlation between regional cerebral blood flow (CBF) and redistribution rate in ischemic lesions. The correlation is significant. Redistribution is noticed at 25-40 mL/100 g of regional CBF per minute and is marked at approximately 30 mL/100 g per minute. (Courtesy of Odano I, Tsuchiya T, Nishihara M, et al: *Stroke* 24:1167-1172, 1993.)

and peri-infarct area—were characterized by regional blood flow averaging 9-20 mL/100 g/min and 22-41 mL/100 g/min. Redistribution was minimally present in the infarct region and markedly enhanced in the peri-infarct region. Blood flow significantly increased in the peri-infarct region after bypass surgery (Fig 9-1).

Conclusion.—The redistribution phenomenon relies on the maintenance of a minimal blood flow that sustains cellular function. This phenomenon is useful for assessing bypass surgery in patients with chronic infarction.

▶ We see the larger question here: Whether the redistribution of this tracer that is seen early on in this study is simply a hallmark for what ultimately becomes luxury perfusion in the penumbra. Others have previously shown the penumbra is an area where precious little neurologic function is regained. However, these folks might have a handle on brain tissue that could be salvaged. They suggest that some salvage is possible and mention that 2 of their patients showed improvement after bypass surgery. The authors further suggest that redistribution as they show it might be related to "neuronal disconnection or diaschesis rather than neuronal loss." We certainly hope so and look forward to further studies from this group that might substantiate this hypothesis.—A. Gottschalk, M.D.

Value of Single-Photon Emission-Computed Tomography in Acute Stroke Therapeutic Trials

Hanson SK, Grotta JC, Rhoades H, Tran HD, Lamki LM, Barron BJ, Taylor WJ

(Univ of Texas, Houston)
Stroke 24:1322–1329, 1993   124-95-9-4

Background.—New treatment approaches for acute ischemic stroke strive to improve cerebral blood flow in the first 3–6 hours after the onset of symptoms. If SPECT is performed in clinical trials, it may improve understanding of the physiologic response to new forms of treatment and influence acute management decisions.

Methods.—Fifteen patients with hemispheric ischemic stroke were prospectively assessed with SPECT within 6 hours of symptom onset and again at 24 hours. The ischemic defect was evaluated semiquantitatively using computer-generated regions of interest.

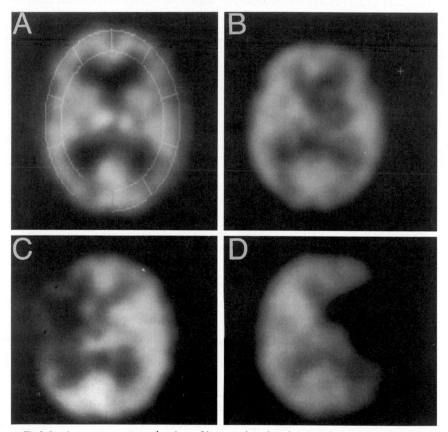

Fig 9–2.—A, computer-generated regions of interest plotted on 4 consecutive transverse images and used for the calculation of the SPECT-graded scale. **B–D,** examples of transverse images from the time O SPECT in patients with mild (**B**), moderate (**C**), and severe (**D**) ischemia. The SPECT-graded scales calculated for these scans were 5, 40, and 70, respectively. The cursor (+) in **B** is adjacent to the abnormal region of interest. (Courtesy of Hanson SK, Grotta JC, Rhoades H, et al: *Stroke* 24:1322–1329, 1993.)

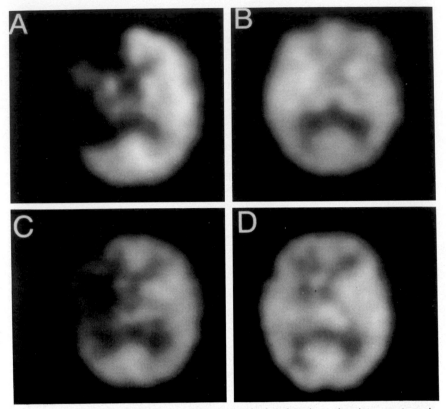

Fig 9–3.—Transverse SPECT images from time O (**left**) and 24 hours (**right**) in a patient who showed no clinical improvement (**A** and **B**), and a patient who demonstrated substantial clinical improvement during the first 24 hours (**C** and **D**). In both patients, there was substantial improvement in the SPECT-graded scale between time O and 24 hours. (Courtesy of Hanson SK, Grotta JC, Rhoades H, et al: *Stroke* 24:1322–1329, 1993.)

Findings.—The severity of the SPECT graded scale on the admission scan was associated with the severity of the neurologic deficit. It was also positively associated with poor long-term outcome as measured with the Barthel Index, the complications of cerebral bleeding, and massive cerebral edema. There was a threshold value for the SPECT-graded scale above which all patients had poor long-term outcomes and cerebral hemorrhage and edema. However, 5 patients showed improvement in SPECT when the initial study was compared with the 24-hour study, but they showed no clinical improvement. (Figs 9–2 and 9–3).

Conclusion.—Measuring ischemic defects using SPECT provides a valid determination of hemispheric stroke severity in the hyperacute setting. It may also be useful for selecting or stratifying patients in clinical treatment trails.

▶ These are the data that make me worry about the previous article (Abstract 124-95-9–3). The authors clearly demonstrate that the delayed SPECT study may show significant improvement without a corresponding clinical improvement in the patient. This then raises the following questions: Is redistribution with iodoamphetamine (IMP) simply a quick way of obtaining the 24-hour SPECT (i.e., it will not be of much prognostic value), or does the redistribution of IMP provide us with "stunned" brain that really can recover?—A. Gottschalk, M.D.

Carbon Dioxide Reactivity by Consecutive Technetium-99m-HMPAO SPECT in Patients With a Chronically Obstructed Major Cerebral Artery

Oku N, Matsumoto M, Hashikawa K, Moriwaki H, Okazaki Y, Seike Y, Handa N, Uehara T, Kamada T, Nishimura T (Osaka Univ, Japan)
J Nucl Med 35:32–40, 1994   132-95-9–5

Background.—Cerebral perfusion reserve is the key to introducing cerebral revascularization surgery in the management of major cerebral artery obstruction. The feasibility of evaluating cerebral perfusion reserve by the consecutive technetium-99m hexamethylpropyleneamine-oxime (^{99m}Tc-HMPAO) SPECT with 5% carbon dioxide (CO_2) inhalation was assessed.

Methods.—Thirty patients with chronic ischemic cerebrovascular disease and unilateral major cerebral artery obstruction and 27 patients without it were studied. The CO_2 reactivity was expressed as the percentage increase of ^{99m}Tc-HMPAO accumulation from the baseline (% change) and as a constant k', the ratio of ^{99m}Tc-HMPAO accumulation per 1–mm Hg change of end-tidal CO_2 tension by exponential curve fitting.

Findings.—The range of mean % change and k' in the middle cerebral artery (MCA) territory on the side without an obstructive lesion or in the cerebellum was 10% to 11.1% and .98% to 1.13% per mm Hg, respectively. Obstructive lesions were found in 5.9% per mm Hg in the MCA territory and in .54% per mm Hg in the contralateral MCA territory. Eleven of the patients with major cerebral artery obstruction had significant asymmetry in the k' value between bilateral MCA territories (Fig 9-4).

Conclusion.—Cerebral perfusion reserve was compromised in the obstructed major cerebral artery territory. The method was clinically useful for assessing cerebral perfusion reserve in patients with unilateral obstruction.

▶ This is a complicated paper that describes an easy intervention. We are not sure the authors have proved this is a clinically useful method, so we will

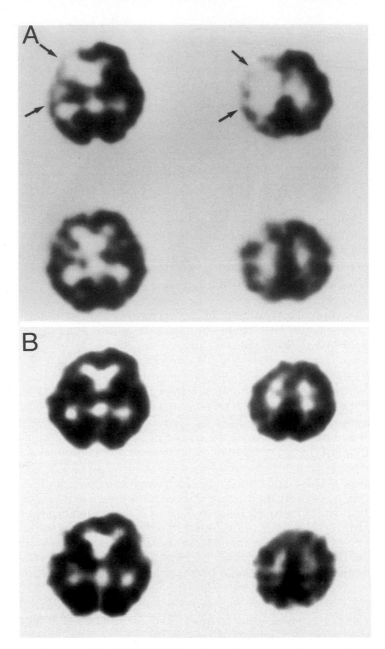

Fig 9–4.—Consecutive ^{99m}Tc-HMPAO SPECT studies performed on a male patient 63 years of age with right internal carotid artery occlusion before (**A**) and after (**B**) external to internal cranial bypass surgery. Preoperative SPECT study (**A**) demonstrated mild hypoperfusion during normocapnia and poor response of regional cerebral blood flow to CO_2 in the right MCA territory (*arrows*) when compared with the left. A postoperative SPECT study (**B**) demonstrated improvement in impaired CO_2 reactivity in the right MCA territory. **Upper row,** brain perfusion images during hypercapnia; **lower row,** those during normocapnia. (Courtesy of Oku N, Matsumoto M, Hashikawa K, et al: *J Nucl Med* 35:32–40, 1994.)

await further studies for assessment. However, there is much potential here.—A. Gottschalk, M.D.

Brain Blood Flow SPECT in Temporary Balloon Occlusion of Carotid and Intracerebral Arteries

Mathews D, Walker BS, Purdy PD, Batjer H, Allen BC, Eckard DA, Devous MD Sr, Bonte FJ (Univ of Texas, Dallas)
J Nucl Med 34:1239–1243, 1993   124-95-9-6

Introduction.—When it seems necessary to sacrifice a carotid artery, it is important to know whether the patient will have a neurologic deficit as a result. Recently, tolerance was tested using a percutaneously placed endovascular balloon catheter. Patients whose perfusion reserve is mar-

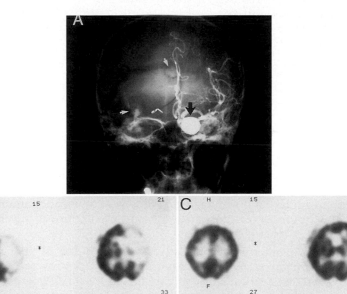

Fig 9–5.—Patient with a large left cavernous carotid aneurysm. **A,** angiogram demonstrates left cavernous carotid aneurysm (*black arrow*). Note also the presence of previously clipped aneurysms (*white arrows*). **B,** representative transaxial slices of technetium-99m hexamethylpropyleneamine oxime (^{99m}Tc-HMPAO) SPECT scan. The patient was injected during trial balloon occlusion of the left internal carotid artery. Note the large perfusion defect involving the anterior and middle cerebral arterial distributions. Note also the crossed cerebellar diaschisis (*arrowhead*). **C,** representative transaxial slices of the ^{99m}Tc-HMPAO SPECT scan demonstrate normal baseline perfusion. (Courtesy of Mathews D, Walker BS, Purdy PD, et al: *J Nucl Med* 34:1239-1243, 1993.)

Summary of Treatment in Patients With Vascular Lesions Undergoing
Trial Balloon Occlusion and SPECT Imaging

	No. of patients
Positive SPECT scan	
ECIC then carotid sacrifice	3
Gradual carotid occlusion	3[†]
Embolization of aneurysm only, carotid spared	2
AVM surgically removed, then carotid sacrifice	1
Carotid endarterectomy, no further surgery at this time	1
Embolization of AVF	1
Patients not operated upon	3
Total	14
Negative SPECT scan	
Permanent carotid occlusion	10
Permanent carotid occlusion, transient symptoms	1
Patients not operated upon	1
Permanent PCA occlusion with AVF resection	1
Total	13

Abbreviations: AVF, arteriovenous fistula; PCA, posterior cerebral artery; ECIC, extracranial-intracranial bypass; AVM, arteriovenous malformation.
Note: All patients were asymptomatic post treatment unless otherwise noted.
† One patient underwent both ECIC and gradual carotid occlusion.
(Courtesy of Mathews D, Walker BS, Purdy PD, et al: *J Nucl Med* 34:1239–1243, 1993.)

---

ginal might be identified by estimating cerebral blood flow during a trail of arterial occlusion.

Objective.—Forty-two patients with a variety of diagnoses underwent trial balloon occlusion of an internal carotid or intracerebral artery in conjunction with blood flow imaging by SPECT. The most common disorders were cavernous carotid aneurysm and squamous-cell carcinoma of the head/neck region.

Procedure.—An internal carotid artery was occluded in 40 patients and an intracerebral artery was occluded in 2. A balloon catheter was introduced through a femoral artery and inflated for 30–45 minutes, and technetium-labeled hexamethylpropyleneamine oxime was injected, either at the time symptoms developed or near the end of the period of occlusion (Fig 9–5). Six patients had dual isotope studies with iodine-123 iodoamphetamine. Single-photon emission CT imaging of the brain used a rotating triple-head scanner with a super-high-resolution fanbeam collimator (energy resolution 9% full width at half maximum).

Observations.—Eight of 27 patients with vascular lesions became symptomatic during arterial occlusion and had marked defects in SPECT images, which in all patients but 1 resolved rapidly after the balloon was deflated; the exception probably had an embolic stroke. In all 8 patients with abnormalities, the treatment plan was adjusted accordingly. Of 19 patients who did not have symptoms during occlusion, 13 lacked significant SPECT defects, and 12 of them had the vessel sacrificed uneventfully; 1 was not operated on. Treatment was modified in the 6 patients who were asymptomatic and had positive SPECT studies. None of the 15 patients with neoplastic disease became symptomatic during arterial occlusion, but 3 had positive SPECT studies (table). Two of these patients required sacrifice of a carotid vessel, and both had neurologic symptoms postoperatively.

Conclusion.—Single-photon emission CT imaging should be performed as part of all trials of temporary carotid or intracerebral arterial occlusion.

▶ These data make sense to me. The interested reader may wish to read the article, "Assessing collateral cerebral perfusion with technetium-99m-HMPAO SPECT during temporary internal carotid artery aclusion" (1).—A. Gottschalk, M.D.

Reference

1. Palestro CJ, et al: *J Nucl Med* 34:1235, 1993.

Variations in Regional Cerebral Blood Flow Investigated by Single Photon Emission Computed Tomography With Technetium-99m-d, I-Hexamethylpropyleneamineoxime During Temporary Clipping in Intracranial Aneurysm Surgery: Preliminary Results
Medina M, Melcarne A, Musso C, Ettorre F, Bellotti C, Papaleo A, Camuzzini G (S Croce Hosp, Cuneo, Italy)
Neurosurgery 33:441–450, 1993   124-95-9–7

Background.—Many neurosurgeons use temporary occlusion of a cerebral artery rather than controlled hypotension in patients with giant aneurysms to control bleeding, for premature rupture of an aneurysm, or to facilitate dissection and permanent clipping of the sac. Tolerance to temporary clipping has been investigated intraoperatively by different methods. Single-photon emission CT with technetium-99m-d, l-hexamethylpropyleneamine oxime (^{99m}Tc-HMPAO) was used to indicate variations in regional cerebral blood flow in ischemic insults of various types. However, this method does not allow intraoperative changes in surgical procedure that may be suggested by real-time analysis.

Methods and Findings.—Variations in regional cerebral blood flow during temporary clipping were assessed in the course of intracranial aneurysm surgery and postoperatively in 20 patients. Fourteen underwent temporary clipping, 9 of whom had aneurysms of the anterior communicating artery; 2, aneurysms of the middle cerebral artery; and 3, aneurysms of the carotid siphon. Temporary clips were applied on the basis of lesion site—the A1 segment of the anterior cerebral artery; the trunk of the middle cerebral artery; or the trunk of the internal carotid artery.

The occlusion time varied from 2 to 31 minutes. Of the 6 patients who did not undergo temporary clipping, 3 had aneurysms of the posterior communicating artery; 1, the anterior communicating artery; 1, the middle cerebral artery; and 1, the internal carotid artery. In all patients who underwent temporary clipping, there was a sharp decline in the perfusion of the territories of the temporarily clipped parent vessel. All had a nearly complete recovery within 2–7 days of the operation, with no significant neurologic symptoms. Patients who did not have temporary clipping had no such disturbances in perfusion.

Conclusion.—Although temporary clipping reduces morbidity and mortality in aneurysm surgery, it changes regional blood flow, sometimes markedly. If this procedure is to be used routinely, patients should undergo careful blood flow studies first to determine the likelihood of effective compensation. Also, any manipulation of the brain to gain access to an aneurysm, whether it involves dissection or retraction, always results in uptake changes in the affected area. With the use of SPECT with ^{99m}Tc-HMPAO, underperfused territories can be precisely identified.

▶ It comes as no surprise that clipping a major artery in the brain causes potentially serious perfusion defects. We were pleased that in most instances, good recovery in the perioperative period was observed. We like the idea of functional assessment of the neurosurgical approach using SPECT techniques. Furthermore, if there is more than 1 possible approach to take from a surgical standpoint, the technique the authors used could be modified by the "before" and "after" method we described last year using iodine-123 iodoamphetamine and ^{99m}Tc-HMPAO (see the 1994 YEAR BOOK OF NUCLEAR MEDICINE, p 277).—A. Gottschalk, M.D.

A Multi-Institutional Study of Interobserver Agreement in the Evaluation of Dementia With rCBF/SPET Technetium-99m Exametazime (HMPAO)
Hellman RS, Tikofsky RS, Van Heertum R, Coade G, Carretta R, Hoffmann RG (Med College of Wisconsin, Milwaukee; Columbia Univ, New York; Univ of California, San Diego; et al)
Eur J Nucl Med 21:306–313, 1994   124-95-9–8

Introduction.—Previous research has described specific patterns of technetium-99m exametazime (^{99m}Tc-hexamethylpropyleneamine oxime [HMPAO]) brain SPECT uptake in dementia. However, no multicenter studies have confirmed interobserver agreement regarding these patterns. Using scans typical of those encountered under clinical conditions, observers from different institutions studied observer agreement on the categorization of ^{99m}Tc-HMPAO brain SPECT uptake patterns in patients with dementia.

Methods.—Included were 50 patients from 4 institutions who had the clinical diagnosis of dementia. The neurologic diagnosis was presumed

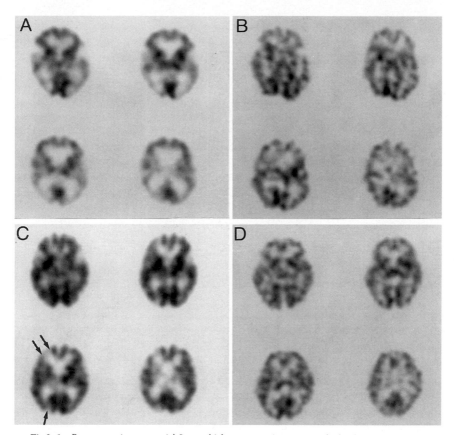

Fig 9–6.—Representative sequential 8-mm-thick transverse images near the level of the basal ganglia for each of the 4 general appearance categories. **A,** global decrease. There is generalized decreased cortical uptake relative to the basal ganglia and occipital cortex. The most marked abnormalities in this patient who has Alzheimer's disease are seen in the temporoparietal regions. **B,** patchy changes. In this HIV-related dementia patient, there is a heterogenous pattern of both increased and decreased uptake in the cortical and subcortical areas. **C,** focal decreases. In this patient with multi-infarct dimentia, there are focal regions of decreased uptake in the right frontal lobe (*double arrow*), the right posterior parietal region (*single arrow*), and the right thalamic nucleus. **D,** normal. The typical pattern of cortical and subcortical uptake is shown. (Courtesy of Hellman RS, Tikofsky RS, Van Heertum R, et al: *Eur J Nucl Med* 21:306-313, 1994.)

Alzheimer's disease in 21 cases, confirmed Alzheimer's disease in 10, multi-infarct dementia in 9, HIV-related dementia in 7, and "mixed" dementia in 3. Five normal scans from each institution were also evaluated. All scans were read in randomized, blinded fashion by 3 observers, each from a different institution. These readers categorized each scan as normal or as showing globally decreased uptake, focal areas of decreased uptake, or patchy changes in uptake (Fig 9-6). They also rated uptake in each of 8 designated regions in both hemispheres (Fig 9-7).

Results.—At least 2 observers agreed about the general appearance of the scan in 94% of cases. Interobserver agreement was strongest for nor-

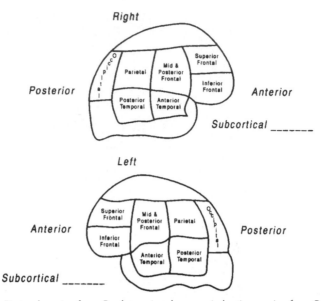

Fig 9–7.—Regional scoring form. Readers assigned a numerical rating ranging from O (absent uptake) to 5 (increased uptake) to each of the regions shown on the form. The *borders* on the form served as a general guide for localizing abnormalities. A sagittal projection was used for its convenient representation of approximate lobar boundaries. (Courtesy of Hellman RS, Tikofsky RS, Van Heertum R, et al: *Eur J Nucl Med* 21:306–313, 1994.)

mal and patchy scans; agreement for the focal and global categories was less strong but still significant. Sensitivity in identifying abnormal scans of demented patients was 72%, with a specificity of 79%. Agreement was also good for ratings of regional uptake.

Conclusion.—Good agreement between observers and institutions regarding the interpretation of regional cerebral blood flow/SPECT images of demented patients was documented. Agreement is not as good on the association of regional abnormalities with various clinical subtypes of dementia. The results apply to most nuclear medicine departments that are capable of performing SPECT, and they suggest that images obtained on similar patient populations can be reliably interpreted.

▶ To put these numbers into some type of perspective, let me point out that in PIOPED, 2 blinded readers reading ventilation-perfusion scans from somebody else's institution and catagorizing the scan as high, intermediate, or low probability agreed with each other about two thirds of the time. If there was disagreement, a third observer was asked to look at the study, and in fewer than 3% of cases was there no agreement between 2 of the 3 observers. In short, in PIOPED, more than 97% of the time 2 of 3 observers concurred. In this study, that happened only 94% of the time. In addition, I have long believed that in any type of difficult imaging situation, an observer who can run a sensitivity and specificity of about 80% when rating normal vs. abnormal is doing well. These numbers certainly suggest this is not a bad rule of thumb.

Finally, for those of you who would point out that I must be balmy to bring up PIOPED, where the sensitivity was about 45% and the specificity 97%, which are a far cry from the numbers presented here, I point out that PIOPED was rated not on a 2 × 2 table (i.e., scan positive vs. scan negative) but on a 2 × 3 table where the intermediate scan was considered a "correct answer" for specificity determination but was a "miss" for sensitivity. In fact, if you take the intermediate studies from PIOPED, you will find sensitivity and specificity numbers that are very close to those presented in this trial.—A. Gottschalk, M.D.

Quantitative Analysis of PET and MRI Data in Normal Aging and Alzheimer's Disease: Atrophy Weighted Total Brain Metabolism and Absolute Whole Brain Metabolism as Reliable Discriminators
Alavi A, Newberg AB, Souder E, Berlin JA (Univ of Pennsylvania, Philadelphia)
J Nucl Med 34:1681–1687, 1993   124-95-9–9

Introduction.—Patients with Alzheimer's disease (AD) and their age-matched controls have no significant difference in average whole-brain metabolic rate, which is corrected for the effects of brain atrophy. With the combination of MRI volumetric data and PET metabolic data, it is theoretically possible to calculate atrophy weighted total-brain metabolism and absolute whole-brain metabolism. Whether the absolute amount of glucose used by the entire brain is a more reliable indicator of AD than the metabolic rate per unit of brain weight was determined.

Methods and Findings.—The participants were 20 patients with probable AD and 17 age-matched controls. Those in both groups underwent both ^{18}F-fluorodeoxyglucose PET and MRI within a few days of each other. Average atrophy-corrected metabolic rates were 3.91 mg/100 mL/min for the patients and 4.43 mg/mL/min for controls. Atrophy-weighted brain metabolism—calculated as brain volume times average metabolic rate—was 29.96 for patients vs. 39.1 for controls, a very significant difference (table). There was very good correlation between atrophy-weighted total-brain metabolism and scores on the Mini-Mental State Examination.

Conclusion.—Significant differences were found between patients with AD and controls in absolute whole-brain metabolism. This measure, as well as the metabolic rate per unit rate of brain, may prove to be a sensitive marker of cognitive dysfunction in patients who are being evaluated for AD. In the future, regional metabolic activities may prove clinically useful.

▶ At the moment, this type of analysis is tedious. However, it is probably no more tedious than it would be to recreate a "bull's-eye" short-access myocar-

Recovered Whole Brain PET Data for Patients With AD and Controls

	Recovered CMRGlc (uncorrected) (mean ± s.d.)	Recovered CMRGlc (corrected) (mean ± s.d.)	Atrophy weighted total brain metab (mean ± s.d.)	Absolute whole brain metab (mean ± s.d.)
AD patients	4.89 ± 1.22*	6.06 ± 1.48[†]	46.61 ± 12.24[‡]	57.86 ± 14.89[§]
Controls	5.38 ± 0.88	6.22 ± 1.07	55.23 ± 9.82	63.73 ± 10.07

Note: Cerebral metabolic rate of glucose (CMRGlc) values in mg glucose/100 cc brain tissue/min; atrophy-weighted total brain metabolism values in mg glucose/brain/min; and absolute whole brain metabolism values in mg glucose/brain/min.
* Not significantly different from controls, P = .17.
† Not significantly different from controls, P = .72.
‡ Significantly different from controls, P = .026.
§ Not significantly different from controls, P = .18.
(Courtesy of Alavi A, Newberg AB, Souder E, et al: J Nucl Med 34:1681–1687, 1993.)

dial perfusion diagram by hand. In other words, I think this type of analysis could be computerized.

It is also possible that subvolumes within the brain might be critical and more important than other volumes. My own guess is that those through the basal ganglia would have the most information on them (i.e., you might not have to analyze the whole brain). If this is true, it might be easy to separate a "normal" from "abnormal" by a numeric analysis. If a similar analysis could be done with SPECT studies, then the observer variability seen in the last paper (Abstract 124-95-9–8) might be reduced.

These data don't tell us whether it is possible to sort out AD from multi-infart dementia and other dementing diseases by this technique. We hope this will be the subject of other papers from these folks.—A. Gottschalk, M.D.

A Method for Assessing the Significance of Abnormalities in HMPAO Brain SPECT Images

Houston AS, Kemp PM, Macleod MA (Royal Naval Hosp, Haslar, Gosport, England)
J Nucl Med 35:239–244, 1994   124-95-9-10

Introduction.—Ordinarily, abnormalities in regional cerebral blood flow (rCBF) are sought by compiling an atlas of normal brain images and then mapping the normal standard deviation or standard error of the mean across the image. It is assumed that deviations in normal images

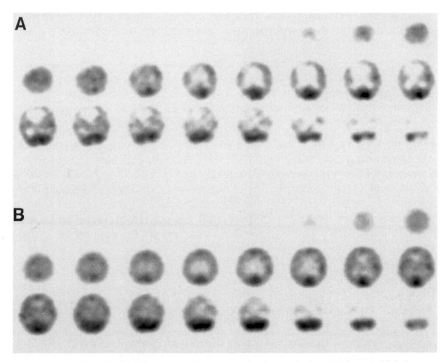

Fig 9–8.—Axial slices of (**A**) the image of a patient with a large right frontal infarct and (**B**) the corresponding "nearest normal equivalent" image. (Courtesy of Houston AS, Kemp PM, Macleod MA: *J Nucl Med* 35:239–244, 1994.)

are noncorrelated voxel by voxel, but there is evidence that this may not be the case for rCBF images.

An Alternative Approach.—A normal atlas of rCBF images acquired by SPECT using hexamethylphenylineamine-oxime was obtained from studies of 53 normal controls. Image registration and normalization were followed by extraction of a mean image. Images representing correlated normal deviants were identified by principal component analysis and formed the basic components of the atlas. The atlas was subsequently used to create a "nearest normal equivalent" image, which was compared with a residual standard deviation image to learn the significance of any deviations in the new image.

Results.—Images from 10 patients who had Alzheimer's disease and 12 who had single or multiple infarcts were analyzed, along with those from 8 normal controls. Image registration proved to be reasonably successful, except at the skull base. It appeared to be no more difficult to register abnormal images than to register normal ones. For normal images, the fitted image generally resembled the original, whereas for abnormal images, the region containing the abnormality appeared normal on the fitted image. All 10 patients with Alzheimer's disease and all but 1 of the 12 with infarcts (Fig 9-8) were correctly identified. There was a single false positive result. Both specificity and sensitivity at the optimal decision level were improved when the nearest normal equivalent images were used, although a larger sample was required to determine the significance of this effect.

Advantages.—This method can identify and evaluate both global and regional abnormalities, provided the latter are large enough to be detected in a low-resolution image. In general, it is equally applicable to high-resolution images obtained using multiheaded and annular systems.

▶ If I take the data from this article and couple it with the 2 preceding articles (Abstracts 124-95-9-8 and 124-95-9-9), I can conclude the following: Even good observers need help analyzing brain SPECT images. Such help is likely to come from a combination of volume-corrected brain metabolism images and an atlas of computerized normal images that provides the nearest normal equivalent image to compare with the patient currently being analyzed. In short, what the computer has helped us do for the heart, it potentially can do for the brain.—A. Gottschalk, M.D.

High-Resolution Technetium-99m-HMPAO SPECT in Patients With Probable Alzheimer's Disease: Comparison With Fluorine-18-FDG PET
Messa C, Perani D, Lucignani G, Zenorini A, Zito F, Rizzo G, Grassi F, Del Sole A, Franceschi M, Gilardi MC, Fazio F (Univ of Milano, Italy)
J Nucl Med 35:210–216, 1994   124-95-9-11

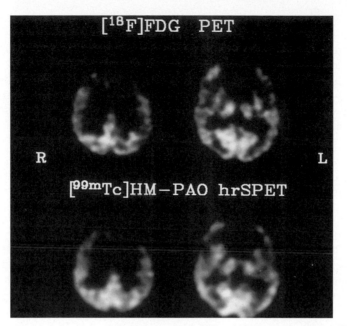

Fig 9–9.—Regional glucose metabolism obtained with PET and [¹⁸F]fluorodeoxyglucose (FDG) (**top row**) and perfusion obtained with high-resolution SPECT and technetium-99m hexamethylpropylenea-mine-oxime (⁹⁹ᵐTc-HM-PAO) (**bottom row**). Two tomographic levels parallel to the orbitomeatal line through the mid- and cranial parts of the brain are represented. Images are displayed with respect to the maximum value of each study (PET and SPECT). Both studies show hypometabolism and hypoperfu-sion bilaterally in the frontal cortex. Hypometabolism of the parietal cortex bilaterally is also shown by PET. (Courtesy of Messa C, Perani D, Lucignani G, et al: *J Nucl Med* 35:210–216, 1994.)

Objective.—The respective merits of PET and SPECT were examined in the same 21 patients with a diagnosis of probable Alzheimer's disease (AD). The 11 women and 10 men had a mean age of 63 years and had been ill for 2 years on average; other causes of dementia were ruled out. Ten normal individuals served as controls for each of the imaging modalities.

Methods.—The PET studies were performed using ¹⁸F-labeled fluoro-deoxyglucose. Images paralleling the orbitomeatal line were acquired 45 minutes after nuclide injection, and axial slices were reconstructed. High-resolution SPECT imaging was done using an annular SPECT system and technetium-labeled hexamethylpropyleneamine-oxime. The regional cerebral glucose utilization (for PET) or counts (for SPECT) in the associative cortices were normalized to average values in the calcarine cortex and basal ganglia.

Results.—Both PET and SPECT demonstrated significant differences between the patients with probable AD and the controls. Positron emission tomography demonstrated significant group differences in the frontal, temporal, and parietal cortices, and SPECT demonstrated significant group differences in the temporal and parietal regions (Fig 9–9). Temporoparietal defects were demonstrated by PET in all patients and in 90% of them by SPECT. Several patients had bilateral abnormalities that were more pronounced on 1 side, but only 1 patient exhibited unilateral involvement of the temporoparietal cortex.

Conclusion.—Positron emission tomography is only marginally more accurate than SPECT in demonstrating temporoparietal abnormality in patients with probable AD. Abnormalities in other associative regions are best evaluated by PET.

▶ In this type of comparison, one of my personal ground rules is that if the authors do not use state-of-the-art equipment for all comparison studies, I throw the article away. In this case, as far as I can tell, the authors are to be congratulated. The PET system used had a spatial resolution of 6.3 mm (full width at half maximum [FWHM]), whereas the SPECT used was Dr. Genna's CERASPECT unit with spatial resolution 8.4 mm (FWHM). Furthermore, the analysis was performed with help from the computer, and the resultant ratios from regions were compared with a numerical atlas. The interested reader may want to look at that atlas, which can be found in *Lesion Analysis in Neuropsychology* (1).—A. Gottschalk, M.D.

Reference

1. Damasio H, Damasio AR: New York, Oxford University Press, 1989.

Dopamine D1 Receptors in Parkinson's Disease and Striatonigral Degeneration: A Positron Emission Tomography Study

Shinotoh H, Inoue O, Hirayama K, Aotsuka A, Asahina M, Suhara T, Yamazaki T, Tateno Y (Chiba Univ, Japan; Natl Inst of Radiological Sciences, Japan)
J Neurol Neurosurg Psychiatry 56:467–472, 1993   124-95-9–12

Study Population.—Agreement is lacking on how the striatal dopamine D1 receptors might be altered in Parkinson's disease (PD). The striatal dopamine D1 receptors were evaluated in 11 patients with PD, 2 of whom had become ill when they were young. All but 2 of the patients had typical parkinsonian findings, including resting tremor and akinetic rigidity. All 6 previously treated patients had responded well to levodopa, and the other patients all responded well to subsequent treatment. Five patients with a diagnosis of striatonigral degeneration (SND) and 6 age-matched normal controls also were studied.

Methods.—Antiparkinsonian therapy was withdrawn at least 48 hours before PET was performed using carbon-11 (^{11}C)–labeled SCH23390. A high-resolution PET system (3.5 to 5.7 mm) was used. Regions of interest were defined in 2 striatal sections, and regional time-activity curves were recorded. All patients except 4 of those with PD also underwent MRI.

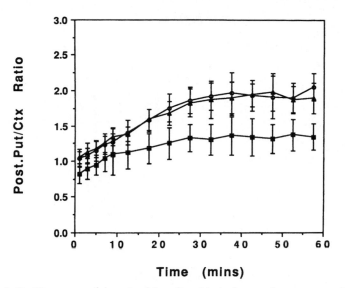

Fig 9–10.—Time course of the ratio of the radioactivity in the posterior putamen to that in the occipital cortex in the control group ($n = 6$, *circles*), in the PD group ($n = 11$, *triangles*), and the SND group ($n = 5$, *squares*) after injection of ^{11}C SCH23390. Values shown are means and standard deviations. (Courtesy of Shinotoh H, Inoue O, Hirayama K, et al: *J Neurol Neurosurg Psychiatry* 56:467–472, 1993.)

Findings.—On MRI, the pars compacta in all patients with PD and SND was narrower than 1 SD of the control mean. Hypointensity was noted in T2-weighted images of the putamen in 2 of the 5 patients with SND, but no striatal atrophy was evident. The PET studies showed mean activity reductions of 12% in the caudate, 21% in the anterior putamen, and 31% in the posterior putamen in patients with SND compared with activity in the occipital cortex (Fig 9–10). No significant changes in activity ratios were noted in the patients with PD.

Conclusion.—Positron emission tomography using ^{11}C-labeled SCH23390 may prove helpful in distinguishing between PD and SND.

► Because patients with SND usually don't respond to levodopa therapy, this differentiation could have therapeutic significance. We hope the authors extend this relatively small series, particularly to look at other PET tracers that might yield the same results.—A. Gottschalk, M.D.

Dopamine Receptor SPET Imaging in Parkinson's Disease: A [^{123}I]-IBZM and [^{99m}Tc]-HM-PAO Study

Pizzolato G, Chierichetti F, Rossato A, Briani C, Dam M, Borsato N, Saitta B, Zanco P, Ferlin G, Battistin L (Univ of Padova, Italy; Hosp of Castelfranco Veneto [TV], Italy)
Eur Neurol 33:143–148, 1993   124-95-9–13

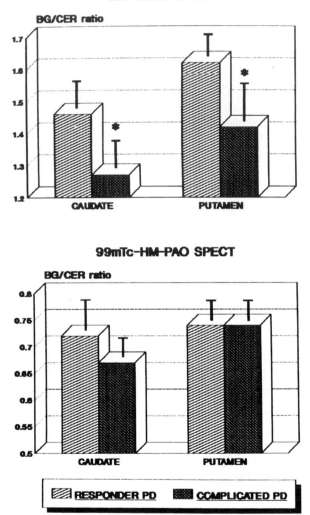

Fig 9–11.—Mean (± 1 SD of the mean) ^{123}I-IBZM and ^{99m}Tc-HMPAO activity (basal ganglia [BG]/ cerebellum [CER] ratios) in caudate and putamen of patients with PD separated on the basis of their response to chronic levodopa therapy. In ^{123}I-IBZM SPECT, the mean values for caudate and putamen of the complicated PD group were significantly (*P < .01) lower than the corresponding values of the responder PD group of patients. No differences were observed between the 2 groups with regard to ^{99m}Tc-HMPAO SPECT values. The mean ^{123}I-IBZM and ^{99m}Tc-HMPAO activity ratios for the responder PD group were not significantly different from the control mean. (Courtesy of Pizzolato G, Chierichetti F, Rossato A, et al: *Eur Neurol* 33:143–148, 1993.)

Study Population.—Eleven patients with idiopathic Parkinson's disease (PD) underwent SPECT using a novel ligand, ^{123}I-labeled IBZM, a D2 receptor ligand, to image the density of central dopamine D2 receptors in the basal ganglia in relation to levodopa therapy. All patients were receiving levodopa at the time of assessment. Six patients had a sustained, stable response to treatment, whereas the other 5 had markedly fluctuating responses with brief periods of motility and prolonged "off" periods. Five age-matched normal controls were also studied.

Methods.—Initially, SPECT studies were performed using technetium-labeled hexamethylpropyleneamine-oxime (HMPAO) to delineate regional perfusion. Patients then underwent SPECT with ^{123}I-IBZM, with images being acquired 2–3 hours after tracer administration.

Findings.—The HMPAO perfusion images failed to show any difference between activity in the caudate and putamen of patients with PD and controls. However, the activity of IBZM in the basal ganglia was significantly less in patients with PD who had responded poorly to levodopa therapy than in those who had responded consistently to treatment (Fig 9–11). In the putamen, D2 receptor activity was 20% lower than control levels in the poor responders, but it slightly exceeded the control mean in patients who responded.

Discussion.—These findings confirm reports of autopsy and in vivo studies showing that basal ganglia dopamine receptors are altered in patients whose response to levodopa is impaired. This alteration appears to be related to progressive PD itself rather than to chronic treatment.

▶ There is obvious potential here for following the therapeutic status of the individual patient. These data also point out that any diagnostic use of IBZM needs to better define the supranormal uptake in the putamen that is seen early in the course of the disease, because early is what we want.—A. Gottschalk, M.D.

Quantification of Technetium-99m Hexamethylpropylene Amine Oxime Brain Uptake in Routine Clinical Practice Using Calibrated Point Sources as an External Standard: Phantom and Human Studies
Dobbeleir A, Dierckx R (Middelheim Hosp, Antwerp, Belgium)
Eur J Nucl Med 20:684–689, 1993   124-95-9–14

Background.—In recent years, various quantitative methods have been proposed for calculating regional cerebral blood flow with technetium-99m hexamethylpropyleneamine-oxime (^{99m}Tc-HMPAO). However, these techniques are very labor-intensive and impractical in routine clinical practice. A simple alternative method has been developed.

Methods and Findings.—The new method uses calibrated point sources as a scaling factor. The tomographic slices are displayed as regional ^{99m}Tc-HMPAO brain uptake per cm^3 of brain tissue in 10^{-6} of the

TABLE 1.—Reproducibility of Point Source Activity, in Counts/μCi, for Repeated HMPAO Brain Studies in 10 Normal Volunteers

Volunteer	Acquisition 1	Acquisition 2
1	29199	27536
2	31132	30674
3	30990	31177
4	31476	30885
5	28940	29230
6	33910	32751
7	31709	32065
8	32498	33512
9	33067	31833
10	31850	31970

(Courtesy of Dobbeleir A, Dierckx R: *Eur J Nucl Med* 20:684–689, 1993.)

TABLE 2.—Reproducibility of Cerebellar Uptake in 10^{-6} of Injected Dose per cm^3 Brain Tissue for Repeated HMPAO Brain Studies in 10 Normal Volunteers and 5 Patients

	Uptake 1	Uptake 2	% change	Heart rate 1	Heart rate 2
Volunteer 1	72.2	65.0	−10.5	74	74
Volunteer 2	42.0	39.7	−5.7	60	60
Volunteer 3	38.6	44.1	13.4	68	68
Volunteer 4	51.0	53.3	4.5	76	72
Volunteer 5	66.6	68.6	3.0	76	80
Volunteer 6	33.3	31.9	−4.4	58	63
Volunteer 7	49.4	60.2	17.6	84	70
Volunteer 8	37.3	55.2	38.7	80	68
Volunteer 9	47.9	55.0	13.8	74	56
Volunteer 10	41.6	56.2	30.0	108	72
Patient 1	36.2	37.1	2.4	77	72
Patient 2	53.3	51.2	−4.0	82	86
Patient 3	48.2	55.0	13.1	88	88
Patient 4	49.7	54.7	9.6	104	105
Patient 5	40.1	46.9	15.6	96	80

(Courtesy of Dobbeleir A, Dierckx R: *Eur J Nucl Med* 20:684–689, 1993.)

injected lipophilic dose. The technique was validated on phantoms with a 3-detector system with high-resolution parallel and high-resolution fan-beam collimators. Under optimal conditions, a measured-to-real ratio activity of 1 was attained. The reproducibility of the cerebellar uptake was then studied in 10 normal volunteers and 5 patients. Intraindividually, the mean deviation for the total group was 12.6%. Those with a heart rate difference of fewer than 5 units between the 2 studies had a mean deviation of 7.2% (Tables 1 and 2).

Conclusion.—This method should be applicable to most SPECT systems after careful phantom work. The main advantages of the technique are its simplicity for clinical use; the same sources used daily for all patient acquisitions; and the final result, which is represented in terms of regional brain uptake.

▶ We are all for simplification and think that this type of approach can certainly help standardization within any 1 facility. However, we remain to be convinced that this will lead to absolute quantification, that is, the same absolute numbers from 1 facility to another with different equipment. We hope we are all wrong, but nuclear medicine history suggests we are not.—A. Gottschalk, M.D.

In Vivo Mapping of Cholinergic Neurons in the Human Brain Using SPECT and IBVM

Kuhl DE, Koeppe RA, Fessler JA, Minoshima S, Ackermann RJ, Carey JE, Gildersleeve DL, Frey KA, Wieland DM (Univ of Michigan, Ann Arbor)
J Nucl Med 35:405–410, 1994   124-95-9–15

Background.—The tracer $(-)$-5-$[^{123}I]$ iodobenzovesamicol (IBVM), an analogue of vesamicol that binds to the acetylcholine transporter in presynaptic vesicles, has been studied in animal models. The use of this tracer was extended to humans in the search for an in vivo marker of cholinergic neuronal integrity.

Methods.—The training agent was prepared with specific activity greater than 1.11×10^9 MBq mmol^{-1}. The $[^{123}I]$IBVM was injected IV into 10 healthy controls, and body distribution and brain SPECT studies were performed. Brain SPECT images were collected sequentially over the first 4.5 hours after injection and again 18 hours later.

Findings.—For as many as 4 hours, dissociation of bound tracer was negligible. The coefficients of variation were about 8% in the cortical regions of interest for the fitted parameters reflecting transport (K_1) and binding site density index (k_3). Relative distributions corresponded well with postmortem immunohistochemical values that have been reported for the acetylcholine-synthesizing enzyme choline acetyltransferase, k_3, and tracer activity distribution 22 hours after injection. These relationships were not observed 4 hours after injection (Fig 9–12).

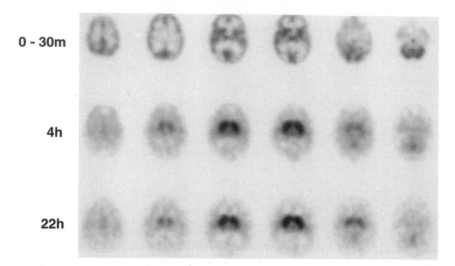

0 - 30m

4h

22h

Fig 9–12.—SPECT images of the human brain with respect to time after IV IBVM injection. The pattern of activity distribution resembles relative perfusion in the earliest images, then progressively striatal concentration dominates. At 22 hours after injection, the relative distribution of count density and IBVM binding site density index are similar. Imaging duration: **top row,** 20 minutes; **middle row,** 30 minutes; **bottom row,** 60 minutes. (Courtesy of Kuhl DE, Koeppe RA, Fessler JA, et al: *J Nucl Med* 35:405–410, 1994.)

Conclusion.—Imaging of [^{123}I]IBVM with SPECT is a useful measure of cholinergic neuronal integrity in vivo. It should be valuable for studying cerebral degenerative processes such as Alzheimer's disease.

▶ We agree and look forward to the first clinical trials in demented patients.—A. Gottschalk, M.D.

Dual Isotope Brain SPECT Imaging for Monitoring Cognitive Activation: Initial Studies in Humans

O'Leary DS, Madsen MT, Hurtig R, Kirchner PT, Rezai K, Rogers M, Andreasen NC (Univ of Iowa, Iowa City)
Nucl Med Commun 14:397–404, 1993   124-95-9–16

Objective.—The value of a dual-isotope SPECT technique for estimating regional cerebral blood flow in relation to cognitive activation was studied. The investigation was conducted in 8 normal young adults, all strongly right-handed, as well as in 3 male inpatients with schizophrenia, aged 21–30 years.

Methods.—The participants received both technetium-99m hexamethylpropyleneamine-oxime (^{99m}Tc-HMPAO) and ^{123}I-labeled iodoamphetamine (IMP), either simultaneously or at different times during performance of the same task. Easy and difficult auditory tasks were carried

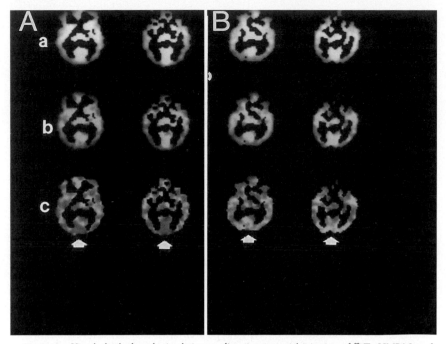

Fig 9–13.—Visual checkerboard stimulation studies. **A,** sequential injection of ^{99m}Tc-HMPAO and ^{123}I-IMP during checkerboard stimulation. Although both the HMPAO (a) and IMP (b) images show increased regional cerebral blood flow in the occipital lobe, the ratio images (c) show no preferential activation. **B,** sequential injection of HMPAO during eyes-closed rest and IMP during checkerboard stimulation. The 2 ratio images (c) illustrate the regional cerebral blood flow was higher in occipital cortex during the IMP-uptake period in which visual stimulation occurred. (Courtesy of O'Leary DS, Madsen MT, Hurtig R, et al: *Nucl Med Commun* 14:397–404, 1993.)

out, with the latter involving the dichotic presentation of 2 streams of words simultaneously to the 2 ears. A visual activation task was also performed.

Findings.—The 2 tracers were similarly distributed in the left and right cerebral hemispheres when they were administered under comparable physiologic conditions. However, there was a significant anteroposterior gradient that appeared to result from partial volume effects related to minor differences in spatial resolution between the 2 agents. The occipital cortex is thinner than the rest of the cortex in the transverse projection, and the resultant reduction in count density is more evident with ^{123}I emissions because system resolution is relatively low. When 2 participants received ^{99m}Tc-HMPAO at rest with their eyes closed and ^{123}I-IMP during visual stimulation, increased occipital activity was evident in the stimulated condition (Fig 9–13).

Conclusion.—The ability of dual-isotope SPECT imaging to localize increased blood flow to the visual cortex during visual stimulation suggests that this method should be useful for monitoring changes in regional cerebral blood flow caused by cognitive activation when they are in the 15% to 20% range.

▶ This is an example of the before-and-after technique we mentioned earlier (see comment after Abstract 124-95-9-7). The authors are trying to fine-tune the system. Frankly, we hope they fine-tune it even more. We are worried that changes of 15% to 20% may not permit subtle but important problems in cognitive activation (e.g., dyslexia) to be studied effectively.—A. Gott-schalk, M.D.

Anatomic Correlates of Memory From Intracarotid Amobarbital Injections With Technetium Tc 99m Hexamethylpropyleneamine Oxime SPECT
Hart J Jr, Lewis PJ, Lesser RP, Fisher RS, Monsein LH, Schwerdt P, Bandeen-Roche K, Gordon B (Johns Hopkins Univ, Baltimore, Md)
Arch Neurol 50:745–750, 1993   124-95-9-17

Background.—Intracarotid amobarbital injections have been used in the treatment of medically intractable seizures. However, memory performance during the injection has been difficult to interpret, because there is no consensus as to what types of memory should be tested or which testing methods should be used. Also, knowledge of which cerebral structures are being irrigated by the amobarbital is speculative.

Methods.—Thirty-nine patients with medically intractable epilepsy were studied. The standard intracarotid amobarbital procedure was modified by adding a radioactive tracer to the injection, which provided a better correlation between behavior and the deactivated brain region. The distribution of amobarbital was measured by SPECT imaging of hexamethylpropyleneamine-oxime (HMPAO). Patient performance on memory tasks was then tested.

Results.—The amobarbital irrigated medial temporal regions in only 28% of patients. The medial temporal and lateral neotemporal cortex appeared to play a role in memory.

Conclusion.—The regions involved in memory function and the distribution of amobarbital vary among individuals. The most accurate way to determine the correlation of a brain region with memory function during intracarotid amobarbital injection involves the use of a tracer (e.g., HMPAO).

▶ We always get nervous with this type of "spin-off" study. Recently (see the 1993 YEAR BOOK OF NUCLEAR MEDICINE, pp 277–279), we noted that patients with strokes could relearn some motor function using neural pathways other than those traditionally accepted (i.e., the precentral gyrus). How do we know that memory for these epileptic patients is not modified by their epilepsy and works by pathways that are unique to this patient group? Thus, we accept the idea that the medial temporal and lateral neotemporal cortex may play a role in memory as a working hypothesis at best. Nevertheless, this is a complicated problem, and we salute the authors for their efforts to elucidate this pathophysiology.—A. Gottschalk, M.D.

High Resolution SPECT With [99mTc]-*d,l*-HMPAO in Normal Pressure Hydrocephalus Before and After Shunt Operation

Waldemar G, Schmidt JF, Delecluse F, Andersen AR, Gjerris F, Paulson OB
(Rigshospitalet, Copenhagen; Hosp Erasme, Brussels, Belgium)
J Neurol Neurosurg Psychiatry 56:655–664, 1993   124-95-9–18

Background.—Normal-pressure hydrocephalus (NPH) is a rare cause of dementia that can be treated. The value of high-resolution SPECT of regional cerebral blood flow (rCBF) using technetium-99m-*d-l*-hexamethylpropyleneamine-oxime (^{99m}Tc-*d,l*-HMPAO) in the diagnosis of NPH, in normal aging, and in the prediction of clinical outcome after shunt surgery in NPH was investigated.

Methods.—Fourteen consecutive patients with dementia and NPH were compared with 14 healthy volunteers of the same age. Patients with NPH had an enlarged subcortical low-flow region, significantly decreased rCBF, enhanced side-to-side asymmetry of rCBF in the central white matter, and increased side-to-side asymmetry in the inferior and midtemporal cortex. Shunt surgery improved 11 patients' clinical status. The area of the subcortical low-flow region correctly classified all 3 unimproved and 10 of the 11 improved patients. In 9 of 10 patients, the shunt operation normalized or reduced the area of the subcortical low-flow region.

Conclusion.—Single-photon emission CT with ^{99m}Tc-*d,l*-HMPAO is a useful supplement for differentiating NPH from normal aging. Single-photon emission CT may also be helpful in identifying patients who are not likely to clinically benefit from surgery.

▶ In the past, we have been less than complimentary about nuclear techniques designed to give diagnoses to patients who are candidates for shunt procedure in NPH. In short, we think routine cisternography is a reasonably lousy test.

These authors have brought in a new, high-technology approach to this problem with apparently good results. However, before getting overly enthusiastic, we should point out that those in the control group—as far as we can tell—did *not* have enlarged ventricles. Is it possible that the subcortical low flow the authors found is related only to ventricular dilatation? Unfortunately, all the data fit this simple hypothesis. In short, we accept this as an interesting idea, but we await additional patient data.—A. Gottschalk, M.D.

Regional Cerebral Blood Flow in Angelman Syndrome

Gücüyener K, Gökçora N, Ilgin N, Buyan N, Sayli A (Gazi Univ, Ankara, Turkey)

Eur J Nucl Med 20:645–647, 1993   124-95-9–19

Introduction.—Angelman, in 1965, described children who were mentally retarded with profoundly delayed speech; seizures; ataxic gait; jerky movements; and paroxysmal, unprovoked laughter. About 150 cases have been reported to date. Most patients appear to have a microdeletion in chromosomal region 15q11–15p13. The defect in speech development is often more marked than would be expected from the degree of retardation. One patient is the first to be examined with SPECT.

Case Report.—Girl, 12 years, was noted at age 8 months to be developmentally delayed. She sat up at age 25 months, stood with support at 3 years, and walked at age 5. When she was 20 months of age, the girl recognized her parents but did not speak. She laughed much more than other children her age and appeared to be very happy. Febrile seizures, which developed at age 3, were controlled by phenobarbital. Examination revealed a grossly retarded child who walked with an ataxic, puppet-like gait and had jerky movements. Paroxysms of laughter occurred without being provoked. The girl understood simple commands, but her speech was unclear and her vocabulary limited. Prognathism and brachymicrocephaly were apparent. An electroencephalogram showed generalized slow activity but no signs of epilepsy. A SPECT study with technetium-labeled hexamethylpropyleneamine-oxime demonstrated a large region of impaired blood flow in the left frontal lobe that extended into the temporal and parietal lobes.

Interpretation.—The hypoactivity seen in the left frontal lobe in this patient may be ascribed to a developmental disorder of the higher-learning centers. Hypoperfusion in the left temporoparietal region reflects a profound delay in language development, overshadowing the mental retardation.

▶ This is certainly an unusual case. It makes me wonder why this child did not redirect her speech to the right temporal lobe and stutter. We also came across some other unusual cases such as cerebral abnormalities in myotonic dystrophia (1), cerebral involvement in McLeod's syndrome (2), familial progressive aphasia and its relationship to other forms of lobar atrophy (3), and increased blood flow in Broca's area during auditory hallucinations in schizophrenia (4).—A. Gottschalk, M.D.

References

1. Chang L, et al: *Arch Neurol* 50:917, 1993.
2. Danek A, et al: *Neurology* 44:117, 1994.
3. Neary D, et al: *J Neurol Neurosurg Psychiatry* 56:1122, 1993.
4. McQuire PK, et al: *Lancet* 342:703, 1993.

**Prognostic Value of Triple Phase Bone Scanning for Reflex Sympa-
thetic Dystrophy in Hemiplegia**
Weiss L, Alfano A, Bardfeld P, Weiss J, Friedmann LW (Nassau County Med
Ctr, East Meadow, NY)
Arch Phys Med Rehabil 74:716–719, 1993   124-95-9-20

Objective.—Reflex sympathetic dystrophy syndrome (RSDS) com-
prises diffuse distal limb pain, hyperesthesia, edema, dystrophic skin
changes, and vasomotor instability. It may result from an abnormal reflex arc that is triggered by stroke or trauma. Triple-phase technetium
bone scanning is a sensitive and specific test to confirm the clinical suspicion of RSDS. Prompted by the clinical observation that many patients
in rehabilitation after cerebrovascular accident (CVA) went on to have
RSDS, a prospective investigation of its incidence after CVA and the
ability of triple-phase bone scanning to predict it was conducted.

Methods.—The participants were 22 patients with CVA, all confirmed
by head CT scanning, on an inpatient rehabilitation unit. Eleven had left
CVAs with right hemiparesis, 11 had left CVA with right hemiparesis,
and 2 had bilateral CVAs. The patients were followed clinically for as
many as 6 months for the development of symptoms of RSDS. In addition, all underwent triple-phase bone scanning within a few months of
their CVAs.

Results.—Bone scans were positive in 73% of patients and negative in
27%. Somewhat more of the patients with a left CVA had positive scans.
None of the patients with negative scans had symptoms of RSDS. Five of
the patients with positive bone scans had symptoms at the time of scanning. Of 11 patients with positive scans but no baseline symptoms, 7
went on to have RSDS. The relationship between a positive bone scan
and the development of RSDS was significant. Among patients who
were asymptomatic when scanned, bone scanning was a good predictor
of the eventual development of RSDS.

Conclusion.—Triple-phase bone scanning may be a good predictor of
risk for clinical RSDS after CVA. Early detection of RSDS and prompt
intervention might help minimize the associated disability, especially in
patients with hemiplegia. Further research is needed to define the characteristics of this postulated preclinical phase.

▶ To be honest, I never realized the incidence of RSDS was so high in stroke
patients. The authors point out that if the results of this study (i.e., a positive
3-phase bone scan before the clinical appearance of RSDS) can be sustained
in a larger series, there is much that rehabilitation workers can do for the
stage 0 RSDS patient. Even before we get these data confirmed, you may
want to share these results with your rehabilitation colleagues.—A. Gottschalk, M.D.

10 Cardiovascular

Introduction

There seemed to be a larger body of literature to draw from this year than in recent past years. Once again, the emphasis is on myocardial perfusion imaging. Almost three fourths of the articles involve perfusion scintigraphy. This year also saw the arrival of a large number of articles dealing with technetium-99m perfusion agents, and the role of sestamibi appears to have been established. In addition, the year marked the arrival of clinical articles involving new technetium agents. The areas of neuro-cardiac imaging and metabolic imaging were also well represented, as was PET investigation that involved perfusion, metabolism, and receptor imaging. This more recent literature appears to be making a real attempt to define the unique aspects of PET, which could help in establishing its place in the imaging spectrum. This year also marks the first time that nuclear cardiology is represented as a field with its own journal—the *Journal of Nuclear Cardiology*. This has been an excellent source for material for the YEAR BOOK OF NUCLEAR MEDICINE.

Barry L. Zaret, M.D.

Prognostic Significance From 10-Year Follow-Up of a Qualitatively Normal Planar Exercise Thallium Test in Suspected Coronary Artery Disease

Steinberg EH, Koss JH, Lee M, Grunwald AM, Bodenheimer MM (The Harris Chasanoff Heart Inst, New Hyde Park, NY; Long Island Jewish Med Ctr, New Hyde Park, NY; Albert Einstein Coll of Med, Bronx, NY)
Am J Cardiol 71:1270–1273, 1993   124-95-10–1

Background.—Many studies have found that patients with normal exercise thallium myocardial perfusion have an excellent prognosis for 1 to 4 years. The likelihood of cardiac death or infarction in such patients is less than 1% a year. However, coronary disease progression may result in cardiac mortality over a longer period.

Methods.—Three hundred nine patients with normal stress thallium myocardial imaging were followed for a mean of 10.3 years. Deaths were categorized as cardiac or noncardiac, and standardized mortality ratios were compared with those from a general population that was matched for age and sex. Complete follow-up data were available on 93% of the group.

Findings.—Only 3 of the 18 deaths that occurred were cardiac; most of the remaining 15 died of cancer. The 10-year total mortality was 6.3%, and the cardiac mortality was 1%. Both rates were significantly lower than would be expected in the general population.

Conclusion.—Normal exercise thallium scintigraphy retains its high negative predictive value for death within 10 years of the initial assessment. Stress thallium imaging can be used to predict which patients with suspected coronary artery disease are at low risk for cardiac death, obviating the need for invasive evaluations.

▶ This important demonstration indicates that the finding of a normal exercise thallium study has substantial clinical impact not only immediately, but over the long term. The 10-year follow-up data set is relatively unique, and the data indicate the profound prognostic importance of a negative exercise perfusion study and support the ongoing clinical use of this technique.—B.L. Zaret, M.D.

Prognostic Value of Thallium-201 Single-Photon Emission Computed Tomographic Myocardial Perfusion Imaging According to Extent of Myocardial Defect: Study in 1,926 Patients With Follow-Up at 33 Months
Machecourt J, Longère P, Fagret D, Vanzetto G, Wolf JE, Polidori C, Comet M, Denis B (Centre Hospitalier Universitaire, Grenoble, France)
J Am Coll Cardiol 23:1096–1106, 1994   124-95-10–2

Background.—Thallium SPECT enables better assessment of the extent of myocardial perfusion defect than planar scintigraphy. However, no previous studies of large patient populations had been done to determine its prognostic value.

Methods.—From 1987 to 1989, 3,193 patients were evaluated; those with unstable angina, myocardial infarction during the previous month, or earlier revascularization were excluded, leaving 1,926 patients in the final group. The mean follow-up after stress thallium SPECT imaging was 33 months. Left ventricle thallium SPECT imaging was divided into 6 segments.

Findings.—After normal thallium SPECT imaging in 715 patients, the annual total and cardiovascular death rates were .42% and .10% per year, respectively. These rates were significantly greater after abnormal thallium SPECT imaging. The number of abnormal segments was significantly related to cardiovascular mortality during follow-up or the occurrence of nonfatal events. The best SPECT variable for long-term prognosis was the extent of the defect on the initial scan. Compared with clinical variables, such as gender and previous myocardial infarction, and

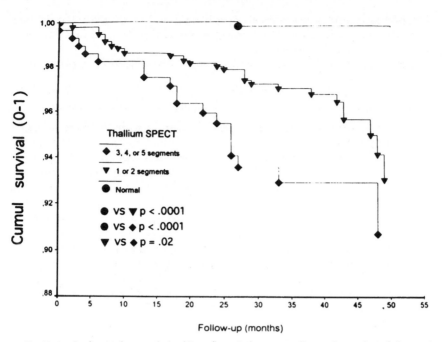

Fig 10–1.—Cardiovascular cumulative (*Cumul*) survival rate according to the number of abnormal segments on initial thallium SPECT imaging. (Courtesy of Machecourt J, Longère P, Fagret D, et al: *J Am Coll Cardiol* 23:1096–1106, 1994.)

exercise ECG results, thallium SPECT imaging provided additional prognostic information (Fig 10–1).

Conclusion.—Normal thallium SPECT imaging indicates a low risk in patients with stable angina. The extent of the myocardial defect is an important prognostic factor.

▶ This article indicates that for thallium-201 SPECT, the magnitude of the perfusion defect has a profound impact on prognosis. It is intuitive that it will be inadequate to simply dichotomize patients into those with merely positive and negative tests. Patients with positive tests will have to be further differentiated, based on the extent of disease. This study illustrates that phenomenon well. It also provides additional evidence regarding the important prognostic impact of a negative study.—B.L. Zaret, M.D.

Independent and Incremental Prognostic Value of Exercise Single-Photon Emission Computed Tomographic (SPECT) Thallium Imaging in Coronary Artery Disease

Iskandrian AS, Chae SC, Heo J, Stanberry CD, Wasserleben V, Cave V (Philadelphia Heart Inst)
J Am Coll Cardiol 22:665–670, 1993   124-95-10-3

Objective.—Whether exercise SPECT imaging with thallium provides more prognostic information than that obtained by clinical, exercise ECG, and cardiac catheterization studies was determined in 316 patients who were managed medically for angiographically confirmed coronary artery disease. Most previous studies of thallium scintigraphy have used planar imaging techniques.

Methods.—The patients performed symptom-limited treadmill exercise using the Bruce protocol. Short-axis slices were acquired at the apical, mid-, and basal levels. Perfusion abnormalities that were at least partially redistributed on the delayed image in 25% or more of the segment were considered to be reversible. Perfusion abnormalities were quantified using polar maps to compare the patient's profile with a gender-matched normal profile.

Results.—Most patients achieved 85% of the maximum predicted heart rate or had ST-segment depression during exercise. Thirty-five patients died of cardiac causes or had a nonfatal myocardial infarction during a mean follow-up of 28 months. Prognostically significant factors in-

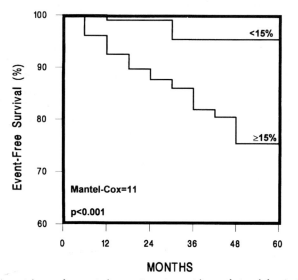

Fig 10–2.—Actuarial event-free survival curves in patients with a perfusion defect ≥ 15% or < 15% of the left ventricular myocardium. (Courtesy of Iskandrian AS, Chae SC, Heo J, et al: *J Am Coll Cardiol* 22:665-670, 1993.)

cluded the exercise workload achieved, the extent of coronary artery disease, the left ventricular ejection fraction, and thallium variables. Data from the SPECT thallium study added prognostic information to that obtained by cardiac catheterization. Patients with a sizable perfusion abnormality that involved 15% or more of the myocardium had a worse outlook than those with a mild abnormality or normal perfusion (Fig 10–2).

Conclusion.—Exercise SPECT thallium imaging provides useful prognostic information beyond that obtained by cardiac catheterization in medically treated patients with coronary artery disease. Those who are found to be at high risk should be considered for coronary revascularization. In many other patients, cardiac catheterization will not be necessary.

▶ This study provides highly relevant data indicating that perfusion scintigraphy adds to the prognostic assessment of patients beyond that obtained from coronary angiography alone. Data such as these must be brought to bear on ongoing debates concerning the utility of perfusion imaging in patients who are undergoing coronary angiography.—B.L. Zaret, M.D.

Quantitative Severity of Stress Thallium-201 Myocardial Perfusion Single-Photon Emission Computed Tomography Defects in One-Vessel Coronary Artery Disease

Matzer L, Kiat H, Van Train K, Germano G, Papanicolaou M, Silagan G, Eigler N, Maddahi J, Berman DS (Cedars-Sinai Med Ctr, Los Angeles; Univ of California, Los Angeles)
Am J Cardiol 72:273–279, 1993   124-95-10–4

Objective.—Quantitative exercise thallium-201 SPECT can accurately delineate the presence, location, and extent of hemodynamically significant coronary artery disease. However, few studies have looked at the relation between the severity of thallium-201 defects and that of the underlying coronary stenoses. A quantitative technique for analyzing the severity of thallium-201 SPECT defects was developed and compared with the degree of stenosis as documented by quantitative coronary angiography.

Methods.—The study sample included 18 patients with single-vessel coronary disease, defined as 50% or greater stenosis, and visually abnormal findings on thallium-201 SPECT. Angiographic-SPECT correlations were performed in 26 vessels, including all 18 diseased vessels, 6 vessels with mild but discrete stenoses, and 2 completely normal arteries. The investigators calculated a thallium-201 SPECT quantitative defect severity score by adding the number of pixels in a coronary territory in which counts fell below the normal mean, then multiplying by the number of standard deviations below the normal mean.

Results.—Significant correlations were noted between the thallium-201 defect severity score and the maximal percentage of luminal diameter narrowing, r = .93; the percentage of area narrowing, r = .89; the absolute stenotic area, r = .79; and the absolute stenotic diameter, r = .81. The low and high ends of the range of coronary stenosis showed the strongest relationship between thallium-201 defect severity and quantitative angiographic variables. Variability was greater and correlation coefficients were lower in the middle ranges of severity, that is, 50% to 80% stenosis.

Conclusion.—For selected patients with coronary artery disease, quantitative thallium-201 defect severity is a potentially useful means of noninvasively characterizing the functional severity of stenoses. As a complementary procedure to coronary angiography, it may prove effective in the prediction of functionally significant stenoses. Correlations between thallium-201 defects and coronary stenosis are weaker in the middle range of stenosis severity, probably because of the complex flow patterns of stenotic lesions.

▶ This article addresses an important issue: the ability of the stress perfusion study to define the magnitude of coronary artery disease. Obviously, this is a complex issue, and it is surprising that the correlations are as good as they are. Many factors must be brought to bear on the physiologic assessment of the magnitude of anatomical disease. Nevertheless, these data are quite encouraging and continue to point out the clinical value of perfusion scintigraphy.—B.L. Zaret, M.D.

Comparative Prognostic Value of Clinical Risk Indexes, Resting Two-Dimensional Echocardiography, and Dipyridamole Stress Thallium-201 Myocardial Imaging for Perioperative Cardiac Events in Major Nonvascular Surgery Patients
Takase B, Younis LT, Byers SL, Shaw LJ, Labovitz AJ, Chaitman BR, Miller DD (St Louis Univ, Mo)
Am Heart J 126:1099–1106, 1993   124-95-10–5

Background.—Resting 2-dimensional echocardiography is a widely available and noninvasive test of global and regional ventricular function. However, there are insufficient data on its preoperative prognostic value in relation to clinical risk analysis and pharmacologic stress perfusion imaging, that is, Goldman risk factor analysis and dipyridamole stress thallium-201 myocardial imaging, in the same population. The prognostic value of 2-dimensional echocardiographic ventricular function data was compared with that of recognized clinical and scintigraphic risk markers in patients with known or suspected ischemic heart disease who were undergoing major nonvascular surgery.

Methods.—Fifty-three consecutive patients, with a mean age of 67 years, were studied retrospectively. All were referred for preoperative evaluation before orthopedic, 30%; intra-abdominal, 23%; thoracic, 9%; and other nonvascular operations, 38%. All had known or suspected coronary artery disease and were unable to perform adequate exercise. Goldman risk factor analysis was performed by a review of the medical records without knowledge of the postoperative outcome. Two-dimensional echocardiography and IV dipyridamole thallium-201 myocardial imaging studies were reviewed as well. The prognostic value of these 3 assessments for perioperative cardiac events was evaluated by multivariate analysis.

Results.—Perioperative cardiac events occurred in 25% of patients, including cardiac death in 4, myocardial infarction in 2, unstable angina in 3, and pulmonary edema in 8. Twenty-eight percent of patients had dipyridamole thallium-201 myocardial redistribution defects, and 40% had resting echocardiographic left ventricular dysfunction. These were the only independent predictors of cardiac events. Cardiac death and myocardial infarction were predicted by the finding of dipyridamole thallium-201 defect redistribution, and perioperative pulmonary edema was predicted by the presence of left ventricular dysfunction on echocardiography. Goldman class or score and other clinical variables did not predict cardiac events.

Conclusion.—For patients undergoing major nonvascular surgery who are at risk for ischemic cardiac events and cannot perform standard exercise stress tests, valuable prognostic information can be obtained by stress thallium-201 perfusion imaging and resting 2-dimensional echocardiography. The combination of these 2 noninvasive studies can predict acute ischemic events and left ventricular decompensation during or immediately after surgery. Clinical risk assessments, such as Goldman risk factor analysis, cannot predict cardiac events in this patient population, although they may be useful in deciding whether to perform noninvasive testing.

▶ This article points out the value of noninvasive risk stratification before noncardiac surgery. When it is done appropriately in the relevant patient populations, it still seems to be a highly relevant clinical study.—B.L. Zaret, M.D.

Separate Acquisition Rest Thallium-201/Stress Technetium-99m Sestamibi Dual-Isotope Myocardial Perfusion Single-Photon Emission Computed Tomography: A Clinical Validation Study

Berman DS, Kiat H, Friedman JD, Wang FP, van Train K, Matzer L, Maddahi J, Germano G (Cedars-Sinai Med Ctr, Los Angeles; Univ of California, Los Angeles)
J Am Coll Cardiol 22:1455–1464, 1993   124-95-10–6

Background.—Standard, same-day rest-stress technetium-99m sestamibi myocardial perfusion SPECT can be time-consuming. It is associated with reduced defect severity and may be unable to differentiate between hibernating and infarcted myocardium. Dual-isotope myocardial perfusion SPECT, using either simultaneous or separate acquisition of rest thallium-201 and stress technetium-99m sestamibi, may be a good alternative that does not have these disadvantages.

Methods.—To determine the sensitivity and specificity for coronary artery disease, the dual-isotope procedure was performed on 63 patients who had no previous myocardial infarctions and were undergoing coronary angiography. To determine the normality rate, the procedure was also performed on 107 patients who had a less than 5% probability of coronary artery disease. A separate group of 31 patients who had previous myocardial infarctions was evaluated to determine defect reversibility. These patients underwent rest thallium-201 and stress technetium-99m sestamibi separate-acquisition dual-isotope myocardial perfusion SPECT. The next day, they received rest technetium-99m sestamibi injections and underwent technetium-99m sestamibi SPECT.

Results.—In angiographic correlations, using the criterion of at least 50% narrowing as significant coronary stenosis, the sensitivity for dual-isotope SPECT was 91%; the specificity for less than 50% was 75%. With the criterion of at least 70% lumen narrowing being significant, the sensitivity of dual-isotope SPECT was 96%; the specificity for less than 70% was 82%. For the 107 patients who had a low probability of coronary artery disease, the normality rate was high. In the group that was tested for defect reversibility in myocardial zones with no previous infarction, the segmental agreement for defect type between rest thallium-201 and rest technetium-99m sestamibi studies was 97%. The segmental agreement for defect type was 98% in myocardial infarct zones. Image quality ranged from good to excellent. In the left anterior descending coronary artery territory of a man 60 years of age with recurrent, typical angina and no previous myocardial infarctions, the stress technetium-99m sestamibi images showed severe defects; the rest thallium-201 images were normal.

Discussion.—For detecting coronary artery disease, the sensitivity of separate-acquisition dual-isotope SPECT is similar to that of SPECT studies using thallium-201 or technetium-99m sestamibi alone. The high values for specificity are insignificant, because few patients had normal coronary arteriograms. The possible higher cost of using 2 radiopharmaceuticals is offset by greater efficiency and productivity, higher-quality images, the potential for first-pass or gated SPECT studies of ventricular function, and improved viability information. Therefore, separate-acquisition dual-isotope SPECT with rest thallium-201 and stress technetium-99m sestamibi is a preferred protocol.

▶ This article presents excellent clinical data indicating the efficacy of a dual-isotope perfusion imaging approach that can take advantage of the attributes of both thallium-201 and technetium-99m sestamibi. This approach may add substantially to throughput in busy clinical laboratories. Further studies in this area surely will be forthcoming soon.—B.L. Zaret, M.D.

Dual-Isotope Myocardial Imaging: Feasibility, Advantages and Limitations: Preliminary Report on 231 Consecutive Patients
Weinmann P, Foult J-M, Le Guludec D, Tamgac F, Rechtman D, Neuman A, Caillat-Vigneron N, Moretti J-L (Avicenne Univ Hosp, Bobigny, France; American Hosp, Paris; Bichat Univ, France)
Eur J Nucl Med 21:212–215, 1994   124-95-10–7

Introduction.—A combination of rest thallium-201 (RT) imaging followed by stress technetium-99m sestamibi (SM) imaging assesses both myocardial viability and ischemia. The procedure was performed on 231 consecutive patients from November 1992 to May 1993.

Patients.—The study population consisted of 134 men and 97 women, with a mean age of 58 years, who came to the nuclear medicine department for myocardial scintigraphy.

Findings.—The duration of the procedure, which was shorter than that of the standard stress-redistribution procedure, permitted improved camera-scheduling flexibility. The different attenuation properties of the 2 radioactive agents enhanced the interpretation of defects because of image attenuation. Maximum crossover was 18% with these 2 agents, and interobserver reproducibility was greater than 97% with this technique.

Conclusion.—The RT-SM procedure is especially useful in patients for whom the assessment of myocardial viability is important, such as those with a history of infarction or those with basal-depressed ventricular function. However, for patients with a lesser chance of coronary artery disease, the extra irradiation dose used in this technique is probably not necessary. More extensive clinical tests are required to determine the optimal acquisition and reconstruction techniques for RT-SM.

▶ I have no comments other than those offered on the preceding article (Abstract 124-95-10–6).—B.L. Zaret, M.D.

Nitrates Improve Detection of Ischemic But Viable Myocardium by Thallium-201 Reinjection SPECT
He Z-X, Darcourt J, Guignier A, Ferrari E, Bussière F, Baudouy M, Morand P (Centre Antoine Lacassagne, Nice, France; Univ of Nice, France)
J Nucl Med 34:1472–1477, 1993   124-95-10–8

Background.—Although thallium-201 (^{201}Tl) reinjection imaging improves myocardial viability detection compared with standard 3- to 4-hour redistribution imaging, it underestimates the extent of ischemic but viable myocardium. Nitrates increase regional blood flow to ischemic myocardial areas. Whether administration of nitrates after exercise increases the sensitivity of reinjection imaging was examined.

Methods.—Twenty patients with coronary artery disease, 11 of whom had a recent myocardial infarction, underwent 2 exercise per 4-hour redistribution ^{201}Tl SPECT protocols. Protocol A measured the effect of reinjection alone; protocol B measured the effect of reinjection and 20-mg isosorbide dinitrate administered immediately after postexercise imaging.

Results.—Protocol A revealed reversible defects in 15 patients, fixed ^{201}Tl defects in 4, and reverse redistribution in 1. In protocol B, 18 patients had reversible defects, 2 had fixed defects, and 1 patient (not the patient in protocol A) had reverse redistribution. Combined, the protocols detected 96 abnormal segments; redistribution patterns were identical for the protocols in 40 reversible and 40 fixed defects. Protocol A revealed 41 reversible segmental defects, 54 fixed defects, and 1 reverse redistribution. Protocol B revealed 54 segmental reversible defects, 41 fixed defects, and 1 reverse redistribution. Only 1 of the reversible myocardial segments in protocol A was not reversible with protocol B. By contrast, 14 of the fixed defects in protocol A were reversible with protocol B. In the 15 patients with reversible defects on both protocols, the mean redistribution extent was significantly higher with nitrates and reinjection: 3.2 segments compared with 2.73 segments with reinjection alone.

Conclusion.—Thallium-201 SPECT with nitrates and reinjection enhances detection of ischemic but viable myocardium compared with SPECT with reinjection alone.

▶ The use of nitrates to augment definition of viability with perfusion imaging is an important and relatively new area. It will be relevant to extend these observations to patients undergoing revascularization surgery so that one can precisely define whether nitrate augmentation of thallium uptake is associated with evidence of reversible left ventricular dysfunction, as judged by improvement following revascularization. Furthermore, the same principles of nitrate augmentation may hold for sestamibi imaging.—B.L. Zaret, M.D.

Immediate Thallium-201 Reinjection Following Stress Imaging: A Time-Saving Approach for Detection of Myocardial Viability
van Eck-Smit BLF, van der Wall EE, Kuijper AFM, Zwinderman AH, Pauwels EKJ (Univ Hosp Leiden, The Netherlands)
J Nucl Med 34:737–743, 1993   124-95-10–9

Background.—Thallium-201 (^{201}Tl) reinjection after 3–4-hour redistribution imaging enhances the identification of viable myocardium. However, the total investigation time is prolonged when using this method.

The results of immediate ^{201}Tl reinjection were compared with 3-hour redistribution imaging to determine whether elimination of the latter images would have a significant impact on detection of myocardial viability and the subsequent diagnosis of myocardial ischemia.

Patients and Methods.—A total of 120 patients aged 30–79 years consecutively undergoing evaluation for myocardial ischemia were investigated. All patients underwent ^{201}Tl reinjection immediately after postexercise image acquisition. Images were acquired 1 hour later and again at the 3-hour redistribution. A total of 960 segments per imaging series were assessed.

Results.—Perfusion defects were noted in 320 segments on the postexercise images. Enhanced thallium uptake was seen in 220 segments on the 1-hour images. Ninety-seven of the segments did not change, and reverse redistribution was noted in 3 segments. Of the 100 persistent defects, fill-in of ^{210}Tl was observed in only 12 segments on the 3-hour redistribution images. Reverse redistribution was seen on a total of 49 segments. Ninety-five patients, 9 of whom had no change on immediate reinjection images, had defects on postexercise images. Diagnosis was changed from myocardial necrosis to myocardial ischemia in only 1 patient after analysis of the 3-hour redistribution images.

Conclusion.—Immediate postexercise reinjection of ^{201}Tl followed by 1-hour image acquisition may be the preferred method for detecting viable myocardium in patients who are assessed for myocardial ischemia. Use of this protocol eliminates the need to obtain an additional series of 3- to 4-hour redistribution images and provides the benefits of decreased total imaging time, improved convenience for the patient, and increased patient processing.

▶ This technique presents yet another option in the thallium protocol cascade. The optimal technique has not as yet been defined. Issues relating to cost-effectiveness and overall laboratory logistics, coupled with the actual scientific data, should be forthcoming in the next year.—B.L. Zaret, M.D.

Comparison of Thallium-201 Single-Photon Emission Tomography After Rest Injection and Fluorodeoxyglucose Positron Emission Tomography for Assessment of Myocardial Viability in Patients With Chronic Coronary Artery Disease
Altehoefer C, vom Dahl J, Buell U, Uebis R, Kleinhans E, Hanrath P (Technical Univ of Aachen, Germany)
Eur J Nucl Med 21:37–45, 1994   124-95-10–10

Background.—Although PET is the preferred imaging modality for evaluation of myocardial viability, it is not widely available. Therefore, SPECT imaging with an optimized protocol was evaluated for its ability to assess viability compared with PET.

Patients and Methods.—Forty-two patients with chronic coronary artery disease and severe wall motion abnormalities (sWMAs), which were confirmed by cineventriculography, were enrolled. The global ejection fraction was 45% ± 13%. Twenty-four patients had previous myocardial infarction that occurred at least 4 weeks before initiation of the study. All patients underwent thallium-201 (^{201}Tl) SPECT and fluorodeoxyglucose (^{18}FDG) PET (after oral glucose load) at rest on the same day or within 3 days. For image analysis, the left ventricle was divided into the supply territory of the left anterior descending coronary artery (LAD) and the lateral wall and posterior territory (inferior, posterior, and posteroseptal segments) because of the high variability of left circumflex and right coronary artery supply territories.

Results.—A close linear relationship in the LAD territory and the lateral wall was noted for segmental ^{201}Tl uptake in SPECT and segmental normalized ^{18}FDG uptake, at r = .79 and .77, respectively. The correlation in the posterior wall was much lower, at r = .52. Thallium-201/^{18}FDG concordance was defined as an ^{18}FDG uptake exceeding ^{201}Tl uptake by less than 20%, whereas discordance was assumed if ^{18}FDG exceeded ^{201}Tl uptake by at least 20%. Concordant results were noted in 81% of segments. In segments with severe ^{201}Tl reduction, defined as 50% and less of peak, discordance was seen in 10% of segments in the LAD territory and lateral wall and in 44% of segments in the posterior territory. In segments with moderate ^{201}Tl reduction, discordance was observed in 12% and 46% of segments, respectively. Discordance was noted in 6 of 43 severe defects, defined as the entire area with ^{201}Tl uptake of 50% or less within a delineated area. Twelve of 90 areas with sWMAs on cineventriculography showed discordant results, 10 of which affected the septum or posterior wall. Discordance occurred in the septum or posterior wall in 22% of areas with normal wall motion or mild hypokinesis only. By comparison, the figure for the anterior or lateral wall was only 2%.

Conclusion.—Viable myocardium can be accurately identified in the supply area of the LAD and in the lateral wall using ^{201}Tl SPECT with a rest protocol. Discordance in the posterior territory may be governed by photon attenuation in the SPECT study as opposed to a pathophysiologic difference.

▶ This study points out some of the known problems with thallium SPECT for assessing viability, especially the possibility of substantial attenuation. This attenuation of the low-energy, low-photon flux thallium uptake is often most marked in the inferior-posterior wall. This diaphragmatic attenuation can be evaluated by comparison of supine and decubitus planar images.—B.L. Zaret, M.D.

Role of Quantitative Planar Thallium-201 Imaging for Determining Viability in Patients With Acute Myocardial Infarction and a Totally

Occluded Infarct-Related Artery

Sabia PJ, Powers ER, Ragosta M, Smith WH, Watson DD, Kaul S (Univ of Virginia, Charlottesville)
J Nucl Med 34:728–736, 1993   124-95-10–11

Introduction.—A number of factors affect the uptake of thallium-201 (^{201}Tl) to the infarct zone after myocardial infarction. These include the blood flow to the infarct zone, which comes only from collateral vessels from other myocardial beds when the infarct-related artery (IRA) is totally occluded, and the mix of normal, ischemic, and necrotic tissue in the IRA bed. Thus, because of redistribution, the relative thallium activity within a hypoperfused but viable zone may only reach its maximal intensity on the delayed image. The relationship between the extent of viable myocardium and thallium uptake on delayed planar images was examined in 57 patients with a recent infarction and an occluded IRA.

Methods.—The patients were all found to have total occlusion of the IRA at cardiac catheterization. Exercise or rest thallium imaging was performed at baseline and exercise thallium imaging was performed 1 month after angioplasty in all patients. Delayed images were obtained 2 hours after thallium injection. Three correlative approaches were used to determine the relation between viable myocardium and delayed thallium uptake: average thallium activity within the occluded bed vs. regional wall motion at baseline, increased thallium uptake in the occluded bed after attempted angioplasty vs. improvement in regional function in the IRA bed, and preangioplasty thallium uptake in the occluded bed vs. wall motion score after attempted angioplasty.

Results.—The mean ^{201}Tl activity in the infarct zone was significantly correlated with regional wall motion in that bed, both at baseline and 1 month after angioplasty, r = −.06 and −.67, respectively. Function was better in patients who had greater thallium uptake in the delayed images. The number of segments showing redistribution was not correlated with the wall motion score. The 10 patients with unsuccessful angioplasty showed no change in the mean wall motion score or the mean thallium activity within the IRA bed, whereas those with successful angioplasty improved significantly in both of these variables.

Conclusion.—There is good correlation between average ^{201}Tl activity within the infarct zone on delayed planar imaging and the extent of viable myocardium in that zone in patients with recent myocardial infarction and complete occlusion of the IRA. The findings of the delayed images are unaffected by the presence or absence of redistribution. Further study is needed to establish the value of delayed planar thallium imaging in the routine management of unselected patients with acute myocardial infarction.

▶ This study provides further corroboration of the value of perfusion imaging in assessing viability in patients after myocardial infarction. This could prove to be of substantial value in the noninvasive definition of collateral flow and residual viability after acute ischemic insults.—B.L. Zaret, M.D.

Concordance and Discordance Between Stress-Redistribution-Reinjection and Rest-Redistribution Thallium Imaging for Assessing Viable Myocardium: Comparison With Metabolic Activity by Positron Emission Tomography

Dilsizian V, Perrone-Filardi P, Arrighi JA, Bacharach SL, Quyyumi AA, Freedman NMT, Bonow RO (Natl Heart, Lung, and Blood Inst, Bethesda, Md; Natl Insts of Health, Bethesda, Md)
Circulation 88:941–952, 1993   1 24-95-10–12

Background.—Impaired left ventricular function at rest is potentially reversible in many patients with chronic coronary artery disease. Such impaired function may improve or normalize after myocardial revascularization. Although it may be more reasonable to perform thallium scintigraphy at rest than during stress to determine whether a region is viable, the finding of exercise-induced ischemia provides valuable diagnostic and prognostic information. Whether stress-redistribution-reinjection imaging provides the same information for identifying viable myocardium as rest-redistribution imaging was studied.

Methods.—Forty-one patients, aged 38 to 76 years, with chronic stable coronary artery disease were included in the study; 38 were men. Stress-redistribution-reinjection and rest-redistribution thallium SPECT imaging was performed with quantitative analysis of regional thallium activity. Thallium reinjection was done just after the 3- to 4-hour redistribution images were obtained. Twenty patients also had PET at rest with [^{18}F]fluorodeoxyglucose and [^{15}O]water.

Findings.—Fifty-nine percent of the 155 myocardial regions with perfusion defects on the stress images were irreversible on conventional 3- to 4-hour redistribution images. Reinjection and rest-redistribution data on myocardial viability were concordant in 79% of the irreversible defects. In the patients undergoing PET imaging, stress-redistribution-reinjection and rest-redistribution imaging data were concordant on myocardial viability in 72% of 594 myocardial regions and discordant in the remainder. When irreversible thallium defects were analyzed according to the severity of the thallium defect in the discordant regions, 89% showed only mild-to-moderate decreases in thallium activity. In addition, PET imaging verified that 98% of these areas were metabolically active and viable. When the severity of thallium activity in irreversible thallium defects was considered, the concordance between stress-redistribution-reinjection and rest-redistribution imaging increased to 94% for myocardial viability.

Conclusion.—Either stress-redistribution-reinjection or rest-redistribution imaging may be used to identify viable myocardium. When stress testing is not contraindicated, stress-redistribution-reinjection imaging can be performed to obtain a more comprehensive picture of the severity and extent of coronary artery disease. Both regional myocardial ischemia and data on myocardial viability can be provided by this modality.

▶ The results are somewhat intuitive, and they corroborate what I suspect has been clinical practice for some time, namely, when dealing with issues of viability and ischemia, a stress study should be done. When the primary clinical question involves viability alone, such as in the heart failure patient, then a rest-redistribution study would be most appropriate.—B.L. Zaret, M.D.

Thallium Reinjection Demonstrates Viable Myocardium in Regions With Reverse Redistribution
Marin-Neto JA, Dilsizian V, Arrighi JA, Freedman NMT, Perrone-Filardi P, Bacharach SL, Bonow RO (Natl Heart, Lung, and Blood Inst, Bethesda, Md; Natl Inst of Health, Bethesda, Md)
Circulation 88:1736–1745, 1993   124-95-10–13

Background.—Reverse redistribution is the worsening of a perfusion defect during the redistribution phase of conventional thallium-201 scintigraphy. It can take the form of a defect worsening that is apparent on the poststress images or the appearance of a new defect on the redistribution images. In patients with chronic coronary artery disease, the clinical significance and pathophysiologic mechanisms of reverse redistribution on stress-redistribution scintigraphy are not understood.

Methods.—Thirty-nine patients with chronic stable coronary artery disease were studied to determine whether thallium reinjection distinguishes viable from nonviable myocardium in areas with reverse redistribution. All patients had reverse redistribution on standard exercise-redistribution thallium SPECT. Reverse redistribution was defined as a reduction of 10% or more in relative thallium-201 activity between stress and redistribution images. Thallium reinjection was done immediately after the 3- to 4-hour redistribution examination.

Findings.—Thirty-two of 39 regions with reverse redistribution, or 82%, showed increased thallium-201 activity after reinjection. The scintigraphic defect persisted after reinjection in the remaining areas. Abnormal Q waves were observed in 25% of the areas with increased thallium-201 uptake after reinjection compared with 71% of the areas that did not respond to reinjection. Nine percent of the areas with enhanced thallium-201 uptake after reinjection showed akinetic or dyskinetic wall motion compared with 71% of those that did not respond to reinjection. Critically stenosed or totally occluded coronary arteries supplied 83% of the areas with increased thallium-201 uptake after reinjection and only 28% of the regions that did not respond to reinjection. Collateral circulation was seen in 79% of the areas with a positive reinjection effect and in only 1 of the 7 other areas.

Conclusion.—Most of the myocardial regions that manifest reverse redistribution have substantial uptake of thallium with reinjection of the tracer at rest. This uptake appears to represent viable myocardium. Thallium reinjection may be a useful method for distinguishing viable from nonviable myocardium in areas with reverse redistribution.

▶ The phenomenon of reverse redistribution continues to be somewhat puzzling. Previous clinical data have indicated that this phenomenon is generally associated with earlier infarction and a patent infarct artery. It has also been associated with a poor clinical outcome. This study demonstrates that reverse redistribution is generally associated with myocardial viability. Such data appropriately lead to a more aggresssive clinical approach in these patients.—B.L. Zaret, M.D.

Impact of Antianginal Medications, Peak Heart Rate and Stress Level on the Prognostic Value of a Normal Exercise Myocardial Perfusion Imaging Study

Brown KA, Rowen M (Univ of Vermont, Burlington)
J Nucl Med 34:1467–1471, 1993   124-95-10–14

Background.—A normal exercise thallium-201 (^{201}Tl) study may underestimate the extent of coronary artery disease and cardiac risk if the patient is taking antianginal medication or achieves only low-level exercise. The impact of antianginal medication and level of stress achieved was assessed with regard to the prognostic value of a normal exercise ^{201}Tl study.

Methods.—Among 261 patients with a normal exercise ^{201}Tl study, 128 were taking antianginal medications. All were followed for a mean of 23 months.

Results.—During exercise, the peak heart rate was 82–217 beats/min; the percentage maximal predicted heart rate was 42% to 136%; the maximal Bruce stage achieved was 0–7. The annual cardiac event rate during follow-up was 1.2%; 3 patients experienced cardiac death and 3 had nonfatal myocardial infarction. The development of a cardiac event did not correlate significantly with use of antianginal medication during the stress test; the frequency of cardiac events was comparable for patients who took antianginal medications and those who did not. The cardiac event rate did not correlate with any measured index of exercise stress, including Bruce stage, peak heart rate, blood pressure, or percentage maximal predicted heart rate achieved. Fourteen patients required revascularization for recurrent chest pain, for a 2.8% annual revascularization event rate. The coronary revascularization rate was higher among patients who took antianginal medications at the stress test and those who did not reach the 85% maximal predicted heart rate.

Conclusion.—The risk of cardiac death or nonfatal myocardial infarction is very low in patients with a normal exercise ^{201}Tl study; concurrent antianginal medication or the level of stress achieved does not affect risk. However, a normal study that is performed while taking multiple antianginal medications or without achieving adequate stress may underestimate the eventual need for revascularization.

▶ This is an important observation. Individuals with negative tests on perfusion scintigraphy clearly have a low cardiac event rate. However, the impact of concomitant therapy has not heretofore been evaluated. This study demonstrates that such therapy does not have a substantial impact on risk stratification in the presence of a normal perfusion study. Such results should provide confidence for the individual who is using these studies for appropriate risk stratification.—B.L. Zaret, M.D.

Myocardial Ischemia Detected by Thallium Scintigraphy Is Frequently Related to Cardiac Arrest and Syncope in Young Patients With Hypertrophic Cardiomyopathy
Dilsizian V, Bonow RO, Epstein SE, Fananapazir L (Natl Heart, Lung, and Blood Inst, Bethesda, Md; Natl Insts of Health, Bethesda, Md)
J Am Coll Cardiol 22:796–804, 1993   124-95-10–15

Introduction.—Patients with hypertrophic cardiomyopathy are at risk of sudden cardiac death and syncope. Among adults, most of these events result from ventricular arrhythmias; the causative mechanism in young patients remains unknown. Myocardial ischemia was studied as a possible mechanism of cardiac arrest and syncope in children and young adults with hypertrophic cardiomyopathy.

Methods.—Twenty-three patients—14 males and 9 females, aged 6–23 years—were studied. Eight had a previous cardiac arrest, 7 had syncope, and 8 had a family history of sudden cardiac death. In addition to history, physical examination, and chest radiography, the patients underwent 24- to 72-hour ECG monitoring to assess the prevalence of spontaneous ambulatory ventricular tachycardia, exercise thallium scintigraphy to assess exercise-induced myocardial ischemia, and electrophysiologic studies to evaluate the inducibility of tachycardia.

Results.—Of the 15 patients with a history of cardiac arrest or syncope, only 3 had ventricular tachycardia on ambulatory ECG monitoring. Inducible ischemia was noted on thallium scintigraphy in all these patients compared with only 3 of 8 patients with no such history. Ventricular tachycardia was inducible in only 27% of the patients with a history of cardiac arrest or syncope—who were treated with an implantable defibrillator, if possible—and in none of the rest. Patients with evidence of ischemia were treated with verapamil with or without β-adrenergic blocking drugs. Of 15 treated patients who had a history of cardiac arrest or syncope, only 4 had further such episodes. All but 1 of these events were related to discontinuation of verapamil. An exercise thallium study was repeated in 8 patients while they were receiving anti-ischemic therapy: 7 showed improvement of regional thallium uptake, and 3 had normal studies.

Conclusion.—Episodes of sudden cardiac arrest in young patients with hypertrophic cardiomyopathy often appear to be related to ischemia. This is in contrast to the situation in adults, in whom these events are most often related to a primary arrhythmogenic substrate. For children and young adults, treatment with verapamil and β-blockers may improve symptoms and reduce the chances of future episodes of cardiac arrest.

▶ This study indicates how perfusion scintigraphy could be used in the clinical evaluation of patients with hypertrophic cardiomyopathy. Clearly, although this technique is not a primary assessment modality for this condition, it can provide highly relevant clinical data concerning risk stratification of patients with hypertrophic cardiomyopathy who are at increased risk of sudden death.—B.L. Zaret, M.D.

Diagnostic Value of ^{123}I-Phenylpentadecanoic Acid (IPPA) Metabolic and Thallium 201 Perfusion Imaging in Stable Coronary Artery Disease
Walamies M, Turjanmaa V, Koskinen M, Uusitalo A (Tampere Univ, Finland)
Eur Heart J 14:1079–1087, 1993   124-95-10–16

Background.—Gamma camera imaging of cardiac diseases with iodine-123 phenylpentadecanoic acid (IPPA) is an interesting modality in nuclear medicine. Despite several sophisticated studies, the clinical usefulness of IPPA imaging is still only promising. The diagnostic value of this modality compared with conventional thallium-201 nuclear perfusion imaging under similar conditions was studied.

Methods.—Twenty-nine patients with angiographically confirmed coronary artery disease (CAD) using SPECT were investigated. A symptom-limited exercise test was done first with IPPA and 2 days later with thallium. Fourteen healthy controls also underwent IPPA, and 15 underwent thallium testing.

Findings.—Data acquisition and output for the 2 modalities were similar. Semiquantitative interpretations were more accurate than visual readings. The best compromise of accuracy with the scored criteria was obtained with IPPA polar tomograms, which had a sensitivity and specificity of 86% each, and thallium, which had a sensitivity of 86% and a specificity of 80%. The sensitivity and specificity of IPPA with visual interpretation alone were 83% and 71%, respectively, compared with 72% sensitivity and 73% specificity with thallium. Exercise ECG alone had a sensitivity of 62%.

Conclusion.—Metabolic imaging with IPPA may be a rational, uncomplicated clinical technique for noninvasively diagnosing CAD. Its diagnostic ability is at least as good as that of thallium. In addition, it is possible to use IPPA and thallium testing in succession.

▶ The use of metabolic imaging with fatty acids during stress either as a complement or alternative to thallium or other perfusion imaging remains an unanswered question. Clearly, it is still an experimental area. I think it is unlikely that fatty acid imaging will supplant perfusion imaging on a routine basis.—B.L. Zaret, M.D.

The Dobutamine Stress Test With Thallium-201 Single-Photon Emission Computed Tomography and Radionuclide Angiography: Postinfarction Study
Coma-Canella I, del Val Gómez Martínez M, Rodrigo F, Beiras JMC (La Paz Hosp, Madrid; Carlos III Hosp, Madrid)
J Am Coll Cardiol 22:399–406, 1993   124-95-10–17

Background.—Stress tests with dobutamine are being used increasingly to detect coronary artery disease. Although high doses of this drug have been assumed to induce the same changes in contractility as physical exercise, some investigators have suggested that ischemic myocardium can respond to dobutamine with increased contractility. Left ventricular wall motion changes were investigated during dobutamine-induced myocardial ischemia.

Methods.—Sixty-three patients who had had infarctions underwent dobutamine assessment twice 1 to 2 days apart. The patients also underwent thallium-201 SPECT and gated equilibrium radionuclide ventriculography at rest and with dobutamine. Sixty patients had coronary cineangiography within 1 week.

Findings.—Forty-five patients showed redistribution, and 22 had no change or a reduction in the global or regional ejection fraction. Overall, the global ejection fraction increased from 46% to 56%. The ejection fraction response to dobutamine in the 6 patients with triple-vessel disease was flat; the rest of the patients had an increase of 11%. The regional ejection fraction of the hypokinetic region increased from 27% to 41%, with no change or a reduction in 13 patients. The regional ejection fraction increase was significantly higher in the 44 patients with peri-infarct redistribution than in those without redistribution. An inverse linear correlation between the redistribution score and the dobutamine-induced regional ejection fraction change was noted in patients with peri-infarct redistribution.

Conclusion.—Mild-to-moderate redistribution in the peri-infarct region appears to respond to dobutamine with increased contractility, whereas severe redistribution responds with wall motion worsening. This can be demonstrated more easily in large infarcts that are less affected by the surrounding contractile myocardium. Further research is needed to assess the prognostic implications of dobutamine-induced peri-infarct redistribution and ejection fraction reduction.

▶ This study indicates that the dobutamine response after myocardial infarction may be quite complicated and does not necessarily result in a simple yes or no response. The contraction response is clearly dependent on the extent of viability and ischemia, as noted by the thallium study. This may provide important data for echographers who are using the dobutamine test on a routine basis.—B.L. Zaret, M.D.

Prognostic Value of Normal Technetium-99m-Sestamibi Cardiac Imaging
Brown KA, Altland E, Rowen M (Univ of Vermont, Burlington)
J Nucl Med 35:554–557, 1994   1-24-95-10–18

Introduction.—Myocardial perfusion imaging with technetium-99m (^{99m}Tc) sestamibi provides results that are superior in quality to thallium-201 (^{201}Tl) imaging. Patients with normal ^{201}Tl imaging have a low rate (less than 1% per year) of myocardial infarction and cardiac death. The prognostic implications of normal ^{99m}Tc-sestamibi cardiac imaging were examined.

Patients and Methods.—The study population consisted of 234 patients (127 men and 107 women; mean age, 55 years) with known or suspected coronary artery disease who were referred for myocardial perfusion imaging. The ^{99m}Tc-sestamibi protocols used were 1-day gated rest-stress planar dipyridamole in 112 patients and symptom-limited exercise in 122 patients. On quantitative analysis, all patients had normal perfusion and wall motion. Patients were followed for a mean of 10 months to determine the incidence of nonfatal myocardial infarction and cardiac death.

Results.—Fifty patients underwent cardiac catheterization before the myocardial perfusion imaging. All but 3 of these patients were found to have angiographically significant coronary disease. Depression of the ST segment or chest pain occurred in 7% and 26%, respectively, of the dipyridamole group and in 16% and 22% of the exercise group. Only 1 patient experienced a primary cardiac event during follow-up—a nonfatal myocardial infarction at 9 months. This patient had not undergone coronary angiography. Only 2 patients had recurrent chest pain that required coronary revascularization.

Discussion.—The recent introduction of ^{99m}Tc-sestamibi provides an alternative to ^{201}Tl myocardial perfusion imaging. Studies performed with ^{99m}Tc-sestamibi have greater count densities and improved imaging quality. The higher count rates allow image acquisition in a gated frame mode, providing analysis of regional and global ventricular function. Normal ^{99m}Tc-sestamibi cardiac imaging in conjunction with dipyridamole or symptom-limited exercise predicts a benign course, at least through an intermediate period of follow-up.

▶ These data are important and indicate that one can substitute a normal sestamibi study for a normal thallium study with respect to outcome analysis. The data here are quite consistent with the previous thallium literature related to the prognostic impact of a normal study.—B.L. Zaret, M.D.

Prognostic Value of Dipyridamole Technetium-99m Sestamibi Myocardial Tomography in Patients With Stable Chest Pain Who Are Unable to Exercise
Stratmann HG, Tamesis BR, Younis LT, Wittry MD, Miller DD (St Louis VA Med Ctr, Mo; St Louis Univ, Mo)
Am J Cardiol 73:647–652, 1994   124-95-10–19

Background.—The ability of technetium-99m sestamibi (MIBI) myocardial imaging to assess the risk of later cardiac events has not been established. The prognostic value of dipyridamole MIBI SPECT for assessing the risk of subsequent events in patients with stable chest pain who were unable to perform diagnostically useful exercise stress levels was evaluated.

Methods and Findings.—Five hundred thirty-four patients were included. During a mean follow-up of 13 months, 58 patients had a major cardiac event; 14 had a nonfatal myocardial infarction, and 44 died of cardiac causes. Univariate and multivariate predictors of increased cardiac risk were a history of congestive heart failure, previous myocardial infarction or diabetes mellitus, and reversible or fixed myocardial perfusion defect on MIBI scans. Cardiac events occurred in 2% of patients with normal MIBI scans, in 15% with abnormal scans, in 17% with reversible perfusion defects, and in 16% with fixed defects. The relative risks associated with an abnormal MIBI scan, a reversible perfusion defect, and a fixed defect were 8.4, 1.9, and 2.4, respectively. The cardiac event-free survival rate was significantly lower in patients with any kind of perfusion abnormality than in those with normal scans (Fig 10–3).

Conclusion.—As with thallium-201 myocardial scintigraphy, a normal MIBI scan is associated with low cardiac risk. Patients with dipyridamole-induced myocardial perfusion defects have a significantly increased risk.

▶ This nice study indicates the prognostic value of dipyridamole sestamibi SPECT in patients who are unable to exercise. It defines both the excellent outcome in those with a negative test and the prognostic value in those with a positive test with respect to future cardiac events.—B.L. Zaret, M.D.

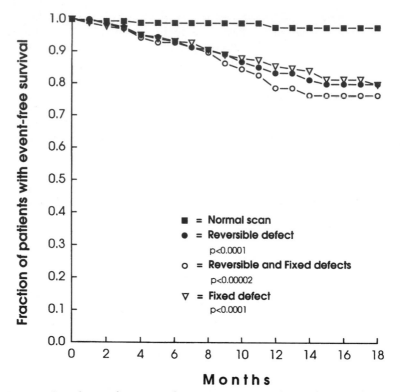

Fig 10–3.—Survival curves for major cardiac events in patients with normal scans and those with specific kinds of perfusion defects. Patients with a reversible defect or a fixed defect, or both, had a significantly decreased event-free survival compared with those with normal scans (all P < .0001). (Courtesy of Stratmann HG, Tamesis BR, Younis LT, et al: *Am J Cardiol* 73:647–652, 1994.)

Exercise Technetium-99m Sestamibi Tomography for Cardiac Risk Stratification of Patients With Stable Chest Pain

Stratmann HG, Williams GA, Wittry MD, Chaitman BR, Miller DD (St Louis VA Med Ctr, Mo; St Louis Univ, Mo)
Circulation 89:615–622, 1994   124-95-10–20

Background.—Exercise stress thallium-201 myocardial imaging provides prognostic information in subsets of patients with coronary artery disease, including those with stable chest pain. However, the prognostic value of symptom-limited maximal exercise treadmill testing with tomographic technetium-99m sestamibi (MIBI) has not yet been determined. This method was used in patients who were referred for evaluation of stable angina to determine its prognostic efficacy.

Patients and Methods.—A total of 548 consecutive patients with stable angina pectoris underwent maximal exercise treadmill stress testing in conjunction with a same-day rest-stress tomographic technetium-99m

MIBI myocardial imaging protocol. Of these, 521 were followed for 13 ± 5 months to determine the univariate and multivariate variables associated with cardiac events and to identify cardiac event-free survival.

Results.—Ten patients were lost to follow-up. In addition, 17 who underwent coronary revascularization within 6 months of testing were excluded. Twenty-four patients experienced major cardiac events, 11 of which were nonfatal myocardial infarctions; the remaining 13 resulted in cardiac death. Significant relative risk and confidence intervals were noted for exercise ST-segment depression, abnormalities on MIBI scan, and a reversible MIBI perfusion defect, as determined by univariate Cox survival analysis. Exercise MIBI perfusion abnormalities and reversible MIBI perfusion defects had an independent predictive value, as demonstrated by multivariate models. Cardiac events occurred in only .5% of patients with normal MIBI scan findings during 1 year of follow-up compared with 7% of those with abnormalities on scans. In patients with reversible MIBI perfusion defects or fixed defects and those with combined reversible and fixed MIBI myocardial perfusion abnormalities, the 12-month cardiac event-free survival was 92%, 96%, and 93%, respectively.

Conclusion.—Exercise stress technetium-99m MIBI myocardial tomography yields significant independent information concerning the subsequent risk of serious cardiac events in patients with stable angina pectoris.

▶ This study is an accompaniment to the preceding paper from the same group (Abstract 124-95-10–19). In this instance, the authors deal with exercise perfusion studies. Again, excellent prognostic data are contained in the perfusion studies. These data point out the continued evidence of the functional value of nuclear cardiology studies for assessing cardiac patients.—B.L. Zaret, M.D.

Gated Technetium-99m Sestamibi for Simultaneous Assessment of Stress Myocardial Perfusion, Postexercise Regional Ventricular Function and Myocardial Viability: Correlation With Echocardiography and Rest Thallium-201 Scintigraphy
Chua T, Kiat H, Germano G, Maurer G, van Train K, Friedman J, Berman D
(Cedars-Sinai Med Ctr, Los Angeles; Univ of California, Los Angeles)
J Am Coll Cardiol 23:1107–1114, 1994   124-95-10–21

Objective.—Assessment of wall motion and thickening was validated by gated SPECT acquisition of stress-injected sestamibi by comparison with echocardiographic assessment. The hypothesis that the combination of stress sestamibi perfusion and rest function with gated SPECT would allow assessment of perfusion defect reversibility with a single injection of the imaging agent was also tested.

Patients and Methods.—The study population included 58 patients who were referred for myocardial perfusion imaging. Twenty-six had historical or ECG evidence of previous myocardial infarction, and 32 had no such evidence. Sixteen patients had previous coronary artery bypass surgery. All underwent rest thallium-201 SPECT, followed by stress sestamibi-gated SPECT. In 43 cases, electrocardiography was performed immediately before or after gated SPECT. Semiquantitative visual scoring was used to analyze all studies.

Results.—Gated SPECT and echocardiography demonstrated a high segmental score agreement for wall motion (91%) and thickening (90%). There was excellent correlation for global wall motion (r = .98) and thickening (r = .96) scores between the 2 modalities. Although there was a high level of agreement (98%) for reversibility between stress sestimibi-gated SPECT and rest thallium-201/stress sestamibi in patients without previous myocardial infarction, discordance between the 2 approaches was frequent in patients with previous infarctions. Twenty of 78 nonreversible defects by stress sestamibi-gated SPECT were reversible by rest thallium-201/stress sestamibi; 23 of 112 reversible defects by the former modality were nonreversible by the latter.

Conclusion.—Visual assessment of global and regional left ventricular function by gated stress-injected sestamibi SPECT correlated well with echocardiography, a widely accepted means of evaluating regional function. Overall, in segments with severe perfusion defects, the agreement between these 2 modalities was 77% for both wall motion and thickening. Because discrepancies with an accepted standard of viability were common, SPECT cannot substitute for rest perfusion studies in patients with previous myocardial infarction.

▶ A major virtue of sestamibi imaging involves its ability to look at both global function with a first-pass ejection fraction measurement and regional function with ECG-gated studies. This is one of the first studies to systematically evaluate the gated technique against the standard of rest perfusion imaging and echocardiography. Clearly, the overall sestamibi study can allow one to come close to the "one-stop shop," involving definition of global and regional ventricular function and myocardial perfusion from a single study.—B.L. Zaret, M.D.

Multicenter Trial Validation for Quantitative Analysis of Same-Day Rest-Stress Technetium-99m-Sestamibi Myocardial Tomograms

Van Train KF, Garcia EV, Maddahi J, Areeda J, Cooke CD, Kiat H, Silagan G, Folks R, Friedman J, Matzer L, Germano G, Bateman T, Ziffer J, DePuey EG, Fink-Bennett D, Cloninger K, Berman DS (Cedars-Sinai Med Ctr, Los Angeles; Univ of California, Los Angeles; Emory Univ, Atlanta, Ga; et al)
J Nucl Med 35:609–618, 1994
124-95-10–22

Introduction.—Technetium-99m (^{99m}Tc) sestamibi, a myocardial perfusion imaging agent that was introduced clinically in 1992, is increasingly being used to evaluate patients with suspected coronary artery disease (CAD). The accuracy of an automated quantitative analysis of same-day rest-stress ^{99m}Tc-sestamibi SPECT images for detection and localization of CAD was assessed.

Patients and Methods.—In a multicenter trial, 161 patients underwent same-day rest-stress ^{99m}Tc-sestamibi SPECT imaging. Thirty-seven consecutive patients were considered normal by having a less than 5% likelihood of CAD. The remaining patients underwent coronary angiography and were found to have less than 50% luminal diameter narrowing (22 patients) or 50% or more coronary luminal diameter narrowing (102 patients) involving 1–3 coronary arteries. An additional group of patients with single-vessel disease was evaluated to determine the optimal criteria for detection of CAD. The objective quantitative analysis method uses gender-specific normal limits.

Results.—The quantitative analysis method had an overall sensitivity of 87% and a specificity of 36%. Its normalcy rate, a true negative rate in low-likelihood patients, was 81%. Some of the 7 participating hospitals used Siemens and others used General Electric camera/computer equipment, but these differences did not significantly affect results. Sensitivity for overall detection of disease was similar in patients with (90%) and without (89%) myocardial infarction. For the identification of disease in individual coronary arteries, the sensitivities and specificities were 69% and 76% for the left anterior descending, 70% and 80% for left circumflex, and 77% and 85% for right coronary artery, respectively.

Conclusion.—This quantitative method offers an objective assessment of a patient's myocardial perfusion based on normal male and female myocardial distribution data bases. A same-day rest-stress imaging protocol can be completed in 5–6 hours, a total time that might be reduced to 2 hours by increasing the stress dose. In addition to its accuracy relative to coronary angiography, the program also correlates well with expert visual interpretation.

▶ This nice multicenter study addresses the issue of quantitative analysis of same-day sestamibi studies. It will be critical for studies to be performed on the same day if an appropriate throughput is to be developed in busy laboratories. Clearly, the use of quantitative data is the future of nuclear techniques.—B.L. Zaret, M.D.

Prevalence of Right Ventricular Perfusion Defects After Inferior Myocardial Infarction Assessed by Low-Level Exercise With Technetium 99m Sestamibi Tomographic Myocardial Imaging

Travin MI, Malkin RD, Garber CE, Messinger DE, Cloutier DJ, Heller GV (Mem Hosp of Rhode Island, Pawtucket; Roger Williams Gen Hosp, Providence, RI; Brown Univ, Providence, RI)

Am Heart J 127:797–804, 1994   124-95-10–23

Introduction.—Right ventricular involvement in patients with inferior wall myocardial infarction is associated with an increase in acute and chronic morbidity. Identification of right ventricular perfusion abnormalities is important in such patients; however, imaging of this chamber with thallium-201 has been difficult. The ability of technetium-99m (^{99m}Tc) sestamibi to evaluate right ventricular perfusion and to determine the prevalence of right ventricular perfusion defects after a recent inferior wall myocardial infarction was assessed.

Patients and Methods.—Thirty-three patients who met study criteria were compared with 22 controls. Patients were evaluated 6 to 14 days after infarction with low-level exercise testing and ^{99m}Tc-sestamibi SPECT myocardial imaging. Controls who had less than a 5% likelihood of coronary artery disease underwent exercise ^{99m}Tc-sestamibi imaging. The right ventricle was isolated by computer from reconstructed transverse cardiac slices for each image. Resultant images were reoriented into oblique slices. All right and left ventricular images from both patients and controls were read visually without knowledge of clinical data. In addition, a quantitative method of defect detection was applied to the right ventricle.

Results.—Stress imaging with ^{99m}Tc-sestamibi provided satisfactory assessment of 98% of the right ventricular images. Ten (30%) of the patients with recent inferior infarction had right ventricular perfusion defects involving at least the inferior segment of the right ventricle. Patients with defects did not differ from those without defects with respect to age, peak creatine kinase value, incidence of Q-wave infarctions, use of thrombolytic therapy, previous myocardial infarction, or incidence of hypotension with clear lungs at admission. Twenty-eight (89%) patients had left ventricular perfusion defects, including all 10 with a right ventricular defect.

Conclusion.—Although poor visualization of the right ventricle with thallium-201 imaging has limited routine assessment of right ventricular perfusion defects, such defects can be adequately evaluated by means of ^{99m}Tc-sestamibi SPECT myocardial perfusion imaging. Defects of the right ventricle often occur after inferior myocardial infarction and are closely associated with left ventricular inferoseptal defects.

▶ The evaluation of right ventricular perfusion with sestamibi has been of interest for a number of years. The first major study that investigated it was by DePuey and associates (1). This technique may be useful in evaluating a variety of patients with right coronary artery disease as well as those with inferior-wall myocardial infarction.—B.L. Zaret, M.D.

Reference

1. DePuey EG, et al: *J Nucl Med* 32:1199, 1991.

Quantitative Same-Day Rest-Stress Technetium-99m-Sestamibi SPECT: Definition and Validation of Stress Normal Limits and Criteria for Abnormality
Van Train KF, Areeda J, Garcia EV, Cooke CD, Maddahi J, Kiat H, Germano G, Silagan G, Folks R, Berman DS (Cedars-Sinai Med Ctr, Los Angeles; Univ of California, Los Angeles; Emory Univ, Atlanta, Ga)
J Nucl Med 34:1494–1502, 1993   124-95-10–24

Background.—The physical and biological characteristics of technetium-99m (^{99m}Tc) sestamibi are such that customized data acquisition and image-processing protocols are needed to take full advantage of it. Initial research geared toward protocol optimization of ^{99m}Tc-sestamibi myocardial SPECT studies has been previously reported. Rest-stress ^{99m}Tc-sestamibi studies from 160 patients were used to develop gender-matched stress normal limits and abnormality criteria for quantitative analysis of rest-stress ^{99m}Tc-sestamibi SPECT.

Methods.—The study patients underwent ^{99m}Tc-sestamibi same-day myocardial perfusion imaging using previously reported optimized acquisition, processing, and quantitative protocols. Data from 35 men and 25 women with less than a 5% likelihood of coronary artery disease were used to compute the gender-matched mean and standard deviation of normal. The criteria for detection of abnormalities were determined by receiver-operating curve analysis, with expert visual interpretation as the gold standard. These criteria were developed in a pilot sample of 35 men and 25 women with a variety of perfusion defects, calculated in terms of the standard deviations from mean and minimum defect size in the 4 major zones of the polar map.

Results.—On comparison of the quantitative measurements with visual analysis for the various segments in the combined male and female pilot samples, optimum standard deviations yielded true positive and true negative rates of 84% and 86%, respectively, for the anterior segment; 70% and 75% for the septal segment; 86% and 76% for the lateral segment; and 69% and 76% for the inferior segment. These criteria were prospectively applied to a sample of 33 men and 7 women. True positive and true negative rates for the overall perfusion abnormalities were 97% and 67%, respectively. Corresponding values were 94% and 73% for the left anterior descending vascular territory, 73% and 90% for the left circumflex territory, and 72% and 91% for the right coronary artery territory.

Conclusion.—Optimized ^{99m}Tc-sestamibi stress normal limits and criteria for abnormality on same-day myocardial perfusion SPECT images are reported. These criteria show good correlation with expert visual interpretation of stress myocardial perfusion defects in a small, prospective pilot population. A large, multicenter validation trial to determine the true accuracy of the criteria is being conducted.

▶ This paper forms the basis for the multicenter trial analysis described in Abstract 124-95-10–22. This technique has been used in multiple laboratories. It points out the need for specific normal gender-matched standard and the use of low-likelihood subjects for defining normal limits.—B.L. Zaret, M.D.

Normal Qualitative and Quantitative Tc-99m Sestamibi Myocardial SPECT: Spectrum of Intramyocardial Distribution During Exercise and at Rest

Lette J, Caron M, Cerino M, McNamara D, Metayer S, D'Aoust S, Eybalin M-C, Levesseur A, Grégoire J, Arsenault A (Maisonneuve Hosp, Montreal; Montreal Heart Inst)
Clin Nucl Med 19:336–343, 1994   124-95-10–25

Background.—Coronary stenoses are routinely investigated with exercise myocardial perfusion imaging with technetium-99m (^{99m}Tc) sestamibi. Ischemia is diagnosed in areas that show reduced tracer uptake during exercise compared with rest. The wide spectrum of normal findings on exercise and rest ^{99m}Tc-sestamibi SPECT assessments was explored.

Methods.—The ^{99m}Tc-sestamibi SPECT images of 42 healthy volunteers were reviewed for potential sources of misinterpretation. Qualitative and quantitative assessments were performed.

Findings.—The most common artifacts on myocardial tomographic slices were diaphragmatic attenuation and bowel interposition, which resulted in fixed or reversible perfusion defects in the inferior and posterior regions. Artifacts related to the presence and shift of hot spots were also common. Such shifts between exercise and rest usually produced pseudoreversible defects in the anterolateral and lateral walls. The quantified polar map display of the myocardium demonstrated a physiologic reduction in sestamibi activity in the basal anterolateral and basal posterolateral regions in men during exercise.

Conclusion.—Many normal variants may mimic coronary artery disease on tomographic sestamibi images. Before a region of reduced activity is reported as a fixed or reversible perfusion defect, the interpreter should make sure that it does not represent an artifact or normal variation in the intramyocardial distribution of sestamibi during exercise.

▶ This paper nicely points out a variety of artifacts associated with sestamibi SPECT imaging. Readers are referred to the original article for review of an interesting set of illustrations.—B.L. Zaret, M.D.

Myocardial Perfusion and Ventricular Function Measurements During Total Coronary Artery Occulusion in Humans: A Comparison With Rest and Exercise Radionuclide Studies
Borges-Neto S, Puma J, Jones RH, Sketch MH Jr, Stack R, Hanson MW, Coleman RE (Duke Univ, Durham, NC)
Circulation 89:278–284, 1994   124-95-10–26

Background.—The diagnostic and prognostic use of radionuclide studies for evaluation of coronary artery disease is based on the concept that the relative deficit of coronary blood flow—induced by exercise and recognized as increased demand—is related to the hazards of decreased or interrupted coronary blood flow. The effects on flow are recognized as a decreased supply associated with coronary stenosis or total occlusion. The magnitude of exercise-induced perfusion and functional abnormalities was compared with that from those induced by total occlusion in 20 patients who were referred for percutaneous transluminal coronary angioplasty (PTCA).

Methods.—The patients underwent a same-day rest-exercise technetium-99m (^{99m}Tc) sestamibi study on the day before PTCA, which was performed regardless of the study results. During the PTCA procedure, 1 minute after the balloon was inflated to totally occlude the vessel, ^{99m}Tc-sestamibi was injected for a first-pass study. One hour after PTCA, tomographic perfusion studies were performed in the nuclear medicine laboratory. The extent of the perfusion and function abnormalities was estimated.

Results.—The mean size of the perfusion defect was 28% during occlusion compared with 13% during exercise. By contrast, the ejection fraction was greater during exercise than during occlusion, 53% vs. 41%. The overall exercise perfusion and functional measurements were not good predictors of the measurements obtained during occlusion. There was also no correlation between the severity of stenosis and functional abnormality, because many of the patients had multivessel disease and/ or a previous myocardial infarction.

Conclusion.—On radionuclide study, the physiologic abnormalities induced by sudden coronary occlusion exceed those induced by exercise, suggesting that stress-induced ischemia does not necessarily reflect the total potential myocardial area endangered by stenotic lesions that become suddenly occluded. A larger and more heterogenous group of patients should be studied to define the relationship between exercise-induced ischemia and interruption of coronary blood flow.

▶ It has long been known that the period of balloon inflation during coronary angioplasty provides a model of acute coronary occlusion. This has been used in a variety of previous studies to demonstrate the effects on ventricular function associated with acute occlusion.

This study very nicely points out differences in the total ischemic risk area that is defined with injection of sestamibi during balloon occlusion in comparison to findings after exercise. Clearly, exercise defects do not represent the total ischemic risk. Further studies in this area would be of interest.—B.L. Zaret, M.D.

Validation of Global and Segmental Left Ventricular Contractile Function Using Gated Planar Technetium-99m Sestamibi Myocardial Perfusion Imaging
Tischler MD, Niggel JB, Battle RW, Fairbank JT, Brown KA (Univ of Vermont, Burlington)
J Am Coll Cardiol 23:141–145, 1994   124-95-10–27

Background.—Technetium-99m sestamibi is a new and recently approved radiopharmaceutical used for myocardial perfusion imaging. Benefits derived from using this agent include a dosimetry that allows use of a dose 10–15 times greater than that of thallium-201. As such, myocardial counts are notably improved. In addition, images can be collected in a gated mode to potentially permit evaluation of global and segmental ventricular function. The reproducibility and accuracy of technetium-99m sestamibi for measurement of global and segmental left ventricular function were studied and the findings were compared with those of a standard technique, such as echocardiography.

Methods.—One hundred thirty-six patients were referred for clinical technetium-99m sestamibi imaging. One-day rest-stress planar technetium-99m sestamibi protocols were used, and stress images were gated. All patients underwent standard rest 2-dimensional echocardiography after technetium-99m sestamibi imaging was performed. A 4-point grading system was used to qualitatively grade global and segmental technetium-99m sestamibi and echocardiographic left ventricular contraction.

Results.—Extremely high interobserver and intraobserver agreement was noted for global and segmental technetium-99m sestamibi wall-motion analysis. Absolute agreements ranged from .92 to 1, with corresponding kappa values of .74 to 1. Similarly high agreement was noted for global and segmental echocardiographic wall motion, with absolute agreements ranging from .93 to 1 and corresponding kappa values of .75 to 1.

Conclusion.—Information concerning rest global and segmental left ventricular systolic function from gated technetium-99m sestamibi cardiac imaging is highly reproducible. In addition, findings obtained when using this method agree very well with those of 2-dimensional echocardiography.

▶ As in previous reviews, sestamibi imaging offers the possibility of the 1-stop shop. These data further support that view.—B.L. Zaret, M.D.

Impact of Regional Ventricular Function, Geometry, and Dobutamine Stress on Quantitative ^{99m}Tc-Sestamibi Defect Size

Sinusas AJ, Shi QX, Vitols PJ, Fetterman RC, Maniawski P, Zaret BL, Wackers FJTh (Yale Univ, New Haven, Conn)
Circulation 88:2224–2234, 1993   124-95-10–28

Introduction.—Initial clinical studies using serial myocardial perfusion imaging with technetium-99m sestamibi (^{99m}Tc-MIBI) suggest that defect size, although unchanged in the presence of an occluded artery, decreases after successful coronary reperfusion. This finding has been inferred to reflect myocardial salvage. However, perhaps the changes in defect size result in part from artifacts caused by changes in regional and global ventricular geometry. Serial ^{99m}Tc-MIBI myocardial perfusion imaging studies were performed in dog models of myocardial stunning and infarction to address this possibility.

Methods.—Twenty-five dogs were thoracotomized, then subjected to left anterior descending artery occlusion, for 15 minutes in group 1 and for 3 hours in group 2, followed by 3 hours of reperfusion. Injection of ^{99m}Tc-MIBI, before occlusion in group 1A and during occlusion in groups 1B and 2, was followed by serial ECG-gated planar imaging. In groups 1B and 2, reperfusion was followed by dobutamine infusion to produce a transient alteration of left ventricular size and function. Serial circumferential profile analyses of end-systolic (ES), end-diastolic (ED), and summed images were used to measure the magnitude (DM) and extent (DE) of perfusion defects. Flow assessments performed with radiolabeled microspheres were correlated with myocardial activity, as shown by the ^{99m}Tc-MIBI images. Myocardial thickening in the area at risk was evaluated using sonomicrometers.

Results.—Large artifactual ^{99m}Tc-MIBI defects produced by ischemic dyskinesis were seen by ES images in group 1A dogs, but were significantly smaller on ED images. An inverse correlation of DM and DE with myocardial thickening was noted on ES and summed images, but not in ED images. An index of defect reduction was derived from summed images that correlated well with thickening fraction in stunned animals, i.e., group 1B, but not in infarcted animals, i.e., group 2, subjected to dobutamine stress.

Conclusion.—In serial ^{99m}Tc-MIBI myocardial perfusion imaging, alterations in left ventricular geometry may affect left ventricular geometry. Analysis of risk and myocardial salvage may be confounded by regional functional changes, which may also affect defect size under dobutamine stress. One potentially useful means of differentiating viable and nonviable myocardium may be dobutamine ^{99m}Tc-MIBI imaging.

▶ The possibility that changes in ventricular geometry may impact on perfusion images has been noted since 1979 (1). Those initial data were obtained with thallium imaging. This study defines this issue for sestamibi imaging. In this experimental model, substantial changes could be induced by altered geometry. This may certainly affect defect size during stress circumstances and may be a significant mechanism with respect to the development of perfusion defects with ischemia and infarction.—B.L. Zaret, M.D.

Reference

1. Gewirtz H, et al: *Circulation* 59:1172, 1979.

---

^{99m}Tc-Sestamibi Uptake and Retention During Myocardial Ischemia and Reperfusion
Beller GA, Glover DK, Edwards NC, Ruiz M, Simanis JP, Watson DD (Univ of Virginia, Charlottesville)
Circulation 87:2033–2042, 1993   124-95-10–29

Background.—Myocardial perfusion imaging with technetium-labeled methoxyisobutyl isonitrile (sestamibi) is a noninvasive means of detecting salvaged myocardium after reperfusion of the coronary vessels in patients with acute myocardial infarction. When the nuclide is given during coronary occlusion, myocardial uptake correlates with blood flow and the area at risk. When it is given 90 minutes or longer after reperfusion, the pattern of activity reflects mainly myocardial viability.

Objective and Methods.—Studies were done in dogs to confirm that the myocardial uptake and retention of sestamibi after myocardial infarction and reperfusion are in fact markers of tissue viability. Sestamibi was injected intravenously into anesthetized dogs 2–5 minutes after reperfusion, which itself followed 3 hours of occlusion of the left anterior descending artery. In addition, the nuclide was given intravenously under normal conditions and the vessel occluded for 3 hours, followed by reperfusion lasting 4 minutes, 30 minutes, or 3 hours. Regional flow was studied by the labeled microsphere technique.

Observations.—Endocardial nuclide activity was 74% of baseline in dogs that were killed 5 minutes after its administration and 31% of nonischemic activity in those that were killed in 3 hours. Regional blood flow was similar in the 2 groups. In animals that were preloaded with sestamibi at baseline, 3 hours of coronary occlusion followed by 3 hours of reperfusion reduced activity in the ischemic endocardium to 40% of the nonischemic level. Coronary sinus activity was increased throughout the period of reflow. Significantly less activity was lost from the myocardium in dogs that were killed 4 or 30 minutes after the start of reperfusion. The extent of the defect increased as reperfusion continued.

Recommendations.—The uptake and retention of technetium-99m sestamibi in the myocardium depend on tissue viability as well as regional myocardial blood flow. If the radiopharmaceutical is given shortly after the start of reperfusion and imaging is performed shortly afterward, the extent of myocardial salvage may be significantly overestimated. It would seem best to delay nuclide administration for at least 2–3 hours after patency is restored. If the nuclide is given sooner, imaging can be delayed for 2–3 hours.

▶ These data suggest that there may indeed be washout of sestamibi after reperfusion. Although this has not been observed to any great extent clinically, these data should be considered in developing infarct-imaging protocols.—B.L. Zaret, M.D.

Myocardial Viability in Patients With Chronic Coronary Artery Disease: Comparison of ^{99m}Tc-Sestamibi With Thallium Reinjection and [18 F]Fluordeoxyglucose
Dilsizian V, Arrighi JA, Diodati JG, Quyyumi AA, Alavi K, Bacharach SL, Marin-Neto JA, Katsiyiannis PT, Bonow RO (Natl Heart, Lung, and Blood Inst, Bethesda, Md; Natl Insts of Health, Bethesda, Md)
Circulation 89:578–587, 1994   124-95-10–30

Background.—When used for diagnostic purposes, technetium-99m (^{99m}Tc) sestamibi and thallium imaging are comparably accurate. However, because there is limited redistribution of sestamibi over time, it may overestimate nonviable myocardium in patients with left ventricular dysfunction whose blood flow may be decreased at rest. Myocardial viability was assessed in patients with chronic coronary artery disease to determine whether sestamibi imaging provides accurate information.

Methods and Findings.—Fifty-four patients with a mean ejection fraction of $34 \pm 14\%$ were investigated. Stress-redistribution-reinfection thallium tomography was performed in all patients. Same-day rest-stress sestamibi imaging using the same exercise protocol (with patients achieving the same exercise duration) was conducted within a mean of 5 days. The redistribution or reinfection studies showed 111 reversible thallium defects. Of these, 40 were determined to be irreversible on the rest-stress sestamibi study. Despite reinfection, only 3 of 63 irreversible thallium defects were classified as reversible by sestamibi imaging. With respect to reversibility of myocardial defects, the agreement between thallium stress-redistribution-reinjection and same-day rest-stress sestamibi imaging was 75%. Positron emission tomography studies were also performed in a subset of 25 patients, using oxygen-15–labeled water and [¹⁸F]fluorodeoxyglucose (FDG) at rest after an oral glucose load. Agreement between thallium and sestamibi imaging that pertained to defect reversibility was noted in 51 of 73 regions. Eighteen of the remaining 22 discordant regions appeared to be irreversible by sestamibi imaging, but they were reversible by thallium imaging. As determined by normal FDG uptake or FDG/blood flow mismatch on PET, myocardial viability was verified in 17 of 18 regions, which were present in 16 of the 25 patients. Methods to improve sestamibi imaging results were also explored. When further analyzing the 18 discordant regions with irreversible sestamibi defects according to severity, 14 showed a mild-to-moderate reduction in sestamibi activity only. This was indicative of predominantly viable myocardium, and the overall agreement between thallium and sestamibi studies increased to 93%. In addition, when another 4-hour redistribution image was obtained in 18 patients after the injection of sestamibi at rest, 6 of 16 discordant irreversible regions on the rest-stress sestamibi study became reversible. The agreement between thallium and sestamibi studies therefore increased to 82%.

Conclusion.—Compared with thallium redistribution-reinfection and PET, same-day rest-stress sestamibi imaging will incorrectly identify 36% of myocardial regions as irreversibly impaired and nonviable. However, the methods discussed for improving the detection of reversible and viable myocardium can greatly improve the results obtained with sestamibi imaging.

▶ The final word on sestamibi as a viability agent is not yet in. These data, which use PET FDG uptake as a gold standard, suggest that sestamibi may underestimate viability. A number of factors may have an impact on this result, including the site of the defect. It is recognized that inferior-posterior defects may actually be caused by diaphragmatic attenuation rather than true ischemia or scarring.—B.L. Zaret, M.D.

Positron Emission Tomography Detects Evidence of Viability in Rest Technetium-99m Sestamibi Defects

Sawada SG, Allman KC, Muzik O, Beanlands RSB, Wolfe ER Jr, Gross M, Fig L, Schwaiger M (Univ of Michigan, Ann Arbor; Veterans Affairs Med Ctr, Ann Arbor, Mich)
J Am Coll Cardiol 23:92–98, 1994   124-95-10–31

Background.—It has recently been reported that thallium-201 reinjection with rest technetium-99m sestamibi imaging may underestimate myocardial viability. The relative value of SPECT imaging at rest using technetium-99m sestamibi with PET was evaluated for its ability to detect viable myocardium.

Patients and Methods.—Rest technetium-99m sestamibi imaging and PET using fluorine-18 (¹⁸F) deoxyglucose and nitrogen-13 (¹³N) ammonia were performed in 20 patients with previous myocardial infarction. A circumferential profile analysis was used to identify technetium-99 sestamibi, ^{18}F-deoxyglucose, and ^{13}N-ammonia activity, which was expressed as the percentage of peak activity, in 9 cardiac segments and in the perfusion defect defined by the area that had technetium-99m sestamibi activity of less than 60%. Moderate technetium-99m sestamibi defects were defined as 50% to 59% of peak activity and severe defects as less than 50% of peak activity. Comparisons of perfusion defect size estimates were made between technetium-99m sestamibi and ^{13}N-ammonia studies.

Results.—Fluorine-18 deoxyglucose activity of 60% or greater, which was considered to be indicative of viability, was noted in 16 of 30 segments with moderate and 16 of 34 segments with severe defects. This viability was still present in 50% of segments with technetium-99m sestamibi activity of less than 40%. No significant difference in the mean technetium-99m sestamibi in viable and nonviable segments was noted. The area of the technetium-99m sestamibi defect was viable in 5 of 18 patients with adequate ^{18}F-deoxyglucose studies. In 16 patients, the perfusion defect size determined via technetium-99m sestamibi exceeded that determined by ^{13}N-ammonia. A significantly greater difference in defect size between technetium-99m sestamibi and ^{13}N-ammonia studies was observed in patients with viable vs. nonviable segments.

Conclusion.—Metabolic evidence of viability is frequently noted in moderate and severe rest technetium-99m sestamibi defects. When using identical threshold values, technetium-99m sestamibi SPECT yields larger perfusion defects than ^{13}N-ammonia PET.

▶ These results are somewhat similar to those described in the preceding review (Abstract 124-95-10–30). In addition, this study indicates a difference between perfusion defect size when sestamibi and ammonia are compared. Further studies are required in this area.—B.L. Zaret, M.D.

Use of Sequential Teboroxime Imaging for the Detection of Coronary Artery Occlusion and Reperfusion in Ischemic and Infarcted Myocardium
Heller LI, Villegas BJ, Weiner BH, McSherry BA, Dahlberg ST, Leppo JA (Univ of Massachusetts, Worcester)
Am Heart J 127:779–785, 1994   124-95-10–32

Background.—Intravenous thrombolytic treatment successfully reperfuses the infarct-related artery in only 50% to 80% of patients with myocardial infarction. A noninvasive method for serially assessing coronary perfusion could identify patients who might benefit from other interventions. Rapid sequential teboroxime imaging was evaluated to determine its value as a noninvasive marker of acute coronary reperfusion in a swine model.

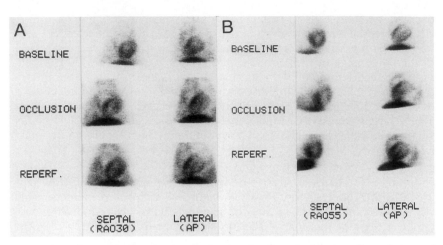

Fig 10–4.—Sequential teboroxime images of a pig at baseline, after left circumflex occlusion, and after reperfusion. **A,** this group A animal did not have a myocardial infarction. The defect is best seen in the septal view during occlusion, and the scan normalizes after reperfusion. **B,** this animal had a myocardial infarction proved by triphenyl tetrazolium chloride staining. The defect is seen in both the septal and lateral views during occlusion. The scans after reperfusion show resolution of the defect. (Courtesy of Heller LI, Villegas BJ, Weiner BH, et al: *Am Heart J* 127:779–785, 1994.)

Methods.—Nine Yorkshire pigs were subjected to coronary artery occlusion and 2 hours of reperfusion. The occlusion time was 15 minutes in 5 pigs (group A) and 1 hour in 4 pigs (group B). Images were acquired after teboroxime administration at baseline, occlusion, and reperfusion. Triphenyl tetrazolium chloride staining was used to determine the infarct size.

Findings.—The mean normalized regional myocardial blood flow, which was determined by radiolabeled microspheres, was .29 and .83 after occlusion and reperfusion, respectively. Significant differences were found between the normal scan ratios on baseline and occlusion scans of the defect, as well as between the occlusion and reperfusion scans (Fig 10-4).

Conclusion.—Rapid sequential teboroxime imaging can detect acute coronary occlusion and reperfusion to both ischemic and infarcted myocardium. Teboroxime may be an excellent tracer for assessing infarct artery patency early in patients who are receiving thrombolytic treatment.

▶ This study forms an experimental basis for sequential teboroxime imaging as it might be applied in the emergency department to detect early reperfusion. Because of the rapid washout of this radiopharmaceutical, sequential measurements can be made in a relatively short time. Because the uptake is primarily flow-related rather than the result of viability, this would appear to be a method of defining the efficacy of reperfusion therapy. Teboroxime could play a relevant and unique role within the radiopharmaceutical-imaging spectrum.—B.L. Zaret, M.D.

Sequential Teboroxime Imaging During and After Balloon Occlusion of a Coronary Artery

Heller LI, Villegas BJ, Weiner BH, McSherry BA, Dahlberg ST, Leppo JA (Univ of Massachusetts, Worcester)
J Am Coll Cardiol 21:1319–1327, 1993   124-95-10–33

Introduction.—Varying but significant proportions of patients who undergo IV thrombolytic treatment for myocardial infarction fail to have the infarct vessel effectively reperfused. A noninvasive means of serially assessing coronary perfusion to identify those patients who might benefit from emergency angioplasty, bypass surgery, or more intensive thrombolysis is needed. Teboroxime is the best available single-photon perfusion-imaging agent. Its short half-life in myocardium and its high initial energy level make rapid sequential imaging possible.

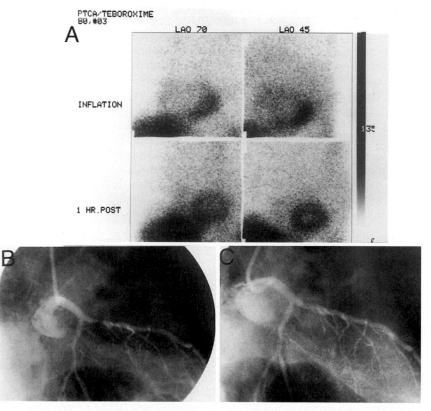

Fig 10–5.—*Abbreviations:* HR. hour; *LAO*, left anterior oblique projection; *POST*, after balloon inflation. **A,** defects are seen in segments 1, 2, 3, 6, 7, and 8. Defects normalize after reperfusion. **B,** before coronary angioplasty; **C,** after coronary angioplasty. (Courtesy of Heller LI, Villegas BJ, Weiner BH, et al: *J Am Coll Cardiol* 21:1319–1327, 1993.)

Methods.—Fifteen patients with stenosis of a single major epicardial coronary artery were studied in conjunction with elective percutaneous transluminal coronary angioplasty. Patients received aspirin, dipyridamole, a calcium channel blocker, and IV heparin before the stenosis was crossed with a guidewire and the vessel was dilated with a balloon catheter. A dose of 20 mCi of teboroxime was injected during the final balloon inflation, and data were recorded in the 45- and 70-degree left anterior oblique projections. The study was repeated after reperfusion was established. An intracoronary ECG was also obtained.

Results.—The number of defects on reperfusion scans was significantly lower than that on initial balloon occlusion scans. At the same time, the ratio of pixel counts in the defect area and normal zone increased significantly. All occlusions, except 1 of 4 involving the left circumflex artery, were correctly identified (Fig 10–5). Scans were totally accurate in distinguishing left anterior descending coronary artery occlusions from those in the left circumflex or right coronary artery; however, the intracoronary ECG was less informative.

Conclusion.—Sequential perfusion imaging with teboroxime reliably identifies the occluded coronary artery in patients with myocardial infarction who undergo balloon inflation in conjunction with thrombolytic treatment. A study comparing this technique with coronary angiography would be of interest.

▶ This article is a clinical extension of the preceding one (Abstract 1 24-95-10–32). Here, the angioplasty model in the cardiac catheterization laboratory was used to permit definition of rapidly changing image patterns after acute coronary occlusion (with the angioplasty balloon inflated) and reperfusion (with the angioplasty balloon deflated). This study provides a good basis for further evaluation of the acute reperfusion phenomenon.—B.L. Zaret, M.D.

Myocardial Single-Photon Emission Computed Tomographic Imaging With Technetium 99m Tetrofosmin: Stress-Rest Imaging With Same-Day and Separate-Day Rest Imaging
Sridhara B, Sochor H, Rigo P, Braat S, Itti R, Martinez-Duncker D, Cload P, Lahiri A (Northwick Park Hosp, Harrow, England; Univ Hosp, Vienna; Centre Hospitalier Universiat, Liege, Belgium; et al)
J Nucl Cardiol 1:138–143, 1994   1 24-95-10–34

Introduction.—The low-energy photons and long half-life (73 hours) of thallium-201 decrease the overall image resolution when this myocardial perfusion agent is used for detecting coronary artery disease. Various technetium-99m (^{99m}Tc) agents have been developed to improve image quality. The newly introduced ^{99m}Tc-tetrofosmin has a short half-life (6 hours) and good uptake by the myocardium, with a relatively slow clearance. Stress-rest SPECT imaging with ^{99m}Tc-tetrofosmin was compared with same-day and separate-day rest imaging to detect myocardial perfusion defects.

Patients and Methods.—Twenty-two patients with stable coronary heart disease were randomly selected. All had undergone planar thallium-201 imaging and coronary angiography. The mean age of those in the group was 62.3 years. Single-day (stress-rest) and separate-day rest ^{99m}Tc-tetrofosmin SPECT protocols were compared in the same patient. A blinded panel evaluated the images to identify myocardial infarction, ischemia, or normal scans.

Results.—Fifteen of the 22 patients had previous evidence of myocardial infarction. During exercise, angina was noted in 15 patients and ST-segment depression (greater than 1 mm) in 9. Nineteen patients were identified with stress perfusion defects by ^{99m}Tc-tetrofosmin imaging, yielding a sensitivity of 86% for both same-day stress-rest and separate-day rest protocols. For individual coronary stenosis with a lesion greater than 50%, the ^{99m}Tc-tetrofosmin SPECT protocols detected 80% of the left anterior descending arteries, 95% of the right coronary arteries, and 75% of the left circumflex coronary arteries.

Conclusion.—This preliminary study indicates that SPECT imaging with ^{99m}Tc-tetrofosmin provides excellent images and has good sensitivity for detecting coronary artery disease. Diagnostic sensitivities were similar for the same-day stress-rest and separate-day rest imaging protocols.

▶ This is a portion of phase II studies involving the new radiopharmaceutical, ^{99m}Tc-tetrofosmin. Good correlations are noted with thallium imaging. This radiopharmaceutical appears to have substantial promise.—B.L. Zaret, M.D.

Myocardial Tomography Using Technetium-99m-Tetrofosmin to Evaluate Coronary Artery Disease

Tamaki N, Takahashi N, Kawamoto M, Torizuka T, Tadamura E, Yonekura Y, Okuda K, Nohara R, Sasayama S, Konishi J (Kyoto Univ, Japan)
J Nucl Med 35:594–600, 1994   124-95-10–35

Introduction.—Several technetium-99m (^{99m}Tc)–labeled compounds have been developed to overcome the physical limitations of thallium-201 (^{201}Tl) imaging for the detection of coronary artery disease (CAD). One new agent, ^{99m}Tc-tetrofosmin, is easy to prepare and permits early imaging. Stress and rest myocardial perfusion images after the administration of ^{99m}Tc-tetrofosmin were compared with those stress and redistribution ^{201}Tl tomography, as well as with those of coronary arteriography.

Methods.—Twenty-five patients with suspected CAD who had undergone coronary arteriography were studied. Those in the group had a mean age of 62.2 years. Patients were studied with both stress tetrofosmin and ^{201}Tl tomography. The stress tetrofosmin perfusion study was performed within 2 weeks of the thallium study. A resting tetrofosmin study was scheduled for 24–72 hours after the stress imaging. All images were separately interpreted by 2 experienced observers.

Results.—The exercise duration was identical for tetrofosmin and thallium studies (8.4 minutes). Tetrofosmin images were superior in quality in all resting studies and in 17 of 25 stress studies. The overall sensitivities for detecting CAD were 95% for ^{201}Tl imaging and 100% for tetrofosmin imaging. The sensitivity and specificity for detecting stenosed vessels were similar for thallium (73% and 77%, respectively) and tetrofosmin (75% and 80%, respectively). Stress distribution tended to be slightly higher with tetrofosmin, indicating less defect contrast. Reversible perfusion abnormalities were observed to be similar between the 2 studies.

Conclusion.—Stress myocardial tomographic imaging with tetrofosmin is a sensitive method for detection of CAD and identification of stenosed coronary arteries. A high concordance rate of the perfusion score was achieved between tetrofosmin and thallium studies. The dose of tetrofosmin that can be administered is 10 times that of ^{201}Tl, resulting in higher-quality perfusion images and a more confident interpretation.

▶ This article represents the first description of tetrofosmin SPECT. As has been shown in other studies, if has substantial potential.—B.L. Zaret, M.D.

Technetium-99m-Tetrofosmin to Assess Myocardial Blood Flow: Experimental Validation in an Intact Canine Model of Ischemia

Sinusas AJ, Shi Q, Saltzberg MT, Vitols P, Jain D, Wackers FJT, Zaret BL (Yale Univ, New Haven, Conn)
J Nucl Med 35:664–671, 1994   124-95-10–36

Objective.—A canine model of ischemia was used to determine whether technetium-99m (^{99m}Tc)–tetrofosmin, a diphosphine compound that can be rapidly prepared from a freeze-dried kit formulation, is a reliable myocardial flow tracer through a pathophysiologic range.

Methods.—Six adult mongrel dogs were subjected to complete left anterior descending coronary artery occlusion. The animals were injected with ^{99m}Tc-tetrofosmin and radiolabeled microspheres during pharmacologic stress. Dynamic planar imaging and arterial sampling were performed coincident with radiotracer injection to assess ^{99m}Tc-tetrofosmin clearance from blood, myocardium, lung, and liver. The hearts were excised 15 minutes later, and myocardial slices were prepared for well counting of myocardial ^{99m}Tc-tetrofosmin activity and flow.

Results.—In each dog, myocardial ^{99m}Tc-tetrofosmin activity 15 minutes after injection correlated linearly with microsphere flow during peak stress. The plot of tetrofosmin activity vs. flow achieved a plateau at higher flow ranges (greater than 2 mL/min/g). Myocardial ^{99m}Tc-tetrofosmin activity appeared to underestimate flow at flows exceeding 1.5–2 mL/min/g and to overestimate flow in lower-flow ranges. The agent cleared rapidly from the blood and was retained in the myocardium. Target-to-background activity ratios were similar to other available ^{99m}Tc-labeled myocardial perfusion tracers.

Conclusion.—In a canine model of ischemia, ^{99m}Tc-tetrofosmin was a reliable flow tracer through a range of flows produced by pharmacologic stress. The data support the use of early poststress ^{99m}Tc-tetrofosmin for assessing myocardial perfusion in humans.

▶ This is the first demonstration of the relationship between myocardial blood flow and regional uptake of tetrofosmin. It behaves much like other perfusion agents in this regard.—B.L. Zaret, M.D.

Comparison of Technetium-99m-Q3 and Thallium-201 for Detection of Coronary Artery Disease in Humans

Gerson MC, Lukes J, Deutsch E, Biniakiewicz D, Washburn LC, Elgazzar AH, Elder RC, Walsh RA (Univ of Cincinnati, Ohio; Mallinckrodt Med Inc, St Louis, Mo)
J Nucl Med 35:580–586, 1994   124-95-10–37

Background.—During the past decade, numerous advances have been made in the development of technetium-99m (^{99m}Tc) myocardial imaging agents. The newer Q series tracers appear to clear more rapidly from the liver, facilitating early myocardial imaging after tracer injection and affording greater convenience to patients. In patients with documented angiographic coronary anatomy, ^{99m}Tc-Q3 images were compared with thallium-201 (^{201}Tl) images. At present, no single-photon–emitting myocardial imaging agent has proven to be more accurate than [201]Tl.

Methods.—Twenty-one patients with known or suspected coronary artery disease (CAD) and 6 healthy volunteers took part. Resting and exercise ^{99m}Tc-Q3 imaging was performed at least 2 days before or after ^{201}Tl imaging in each participant. The ^{99m}Tc-Q3 studies were performed with a high-resolution technetium collimator, using the same gamma camera and nuclear medicine computer as the thallium studies. A modification of the method of Wackers and colleagues was used to calculate heart-to-organ radioactivity ratios.

Results.—The overall accuracy of ^{99m}Tc-Q3 tomographic imaging for detection of CAD was 89%; tomographic thallium imaging had an accuracy of 78% in this series. The 2 imaging agents were also similarly accurate for detection of individual coronary stenoses: 83% for ^{99m}Tc-Q3 imaging and 75% for ^{201}Tl imaging. Heart-to-liver ratios of ^{99m}Tc-Q3 activity acquired 20 minutes after Q3 injection compared favorably with corresponding 60-minute postinjection ratios that previously had been reported for ^{99m}Tc-sestamibi.

Conclusion.—Technetium-99m–Q3 provided diagnostic accuracy comparable to ^{201}Tl for overall coronary disease detection and the detection of individual coronary artery stenoses. The myocardial tomograms acquired after ^{99m}Tc-Q3 injection were of excellent technical quality. Fewer than 100 minutes were required to complete the rest and exercise sequence. A favorable early ratio of heart-to-liver activity after administration of this agent suggests that a relatively condensed imaging sequence may be possible.

▶ This is one of the first studies on a new diphosphine complex for myocardial perfusion imaging. In these preliminary results, ^{99m}Tc-Q3 looks quite good using thallium data as a means of comparison. How it will fare in relation to the more established ^{99m}Tc-sestamibi and the somewhat newer ^{99m}Tc-tetrofosmin remains to be determined.—B.L. Zaret, M.D.

Bis(Dithiocarbamato) Nitrido Technetium-99m Radiopharmaceuticals: A Class of Neutral Myocardial Imaging Agents

Pasqualini R, Duatti A, Bellande E, Comazzi V, Brucato V, Hoffschir D, Fagret D, Comet M (CIS Bio International, Gif-sur-Yvette, France; Università di Bologna, Italy; LRT/DPTE C.E.A., Bruyere-le-Chatel, France; et al)
J Nucl Med 35:334–341, 1994   124-95-10–38

Background.—An efficient method for the preparation of technetium-99m (^{99m}Tc) radiopharmaceuticals containing the Tc $\equiv$ N multiple bond under sterile and apyrogenic conditions was described. A wide category of radiopharmaceuticals characterized by the presence of this terminal multiple bond can now be explored. The synthesis and biodistribution of ^{99m}Tc radiopharmaceuticals containing the Tc $\equiv$ N multiple bond were examined in various animal models, including a rat, dog, pig, and monkey.

Methods.—The complexes are represented by the general formula ^{99m}TcN(L)$_2$. In this formula, L is the monoanionic form of a dithiocarbamate ligand of the type [R^1(R^2)-N-C(=S)S]$^-$, and R^1 and R^2 are variable, lateral groups. The preparations were performed both as a liquid and freeze-dried formulation using a simple procedure. This involved the initial reaction of [^{99m}TcO$_4$]$^-$ with S-methyl N-methyl dithiocarbazate [H$_2$NN(CH$_3$)] in the presence of tertiary phosphines or Sn^{2+} ion as reductants. Next, the sodium salt of the ligand (NaL) was added to provide the final product. The chemical identity of the ensuing complexes was determined by comparing their chromatographic properties with those of the corresponding ^{99m}Tc analogues characterized by spectroscopic and x-ray crystallographic techniques. The complexes are neutral and have a distorted, square pyramidal geometry.

Results.—No decomposition of the complexes in physiologic solution was noted during a 6-hour interval. Imaging and biodistribution investigations showed that these radiopharmaceuticals localized selectively in rat, dog, and primate myocardium, but they failed to visualize the pig heart. After studying the kinetics of heart intake and clearance in rats and dogs, these factors were heavily influenced by variation of the lateral R^1 and R^2 groups.

Conclusion.—The high quality of myocardial images obtained in dogs and monkeys indicates that the derivative $^{99m}TcN[E-t(EtO)NCS_2]_2$ demonstrates the most favorable distribution properties for further studies in humans.

▶ These new compounds, which have the potential for visualizing ischemic tissue, are of substantial interest. Although a large amount of work is required, the potential for visualizing the hypoxic or ischemic zone as a hot spot is extremely appealing. This could enable definition of relatively small zones of ischemia, because they would appear as positive zones within the total image field.—B.L. Zaret, M.D.

Characterization of Iodovinylmisonidazole as a Marker for Myocardial Hypoxia
Martin GV, Biskupiak JE, Caldwell JH, Rasey JS, Krohn KA (Veterans Affairs Med Ctr, Seattle; Univ of Washington, Seattle)
J Nucl Med 34:918–924, 1993   124-95-10–39

Background.—As a result of reduced cellular partial pressure of oxygen, misonidazole and related compounds are trapped metabolically in viable cells. The binding of iodovinylmisonidazole (IVM) in ischemic myocardium in vivo was characterized in a canine model, and its deposition was compared with myocardial flow measured with radiolabeled microspheres.

Methods.—Two groups of dogs were studied. The 6 dogs in group 1 had partial occlusion of the left anterior descending (LAD) coronary artery. In the 4 dogs in group 2, demand ischemia was produced through atrial pacing and catecholamine infusion in the presence of a LAD stenosis. Iodine-131–labeled IVM was administered after ischemia onset. The dogs were killed, and trace deposition was measured by tissue sampling 4 hours after injection. These data were compared with microsphere myocardial blood flow measures that were obtained at baseline and 2 hours after injection.

Findings.—Regional IVM deposition in group 1 heart samples in the ischemic region was inversely associated with myocardial blood flow. The maximum ratio of tissue to blood was 3.2. For a given level of decreased blood flow, the IVM uptake was greater in the subendocardium, indicating a higher vulnerability of the subendocardium to decreases in oxygen delivery. Increased IVM deposition was found in group 2 that resulted from demand ischemia, even in some areas in which absolute flow was normal or increased compared with baseline values, indicating that flow per se is not the main factor in tracer uptake.

Conclusion.—Hypoxia tracers such as IVM may play an important role in the assessment of patients with ischemic heart disease. Such tracers may provide information that cannot be obtained from flow tracers alone. Noninvasive assessment of myocardial oxygen status can be facilitated by the use of iodine-131–labeled IVM.

▶ The comments made regarding the preceding article (Abstract 124-95-10–38) are relevant here as well. The potential excitement generated by these new compounds is substantial. However, whether this can be translated into a logistically feasible imaging technique remains to be seen.—B.L. Zaret, M.D.

Regional Myocardial Sympathetic Dysinnervation in Arrhythmogenic Right Ventricular Cardiomyopathy: An Analysis Using 123I-Meta-Iodobenzylguanidine Scintigraphy
Wichter T, Hindricks G, Lerch H, Bartenstein P, Borggrefe M, Schober O, Breithardt G (Hosp of the Westfälische Wilhelms-University, Münster, Germany)
Circulation 89:667–683, 1994   124-95-10–40

Introduction.—The presence, extent, and location of impaired myocardial innervation in patients with arrhythmogenic right ventricular cardiomyopathy (ARVC) were examined using iodine-123 meta-iodobenzylguanidine (^{123}I-MIBG) scintigraphy.

Patients and Methods.—Forty-eight patients with ARVC were studied with ^{123}I-MIBG scintigraphy. Nine patients with idiopathic ventricular tachycardia and 7 controls were also examined for comparison.

Results.—Clinically sustained or nonsustained ventricular tachycardia originated in the right ventricular outflow tract in 38 of the 48 patients with ARVC. In the other 10 patients, the site of origin was the apical or inferior right ventricle. Nonsustained or sustained ventricular tachycardia was provocable by exercise and/or by isoproterenol infusion in 33 patients, whereas programmed ventricular stimulation induced sustained or nonsustained ventricular tachycardia in 16 patients each. The right ventricle was not visible in any patient with ^{123}I-MIBG scintigraphy, and no areas of intense uptake were noted. All 7 controls and 7 of 9 patients with idiopathic ventricular tachycardia showed a uniform tracer uptake in the left ventricle. By contrast, only 8 of the 48 with ARVC showed a homogenous distribution of ^{123}I-MIBG uptake. The other 40 showed regional inductions or defects of tracer uptake. Thirty-eight of the 40 with abnormal scans showed reduced tracer uptake in the basal posteroseptal left ventricle, involving the adjacent lateral wall, the anterior wall, or the apex. Isolated defects of the anterior or lateral wall, 1 of which involved the apex, were seen in only 2 patients. In all patients, perfusion abnormalities in the areas of ^{123}I-MIBG defects were excluded by stress-redistribution thallium-201 SPECT scintigraphy and normal coronary angiograms. In patients with ARVC, abnormalities on ^{123}I-MIBG scans correlated with the site of origin of ventricular tachycardia, showing a regionally reduced tracer uptake in 36 of 38 patients with right ventricular outflow tract tachycardia compared with only 4 of 10 patients with other right ventricular origins of tachycardia. No association between ^{123}I-MIBG scintigraphy findings and the extent of right ventricular contraction abnormalities, right ventricular ejection fraction, biopsy specimen results, coronary anatomy, or left ventricular involvement in ARVC was noted.

Conclusion.—Regional abnormalities of sympathetic innervation are frequent in patients with ARVC and can be detected by ^{123}I-MIBG scintigraphy. Sympathetic denervation appears to be the underlying mechanism of reduced uptake, which is possibly related to frequent provocation of ventricular arrhythmias by exercise or catecholamine exposure in ARVC.

▶ The imaging of the sympathetic nervous system in cardiac arrhythmias should be an increasingly important area. This particular technique provides unique information that is not available by other means. It is also one of the strengths of the nuclear approach.—B.L. Zaret, M.D.

Risk Stratification in the Elderly Patient After Coronary Artery Bypass Grafting: The Prognostic Value of Radionuclide Cineangiography

Supino PG, Wallis JB, Chlouverakis G, Borer JS (Cornell Univ, New York)
J Nucl Cardiol 1:159–170, 1994   124-95-10–41

Introduction.—No previous study of late postoperative prognosis after coronary artery bypass grafting (CABG) in the elderly has assessed risk factors measured after hospital discharge. Recent data indicate that left ventricular function, as determined by radionuclide cineangiography (RNCA), predicts survival and cardiac events among non–age-selected patients. The postoperative course was assessed in 41 patients 65 years of age and older who had undergone RNCA 1 month or more after CABG.

Patients and Methods.—The 41 patients were drawn from a group of 325 patients who had undergone CABG and RNCA between August 1979 and February 1983. Their mean age at surgery was 67.8 years; 80% received between 2 and 4 grafts. None had previously undergone coronary bypass surgery. Gated equilibrium RNCA was performed in the supine position at rest in all patients and at maximal symptom-limited bicycle exercise in 38 of 41. The mean interval between CABG and postoperative testing was 2.3 years. The average follow-up among patients with event-free survival was 8.8 years after the index RNCA.

Results.—Thirteen patients died during follow-up with no known intercurrent event; 5 had nonfatal myocardial infarctions, and 5 underwent repeat CABG or percutaneous transluminal coronary angioplasty 3 months or more after RNCA. The only significant predictor of survival, based on log-rank comparisons of Kaplan-Meier product limit estimate curves, was left ventricular ejection fraction (LVEF) at rest. The average annual mortality risk was 2.3% for patients with normal resting function vs. 7.8% for those with LVEF at rest of less than 45%. A number of factors exhibited a statistical trend toward prognostic value, including completeness of revascularization, extent of anatomical disease, and age at index RNCA.

Conclusion.—As with non–age-selected patients, assessment of LVEF at rest was prognostically useful for elderly patients who had undergone CABG. With confirmation of this approach in a larger population, RNCA may help determine the need for additional evaluation and treatment in LVEF-depressed patients.

▶ It is refreshing to note that over the years, ejection fraction continues to be perhaps the most relevant measure of outcome in patients under a variety of clinical circumstances.—B.L. Zaret, M.D.

Left Ventricular Dysfunction During Exercise in Patients With Angina Pectoris and Angiographically Normal Coronary Arteries (Syndrome X)
Taki J, Nakajima K, Muramori A, Yoshio H, Shimizu M, Hisada K (Kanazawa Univ, Japan)
Eur J Nucl Med 21:98–102, 1994   124-95-10–42

Objective.—A continuous left ventricular function monitor with a cadmium telluride detector (CdTe-VEST) was used to evaluate left ventricular function during exercise and recovery in patients with angina pectoris, ST-segment depression during exercise, and angiographically normal coronary arteries (syndrome X). Such patients have been clinically indistinguishable from patients with atherosclerotic coronary artery disease.

Methods.—The study group consisted of 28 patients with normal coronary arteriography. Half had syndrome X, and half were controls with atypical chest pain, a normal exercise test, and angiographically normal coronary arteries. The 2 groups were similar in terms of age and gender distribution. Patients performed supine ergometric exercise after administration of 740–925 MBq of technetium-99m–labeled red blood cells. Left ventricular function was monitored every 20 seconds using the CdTe-VEST.

Results.—All patients with syndrome X but none of the controls showed ST-segment depression during exercise. The ST depression appeared 3.4 minutes after the start of exercise and persisted until 4.8 minutes after its conclusion. Exercise was terminated because of chest pain in 12 patients with syndrome X and because of fatigue in all other patients. At peak exercise, the heart rate was higher in patients with syndrome X than in controls, but systolic blood pressure was similar in the 2 groups. All control patients, but only 3 patients with syndrome X, showed a type 1 ejection fraction (EF) response pattern during exercise. The EF increase from rest to peak exercise was lower for syndrome X. The end-systolic volume increased at peak exercise in patients with syndrome X (mean, 116% of resting value) and decreased in control patients (mean, 65% of resting value).

Conclusion.—Despite normal epicardial coronary arteries, left ventricular dysfunction during exercise and a lower EF overshoot during recovery were frequently observed in patients with syndrome X. The cause of delayed and low EF overshoot in syndrome X may be ventricular dysfunction induced by ischemia during exercise.

▶ This is a nice demonstration of the functional evidence of ischemia in patients with syndrome X. The ambulatory ventricular function monitor provided highly relevant clinical data.—B.L. Zaret, M.D.

Left Ventricular Systolic and Diastolic Function Measurements Using an Ambulatory Radionuclide Monitor: Effects of Different Time Averaging on Accuracy

Pace L, Cuocolo A, Mangoni di S Stefano ML, Nappi A, Nicolai E, Imbriaco M, Trimarco B, Salvatore M (Università degli Studi Federico II, Naples, Italy; Istituto Nazionale Tumori Fond Sen G Pascale, Naples, Italy)
J Nucl Med 34:1602–1606, 1993   124-95-10–43

Objective.—Radionuclide techniques have recently been developed for the continuous ambulatory evaluation of left ventricular (LV) function. These devices, which work by simultaneous and continuous acquisition of nuclear and ECG data in an ambulatory setting, may be especially valuable in the detection of silent myocardial ischemia during ambulatory activities or after intervention. Changes in the ejection fraction (EF) and peak filling rate (PFR) are useful markers of LV functional impairment suggesting ischemia. The accuracy of the VEST, a commercially available ambulatory radionuclide detector, was evaluated in the measurement of EF and PFR, including the influence of different time-averaging techniques.

Methods.—Fifty-one consecutive patients, most with coronary artery disease, underwent a total of 67 studies with both equilibrium radionuclide angiography (RNA) and the VEST. The RNA studies were performed immediately before the VEST studies. Both single-beat analysis and different time-averaging intervals—5, 10, 15, 30, and 60 seconds—were used to analyze the VEST data. The limits of agreement (LAs) were computed to evaluate agreement between the 2 studies in estimating EF and PFR. The method used to compute LAs was 1.96 times the standard deviation of the mean differences between the 2 methods, expressed in the same units of parameters evaluated for both EF and PFR. To study possible relationships between measurement error and the true value, i.e., the mean between the 2 methods, the differences between the 2 methods were plotted against their mean.

Results.—The LAs for EF measurement by VEST were −10.4:8.8 on single-beat analysis, 11.2:9.9 on 5-second averaging, −5.4:4.8 on 10-second averaging, 4.9:4.5 on 15-second averaging, −6.2:5.6 on 30-second averaging, and 6.9:4.5 on 60-second averaging. Thus for time averaging of 10 seconds or greater, VEST and RNA had good agreement in measuring EF. For PFR measurement, the LAs ranged from −.6:.6 on single-beat analysis to 1:.6 on 60-second averaging, which constituted a clinically acceptable level of agreement between VEST and RNA. Neither parameter indicated any relationship between measurement error and true value.

Conclusion.—The commercially available VEST device appears to provide an accurate method of evaluating LV function, capable of assessing both systolic and diastolic performance in the form of EF and PFR, respectively. For time averaging of 10 seconds or greater, the results are unaffected by time averaging; thus short period-of-time summing is indicated for the detection of transient phenomena.

▶ This nice technical study indicates relevant temporal ranges within which the ambulatory ventricular function monitor can be used. This study forms a basis for further applications.—B.L. Zaret, M.D.

Role of Behavioral and Psychological Factors in Mental Stress–Induced Silent Left Ventricular Dysfunction in Coronary Artery Disease

Burg MM, Jain D, Soufer R, Kerns RD, Zaret BL (Veterans Affairs Med Ctr, West Haven, Conn; Yale Univ, New Haven, Conn)
J Am Coll Cardiol 22:440–448, 1993   124-95-10-44

Purpose.—Although the concept is somewhat controversial, the psychological profile has been suggested as a potential factor in the phenomenon of silent myocardial ischemia. The role of the type A psychological profile—characterized by a hostile, angry response style and associated behavioral reactivity—in mental stress–provoked silent myocardial ischemia was ivestigated by using serial radionuclide assessment of left ventricular function.

Methods.—The study sample comprised 30 patients with chronic stable coronary artery disease and a reversible defect on stress thallium-201 imaging. Each patient completed a psychological assessment with a questionnaire and structured interview, a serially administered mental stress, and a brief walking exercise. Ambulatory serial radionuclide ventriculography was used to determine blood pressure, ECG, and left ventricular indexes. The study definition of a silent ventricular dysfunction was a .05- or more decrease in the ejection fraction or a 1-mm or more decrease in the ST segment with no accompanying symptoms.

Results.—Fifteen patients, composing group I, showed evidence of silent left ventricular dysfunction during a mental arithmetic task, whereas the other 15, composing group II, showed no such change. Dysfunction was noted during the structured interview in 18 patients. Heart rate and blood pressure increased significantly and comparably in both groups. Group I patients scored higher for aggressive responses, trait anger, hostile affect, and behavioral reactivity and lower for anger control. No historical, clinical, or other variables distinguished between the 2 groups.

Conclusion.—Among patients with coronary artery disease, mental stress–provoked silent ventricular dysfunction is associated with a psychological profile of emotional reactivity to social interaction and mental provocation. Anger is the predominant affective state in these individuals, who may experience frequent episodes of silent left ventricular dysfunction. Mental stress can cause significant myocardial wall motion abnormalities, perfusion abnormalities, and decreased global left ventricular ejection fraction; the exact mechanism of these effects remains to be determined.

▶ Mental stress may be a potential provocateur for myocardial ischemia. Further studies are clearly needed in this area. By studying the ventricular response to mental stress in the laboratory in patients with coronary artery disease, relationships were noted between various psychological indices and an abnormal response. It is conceivable that mental stress testing could become an important aspect of the evaluation of patients with coronary artery disease.—B.L. Zaret, M.D.

Feasibility of Assessing Regional Myocardial Uptake of ^{18}F-Fluorodeoxyglucose Using Single Photon Emission Computed Tomography

Bax JJ, Visser FC, van Lingen A, Huitink JM, Kamp O, van Leeuwen GR, Visser GWM, Teule GJJ, Visser CA (Free Univ, Amsterdam; RadioNuclide Centre, Amsterdam)
Eur Heart J 14:1675–1682, 1993   124-95-10–45

Background.—Differentiation of viable myocardium and scar tissue in areas of abnormal contractility has important consequences in the clinical management of patients with coronary artery disease. Positron emission tomography with fluorine-18 fluorodeoxyglucose (FDG) can identify viable tissue, but high costs and limited availability prevent its routine use. The clinical usefulness of FDG uptake with SPECT was evaluated.

Methods.—Nine patients with wall motion abnormalities underwent resting thallium-201 (^{201}Tl) and FDG SPECT. The scintigraphic findings were related to 2-dimensional ECG regional wall motions. Reconstructed data were analyzed visually and semiquantitatively using circumferential profiles.

Results.—Thallium-201 SPECT images found 14 tracer defects in 8 patients. The focus of scintigraphic infarction was in agreement with the ECG infarction site in 6 infarcts in which ECG localization was possible. The FDG uptake was decreased concordantly, indicating a match in 8 perfusion defects. In 6 areas of hypoperfusion, normal or increased FDG uptake occurred, indicating a mismatch. Comparison of regional wall motion in matched or mismatched segments revealed akinetic regions in 7 of 8 matching defects, and hypo- or normokinetic regions in 5 of 6 mismatched segments. Semiquantitative analysis confirmed visual analysis results. The mean ^{201}Tl and FDG activities were comparable in matching defects, but the mean FDG activity was significantly higher in the mismatches.

Conclusion.—Myocardial FDG uptake can be visualized with SPECT. This approach can identify viable myocardial tissue in patients with coronary artery disease.

▶ If FDG could be imaged effectively and consistently with SPECT equipment, it would be a major attribute and could substantially enhance the use of metabolic imaging on a wider basis. Further approaches in this area using a variety of collimating systems will be necessary. However, it should be noted that even using conventional equipment, regional cyclotrons will be needed to provide the radiopharmaceutical.—B.L. Zaret, M.D.

Value of Metabolic Imaging With Positron Emission Tomography for Evaluating Prognosis in Patients With Coronary Artery Disease and Left Ventricular Dysfunction

Di Carli MF, Davidson M, Little R, Khanna S, Mody FV, Brunken RC, Czernin J, Rokhsar S, Stevenson LW, Laks H, Hawkins R, Schelbert HR, Phelps ME, Maddahi J (Univ of California, Los Angeles)

Am J Cardiol 73:527–533, 1994   124-95-10–46

Background.—The annual mortality rate among patients with coronary artery disease (CAD) and severe left ventricular dysfunction is high but variable. Some patients may benefit from myocardial revascularization. The prognostic value of PET and its relationship to the choice of medical therapy or revascularization for predicting survival and heart failure symptom improvement in patients with CAD and left ventricular dysfunction were studied.

Methods.—Ninety-three consecutive patients with angiographic CAD and a mean left ventricular ejection fraction of .25 were evaluated. The patients underwent cardiac PET studies for the assessment of hypoperfused but viable myocardium using nitrogen-13 ammonia and fluorine-18 deoxyglucose. The mean follow-up was 13.6 months. Fifty patients were treated medically, and 43 had revascularization.

Findings.—In a Cox model analysis, the extent of mismatch had a negative effect on survival, whereas revascularization had a positive effect. Patients with mismatch who were receiving medical treatment had a lower annual survival probability than those without a mismatch. Patients with a mistmatch who were undergoing revascularization had a greater survival rate than patients who were treated medically. Mismatch also predicted improvement in heart failure symptoms after revascularization.

Conclusion.—The presence of mismatch in patients with CAD and severe left ventricular dysfunction may be associated with the poor annual survival rate with medical treatment. Improved survival and heart failure symptoms are associated with revascularization in patients with PET mismatch.

▶ This is an important study, even though it is a retrospective analysis and there is a possibility that PET results have an impact on care. The results are significant because they indicate that a particular PET finding, namely mismatch, can be an entry step into a therapeutic pathway that is associated with a more favorable outcome. This kind of outcomes research will be required of all techniques in the future to justify their real clinical utility.—B.L. Zaret, M.D.

Quantitative Relation of Myocardial Infarct Size and Myocardial Viability by Positron Emission Tomography to Left Ventricular Ejection Fraction and 3-Year Mortality With and Without Revascularization
Yoshida K, Gould KL (Univ of Texas, Houston)
J Am Coll Cardiol 22:984–997, 1993   125-95-10–47

Background.—After successful revascularization procedures, areas of poorly contracting but viable myocardium show recovery of contractile performance. However, no previous studies have examined the relation of quantitative infarct size and myocardial viability, as measured by PET, to left ventricular ejection fraction and long-term mortality. This was addressed in a 3-year follow-up analysis of patients with myocardial infarction.

Methods.—The patients were studied over a 3-year period by PET using generator-produced rubidium-82 to objectively quantify infarct size and viability by automated software. The PET measurements were correlated with the findings of coronary angiography, left ventricular ejection fraction, revascularization, and 3-year mortality.

Results.—Patients with myocardial infarction or scarring of 23% or greater of the left ventricle had a 3-year mortality of 43%, compared with 5% for patients with less than 23% scarring of the left ventricle. Patients with an ejection fraction of 43% or less had a 3-year mortality of 38%, compared with 6% for those with a higher ejection fraction. A large left ventricular infarct of 23% or greater was associated with a low ejection fraction of 43% or less. The presence of such a low ejection fraction or large infarct size did not predict mortality; however, patients with a low ejection fraction and no viable myocardium in arterial zones at risk had a mortality of 63%, compared with 13% in patients with viable myocardium. There was just a 6% probability that this difference resulted from chance alone.

Mortality was 8% for patients with viable myocardium in arterial zones at risk; over 3 years' follow-up, 80% of these patients underwent revascularization. In contrast, mortality was 50% for patients with only fixed scar in arterial zones at risk. Just 40% of these patients underwent revascularization, which made no difference in mortality.

Conclusion.—Positron emission tomography measurements of scar size and viable myocardium in arterial zones at risk are good predictors of the 3-year mortality. The infarct scar or size determines the ejection fraction, so the PET measurements provide a primary prognostic indicator that explains the association of impaired ejection fraction with reduced survival. These measurements can be used to identify patients who are suitable candidates for revascularization.

▶ This paper presents interesting data relating viability determined by PET to the extent of the perfusion defect as well as ventricular function. Again, these types of data are quite important in determining the viability of a technique as well as that of the myocardium studies.—B.L. Zaret, M.D.

Positron Emission Tomographic Measurements of Absolute Regional Myocardial Blood Flow Permits Identification of Nonviable Myocardium in Patients With Chronic Myocardial Infarction
Gewirtz H, Fischman AJ, Abraham S, Gilson M, Strauss HW, Alpert NM (Brown Univ, Providence, RI; Harvard Med School, Boston; Bristol-Myers Squibb Pharmaceutical Research Inst, New Brunswick, NJ)
J Am Coll Cardiol 23:851–859, 1994   124-95-10–48

Background.—At basal steady state, blood flow of approximately 1 mL/min/g is required to maintain myocardial cell membrane integrity and myocardial contraction. Maintenance of membrane integrity alone requires much less blood flow; as a result, areas of chronic infarction with very low flow may be composed of inelastic scar tissue. Areas of nonviable myocardium were identified by quantifying regional myocardial blood flow.

Methods.—Basal regional myocardial blood flow was measured in 26 patients with chronic myocardial infarction using PET imaging with nitrogen-13 ammonia and fluorine-18 (^{18}F) fluorodeoxyglucose. Blood flow measurements were correlated with information about coronary anatomy and regional wall motion to assess myocardial viability.

Results.—The mean absolute blood flow in normal myocardial segments was .81 mL/min/g, significantly greater than that of infarct zones at .27 mL/min/g or border zones at .59 mL/min/g. Revascularized infarct and border segments had greater blood flow and better wall motion. Relative ^{18}F-fluorodeoxyglucose uptake and relative regional myocardial blood flow correlated significantly in all zones. With only 1 exception, blood flow and ^{18}F-fluorodeoxyglucose uptake matched in segments with blood flow less than .25 mL/min/g. Dyskinetic segments had blood flow less than .25 mL/min/g and no ^{18}F-fluorodeoxyglucose–blood flow mismatch. Flow exceeded .39 mL/min/g in 96% of myocardial segments with normal contraction or mild hypokinesia; 74% of these segments exhibited normal or only mildly abnormal regional wall motion.

Conclusion.—Positron emission tomographic measurement of regional myocardial blood flow can identify nonviable myocardium in patients with chronic myocardial infarction. Myocardial viability requires basal regional myocardial blood flow greater than .25 mL/min/g. The average basal flow in zones with normal or nearly normal wall motion is .78 mL/min/g.

▶ A major attribute of PET is the ability to measure myocardial blood flow in absolute terms. These data demonstrate how such measurements can be used to assess myocardial viability. I believe there is a substantial future in absolute flow measures defined by PET.—B.L. Zaret, M.D.

Factors Affecting Myocardial 2-[F-18]Fluoro-2-Deoxy-D-Glucose Uptake in Positron Emission Tomography Studies of Normal Humans
Choi Y, Brunden RC, Hawkins RA, Huang S-C, Buxton DB, Hoh CK, Phelps ME, Schelbert HR (Univ of Calif, Los Angeles)
Eur J Nucl Med 20:308–318, 1993   124-95-10–49

Purpose.—In patients with coronary artery disease, regional myocardial glucose metabolism can be noninvasively assessed by means of PET with 2-[F-18]fluoro-2-deoxy-D-glucose (FDG). However, there is evidence that a number of different factors may affect the interpretation of these metabolic studies. The anatomical and physiologic factors affecting left ventricular myocardial FDG uptake and myocardial glucose use rates (MRGlc) were examined in a population of normal young men.

Methods.—The FDG PET studies were performed in 18 healthy volunteers (mean age, 23 years). The participants were studied both after a fast of 4–19 hours and 16 hours after oral glucose loading with 100 g of dextrose. Substrate and hormone concentration measurements were obtained during each study. Both a 3-compartment model and Patlak graphic analysis were used to analyze the kinetics of myocardial FDG uptake.

Results.—The fasting and postglucose states were associated with similar systolic blood pressures and rate pressure products. The average MRGlc was .24 μmol/min/g in the fasting studies and .69 μmol/min/g in the glucose-loading studies. A linear relation was noted between phosphorylation rate constant and MRGlc. Factors correlated with increased MRGlc after glucose loading included plasma glucose, insulin and free fatty acid concentrations, insulin-glucagon ratios, and FDG influx rate constants.

Tracer cleared more rapidly from the blood and myocardial FDG uptake was higher with glucose loading, improving the quality of the diagnostic images. Myocardial FDG uptake was always sufficient for diagnostic imaging when the MRGlc exceeded .2 μmol/min/g, glucose concentration exceeded 100 mg/dL, insulin concentration exceeded 19 μU/mL, and insulin-glucagon ratio exceeded .2 μU/pg. There were no significant differences in FDG image quality and MRGlc after short vs. overnight fasts. Myocardial FDG uptake and MRGlc exhibited significant regional heterogeneity in both the fasting and glucose studies, with both values being greater in the posterolateral wall than in the anterior wall and septum.

Conclusion.—In FDG PET studies in normal humans, both 6-hour and overnight fasts are associated with similarly low MRGlc. Plasma glucose, free fatty acid, and insulin concentrations all affect MRGlc and myocardial FDG uptake; plasma glucagon levels may have a significant effect as well. Also, regardless of the individual's dietary status, significant regional heterogeneities in myocardial FDG uptake and MRGlc are present and should be kept in mind in the interpretation of clinical studies in patients with cardiac disease.

▶ As the FDG literature has developed, it has become clear that there can be major heterogeneity in results depending on the metabolic state of the patient. This paper helps define those issues relevant to obtaining data that can be transposed from 1 environment to another.—B.L. Zaret, M.D.

Myocardial Glucose Uptake in Patients With Insulin-Dependent Diabetes Mellitus Assessed Quantitatively by Dynamic Positron Emission Tomography

vom Dahl J, Herman WH, Hicks RJ, Ortiz-Alonso FJ, Lee KS, Allman KC,

Wolfe ER Jr, Kalff V, Schwaiger M (Univ of Michigan, Ann Arbor)
Circulation 88:395–404, 1993   124-95-10–50

Introduction.—Myocardial glucose use is reduced in diabetic animals, suggesting abnormal glucose transport. Myocardial glucose uptake was studied by PET with 2-fluoro-deoxy-D-glucose (FDG) in patients with insulin-dependent diabetes (IDDM) under standardized metabolic conditions.

Methods.—Dynamic PET imaging was performed in 7 young male patients with IDDM and 9 healthy controls who had normal glucose tolerance. All patients had had diabetes for fewer than 5 years and were receiving only human insulin. Oxidative metabolism was studied using carbon-11 (^{11}C) acetate, and glucose uptake was studied using FDG. A hyperinsulinemic-euglycemic clamp technique was used as PET data were acquired.

Results.—Global clearance rates of ^{11}C acetate were slightly higher in the diabetic patients than in the controls, but the difference was not significant. Myocardial glucose uptake was nearly identical in the 2 groups, as were the ratios of peak blood nuclide activity to activity 1 hour after tracer injection. The ratio of ^{18}F activity between the myocardium and blood pool averaged 7.2 in normal hearts and 7.5 in diabetic hearts.

Implications.—Individuals with diabetes and other patients with a markedly increased plasma glucose now receive IV insulin before FDG. This form of metabolic standardization optimizes image quality when diabetic patients undergo PET imaging with FDG.

▶ The question of how best to approach FDG studies in diabetics is addressed in part by this study. As in the preceding paper (Abstract 124-95-10–49), it is vital to have all metabolic issues defined and standardized so that results are transferable from 1 laboratory to another.—B.L. Zaret, M.D.

Myocardial Substrate Utilization and Left Ventricular Function in Adriamycin Cardiomyopathy

Wakasugi S, Fischman AJ, Babich JW, Callahan RJ, Elmaleh DR, Wilkinson R, Strauss HW (Massachusetts General Hosp, Boston; Harvard Medical School, Boston)
J Nucl Med 34:1529–1535, 1993   124-95-10–51

Background.—Adriamycin cardiotoxicity, a dose-dependent process, damages myocytes and culminates in congestive heart failure. If these cytotoxic effects are important factors in subclinical myocardial injury, alterations in myocardial metabolism may precede the changes observed in cardiac function and provide a useful clinical marker of cardiotoxicity. The relationship between changes in myocardial substrate use and left ventricular function was studied in a rat model of adriamycin cardiomy-opathy.

Methods.—Rats were given with adriamycin, 2 mg/kg, every week for 6, 8, 9, and 10 weeks. Fluorine-18 fluorodeoxyglucose (^{18}F-FDG) and ^{125}I-beta-methyl-branched fatty acid (^{125}I-BMIPP) were used as tracers of glucose and fatty acid metabolism. Technetium-99m hexakis (^{99m}Tc-MIBI) was used as a myocardial blood flow tracer. The left ventricular ejection fraction (LVEF) was calculated from gated blood pool images to serve as an indicator of cardiac function.

Findings.—The LVEF was normal in the 6-week group, but it declined abruptly in the 8-week group and deteriorated further in the 9-week group. The accumulation of ^{18}F-FDG in the hearts of rats given adriamycin declined progressively compared with that in control animals, occurring earlier than the LVEF deterioration. Myocardial accumulation of ^{125}I-BMIPP was reduced in the advanced stages of adriamycin cardiomyopathy, and it correlated well with the reduction in ^{18}F-FDG accumulation. However, this reduction was less marked for ^{18}F-FDG. The accumulation of ^{99m}Tc-MIBI between the control and adriamycin groups was comparable. In addition, no differences were noted in blood glucose levels between these 2 groups.

Conclusion.—Myocardial ^{18}F-FDG accumulation may be a useful clinical marker for identifying adriamycin cardiotoxicity, in which both glucose and fatty acid use appear to be reduced. Critical impairments in myocardial energy metabolism seem to occur before mechanical function is markedly decreased.

▶ Although this article is of interest experimentally, I doubt it will ever have a clinical expression. Substantial data indicate the value of simple left ventricular function analysis in defining adriamycin cardiotoxicity. I suspect that ejection fraction monitoring will be the most cost-effective method of evaluating such patients and doubt that metabolic imaging with FDG will play a significant clinical role.—B.L. Zaret, M.D.

Comparison of Carbon-11-Acetate With Fluorine-18-Fluorodeoxy-glucose for Delineating Viable Myocardium by Positron Emission Tomography
Gropler RJ, Geltman EM, Sampathkumaran K, Pérez JE, Schechtman KB, Conversano A, Sobel BE, Bergmann SR, Siegel BA (Edward Mallinckrodt Inst of Radiology, St Louis, Mo; Washington Univ, St Louis, Mo)
J Am Coll Cardiol 22:1587–1597, 1993   124-95-10-52

Background.—Accurately differentiating myocardium that is hibernating or stunned but is still viable from tissue that is irreversibly damaged and nonviable is necessary to identify patients with impaired left ventricular systolic function who would benefit from coronary revascularization. Such differentiation may be better accomplished using PET with carbon-11 (^{11}C)-acetate than by PET with fluorine-18 (^{18}F) fluorodeoxyglucose.

Methods.—In 34 patients, myocardial oxidative metabolism was quantified before revascularization by analyzing the rate of myocardial ^{11}C-acetate clearance. Glucose metabolism was determined by analyzing ^{18}F-fluorodeoxyglucose uptake.

Findings.—Receiver operating characteristic curve analysis showed that estimates of oxidative metabolism more robustly predicted functional recovery than estimates of glucose metabolism. Positive and negative predictive values were superior with threshold criteria with ^{11}C-acetate than with ^{18}F-fluorodeoxyglucose criteria, those values being 67% and 89%, respectively, compared with 52% and 81%. Estimates of oxidative metabolism in segments with initially severe dysfunction tended to be more robust than estimates of glucose metabolism in predicting functional recovery. Also, the threshold criteria with ^{11}C-acetate in such segments tended to show superior positive and negative predictive values, although nonsignificant, compared with ^{18}F-fluorodeoxyglucose criteria.

Conclusions.—In patients with left ventricular dysfunction from mostly chronic coronary artery disease, regional estimates of overall myocardial oxidative metabolism by PET with ^{11}C-acetate can accurately identify myocardium that is dysfunctional but still viable and able to recover systolic function after coronary revascularization. These estimates are more robust and better than those obtained with a tracer that is not specific for oxidative metabolism.

▶ The concept of using acetate clearance to assess viability is appealing. It is conceivable that one could look at initial uptake patterns for evaluating perfusion and then follow that with a kinetic analysis for metabolic assessment. Further studies comparing this approach to that of fluorodeoxyglucose imaging are indicated.—B.L. Zaret, M.D.

Time Dependence of Residual Tissue Viability After Myocardial Infarction Assessed by [^{18}F]Fluorodeoxyglucose and Positron Emission Tomography

Fragasso G, Chierchia SL, Lucignani G, Landoni C, Conversano A, Gilardi MC, Colombo F, Rossetti C, Fazio F, Striano G (Univ of Milan, Italy; Istituto Scientifico H San Raffaele, Milan, Italy)
Am J Cardiol 72:131G–139G, 1993   124-95-10–53

Background.—Regions of myocardial infarction may retain glycolytic activity. This finding indicates that tissue is viable and predicts functional recovery after revascularization. The presence of myocardial metabolic activity in relation to the time elapsed since the acute coronary artery thrombosis has not been studied. In addition, the relationship between increased glucose uptake and patency of the infarct-related coronary artery or the presence of collateral vessels has never been investigated in a large series.

Methods.—Sixty-five patients (mean age, 56 years) who had previously sustained myocardial infarction were studied prospectively. Coronary angiography and contrast left ventriculographic assessment of regional myocardial glucose metabolism by PET with 2-[¹⁸F]fluoro-2-deoxy-D-glucose ([¹⁸F]FDG) and evaluation of myocardial perfusion using SPECT with technetium-99m methoxyisobutyl isonitrile (⁹⁹ᵐTc-MIBI) were performed in all patients.

Findings.—Uptake of [¹⁸F]FDG in the underperfused regions was not observed in 26 patients who composed group 1, but it was seen in 39 patients, who composed group 2. All patients had regions of underperfusion at rest that were consistent with the myocardial infarction site identified clinically. The severity of coronary artery disease, the presence of collateral vessels, the number of hypocontractile segments, and wall motion scores were comparable in the 2 groups. The median time since infarction was 1,860 days in group 1 and 92 days in group 2, a significant difference. Exercise increased the severity and/or extent of resting perfusion abnormalities in 53% of group 1 patients and 23% of group 2 patients. Those in group 2 had a higher prevalence of exercise-induced ST-segment increases.

Conclusion.—Most recently infarcted myocardial areas retain residual metabolic activity. The extent of this is related inversely to the time that has elapsed since the acute event, which may suggest that the myocardium surviving the initial insult but remaining severely underperfused for prolonged periods may eventually become necrotic and be replaced by scar tissue. However, PET scanning with [¹⁸F]FDG in the assessment of myocardial metabolism may trace only postischemically stunned myocardium.

▶ This article addresses some issues relating to the temporal sequence of FDG assessment of viability. However, it deals with a period that is relatively late after infarction. It will be very interesting to assess individuals in the first week of infarction, because there has been speculation concerning the use of FDG for detecting stunned myocardium soon after infarction.—B.L. Zaret, M.D.

Assessment of Coronary Reserve in Man: Comparison Between Positron Emission Tomography With Oxygen-15-Labeled Water and Intracoronary Doppler Technique

Merlet P, Mazoyer B, Hittinger L, Valette H, Saal JP, Bendriem B, Crozatier B, Castaigne A, Syrota A, Randé JLD (Service Hospitalier Frédéric Joliot, CEA,

Orsay, France; Centre Hospitalo-Universitaire Henri Mondor, Créteil, France)
J Nucl Med 34:1899–1904, 1993   124-95-10–54

Introduction.—Significant advances have been made in the measurement of regional myocardial perfusion in patients with coronary artery disease and other conditions. These advances include PET as a noninvasive means of quantifying myocardial blood flow. Of the various available PET tracers, oxygen-15–labeled water offers many important advantages and can be combined with a metabolic ¹⁸F-fluorodeoxyglucose (FDG) study to define regions of interest (ROIs). This combined method was compared with the findings of intracoronary Doppler in the assessment of coronary reserve under dipyridamole stress.

Patients.—Three groups were studied: 8 patients with 70% to 90% stenosis of the left anterior descending artery, confirmed by coronary angiography; 6 patients with at least 1 episode of congestive heart failure associated with idiopathic dilated cardiomyopathy; and 6 controls with no coronary lesions and a coronary reserve of greater than 3, as assessed by intracoronary Doppler.

Methods.—All patients underwent direct ultrasonic measurement of coronary reserve the day before PET. For this study, a Doppler catheter in the proximal left anterior descending artery was used to record the mean velocity at baseline and after dipyridamole infusion. The PET studies were performed using a time-of-flight system. Patients received an IV bolus of oxygen-15–labeled water at baseline and 4–6 minutes after infusion of dipyridamole, which was given by the same protocol as in the Doppler study. They also underwent FDG myocardial imaging. Myocardial ROIs were drawn on a static FDG image, and oxygen-15 time-activity curves were recorded in these ROIs. A standard model was fitted with a single-tissue compartment to the PET data, with the left ventricular time-activity curve used as an input function and myocardial blood flow estimated as the blood-to-tissue transfer rate constant.

Results.—The mean coronary reserve as measured by intracoronary Doppler was 4.13 in the controls, 1.8 in those with left anterior descending stenosis, and 2.37 in those with dilated cardiomyopathy. Corresponding values measured by PET in the anteroseptal myocardium were 3.99, 1.83, and 2.3. Good correlation was noted between the PET and intracoronary Doppler measurements of coronary reserve in the group overall, r = .98, and in each of the 3 subgroups.

Conclusion.—The combination of PET using oxygen-15–labeled water and FDG myocardial imaging provides an accurate, reliable, and noninvasive technique for measuring coronary reserve. This is true even in patients with left ventricular dysfunction. For patients with coronary obstructions of doubtful physiologic significance, measurement of coronary blood flow reserve may have an important impact on the diagnosis and clinical management.

▶ The use of absolute flow measurements allows the most accurate noninvasive assessment of coronary flow reserve. Correlation with intracoronary Doppler measurements is valuable and has been used in other studies involving single-photon agents as well.—B.L. Zaret, M.D.

Noninvasive Assessment of Cardiac Diabetic Neuropathy by Carbon-11 Hydroxyephedrine and Positron Emission Tomography
Allman KC, Stevens MJ, Wieland DM, Hutchins GD, Wolfe ER, Greene DA, Schwaiger M (Univ of Michigan, Ann Arbor)
J Am Coll Cardiol 22:1425–1432, 1993   124-95-10–55

Background.—Little is known about the pathophysiology of cardiac sympathetic denervation in patients with diabetes, because methods for directly assessing damage to sympathetic neurons in the living heart have been lacking. In patients with autonomic neuropathy, cardiac carbon-11 (^{11}C) hydroxyephedrine uptake was quantitatively assessed as a marker for the integrity of sympathetic nerve terminals, and scintigraphic findings were correlated with conventional markers of sympathetic and parasympathetic dysfunction.

Methods.—Fourteen healthy controls, 5 controls with type 1 diabetes and no evidence of autonomic neuropathy, and 8 patients with type 1 diabetes with 2 or more abnormal findings on standardized autonomic function testing were included in the study. All underwent PET imaging with ^{11}C-hydroxyephedrine and rest myocardial blood flow imaging with nitrogen-13 ammonia.

Findings.—Seven patients with autonomic neuropathy had abnormal regional ^{11}C-hydroxyephedrine retention. In apical, inferior, and lateral segments, relative tracer retention was decreased significantly. The extent of the abnormality was associated with the severity of conventional autonomic dysfunction markers. Measures of absolute myocardial tracer retention index showed that distal myocardial segments in autonomic neuropathy were reduced 45% compared with proximal segments.

Conclusion.—Patients with diabetic cardiac neuropathy have a heterogenous pattern of neuronal abnormalities. Additional research involving larger groups of patients is needed to define the relative sensitivity of this imaging approach in the detection of cardiac neuropathy and to establish the clinical significance of these scintigraphic findings compared with that for conventional autonomic innervation markers.

▶ This is a nice demonstration of potential neuropathic findings in the myocardium of diabetics. Further studies in this area are clearly indicated.—B.L. Zaret, M.D.

Correlation Between Scintigraphic Evidence of Regional Sympathetic Neuronal Dysfunction and Ventricular Refractoriness in the Human Heart
Calkins H, Allman K, Bolling S, Kirsch M, Wieland D, Morady F, Schwaiger M
(Univ of Michigan, Ann Arbor)
Circulation 88:172–179, 1993 124-95-10–56

Objective.—Denervation supersensitivity has been invoked to explain the association between ventricular arrhythmias and the sympathetic nervous system. Whether sympathetic neuronal dysfunction correlates with ventricular refractoriness was studied.

Methods.—The pattern of sympathetic innervation was examined using the norepinephrine analogue carbon-11 hydroxyephedrine (HED) in 9 patients who were seen at the time of sudden cardiac death and 2 others who had ventricular tachycardia and hemodynamic instability. Positron emission tomography was done using 20 mCi of HED. Polar maps of relative nuclide activity were generated from short-axis blood flow and 30–40-minute HED images. In addition, electrophysiologic testing was performed after withdrawing all antiarrhythmic drugs, and refractoriness was estimated intraoperatively. The effective refractory period was determined in areas of normal and reduced HED retention under baseline conditions and during norepinephrine infusion.

Results.—Areas in which retention of HED activity was reduced were found in each patient. The effective refractory period was significantly longer in those areas than in areas where nuclide retention was normal. Infusion of norepinephrine shortened the effective refractory period to a similar degree both in myocardial areas with normal retention and in those with reduced retention of activity.

Conclusion.—Scintigraphic findings of sympathetic neuronal dysfunction correlate with ventricular refractoriness in humans with cardiac arrest or ventricular tachycardia.

▶ It is highly relevant to evaluate sympathetic function in patients with cardiac arrhythmias. This study involves PET technology using HED as the radiopharmaceutical. The relationship between these studies and those obtained with meta-iodobenzylguanidine and SPECT requires further definition.—B.L. Zaret, M.D.

Carbon-11 Hydroxyephedrine With Positron Emission Tomography for Serial Assessment of Cardiac Adrenergic Neuronal Function After Acute Myocardial Infarction in Humans
Allman KC, Wieland DM, Muzik O, Degrado TR, Wolfe ER Jr, Schwaiger M
(Univ of Michigan, Ann Arbor)
J Am Coll Cardiol 22:368–375, 1993 124-95-10–57

Background.—Previous experimental studies have reported ischemic injury to sympathetic neurons surpassing the area of myocardial necrosis. Carbon-11 (^{11}C) hydroxyephedrine (HED), a norepinephrine analogue, can be used to evaluate neuronal integrity noninvasively with PET. The extent and reversibility of neuronal abnormalities were assessed in patients with acute myocardial infarction.

Patients and Methods.—Fourteen volunteers and 16 patients with a first-time acute myocardial infarction were studied. Positron emission tomography imaging was used to quantitatively compare regional perfusion, as determined by nitrogen-13 ammonia, with myocardial retention of ^{11}C-HED soon after myocardial infarction and more than 6 months after the acute incident.

Results.—The ^{11}C-HED and flow images showed homogenous tracer retention in the 14 volunteers, but they were abnormal in the patient group. The ^{11}C-HED abnormalities were more extensive compared with those for blood flow evaluated using semiquantitative polar map analysis. This was particularly noteworthy in 5 patients with non–Q-wave infarction. Matched defects were seen in 11 patients with Q-wave infarction. The ^{11}C-HED tissue fraction was quantified in 3 tissue zones. Zone 1 (abnormal rest flow), zone 2 (normal rest flow but reduced ^{11}C-HED retention), and zone 3 (normal flow and ^{11}C-HED retention) had retention fractions of .037 $\pm$ .022, .068 $\pm$ .034, and .087 $\pm$ .041^{-min}, respectively. Eight patients undergoing follow-up studies at 8 $\pm$ 3 months had no change in the extent of abnormalities or absolute tissue tracer retention in infarct and peri-infarct territories.

Conclusion.—The findings of abnormal regional sympathetic innervation in patients with infarction verify previous experimental results. In addition, these results suggest persistent neuronal damage in infarct and peri-infarct regions, without evidence of reinnervation of reversibly injured myocardium.

▶ This study, which is similar to the preceding one from the same group (Abstract 124-95-10–56), emphasizes the potentially relevant physiologic information that can be extracted from unique PET studies involving the combined assessment of sympathetic function and myocardial perfusion. Further studies in this area are certainly of interest. It would be relevant to compare these data with similar data that could be generated by SPECT using meta-iodobenzylguanidine and sestamibi.—B.L. Zaret, M.D.

Quantification of Myocardial Muscarinic Receptors With PET in Humans

Delforge J, Le Guludec D, Syrota A, Bendriem B, Crouzel C, Slama M, Merlet P (Service Hospitaliér Frédéric Joliot, Orsay, France; Hôpital Bichat, Paris;

Hôpital Béclère, Clamart, France)
J Nucl Med 34:981–991, 1993   124-95-10–58

Background.—Previous studies in dogs have shown the potential for noninvasive quantification of myocardial muscarinic receptors using PET data, a mathematical model, multi-injection protocols, and carbon-11–labeled methylquinuclidinyl benzilate (MQNB) as a radioligand. The possibility of maximizing the experimental protocol to make it suitable for human studies was examined.

Methods and Findings.—Thirteen normal, healthy volunteers, aged 24–44 years, participated. Three protocols were examined. The first included 6 participants who were given 3 injections. A tracer injection was administered first, followed 30 minutes later by an injection of an excess of unlabeled MQNB (displacement). After another 30 minutes, a simultaneous injection of unlabeled and labeled MQNB (co-injection) was given. Estimates of the model input function were made using PET data that corresponded to the left ventricular cavity. This protocol enabled a separate assessment of all parameters of a ligand-receptor model, which included 3 compartments and 7 parameters. However, the complexity of this 3-injection protocol seems to make it inconvenient for clinical use. Another simplified 2-injection protocol was assessed in 5 other participants. Tracer injections were given first, followed 30 minutes later by a simultaneous injection of labeled and unlabeled MQNB (co-injection). The results were compared with those obtained using the 3-injection method. The mean value of the receptor concentration B_{max} and the equilibrium dissociation constant K_d were 26 ± 7 and $2 \pm .5$ pmol mL of tissue, respectively, in regions of interest over the left ventricle. The possible existence of nonspecific binding was evaluated in the remaining 2 participants, using a double-displacement protocol. Initial tracer injections were first administered, followed by 2 injections of unlabeled MQNB at 30 and 60 minutes, respectively. The corresponding rate constant was very low, at .03 minutes^{-1}.

Conclusion.—It is now possible to noninvasively quantify myocardial muscarinic receptors in the human heart using PET with a simplified 2-injection protocol.

▶ This PET protocol identifies another entire class of receptors that could be imaged using PET. No doubt this will provide highly relevant pathophysiologic data. Whether they will ever play a clinical role remains to be defined.—B.L. Zaret, M.D.

Diffuse Reduction of Myocardial Beta-Adrenoceptors in Hypertrophic Cardiomyopathy: A Study With Positron Emission Tomography

Lefroy DC, De Silva R, Choudhury L, Uren NG, Crake T, Rhodes CG, Lammertsma AA, Boyd H, Patsalos PN, Nihoyannopoulos P, Oakley CM, Jones T, Camici PG (Royal Postgraduate Medical School, London)

J Am Coll Cardiol 22:1653–1660, 1993   124-95-10–59

Introduction.—Most cases of hypertrophic cardiomyopathy are familial in nature, with an autosomal dominant pattern of inheritance. However, many affected patients have neither a family history nor any identifiable genetic abnormality. For these patients, the phenotypic expression of hypertrophic cardiomyopathy may rely on additional genetic and acquired abnormalities. Clinical and metabolic evidence suggests that sympathetic nervous system activity can be increased in this disease. Tracer studies were performed to evaluate myocardial β-adrenoreceptor density as a marker of sympathetic function in individuals with and without hypertrophic cardiomyopathy.

Methods.—Eight patients with hypertrophic cardiomyopathy, with a mean age of 37 years, and 8 normal controls were studied. The patients had received no previous treatment with β-blocking drugs. Both groups underwent PET for assessment of regional left ventricular β-adrenoreceptor density and myocardial blood flow. The tracers used were carbon-11–labeled CGP 12177 and oxygen-15–labeled water. In addition, plasma catecholamine measurements were performed.

Results.—The patients with hypertrophic cardiomyopathy had a mean myocardial β-adrenoreceptor density of 7.7 pmol/g of tissue, significantly less than the 11.5 pmol/g level in controls. There was no difference in myocardial blood flow (mean, .91 mL/min/g in both groups). The left ventricular distribution of β-adrenoreceptor density was uniform in both groups. The patients showed no correlation between regional wall thickness and myocardial β-adrenoreceptor density, and there were no differences in plasma norepinephrine or epinephrine concentrations between groups.

Conclusion.—Patients with hypertrophic cardiomyopathy demonstrate diffuse reductions in myocardial β-adrenoreceptor density, with no significant elevations in circulating catecholamines. This finding, which supports the hypothesis that cardiosympathetic drive is increased in hypertrophic cardiomyopathy, probably reflects downregulation of myocardial β-adrenoreceptors resulting from increased myocardial norepinephrine concentrations. A greater understanding of the role of sympathetic function abnormalities in hypertrophic cardiomyopathy may eventually lead to rational treatment strategies aimed at modulating sympathetic function to improve clinical outcome.

▶ Here is yet another example of how PET can be used to provide innovative and highly relevant pathophysiologic insights. In this instance, it involved the study of the β-receptor. This particular approach could play a role in identifying high-risk patients with hypertrophic cardiomyopathy who would be in danger of sudden death. It would be interesting to use these kinds of studies in relation to electrophysiologic data in hypertrophic cardiomyopathy.—B.L. Zaret, M.D.

Call Mosby Document Express at **1 (800) 55-MOSBY** to obtain copies of the original source documents of articles featured or referenced in the YEAR BOOK series.

11 Correlative Imaging

Introduction

This is the first year this chapter has appeared. It contains a potpourri of various subjects that either relate the nuclear medicine technique to other imaging modalities or contain information about other modalities that may relate to the nuclear medicine technique. Because bone scanning is a major aspect of the current practice of nuclear medicine, it is not surprising that a majority of these selections deal with bone.

Alexander Gottschalk, M.D.

Magnetic Resonance Imaging of Occult Fractures of the Proximal Femur
Haramati N, Staron RB, Barax C, Feldman F (Albert Einstein College of Medicine and Montefiore Med Ctr, Bronx, NY; Columbia Univ, New York)
Skeletal Radiol 23:19–22, 1994   124-95-11–1

Background.—Painful hip in the elderly patient is often a result of bone fracture, which can have serious complications. However, not all fractures can be seen on radiographs, and in such cases, diagnosis and treatment can be difficult, resulting in longer hospital stays. Bone scans are helpful but may not provide accurate results until some time after the patient is first scanned. At times after a positive diagnosis of fracture, more information is needed and more expensive methods of imaging may be used in planning treatment. The use of MRI as an initial step in diagnosing hip fracture in the elderly was evaluated.

Materials and Methods.—A 1.5-tesla MRI unit was used to generate 5-mm slices. Imaging took place within 24 hours of the patient's being seen. Patients with positive radiography results were excluded from the study.

Results.—In 10 of 15 patients with negative results at radiography but for whom there was a strong clinical suspicion of femur fracture, MRI clearly delineated a fracture (Fig 11–1). The images were additionally used in the treatment of fractures. In 2 other patients, MRI provided evidence of synovitis; those patients were successfully treated. Patients who were found not to have fracture by MRI were followed up for 3 months, and no fractures were subsequently diagnosed.

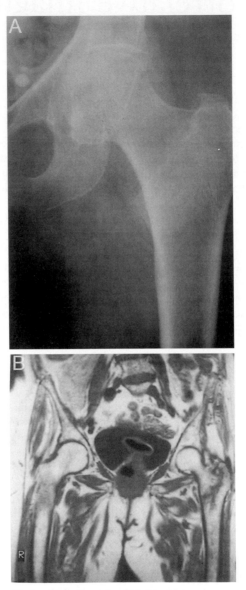

Fig 11–1.—Woman, 84. **A,** plain radiograph of left hip demonstrates osteopenia and no radiographic sign of fracture. **B,** coronal T1-weighted MR image demonstrates nondisplaced intertrochanteric fracture. (Courtesy of Haramati N, Staron RB, Barax C, et al: *Skeletal Radiol* 23:19–22, 1994.)

Discussion.—Significant morbidity is associated with hip fracture, although early treatment can help to reduce the toll. The alternatives of MRI, radionuclide bone scans, and CT can all help in making treatment decisions when radiographs do not reveal fractures. A bone scan is a good method, but it may take 2–3 days to demonstrate a fracture in the elderly, and a variety of other variables can dictate its accuracy. Magnetic resonance imaging provides information about the conformation of the fracture that can help in making treatment decisions. The T1-weighted images may be the best to use in this setting, and both coronal and axial scans should be performed.

▶ All I know about this topic I learned from Dr. Lawrence E. Holder. Dr. Phil Matin (1) has stated that older patients might well have a negative bone scan if they are examined very shortly (up to 3 days) after a fracture and that one should wait 1 week before making a definitive nuclear medicine bone scan diagnosis. Larry Holder and colleagues (2), in a very important 1990 article, point out that this is not the case with current techniques. In a group of 28 patients older than 70 years who were examined within the first 24 hours, these authors had only 1 false negative examination, 1 false positive examination, 12 true negative examinations, and 14 true positive examinations—for an accuracy rate of 93%.

I do not think there is any argument that occult fractures can be easily visualized by MRI and will yield the diagnosis. However, it is not always easy to get an elderly patient in pain into an MRI magnet. They can be claustrophobic, they may not hold still, and they may have on board paraphernalia (such as multiple IVs and other devices) that make imaging with MRI quite complicated.

If you have available time to use MRI and the patient is cooperative, MRI is an excellent test, and it will virtually always provide the diagnosis of occult hip fracture.

However, Holder and colleagues have shown that you can do very well with a gamma camera, imaging patients where they lie in a bed or gurney. Usually, you are much more likely to be able to do this in a timely manner in the nuclear medicine suite than in the MRI magnet.

Remember that the classic teaching of Matin needs revision. Most patients—and this includes the elderly—can have their occult fracture well imaged by nuclear medicine bone scanning.—A. Gottschalk, M.D.

References

1. Matin P: *J Nucl Med* 20:1227, 1979.
2. Holder LE, et al: *Radiology* 174:509, 1990.

Negative Scintigraphy Despite Spinal Fractures in the Multiply Injured

Hildingsson C, Hietala S-O, Toolanen G, Björnebrink J (Univ of Umeå, Sweden)
Injury 24:467–470, 1993   124-95-11–2

Background.—Musculoskeletal injuries are frequently overlooked in patients with multiple injuries, particularly those who have experienced head trauma. The diagnostic value of scintigraphy, a well-established indicator of skeletal injuries, was evaluated in a series of multiply injured patients.

Patients and Methods.—Twenty patients, aged 20 to 81 years, were studied. All had experienced multiple injuries that required hospitalization. Each patient received an IV injection of 550 MBq of technetium-99m methylene disphosphonate 3 to 4 hours before scintigraphy. After scintigraphy, findings of focally increased activity were compared with available skeletal radiographs.

Results.—Overall, 38 fractures diagnosed by plain skeletal radiography were also identified during scintigraphy. Moreover, scintigraphic evaluation showed a pelvic fracture in 1 patient and a tibial plateau fracture in another. However, scintigraphy did not demonstrate increased activity in 3 patients with radiographically confirmed fractures of the vertebral column. Of these, 1 patient had fractures of the transverse processes in all lumbar vertebrae. The second patient had fractures of the transverse processes and a traumatic spondylolisthesis of the fifth lumbar vertebra, and the third had a cervical spine fracture of the articular processes with dislocation.

Conclusion.—In patients with multiple injuries, scintigraphy may be useful in identification of skeletal trauma. In this experience, however, vertebral fractures were not always detected, possibly because of technically inadequate examinations in patients who were not able to cooperate.

▶ I agree with these authors that these may not be the best technical bone scans I have ever seen. They look like they need more counts per image. In addition, spondylolisthesis might be suggested by a comparison of anterior and posterior views, which the authors do not provide.

On the anterior projection in a patient with significant spondylolisthesis, the vertebra that has slipped forward may appear to be more active than it has any right to be in a normal study, in which the anterior views of the vertebrae ordinarily show decreased uptake. This could then lead to the use of regional oblique views, which might be very helpful (assuming SPECT was not available).

Finally, I believe that reading the bone scan in isolation from the regional radiographs is a major mistake. In this case, an entirely different set of exposure factors might have been required to see the transverse process fractures that were present. However, the message that transverse process fractures of the lumbar vertebrae may be difficult to see on a bone scan is one worth filing away in your memory bank.—A. Gottschalk, M.D.

The Value of Radiographs and Bone Scintigraphy in Suspected Scaphoid Fracture: A Statistical Analysis

Tiel-Van Buul MMC, Van Beek EJR, Borm JJJ, Gubler FM, Broekhuizen AH, Van Royen EA (Univ of Amsterdam)
J Hand Surg (Br) 18B:403–406, 1993   124-95-11–3

Background.—Scaphoid fracture can be difficult to diagnose via radiography. Early bone scintigraphy, suggested as the next diagnostic test, has been shown to have good positive predictive value, high intraobserver and interobserver agreement, and nearly 100% sensitivity. The 2 strategies for the detection of suspected scaphoid fracture after carpal injury in patients with initial negative radiographs—repeat radiography vs. selective bone scintigraphy—were assessed.

Methods.—A total of 78 consecutive adult patients with suspected scaphoid fracture after a recent carpal injury were evaluated; their mean age was 42 years. If initial radiographs did not show a fracture, the patients were referred for three-phase bone scintigraphy from 72 hours after trauma. The bone scans were interpreted in blinded fashion by experienced nuclear physicians, and they were interpreted as positive if they showed focal increased activity in the scaphoid region. Radiography was repeated at 10 to 14 days and, if necessary, 6 weeks after trauma. The radiographs were independently reviewed by 3 radiologists. Kappa statistics were used to assess agreement between these observers.

Results.—Of 60 patients with negative initial radiographs, 15 had positive bone scans. The initial radiographs had a kappa value of .76, which decreased to .5 for subsequent radiographs. Sensitivity decreased from 64% for initial radiographs to 30% for follow-up radiographs. Bone scanning had a specificity of 98% and a sensitivity of 100%.

Conclusion.—In patients with suspected scaphoid fracture after wrist injury, the diagnostic approach begins with radiography. If these initial films are negative, bone scintigraphy is more sensitive and specific than repeated radiography. For repeated radiographs, interobserver agreement and sensitivity are unacceptably low.

▶ This makes sense to me. You might seriously think about circulating this article to your sports medicine and orthopedic colleagues.—A. Gottschalk, M.D.

Magnetic Resonance Imaging for the Diagnosis of Osteomyelitis in the Diabetic Patient With a Foot Ulcer

Levine SE, Neagle CE, Esterhai JL, Wright DG, Dalinka MK (Hosp of the Univ of Pennsylvania, Philadelphia; Southwest Orthopaedic Inst, Dallas)
Foot Ankle 15:151–156, 1994   124-95-11–4

Introduction. —It is often difficult to distinguish between osteomyelitis and other pathologic conditions in the diabetic foot. Both plain film radiography and scintigraphic methods are limited in their ability to yield a positive diagnosis. However, MRI is reported to be useful in such cases. The results of MRI, plain film radiography, indium-111 (^{111}In)–labeled leukocyte scintigraphy, and technetium-99m bone scans in the diagnosis of osteomyelitis of the diabetic foot were compared.

Patients and Methods. —Twenty-seven diabetic patients with clinically suspected osteomyelitis underwent 30 MRI studies. Routine radiographic studies were performed in 25 patients, indium scintigraphy in 12, and technetium bone scans in 11. A definitive diagnosis was obtained in all patients. Osteomyelitis was confirmed by pathologic evidence in 13 patients. Affected regions of the foot included the phalanges (5), metatarsal and phalanx (1), metatarsal (6), and calcaneus (1). The site of the soft tissue ulcer without bony involvement was the toes (4), forefoot (7), dorsum of the foot (2), region of tarsometatarsal joint (2), and toes and forefoot bilaterally (1).

Results of Imaging. —In 10 of 13 histologically proven cases, the MRI diagnosis concurred with the final diagnosis. Magnetic resonance imaging had a sensitivity of 77%, a specificity of 100%, and an accuracy of 90%. Osteomyelitis was identified when an area of abnormal marrow with decreased signal intensity on T1-weighted images corresponded with an area of high signal intensity on T2-weighted images. Two of the 3 cases in which MRI yielded false negative results were also false negative on radiographs. Two of these 3 cases were correctly diagnosed with ^{111}In-labeled leukocyte scintigraphy. Technetium bone scans demonstrated a sensitivity of 100%, a specificity of 25%, and an accuracy of 45%. For ^{111}In-labeled leukocyte scintigraphy, these values were 80%, 29%, and 50%, respectively. Plain film radiography had a sensitivity of 60%, a specificity of 81%, and an accuracy of 73%.

Conclusion. —The diabetic foot is at risk for development of a number of bone and soft tissue abnormalities. Proper therapeutic planning depends on an accurate diagnosis. The findings show MRI to be a powerful, noninvasive method for defining the presence or absence of osteomyelitis. With MRI the marrow can be visualized directly, revealing the extent of the disease and amount of resection required. Because osteomyelitis is diagnosed earlier with MRI, more timely intervention is possible.

▶ I am delighted to see these results. The many years I spent using various types of tracers to make a diagnosis of osteomyelitis vs. overlying toe ulcer could probably have been spent doing virtually anything else. Nevertheless, I note that although MRI correctly diagnosed 10 of the 13 patients with proven osteomyelitis, 2 of the 3 proven cases that MRI missed were diagnosed with ^{111}In-labeled white cells. Surely, some type of algorithm to relate the 2 examinations will have to be devised.

These authors also suggest that the patient be screened with a routine bone scan, because if the result is negative, the possibility of osteomyelitis seems remote. I suggest that these authors not hold their breath. I cannot remember the last time I saw a negative bone scan result in a diabetic patient who had a soft tissue ulcer and was suspected of having osteomyelitis.

These data suggest that if a serious clinical concern for osteomyelitis in the diabetic foot exists, MRI is the best initial test. If the marrow is involved, you can stop and provide treatment. If MRI is negative, labeled leukocytes seem like the next step. I hope this concept is tested in a future series, because some of the numbers here need to be larger.—A. Gottschalk, M.D.

Comparison of Radionuclide Bone Scans and Magnetic Resonance Imaging in Detecting Spinal Metastases

Gosfield E III, Alavi A, Kneeland B (Univ of Pennsylvania, Philadelphia)
J Nucl Med 34:2191–2198, 1993   124-95-11–5

Objective.—A retrospective comparison between radionuclide bone scans using technetium-99m–labeled phosphates and MRI of the spine was conducted in patients with suspected metastases to the spine to evaluate the complementary role of MRI to that of bone scintigraphy.

Methods.—Thirty-five patients with cancer previously diagnosed by bone scans and MRI spinal studies done within 2 months of each other were evaluated. Cancer diagnoses included 14 prostate, 12 breast, 1 bladder, 2 renal, 2 lung, and 1 each of esophagus, melanoma, myeloma, and adenocarcinoma of unknown primary cancer. Bone scans were performed with planar imaging of the entire body, and MRI was performed with a 1.5-tesla signal scanner using standard techniques with T1- and T2-weighted images. The studies were read blindly and independently by an experienced orthopedic radiologist and a nuclear physician.

Findings.—Of the 157 technically comparable regions, 69 (44%) were positive for bony metastases by MRI, and 63 (40%) regions were positive by bone scan. Thirty-eight regions read positive on both MRI and bone scan, and 56 regions were concordantly negative. None of the patients with entirely positive bone scans had negative findings on MRI, but 1 patient who had an entirely positive MRI had a negative bone scan. Twenty-one (60%) patients had at least 1 discordantly read region. The distribution of positive regions was similar on bone scans and MRI, with the greatest number in the lower thoracic region. The greatest number and proportion of discordant readings were obtained in the lower lumbar regions, usually in patients with prostate cancer. In 2 patients with Schmorl's nodes in renal cancer, MRI provided an accurate diagnosis, whereas a bone scan read positive or questionable for metastasis.

Conclusion.—Radionuclide bone scans remain the study of choice for the initial screening for metastases, considering their higher sensitivity, lower cost, widespread availability, and ability to assess the entire body conveniently. However, MRI is an excellent complementary study in patients with equivocal or negative bone scan findings in the presence of high clinical suspicion or in patients with a positive bone scan but a low clinical suspicion for metastases. In certain locations in the spine, MRI appears to be quite sensitive and is probably more specific for metastasis.

▶ These authors present the nuclear medicine side of the coin. You may be interested in looking at the article written by Pomeranz, Pretorius, and Ramsingh (1) in the July 1994 *Seminars in Nuclear Medicine*, who take a different point of view and argue that if a patient with a known primary tumor has localized back pain, he or she should undergo imaging of the axial skeleton with MRI first. This can be done with a 20- to 30-minute survey using only the T1-weighted images and the rapid new specialized sequences, such as the fast T2-weighted inversion recovery.

However, you must be able to accept these patients quickly, otherwise time in the MRI unit seems to drag, and the 30-minute screen can be more difficult than it would seem in most cases.—A. Gottschalk, M.D.

Reference

1. Pomeranz JP, et al: *Semin Nucl Med* July, 1994.

Clinical Value of Combined Contrast and Radionuclide Arthrography in Suspected Loosening of Hip Prostheses
Köster G, Munz DL, Köhler H-P (Georg-August-Universität, Göttingen, Germany)
Arch Orthop Trauma Surg 112:247–254, 1993   124-95-11–6

Background.—In patients with loose hip prosthesis components, early diagnosis and reoperation are essential to avoid the further complication of osteolysis. In the patient with a painful hip after arthroplasty, conventional radiography will not reveal the problem until radiolucency or obvious migration exists. Previous studies of combined contrast and radionuclide arthrography for evaluation of these patients have yielded mixed results. Improvement of the technique of combined contrast and radionuclide arthrography for the diagnosis of loosened acetabular component was attempted.

Methods.—The study material comprised 71 artificial hip arthroplasties in 61 patients with a mean age of 70 years. There were 36 uncemented, 28 cemented, and 7 hybrid arthroplasties. Thirty-one joints had clinically or radiographically obvious loosening of 1 or 2 components, which was confirmed at reoperation. In the remaining 40 joints, the clinical and radiographic findings disagreed. Those in both groups underwent combined contrast and radionuclide arthrography, which were compared with sequential plain radiographs for their sensitivity, specific-

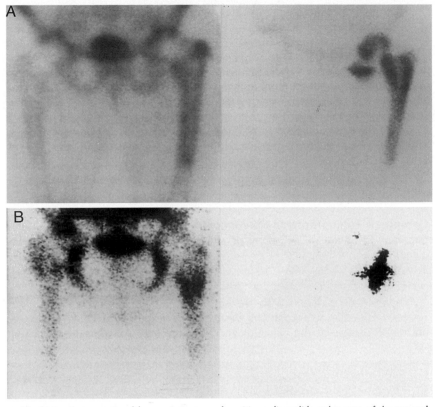

Fig 11–2.—**A,** conventional bone scintigram and positive radionuclide arthrogram of the cup and stem. Note the distribution of increased activity along the stem and up to the bottom of the socket. **B,** conventional bone scintigram and negative radionuclide arthrogram of the cup and stem. There is an increase in activity in the region of the neocapsule without further distribution. (Courtesy of Köster G, Munz DL, Köhler H-P: *Arch Orthop Trauma Surg* 112:247-254, 1993.)

ity, and predictive accuracy in detecting component loosening (Fig 11–2).

Results.—The results of the combined arthrographic studies supported the intraoperative findings in 91% of cases. Sensitivity, specificity, and predictive accuracy were high for both the acetabular and femoral components. For the acetabular components, combined arthrography was considerably more sensitive and accurate than plain radiography. When the clinical and radiographic findings conflicted, combined arthrography permitted a conclusive diagnosis. Both arthrographic studies were positive in 25 patients in this group: all 15 who have had surgery so far were found to have had loosening.

Conclusion.—Combined contrast and radionuclide arthrography, together with routine sequential plain radiographs, is valuable for the conclusive diagnosis in patients with questionable loosening of their hip arthroplasty components. In these patients, it may enable diagnosis of early loosening, permitting prompt intervention. Radionuclide angiography is particularly sensitive and accurate on the acetabular side.

▶ These data appear very promising. These authors use a combination of radiographic contrast material and radiocolloid. If your orthopedist is going to inject a joint anyway, why not show him/her this article and have him/her inject the radiocolloid as well.

The authors considered the radionuclide portion to be positive if the tracer was seen at the prosthesis-bone interface in the lower two thirds of the femoral stem. This could be either spotty or continuous activity.—A. Gottschalk, M.D.

Computed Tomography in Sternocostoclavicular Hyperostosis
Economou G, Jones PBB, Adams JE, Bernstein RM (Univ of Manchester, England)
Br J Radiol 66:1118–1124, 1993   124-95-11-7

Purpose.—In patients with the uncommon condition known as sternocostoclavicular hyperostosis, ossification of the peristernal ligaments and hyperostosis of the clavicles and sternum lead to limited mobility of

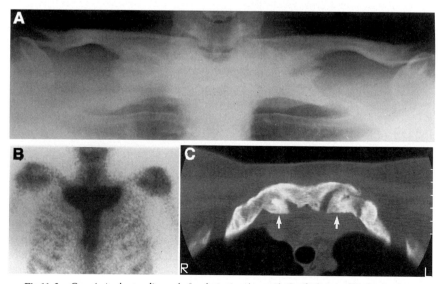

Fig 11–3.—Case 4. **A,** chest radiograph. Lordotic view (stage 2). Ossified tissue fills the gap between the medial end of the clavicles and the first ribs. **B,** radionuclide bone scan shows increased uptake over the manubrium sterni, extending to the body and medial parts of the clavicles. **C,** computed tomography (stage 3). Anterior bony bridging of the sternoclavicular joints. Abnormal texture of the medial ends of the clavicles (*arrows*). New bone on the posterior surface of the manubrium. (Courtesy of Economou G, Jones PBB, Adams JE, et al: *Br J Radiol* 66:1118–1124, 1993.)

the sternoclavicular joints. The cause is unknown. Pain and swelling are the major complaints, and although radiography is diagnostic, the diagnosis is often delayed, either because of lack of suspicion or inadequate radiographic studies. Four cases that illustrate the diagnostic value of radionuclide bone scanning and CT in this condition were presented.

Case Report.—Woman, 43, had a 5-year history of shoulder and sternal pain with progressive loss of movement. No diagnosis had been reached, despite multispecialty consultation; treatment, including prednisolone, was ineffective. The only radiographic abnormality of the chest was some increased density in the sternoclavicular area, but a lordotic view of the clavicles showed hyperostosis in the sternoclavicular and first sternocostal junction. On radionuclide bone scanning, there was increased uptake in the medial ends of the clavicles and in the manubrium (Fig 11-3). A bone biopsy specimen revealed evidence of very active remodeling and apposition of new bone, with fibrotic marrow cavities and nonspecific acute and chronic inflammatory cells. The CT scan demonstrated ossification of the costal cartilage surfaces, with bridging of the sternocostal junctions; sclerosis of the costochondral junctions of the first ribs; and expansion, with areas of lysis and sclerosis, of the medial ends of the clavicles. A diagnosis of stage 3 sternoclavicular hyperostosis was made. The patient showed no response to conservative management and was scheduled for surgical excision.

Discussion.—The clinical and radiologic findings of sternoclavicular hyperostosis were outlined. Radionuclide bone scanning is a very sensitive, although nonspecific study for such patients. High-resolution, thin-section CT is the examination of choice for depicting the characteristic features of this disease. This approach, along with heightened awareness of the problem, can enable early recognition and management.

▶ I saw such a case recently, and if it was any indication, the problem lies in the inability of anyone caring for the patient to label the condition. Please engrave Figure 11–3 on your mind.

My case looked very similar, except that there was a little more clavicular uptake that was symmetric bilaterally. If you can label the disease properly and direct the patient to your CT section for thin-section bone studies (such as those described above), you will save yourself, your colleagues, and the patient a lot of needless diagnostic expense and probably ensure that the patient gets the best possible care, although it may be nonspecific and not very effective.—A. Gottshalk, M.D.

Calcific Tendinitis in the Proximal Thigh
Hodge JC, Schneider R, Freiberger RH, Magid SK (Hosp for Special Surgery, New York)
Arthritis Rheum 36:1476–1482, 1993   124-95-11–8

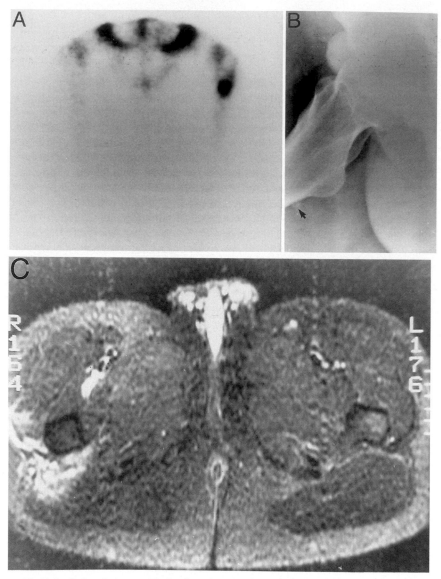

Fig 11–4.—Patient 2. **A,** posterior view from the static phase of a 3-phase bone scan, demonstrating a focal area of increased radiotracer activity in the proximal right thigh. **B,** "frog" lateral radiograph of the right thigh, revealing a small globular calcification in the posterior soft tissues (*arrow*). No abnormalities were found on the anteroposterior view (not shown). **C,** axial MR image of the proximal thighs, with fat suppression (repetition time, 2,000 ms; echo time, 70 ms). Increased signal intensity extends into the vastus lateralis and gluteal muscles (*arrows*). The signal arising from the femur is normal. (Courtesy of Hodge JC, Schneider R, Freiberger RH, et al: *Arthritis Rheum* 36:1476–1482, 1993.)

Background.—Calcific tendinitis, which commonly occurs in the shoulder, is uncommon in other sites. It has been reported in the tendons of the deltoid, pectoralis major, piriformis, and rectus femoris muscles, and in the thigh in the gluteus maximus and vastus lateralis muscles. Dramatic clinical improvement can result from percutaneous steroid injection. Computed tomography guidance is recommended for precisely localizing calcifications to avoid the sciatic nerve.

Methods and Findings.—Five patients, aged 31–57 years, with calcific tendinitis of the proximal thigh were assessed. Calcification was found on the anteroposterior radiographs in 3 patients and on frog lateral radiographs in all 5 (Fig 11-4). The patient who had a whole body bone scan showed increased radiotracer activity in the thigh. Only the delayed phase showed an abnormal radiotracer activity focus in the 2 patients who had three-phase bone scintigraphy. In both patients, soft tissue calcifications in the posterolateral thigh were seen on CT scans. The findings of the 2 MR assessments were positive: in 1, there was an area of signal void, and in the other there was an area of soft tissue edema in the posterolateral thigh. In 2 patients, percutaneous CT-guided injection of steroids completely alleviated pain in 1–2 weeks.

Case Report.—Man, 57, sought medical attention for progressive posterolateral hip pain. He reported having intermittent pain in the right greater trochanter for 1 year. On physical assessment, he had a full range of active and passive motion with no focal tenderness. He was hospitalized and was found to have a mildly increased white blood cell count and a normal erythrocyte sedimentation rate. A frog lateral radiographic view showed a posterolateral location of the calcifications and a smooth erosion of the adjacent femoral cortex. Computed tomography confirmed the soft tissue calcifications and a saucer-shaped erosion of the femoral cortex.

Conclusion.—Calcific tendinitis of the proximal thigh, a benign entity that can cause significant pain, must be distinguished from chronic or malignant diseases (e.g., arthritis, infection, and soft tissue/cortical neoplasms). It may be self-limited, but medical intervention can help in some cases. Computed tomography–guided percutaneous injection of steroids is recommended for these patients.

▶ Calcific tendinitis is a strange entity. In recent years, this once common shoulder disease has been hard to find on plain radiographs. If it starts cropping up in unusual places, as indicated in this article, it would become even more enigmatic.

As always, however, there is a place for the bone scan to localize the site of bone pain and permit other modalities to zero in for an occasional definitive diagnosis as a result of higher resolution. Most often, however, they simply localize the appropriate site for a bone biopsy.—A. Gottschalk, M.D.

Communicating Intraosseous Ganglion of the Lunate

Luke DL, Pruitt DL, Gilula LA (Washington Univ, St Louis, Mo)
Can Assoc Radiol J 44:304–306, 1993   124-95-11–9

Background.—Intraosseous ganglia usually involve the lunate or the scaphoid, and communication between the ganglion and the joint space is rare. A patient was seen with a physiologically active intraosseous ganglion of the lunate that communicated with the scapholunate joint.

Case Report.—Woman, 24, was examined 5 days after experiencing blunt trauma to the dorsum of the right wrist. Diffuse tenderness, limited active range of motion, and minimal soft tissue swelling were noted. A radiolucent defect on the radial side of the lunate was demonstrated radiographically (Fig 11-5). The patient had a soft tissue injury diagnosed, and conservative treatment was rendered. Four weeks later, the patient was reevaluated for persistent pain at wrist dorsiflexion and ulnar deviation. Radiography showed no changes, although bone scanning revealed increased uptake localized to the lunate (Fig 11-6). Arthrography was performed to exclude a ligamatous injury. The midcarpal compartment was opacified with dilute water-soluble contrast agent, which collected inside the lunate defect. A bone defect in the radial side of the lunate that connected to the scapholunate joint was demonstrated with CT (Fig 11-7). The patient subsequently had a previously asymptomatic intraosseous ganglion of the lunate diagnosed, which became symptomatic after trauma. The patient under-

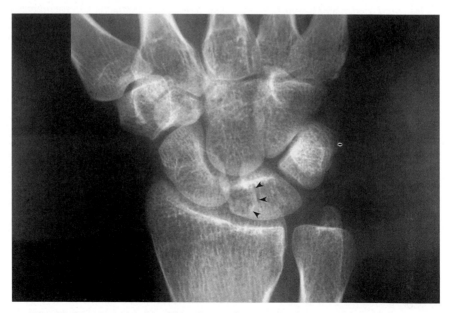

Fig 11–5.—Posteroanterior view of the right wrist shows a lucent defect, appearing to have thin sclerotic borders (*arrowheads*), involving the radial side of the lunate. (Courtesy of Luke DL, Pruitt DL, Gilula LA: *Can Assoc Radiol J* 44:304–306, 1993.)

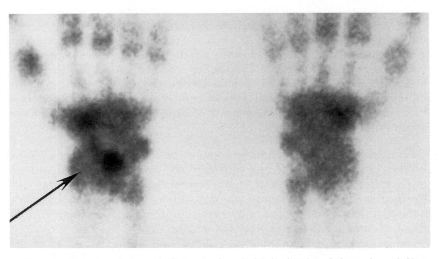

Fig 11–6.—Bone scan shows markedly increased uptake localized to the right lunate (*arrow*). (Courtesy of Luke DL, Pruitt DL, Gilula LA: *Can Assoc Radiol J* 44:304-306, 1993.)

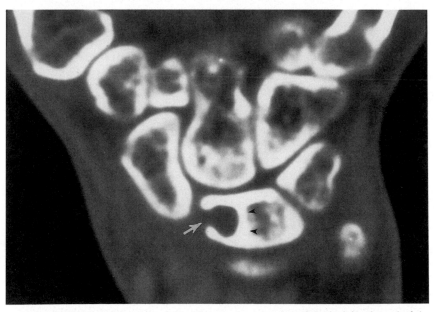

Fig 11–7.—Coronal CT sections of the right wrist show that the radial-side defect (*arrow*) of the lucent lesion connects to the scapholunate joint. The sclerotic margin of the defect is indicated (*arrowheads*). (Courtesy of Luke DL, Pruitt DL, Gilula LA: *Can Assoc Radiol J* 44:304-306, 1993.)

went conservative treatment for 8 weeks, but symptoms failed to resolve. Exploration, curettage, and bone grafting were performed. By using a dorsal approach, the cavity was entered through a drill hole in the intact dorsal cortex. A yellow, viscous, mucoid material was removed, and the lesion walls were curetted. A cancellous bone graft from the distal radius was then packed into the defect. Histologic examination verified an intraosseous ganglion. The bone graft was incorporated at 12 weeks, and the patient's pain and tenderness resolved. However, range of motion remained limited at 45 degrees of dorsiflexion and 40 degrees of volar flexion.

Conclusion.—This patient is believed to be the first in whom an intraosseous connection of the cyst with the joint was demonstrated with arthrography. Demonstration of such a communication precludes the need for further diagnostic imaging. Surgery, which consists of curettage and bone graft, is recommended only when symptoms are persistent and extreme. Reports of cyst recurrence are uncommon.

▶ This is a nice imaging modality correlative case. From the nuclear medicine standpoint, perhaps its most important aspect is the authors' belief that a tender wrist lesion that is seen as a focal carpal defect on x-ray examination should first be evaluated with radionuclide bone scanning. If this produces a significant hot spot, the common benign defects often seen (such as subcortical cysts) can probably be dismissed. Once the defect has been localized, a follow-up CT scan can be used to provide the best bony anatomical information possible, enabling diagnostic possibilities that include entities like giant-cell tumor, chondroblastoma, and endochondroma to be differentiated.—A. Gottschalk, M.D.

Intraoperative, Probe-Guided Curettage of Osteoid Osteoma
Kirchner B, Hillmann A, Lottes G, Sciuk J, Bartenstein P, Winkelmann W, Schober O (Westfälische Wilhelms-Universität Münster, Germany)
Eur J Nucl Med 20:609–613, 1993   124-95-11–10

Introduction.—Osteoid osteoma is characterized by its nidus—a spongy hypervascularized focus up to 1.5 cm in diameter. When surgical intervention is required, it may be difficult to localize the nidus preoperatively using plain radiography. Although tomographic imaging procedures provide preoperative proof of the nidus, intraoperative localization is a greater challenge. Success with a simple probe-guided operative procedure using technetium-99m (^{99m}Tc) methylene diphosphonate (MDP) was described.

Patients and Methods.—Twelve patients with a mean age of 22 years and a mean duration of disease of 5.6 months were studied. All reported a recent increase in pain. Localization of the nidus was in the tibia in 7 patients and the femur in 2; the humerus, the radius, and the head of the fibula were the locations in the remaining 3 patients. In 3 patients, a previous operation had failed to remove the nidus completely. Surgery was started 45–180 minutes after injection of age- and weight-related amounts of ^{99m}Tc-MDP. A TEC-PROBE 2000 with a CsI crystal was used to detect accumulation of activity in the lesion. The count rates 3 cm proximal and distal to the zone of sclerosis were first determined as a baseline. Starting from baseline areas and moving slowly horizontally and vertically over the lesion, the probe localized the point of maximal count rate. Operative removal was started from the area of maximum count rate.

Results.—The probe easily located a distinct maximum of activity in all patients, even those who had previously undergone surgery and in whom the blood pool phase of the bone scans did not reveal focal accumulation. In 11 of 12 patients, a decrease in the count rate of at least 80% relative to reference count rates was seen postoperatively in the region of the lesion. All patients were free of pain 7 days after the operation and were discharged on the tenth postoperative day. At at least 10 months of follow-up, all are free of relapse of osteoid osteoma.

Conclusion.—Use of the high-resolution probe facilitated intraoperative localization of osteoid osteoma. The probe is safe, is easy to use, and minimizes the risk of incomplete excision of the nidus.

▶ What a neat trick! This certainly seems easier than CT-guided insertion of wire into the nidus of the osteoid osteoma. If you are interested in doing this, you will probably want to order the probe before the Food and Drug Administration decides it is a device worth looking into, which would take the probe off the market for the foreseeable future.—A. Gottschalk, M.D.

Normal Brain F-18 FDG-PET and MRI Anatomy

Schifter T, Turkington TG, Berlangieri SU, Hoffman JM, MacFall JR, Pelizzari CA, Tien RD, Coleman RE (Duke Univ, Durham, NC; Univ of Chicago)
Clin Nucl Med 18:578–582, 1993   124-95-11–11

Introduction.—The use of PET F-18 fluorodeoxyglucose (FDG) metabolic imaging complements MRI findings in the evaluation of multiple neurologic disorders. Adequate interpretation of clinical PET studies depends on a knowledge of normal correlative structural and functional anatomy. A registered brain atlas of PET and MRI using studies obtained in a normal volunteer was developed.

Methods.—The MR images were acquired on a General Electric Signa 1.5-tesla system using T1-weighted and T2-weighted images, both consisting of contiguous 5-mm-thick slices. A General Electric 4096-Plus 8-ring PET system was used to obtain the high-resolution (FWHM 6.5 mm) 15-slice F-18 FDG PET images. In the registration technique, brain outlines were determined for all slices of both MR and PET image sets. The resultant surfaces were then used to find a transformation from 1 image set to the other that would make the surfaces fit. The final step uses this transformation, reslicing the MR images to match the PET slices. The MR brain edges were determined using the T2 images by setting a threshold of two thirds of the average brain matter pixel value. To prevent serious degradation of the MR image when it was resliced to match the PET, the PET images were zoomed by bilinear interpolation using a factor of 2, yielding 1-mm pixels. Appropriate rotation and translation to make the set of points defining the PET brain edge match the MR brain surface as closely as possible were achieved with the SurfaceFit program. After the transformation parameters were determined, both T1 and T2 MR images were resliced to match the PET slices. Brain structures were identified and marked with an X window image display and analysis program (SPECTER), using the resliced T1 and T2 data. A mark was made for a structure in 1 image set (T1 or T2), and then the corresponding pixel was marked in the other sets (T1 or T2 and PET). A number was then placed on the marked pixels of all 3 sets, and the marked images were transformed to PICT format for transfer to a Macintosh computer.

Results.—Normal FDG metabolism was greater in cortical gray matter and basal ganglia than in white matter structure, and it was greatest in the occipital cortex. In comparison with surrounding frontal cortical gray matter, the primary motor cortex and primary somesthetic cortex demonstrate relatively increased FDG uptake. The registered brain atlas enables the clinician to refer to a structural abnormality on MRI or a metabolic abnormality on PET and correlate it neuroanatomically.

▶ I included this article to provide you with a ready reference if you need it. To use this information you must refer to the original paper.

In my experience, the first major integration of all these images was done by Dr. Allen Lechter's therapy group at the University of Michigan. Lechter, a pioneer in conformal therapy, molded together all the diagnostic images he could find to get as precise a definition of tumor boundaries as possible to make his high-dose conformal therapy as accurate as the machines allow.—A. Gottschalk, M.D.

Neuroimaging of Juvenile Pilocytic Astrocytomas: An Enigma
Fulham MJ, Melisi JW, Nishimiya J, Dwyer AJ, Di Chiro G (Natl Inst of Neurological Diseases and Stroke, Bethesda, Md)
Radiology 189:221–225, 1993   124-95-11–12

Background.—With both CT and MRI studies, marked enhancement in a brain tumor after administration of contrast medium usually suggests an aggressive lesion. Similarly, brain tumors that exhibit increased glucose utilization relative to white matter at PET with fluorine-18 fluorodeoxyglucose (FDG) are associated with a poor prognosis. Paradoxical neuroimaging findings in 5 patients with juvenile pilocytic astrocytomas

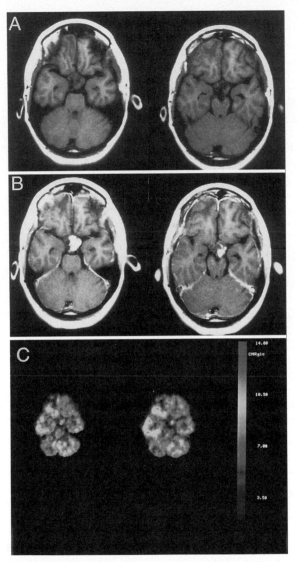

Fig 11–8.—A, T1-weighted (600/16) MR images, obtained at .5 tesla when the patient was 32 years of age, reveal a large heterogeneous suprasellar mass in the midline and left of the midline. Hypointensity in the right inferior frontal lobe is also evident. **B,** T1-weighted MR images (600/16) obtained after intravenous administration of gadopentetate dimeglumine show heterogeneous enhancement in the suprasellar mass and meninges. **C,** FDG PET images (color scale indicates glucose utilization in milligrams of glucose per 100 g of tissue per minute) show a close correspondence between increased glucose utilization in the suprasellar mass and gadolinium enhancement. In addition, hypometabolism is seen in the left orbitofrontal and temporal lobes, and right cerebellar hemisphere (crossed cerebellar diaschisis), with preserved glucose metabolism in the right dentate nucleus. (Courtesy of Fulham MJ, Melisi JW, Nishimiya J, et al: *Radiology* 189:221–225, 1993.)

(JPAs) that were considered low grade, showed intense enhancement on MR contrast images, and demonstrated higher-than-expected glucose utilization with FDG were analyzed.

Patients and Methods.—The patients—4 women and 1 man, with a mean age of 32 years—underwent 8 FDG PET studies. The pathologic diagnosis of JPA had been made on the basis of distinctive histologic findings. Normalized glucose utilization rates (GURs) in the tumors were compared with GURs in histopathologically verified low-grade astrocytomas and high-grade tumors according to the World Health Organization classification. T1-weighted, T2-weighted, and T1-weighted gadolinium-enhanced clinical MR images were obtained in all patients at .5 tesla. One patient had CT studies before and after IV contrast medium.

Results.—Marked contrast enhancement was seen on structural images in all 5 patients. There was a close correspondence between the region of enhancement and the location of increased glucose utilization seen at FDG PET (Fig 11-8). The glucose metabolism of the JPAs was significantly higher than that of low-grade astrocytomas and similar to that of anaplastic astrocytomas. At the time of publication, all patients were alive and in stable condition; 4 were able to work on either a full-time or part-time basis. There was no evidence of disease progression in these patients, despite contrast enhancement and high tumoral glucose metabolism.

Conclusion.—The findings prompt a number of questions about the nature of JPAs and suggest that their prognosis may not always be benign. Some tumors may undergo malignant degeneration and metastasize without a change in histologic appearance. The paradoxical FDG PET findings and enhancement at structural imaging could reflect the unusual vascularity of JPAs, whereas the increased GUR may be related to expression of the glucose transporter.

▶ Although personal experience has suggested that many relatively indolent brain tumors soak up contrast material (e.g., the often indolent acoustic neuroma usually shows lightbulb-type enhancement with gadolinium contrast on MRI), the functional PET data in this article are convincing and surprising. I certainly hope exceptions such as juvenile pilocytic astrocytoma are rare; however, I applaud these authors for bringing this exception to our attention.—A. Gottschalk, M.D.

Intracranial Hypertension After Resection of Cerebral Arteriovenous Malformations: Predisposing Factors and Management Strategy

Awad IA, Magdinec M, Schubert A (Yale Univ, New Haven, Conn; Cleveland Clinic Found, Ohio)

Stroke 25:611–620, 1994   124-95-11–13

Objective.—In patients who undergo surgery for cerebral arteriovenous malformations (AVMs), postoperative breakthrough edema with hemorrhage and elevated intracranial pressure (ICP) are potentially devastating complications. Risk has been reduced, but not eliminated, by such measures as embolization, staged resection, and meticulous surgical technique. The prevalence of intracranial excision was documented in a series of 32 patients undergoing excision of cerebral AVMs. Predisposing factors and the results of aggressive monitoring and treatment of elevated ICP were also identified.

Methods.—The patients underwent surgery consecutively, over 4 years. All operations were performed at least 1 month after overt cerebral hemorrhage, and most patients underwent preparatory embolization, especially those with larger lesions. Postoperative management included ICP monitoring and a standard protocol for management of elevated ICP, including barbiturate therapy for those with intractable intracranial hypertension. Perfusion SPECT was performed before embolization or resection in 17 patients and after embolization but before resection in 11.

Results.—Intractable elevated ICP—defined as a sustained symptomatic pressure of more than 30 mm Hg—developed in 28% of patients overall, including 15% of those with AVMs that had a maximum diameter of 6 cm or less and half of those that measured more than 6 cm. All such cases involved lesions that were located in distal or border-zone locations or those arising directly from proximal cerebral arteries. Ten of the patients who underwent preoperative SPECT had AVMs measuring 6 cm or less. Five of these patients, none of whom had intractable elevated ICP develop, showed parenchymal hypoperfusion beyond the AVM nidus. All 7 scanned patients who had larger AVMs showed hypoperfusion, and 5 of them had intractable intracranial hypertension. None of the 11 patients who received barbiturate therapy had uncontrollable intracranial hypertension or breakthrough edema during treatment. Barbiturate therapy caused no permanent morbidity, new disabling morbidity, or mortality.

Conclusion.—Even with the most up-to-date surgical and critical care techniques, intractable intracranial hypertension remains a common complication among patients with some types of cerebral AVMs. Preoperative SPECT can be a sensitive marker of hemodynamic features that predispose to this complication, although SPECT abnormalities do not necessarily predict uncontrollable ICP. For patients who have this complication, barbiturate therapy is a safe and effective form of management.

▶ If you have a neurosurgical or neurointerventional service, or even if you are going to refer your patient to one, it would seem to be a very good indication for cerebral SPECT. The authors used IMP, but I would imagine that hexamethylpropyleneamine-oxime would work just as well.—A. Gottschalk, M.D.

Cognitive Functions and Brain Structures: A Quantitative Study of CSF Volumes on Alzheimer Patients and Healthy Control Subjects

Wahlund L-O, Andersson-Lundman G, Basun H, Almkvist O, Björkstén KS, Sääf J, Wetterberg L (Karolinska Inst, Stockholm)

Magn Reson Imaging 11:169–174, 1993   124-95-11–14

Background.—Many investigators have been interested in brain atrophy in patients with Alzheimer's disease. Magnetic resonance imaging was used to estimate the CSF volumes in patients with senile dementia of the Alzheimer type (SDAT) and in healthy elderly persons. The relationship between the CSF volumes and cognitive impairment was also investigated.

Methods.—The study group included 8 men and 6 women with SDAT, aged 57–87 years, and 10 healthy women and 8 healthy men aged 77–87 years. Volumes of CSF were measured using a low-field MRI technique. Cognitive functions were assessed with a battery of psychometric tests.

Findings.—The patients with SDAT had significantly larger relative volumes in all CSF spaces examined. The greatest between-group differences were in the temporal horn volumes. The relative CSF volumes in the basal parts of the brain correlated significantly with episodic memory tests. The relative volumes of the lateral ventricles were significantly associated with the degree of dementia. The relative volumes of the lateral ventricles and episodic memory tests were also related (Fig 11-9, table).

Conclusion.—Measurement of temporal horn volumes may be a reliable diagnostic indicator of Alzheimer's disease and disease severity. Further research is needed to determine the usefulness of such volume measures as a differential diagnostic tool.

▶ Although this is not a comparison study, I will also try to let you know what the opposition is doing. Looking at relative CSF volumes in different portions of the brain is not a new MRI approach to assessing Alzheimer's disease. However, as time goes on, it gets easier and easier to do. This particular study was done on an MRI unit that was old by current standards, but the processing equipment seems to be state of the art.

This work should be considered simply a hypothesis. I suspect that the patients selected were probably those with advanced Alzheimer's disease. We don't know how well this type of analysis will separate patients with Alzheimer's disease from those with other forms of dementia. In all fairness, the authors acknowledge that this is a series of early observations and that there is much to do before clinical utility is achieved.—A. Gottschalk, M.D.

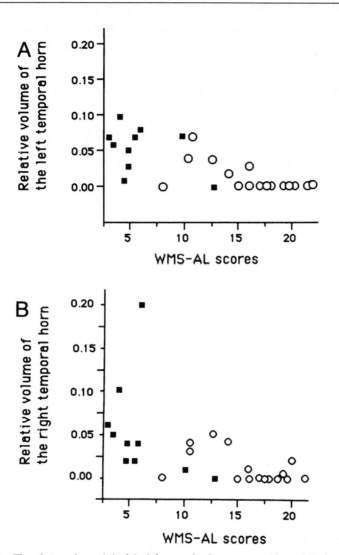

Fig 11–9.—The relative volumes (%) of the left **(A)** and right **(B)** temporal horn plotted against the raw scores from the Wechsler memory subtest: associative learning (WMS-AL). *Squares* represent pa- tients with SDAT; *circles,* healthy controls. (Courtesy of Wahlund L-O, Andersson-Lundman G, Basun H, et al: *Magn Reson Imaging* 11:169–174, 1993.)

Relative Volumes of CSF in Controls and Patients With SDAT

Relative volume (%)

Structure	Controls (n = 18)	SDAT (n = 14)	p (C vs SDAT)
Left ventricle	1.55 ± 0.69**	2.26 ± 0.86***	0.01
Right ventricle	1.41 ± 0.62	1.95 ± 0.68	0.02
Third ventricle	0.15 ± 0.05	0.19 ± 0.03	0.01
Left Sylv. fiss.	0.54 ± 0.1	0.71 ± 0.25*	0.02
Right Sylv. fiss.	0.49 ± 0.17	0.59 ± 0.17	0.09
Left cistern	0.06 ± 0.03	0.10 ± 0.05	0.03
Right cistern	0.06 ± 0.03	0.10 ± 0.04	0.03
Left temp. horn	0.01 ± 0.02	0.05 ± 0.03	0.0005
Right temp. horn	0.01 ± 0.02	0.07 ± 0.06	0.002

Note: Significantly different from the right side at *P < .05, **P < .01, and ***P < .001, respectively. The volumes are given in percentage of intracranial volume and expressed as means ± 1 SD. Mean differences were evaluated with unpaired t-test.
(Courtesy of Wahlund L-O, Andersson-Lundman G, Basun H, et al: *Magn Reson Imaging* 11:169–174, 1993.)

Hepatic Cavernous Hemangiomas: Lack of Enlargement Over Time
Mungovan JA, Cronan JJ, Vacarro J (Rhode Island Hosp, Providence; Oregon Health Sciences Univ, Portland)
Radiology 191:111–113, 1994   124-95-11–15

Background.—Today, it is common to discover an asymptomatic cavernous hemangioma of the liver during routine abdominal ultrasonography or CT scanning. A follow-up study after 4–6 months often is suggested to document the lack of growth expected from a malignancy, but long-term longitudinal studies of pathologically proven hemangiomas are lacking.

Objective and Methods.—Follow-up imaging studies were performed in 21 patients who had biopsy-proven cavernous hemangiomas. The patients all had initially undergone imaging-guided percutaneous fine-needle biopsy of the liver. Both ultrasonography and MRI were done at follow-up in 17 patients. Two patients had a CT examination only, one on an emergency basis because of presumed rupture and one who refused MRI. Two other patients were followed by ultrasonography only.

Findings.—Initially, the hemangiomas had a mean diameter of 5.3 cm. Thirteen of the 21 lesions were giant hemangiomas of more than 4 cm in diameter. None of the 8 hemangiomas smaller than this changed in size during follow-up examination. The mean follow-up interval in all patients was 26 months; 2 of the 13 giant lesions increased in size, and 1 of them ruptured spontaneously.

Implications.—Cavernous hemangiomas of the liver do not appear to enlarge over time, particularly those that initially are less than 4 cm in diameter. A majority of these lesions were giant hemangiomas, however, including both of those that enlarged, so this conclusion may not be applicable to all cavernous hemangiomas.

▶ There is plenty of competition in the hemangioma detection business these days, particularly from MRI. Consequently, I think it might be to your advantage to be as helpful as possible when diagnosing a cavernous hemangioma of the liver. If you find that you can measure the lesion or if a correlative cross-sectional imaging study that you have available (probably ultrasound but possibly CT) shows the lesion to be less that 4 cm in diameter, spread the message that is nicely illustrated in this article. It may help with the management of the patient you are examining.—A. Gottschalk, M.D.

Liver/Spleen Scintigraphy for Diagnosis of Splenic Infarction in Cirrhotic Patients
Chin JKT, McCormick PA, Hilson AJW, Burroughs AK, McIntyre N (Royal Free Hosp, London)
Postgrad Med J 69:715–717, 1993   124-95-11–16

Background.—Patients with cirrhosis rarely have splenic infarction. Diagnosis of this condition relies on clinical findings and splenic imaging. Recently, ultrasonography and CT scanning have become more popular than classic scintigraphy in diagnosing splenic infarction. Three cases of splenic infarction in patients with cirrhosis and portal hypertension were diagnosed with the aid of liver-spleen scintigraphy.

Case Report.—Woman, 24, with cirrhosis caused by Wilson's disease, was hospitalized for a few months' history of left upper quadrant pain. The pain had gotten worse in the 2 days preceding admission. She also reported nausea and heartburn. A CT scan with contrast enhancement of the abdomen was obtained, and massive splenomegaly with collaterals and varices was observed. Although the spleen showed regions of heterogeneous attenuation, there were no definite signs of splenic infarction. These findings were confirmed by ultrasonography and angiography. On technetium scintigraphy with tomography, a wedge-shaped defect was seen laterally in the midportion, which was consistent with a splenic infarction.

Conclusion.—In the cases described, CT scanning, angiography, and ultrasonography failed to identify the lesions. The diagnosis was finally established by liver-spleen scintigraphy. Scintigraphy appears to be the examination of choice in patients with congestive splenomegaly secondary to liver cirrhosis with suspected splenic infarction.

▶ This is a new twist. I used to do a lot of liver-spleen scans, but they were upstaged by CT and echocardiography, so that in most institutions the number of liver-spleen scans being done has precipitously fallen. It is nice to see the pendulum swing back the other way, even in this small group of patients.—A. Gottschalk, M.D.

The Radiological Features of Adult T-Cell Leukaemia/Lymphoma
George CD, Wilson AG, Philpott NJ, Bevan DH (St George's Hosp, London)
Clin Radiol 49:83–88, 1994   124-95-11–17

Background.—Adult T-cell leukemia/lymphoma (ATLL), once thought to be specific to certain regions of Japan, has since been found among Afro-Caribbeans in the United Kingdom and the United States. The causative agent is human T-cell lymphotropic virus type 1 (HTLV-1), which causes monoclonal expansion of infected lymphocytes. Some of the radiologic features of ATLL are unlike those of other lymphomas and leukemias and may suggest the diagnosis.

Patients.—The radiologic findings in 6 patients with ATLL were reviewed. There were 3 men and 3 women, who had a mean age of 55 years. All were Caribbean immigrants to the United Kingdom. Clinical findings included malaise, weight loss, skin lesions, dysphagia, and abdominal pain, with lymphadenopathy in all peripheral node groups. Mean survival was 7 months.

Findings.—Four generally asymptomatic patients showed radiographic bone lesions. These included multiple lytic lesions in 4 patients, involving both the axial and appendicular skeleton, and subperiosteal bone resorption in 1. Two patients had numerous well-defined lesions of the skull, with no sclerotic rim; bone scans were normal. One patient had large lytic areas of the proximal tibia and fibulae (Fig 11–10); the only abnormal bone scan finding was a pathologic fracture of the proximal left fibula (Fig 11–11). There was 1 patient with the previously unreported finding of mediastinal adenopathy.

Conclusion.—In addition to the bone changes, the wide spectrum of radiologic changes in patients with ATLL was shown. The major bone abnormality was lytic lesions of the skull and long bones. Gastrointestinal, pancreatic, and cutaneous changes may be noted as well.

▶ For radionuclide bone scanning purposes, this is a clone of a multiple myeloma.—A. Gottschalk, M.D.

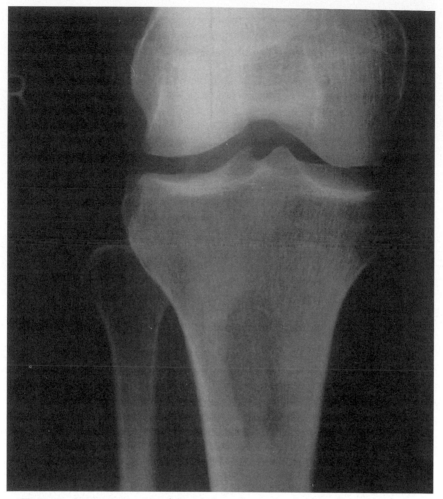

Fig 11–10.—Anteroposterior view of the right knee, showing lytic lesions in the upper tibia. (Courtesy of George CD, Wilson AG, Philpott NJ, et al: *Clin Radiol* 49:83–88, 1994.)

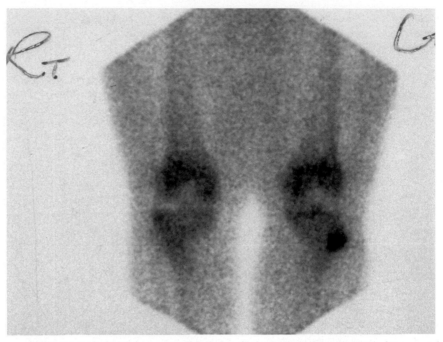

Fig 11–11.—Radionuclide bone scans of the knees of same patient in **Figure 11–10.** The lytic areas in the right knee do not show increased uptake. The hot spot in the upper left fibula corresponds to a pathologic fracture through a small lytic lesion. (Courtesy of George CD, Wilson AG, Philpott NJ, et al: *Clin Radiol* 49:83–88, 1994.)

Prone Scintimammography in Patients With Suspicion of Carcinoma of the Breast

Khalkhali I, Mena I, Jouanne E, Diggles L, Venegas R, Block J, Alle K, Klein S (Harbor-UCLA Med Ctr, Torrance, Calif)
J Am Coll Surg 178:491–497, 1994   124-95-11–18

Introduction.—The sensitivity of mammography plus physical examination for detecting breast carcinoma is 85%, whereas mammography has a positive predictive value of 15% to 30%. Abnormal screening stud-

Fig 11–12.—**A,** screening mammogram of a cone-compression magnified view of the left breast shows a cluster of microcalcifications suspicious for malignancy that are linearly arrayed. No mass is seen. Lead markers on the film denote scars from an old biopsy. **B,** magnified radiograph of a biopsy specimen demonstrates multifocal microcalcifications that are linearly arrayed and suspicious for carcinoma. **C,** scintimammogram of the left lateral prone projection shows a focal area of moderate increased ^{99m}Tc-sestamibi uptake corresponding to mammographic abnormality. Pathologic diagnosis was comedocarcinoma in situ. This was a nonpalpable lesion. Note that the extent of ^{99m}Tc-sestamibi uptake exceeds that of mammographic abnormality, which correlated better with pathologic findings. (Courtesy of Khalkhali I, Mena I, Jouanne E, et al: *J Am Coll Surg* 178:491–497, 1994.)

(continued)

Fig 11–12 (cont).

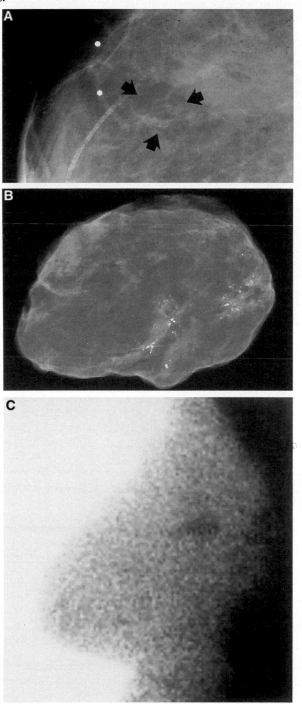

ies often lead to breast biopsy, with its attendant side effects and costs. Some better noninvasive test to select patients who could receive the greatest potential benefit from biopsy could decrease the number of negative biopsies. The use of scintimammography (SMM) with technetium-99m (^{99m}Tc) sestamibi was evaluated.

Methods.—The participants were 59 women with abnormal mammographic and physical examination findings that necessitated biopsy or fine-needle aspiration cytology of the breast. All patients were studied 5 and 60 minutes after IV injection of 20 mCi of ^{99m}Tc-sestamibi. The SMM examination included planar breast images in the lateral and posterior oblique views.

Results.—The SMM was positive in 23 patients with biopsy-proven breast carcinoma and negative in 33 patients with benign lesions (Fig 11–12). In 5 patients with benign breast lesions, SMM gave a false positive result. There was 1 false negative result in a patient with intraductal carcinoma, a cluster of microcalcifications seen on mammography, and no associated mass. As a result, the sensitivity of SMM was 96%, the specificity 87%, the positive predictive value 82%, and the negative predictive value 97%.

Conclusion.—This pilot research suggests that SMM is a potentially useful screening test for the detection of breast carcinoma. It is highly sensitive and more specific than conventional mammography. Further research will determine whether SMM can reduce the number of negative biopsies for breast carcinoma.

▶ From where I sit, the step between the screening mammogram and the surgical biopsy is either the stereotactic core biopsy or the stereotactic fine-needle aspiration. However, if neither of these techniques is available where you work, scintimammography, as these authors describe it, may be a good next step after the radiographic mammogram.—A. Gottschalk, M.D.

Hiatal Hernia on Whole-Body Radioiodine Survey Mimicking Metastatic Thyroid Cancer

Schneider JA, Divgi CR, Scott AM, Macapinlac HA, Sonenberg M, Goldsmith SJ, Larson SM (Mem Sloan-Kettering Cancer Ctr, New York)
Clin Nucl Med 18:751–753, 1993   124-95-11–19

Objective.—Identification of sites of false positive uptake requires knowledge of the physiologic routes of secretion of elemental iodine and an awareness of pathologic conditions that may suggest radioiodine concentration. A case in which a hiatal hernia appeared as metastasis from thyroid cancer at total body iodine-131 scanning was presented.

Case Report.—Woman, 67, was seen with a neck swelling in 1984 and eventually had surgery 2 years later. Follicular carcinoma was demonstrated after a thyroid lobectomy. The patient was treated with a cumulative dose of 806 mCi of iodine-131 during a 5-year period, when increased uptake was observed in the left neck and midthorax at follow-up iodine-131 scans. Multiple chest radiographs and an MRI showed a hiatal hernia but no evidence of skeletal, mediastinal, or pulmonary metastasis. The patient had repeatedly normal thyroglobulin levels. Approximately 8 years after she was first seen, she was referred for follow-up iodide scanning and dosimetry. A large collection of tracer was observed in the mid-thorax at total body iodine-131 scanning. However, SPECT images revealed the uptake to be contiguous with the uptake in the stomach, which was consistent with a hiatal hernia. Orally administered technetium-99m sulfur colloid (SC) in water confirmed the alimentary tract location of the radioiodine.

Discussion.—Secretion of radioiodine by gastric mucosa can lead to accumulation within a hiatal hernia. Although hiatal hernia is very common, it is rarely seen on iodine-131 images. The oral technetium-99m SC study has limited resolution, but it provides directly comparable images of alimentary tract uptake. Internal artifacts are more readily identified with SPECT images than with planar images, because of SPECT's better image contrast and superior 3-dimensional information.

▶ This case conveys an important message. I am intrigued that it was an MRI image that proved the activity in the chest was stomach fundus. However, once you have been warned about this entity, a plain posteroanterior lateral chest radiograph may be much cheaper.

I also firmly believe in giving a little oral technetium-99m–labeled colloid to locate the stomach. I have done this from time to time on confusing hepatobiliary studies, and it is another good indication. The authors are to be congratulated for thinking of it.

Incidentally, the idea of multitracer multiorgan nuclear medicine imaging, in my experience, goes back to Dr. Ben C. Berg, who used to do this regularly when analyzing his patients with trauma. It was common for him to image the kidneys along with doing liver and spleen scanning. Occasionally, he would also add ingested sulfur colloid to look at the stomach as well.—A. Gottschalk, M.D.

Intracardiac Ectopic Thyroid: Conservative Surgical Treatment
Polvani GL, Antona C, Porqueddu M, Pompilio G, Cavoretto D, Gherli T, Sala A, Biglioli P (Univ of Milan, Italy)
Ann Thorac Surg 55:1249–1251, 1993   124-95-11–20

Introduction.—Intracardiac masses are rare, occurring in less than .5% of the population. Rarer still is intracardiac ectopic thyroid, which has been reported only 8 times in living patients. An additional case of intracardiac ectopic thyroid was reported.

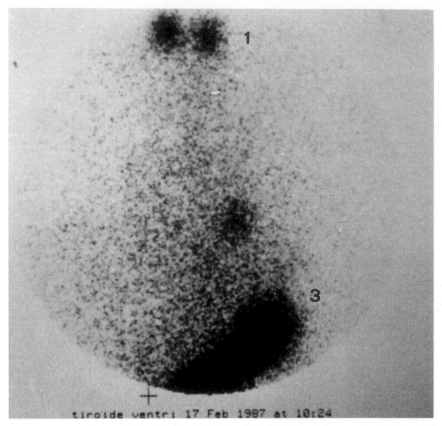

Fig 11–13.—Oval areas fixing iodine-123 in cardiac, thyroid, and gastric locations 5 days after the surgical treatment. (Courtesy of Polvani GL, Antona C, Porqueddu M, et al: *Ann Thorac Surg* 55:1249–1251, 1993.)

Case Report.—Woman, 66, with no history of cardiac disease, complained of palpitations, fatigue, and occasional dizziness. She had a systolic murmur suggesting an ejection murmur, ECG findings of sinus rhythm with complete right bundle-branch block and left posterior hemiblock, and a cardiac shadow with an enlarged right inferior arch on chest radiography. An intracavitary mass was noted encroaching on the right ventricular outflow tract on two-dimensional echocardiography. The patient underwent surgery for suspected neoplasm. On biopsy, the 8.5-cm mass showed thyroid micro-mid follicles filled with colloid on histologic examination. The mass was left in place because of its size, location, and relationship to adjacent structures. Postoperative thyroid scintigraphy demonstrated the thyroid gland in its normal location, as well as an oval area in a cardiac location fixing iodine-123 (Fig 11–13). The patient remained in good clinical condition 5 years later.

Discussion.—A patient with intracardiac ectopic thyroid, which was successfully managed with conservative surgery, was reported. Of the 8 similar patients reported since 1986, 7 had ectopic thyroid in the right ventricle and 1 in the left ventricular outflow tract. The tissue was morphologically identical to normal thyroid tissue. Such aberrant thyroid migration may result from persistence of very early embryonic contact between the thyroid primordium and bulbus cordis.

▶ I hope you have been paying attention. The differential diagnosis for this case is obviously hiatal hernia.—A. Gottschalk, M.D.

Preoperative Localization of Gastrointestinal Endocrine Tumors Using Somatostatin-Receptor Scintigraphy
Weinel RJ, Neuhaus C, Stapp J, Klotter HJ, Trautmann ME, Joseph K, Arnold R, Rothmund M (Phillips-Univ Marburg, Germany)
Ann Surg 218:640–645, 1993   124-95-11-21

Background.—High-affinity somatostatin receptors are found in most endocrine tumors. With pentatreotid, a stable, indium-111–labeled somatostatin analogue that binds to these receptors, somatostatin receptor–positive tumors can be detected scintigraphically. The value of somatostatin receptor scintigraphy (SRS) in the preoperative localization of gastrointestinal endocrine tumors was investigated.

Methods.—Nine patients with various gastrointestinal endocrine tumors underwent SRS, CT, and ultrasound before surgery. The results of

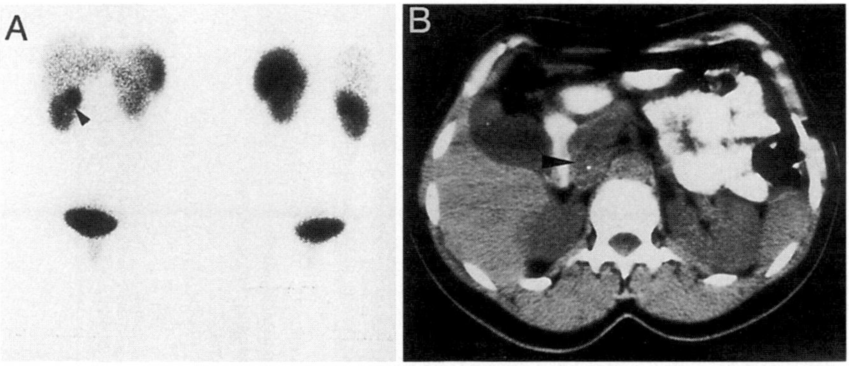

Fig 11–14.—**A,** whole body SRS in a patient with Zollinger-Ellison syndrome. Left ventral view and right dorsal view. There is nonspecific enhancement to the liver, spleen, kidneys, and bladder. The gastrinoma (diameter, 14 mm) localized within the pancreatic head can be seen at the **left,** near the upper pole of the right kidney (*arrowhead*). **B,** corresponding CT scan of the pancreatic head showing the area where the gastrinoma was found at surgery (*arrowhead*). No suspicious lesions in the area of the pancreatic head could be identified on the CT scan. (Courtesy of Weinel RJ, Neuhaus C, Stapp J, et al: *Ann Surg* 218:640–645, 1993.)

Results of Different Methods in the Preoperative and Intraoperative Localization of Endocrine Gastrointestinal Tumors

Patient No.	Diagnosis	Localization of Primary Tumor					Localization of Metastases				
		SRS	CT	US	IOUS	Surgical Exploration	SRS	CT	US	IOUS	Surgical Exploration
1	2 metastases of a functionally inactive endocrine pancreatic tumor	+	–	+	+		+	(+)	(+)	ND	+
2	Solitary pancreatic gastrinoma	+	+	–	+	+					
3	Carcinoid tumor in terminal ileum with liver metastases	+	+	+	ND	+	+	+	+	+	+
4	Paraduodenal carcinoid tumor with 2 local metastases	+	+	+	ND	+	+	+	+	ND	+
5	Carcinoid tumor in ascending colon with small liver metastases and local metastases	+	+	+	ND	+	(+)	+	(+)	ND	+
6	ZES, gastrinoma not identified at surgical exploration	–	–	–	–	–					
7	Gastrinoma in duodenal wall	–	–	+	–	+					
8	Insulinoma	–	–	+	+	+					
9	MEN I, 5 functionally inactive tumors	+	(+)	(+)	(+)	+					

Abbreviations: minus, tumor not localized; *(+)*, some, but not all tumors localized; *plus*, all tumors localized; ND, procedure not done; US, percutaneous ultrasound; IOUS, intraoperative ultrasound; ZES, Zollinger-Ellison syndrome; MEN I, multiple endocrine neoplasia type I. (Courtesy of Weinel RJ, Neuhaus C, Stapp J, et al: *Ann Surg* 218:640–645, 1993.)

preoperative imaging studies and intraoperative ultrasound were compared with surgical findings.

Findings.—At surgical exploration, 12 primary tumors were found in 8 patients. These tumors were correctly identified by SRS in 5 patients, by ultrasound in 4, and by CT in 3. In 1 patient with Zollinger-Ellison syndrome, scintigraphic findings suggested a tumor in the hepatoduodenal ligament region (Fig 11–14). The results of CT and ultrasound in this case were negative. In 4 patients with metastases, scintigraphy, CT, and ultrasound were comparable (table).

Conclusion.—Somatostatin receptor scintigraphy appears to be useful in preoperatively localizing gastrointestinal endocrine tumors. However, the technique has some disadvantages. It seems unlikely to reach a sensitivity and specificity that is high enough to replace conventional imaging methods; instead, SRS can serve as a complement to such methods.

▶ I do not want to belittle somatostatin analogue tracers in any way. However, I want to warn that there may be some very glowing reports in literature from time to time that do not deserve the attention they are likely to receive. It is tempting to discuss the results in terms of patient success rather than the more appropriate site-by-site success of the diagnostic tracer. I went through this with gallium in its early days, and it is important to reiterate the concept.

These authors point out that although somatostatin analogues worked better than ultrasound or CT, only 5 of 8 primary tumors were correctly localized. They believe these data indicate that no single technique is effective by itself for localization of gastrointestinal endocrine tumors. However, in this small group of patients, somatostatin receptor tracers were superior to CT and ultrasound in detecting the primary tumors. All 3 methods were equal in the detection of metastases. I again point out that this tracer gives a positive signal, which is always a major detection advantage. We should do well with endocrine lesions that have somatostatin receptors. Unfortunately, as the authors note, about 10% of carcinoids and 40% of insulinomas apparently are receptor-negative.—A. Gottschalk, M.D.

Scintigraphy and Sonography in Reflux Nephropathy: A Comparison
Riccabona M, Ring E, Maurer U, Güger G, Nicoletti R (Univ Hosp Graz, Austria)
Nucl Med Commun 14:339–342, 1993   124-95-11–22

Background.—Assessing reflux nephropathy (RNP) in children who are followed for vesicoureteral reflux (VUR) is a major task. The adequate monitoring of RNP development requires the frequent use of sonographic and scintigraphic studies. The accuracy of sonography in detecting and staging RNP was determined by comparing sonographic findings with those from static and dynamic renography.

RELATIVE KIDNEY VOLUME (%)

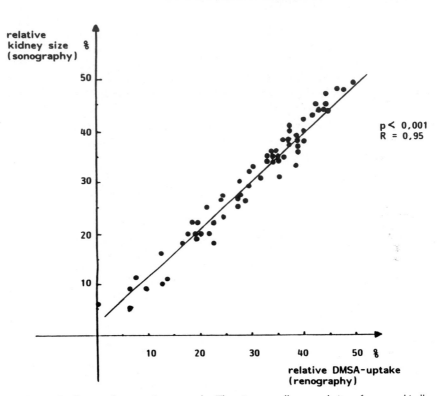

Fig 11–15.—Sonography vs. static renography. There is an excellent correlation of sonographically obtained relative renal volume with relative DMSA uptake on static renography (R = .95, P < .001). (Courtesy of Riccabona M, Ring E, Mauer U, et al: *Nucl Med Commun* 14:339-342, 1993.)

Methods.—Sixty-three patients with VUR were enrolled in the prospective study. The children ranged in age from newborn to 18 years, with a mean age of 8.8 years. Renal size was calculated sonographically and compared with static and dynamic renographic findings.

Findings.—There was a good correlation between relative DMSA uptake and sonographically estimated relative renal size (Fig 11–15). Not surprisingly, the correlation between relative kidney function and sonographically estimated renal size was poor.

Conclusion.—In monitoring children with VUR, sonography provides accurate information about renal size, renal parenchymal structure, and pelvic distention. Scintigraphy was superior in patients with very small or severely dilatated kidneys and for assessing renal function.

▶ These results are good news for us in nuclear medicine, but they are not unexpected. At first glance, it seems surprising that the radionuclide studies did as well at assessing renal volume. However, this is not an absolute volume but, rather, a relative volume. These authors are assessing relative counts in each kidney vs. the total number of counts in both kidneys. In short, calculation of renal dimensions down to the millimeter (or fraction thereof), which is potentially possible with ultrasound, did not come into play in this study. Finally, I would prefer to see comparisons made with state-of-the-art equipment for all the modalities compared. As the authors point out, color Doppler sonography was not performed in these studies. Consequently, the idea that the functional evaluation of the kidneys was far superior with the radionuclide study may have to be amended. Color Doppler provides sonography with a major functional probe that was not tested in this study.—A. Gottschalk, M.D.

Call Mosby Document Express at **1 (800) 55-MOSBY** to obtain copies of the original source documents of articles featured or referenced in the YEAR BOOK series.

12 Radiopharmaceutical

Introduction

It now takes about 231 million dollars and 12 years to develop a new drug, and only 1 in 5 is eventually approved by the United States Food and Drug Administration. New drug applications typically run 100,000 pages or more (1). In the decade that began in 1963, it took only 4.5 years to obtain a new drug application for a new respiratory drug from the time of synthesis; however, in the decade beginning in 1983, it took 16.7 years (2). What chance do new radiopharmaceuticals have?

The big news in radiopharmaceutical development in recent years is [^{111}In-DTPA-D-Phe^1]-octreotide (^{111}-In-Octreoscan or ^{111}In-Pentetreotide), which was developed by a team of scientists at the University of Rotterdam, The Netherlands; the Institute of Pathology, Berne, Switzerland; and Sandoz, Basel, Switzerland. Octreotide is an 8–amino acid cyclic peptide containing a critical 4-membered sequence of Phe-D-Trp-Lys-Thr, which is identical to that of somatostatin, for binding somatostatin receptors. However, there are at least 5 different subtypes of somatostatin receptors (3).

Octreotide images a variety of neuroendocrine gastroenteropancreatic tumors (4), including gastrinomas, polypeptide-producing islet cell tumors (PPomas), insulinomas, and rare tumors such as pancreatic islet G-cell tumors (VIPomas), glucagonomas, and somatostatinomas. Gastrinomas that hypersecrete gastrin are often pancreatic non–β-islet tumors that produce the Zollinger-Ellison (ZES) syndrome and are frequently malignant, with liver, skeletal, and regional lymph node metastases. About 50% are small tumors of the duodenum that are detectable only by duodenostomy. It is questionable whether these can be detected with octreotide. About 20% to 25% of patients with ZES have multiple endocrine neoplasia type 1.

Pituitary tumors that can be demonstrated by octreotide include growth hormone– and thyroid-stimulating hormone–secreting tumors, most nonfunctioning adenomas, eosinophilic adenomas that produce acromegaly, parasellar meningiomas, lymphomas, metastases from somatostatin receptor–positive malignancies, gonadotropinomas (3), and probably some infiltrating adrenocorticotropic hormone (ACTH)–secreting tumors after bilateral adrenalectomy (Nelson's syndrome). Pituitary adenomas associated with Cushing's syndrome and prolactinomas are not demonstrated. However, some autonomous cortisol-secreting adrenal adenomas in Cushing's patients and ectopic ACTH-secreting tumors are imaged. Most bronchial carcinoids are small (mean diameter, 11 mm) and may not be detectable with octreotide (5).

It is likely that more experience is needed to judge the efficacy of octreotide imaging in such "non-neuroendocrine tumors" as breast carcinoma, small-cell carcinomas of the lung, and neuroblastoma.

What other peptides look promising for tumor imaging? Bombesin analogues and vasoactive intestinal peptide are likely candidates. Bombesin itself does not work because its plasma clearance is too rapid, like that of somatostatin. However, analogues with slower clearance have been formulated (6). The Rotterdam group (Abstract 124-95-12-1) suggests substance P as well.

John G. McAfee, M.D.

References

1. Jukes TH: Consumable evils; Book Review of Burkholz H (ed): *The FDA Follies: An Alarming Look at Our Food and Drugs in the 1980's.* New York, Basic Books, 1994.
2. Di Masi JA, Seibring MA, Lasagna L: New drug development in the United States from 1963 to 1992. *Clin Pharmacol Ther* 55:609–622, 1994.
3. Lamberts SWJ, Reubi J-C, de Herder WW, et al: Editorial: A role of (labeled) somatostatin analogues in the differential diagnosis and treatment of Cushing's syndrome. *J Clin Endocrinol Metab* 78:17–19, 1994.
4. Jensen RT, Fraker DL: Zollinger-Ellison syndrome: Grand rounds at the clinical center of the NIH. *JAMA* 271:1429–1435, 1994.
5. Doppman JL: Editorial: Somatostatin receptor scintigraphy and the ectopic ACTH syndrome—The solution or just another test? *Am J Med* 96:303–304, 1994.
6. Moody TW, Cuttitta F: Growth factor and peptide receptors in small cell lung cancer. *Life Sci* 52:1161–1173, 1993.

Somatostatin Receptor Scintigraphy With [^{111}In-DTPA-D-Phe^1]- and [^{123}I-Tyr^3]-Octreotide: The Rotterdam Experience With More Than 1000 Patients

Krenning EP, Kwekkeboom DJ, Bakker WH, Breeman WAP, Kooij PPM, Oei HY, van Hagen M, Postema PTE, de Jong M, Reub JC, Visser TJ, Reijs AEM, Hofland LJ, Koper JW, Lamberts SWJ (Univ Hosp Dijkzigt, Rotterdam, The Netherlands; Univ of Berne, Switzerland)

Eur J Nucl Med 20:716–731, 1993   124-95-12-1

Background.—A number of neuroendocrine and other tumors contain many somatostatin receptors, allowing their in vivo localization by scintigraphy with a radiolabeled somatostatin analogue, octreotide (Fig 12–1). Granulomas and autoimmune diseases also can be visualized in this way. The previous preparation, iodine-123–labeled Tyr^3-octreotide, proved to have several drawbacks for use in in vivo scintigraphy. It now has been replaced by indium-111–labeled DTPA-D-Phe^1-octreotide.

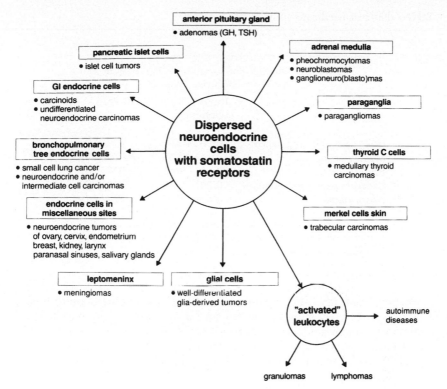

Fig 12–1.—Tumors and diseases with neuroendocrine cells and/or activated leukocytes with increased density of somatostatin receptors, which can be visualized with [¹¹¹In-DTPA-ᴅ-Phe¹]-octreotide scintigraphy. (Courtesy of Krenning EP, Kwekkeboom DJ, Bakker WH, et al: *Eur J Nucl Med* 20:716–731, 1993.)

TABLE 1.—Incidence of Somatostatin Receptors in Neuroendocrine Tumors

	In vivo scintigraphy		In vitro receptor status	
GH-producing pituitary tumour	7/10	70%	45/46	98%
TSH-producing pituitary tumour	2/2	100%	–	–
Non-functioning pituitary tumour	12/16	75%	12/22	55%
Gastrinoma	12/12	100%	6/6	100%
Insulinoma	14/23	61%	8/11	72%
Glucagonoma	3/3	100%	2/2	100%
Unclassified APUDoma	16/18	89%	4/4	100%
Paraganglioma	33/33	100%	11/12	92%
Medullary thyroid carcinoma	20/28	71%	10/26	38%
Neuroblastoma	8/9	89%	15/23	65%
Phaeochromocytoma	12/14	86%	38/52	73%
Carcinoid	69/72	96%	54/62	88%
Small cell lung cancer	34/34	100%	4/7	57%

Note: Results of [¹¹¹In-DTPA-ᴅ-Phe¹]-octreotide scintigraphy, as compared with in vitro somatostatin receptor autoradiography. In vivo and in vitro data are from different patient groups.
(Courtesy of Krenning EP, Kwekkeboom DJ, Bakker WH, et al: *Eur J Nucl Med* 20:716–731, 1993.)

TABLE 2.—Incidence of Somatostatin Receptors in
Non-Neuroendocrine Tumors

	In vivo scintigraphy		In vitro receptor status	
Non-small cell lung cancer	36/36	100%	0/17	0%
Meningiomas	14/14	100%	54/55	98%
Breast cancer	37/50	74%	33/72	46%
Exocrine pancreatic tumours	0/24	0%	0/12	0%
Astrocytoma	4/6	67%	14/17	82%

Note: Results of [^{111}In-DTPA-D-Phe^1]-octreotide scintigraphy as compared with in vitro somatostatin receptor autoradiography. In vivo and in vitro data are from different patient groups.

(Courtesy of Krenning EP, Kwekkeboom DJ, Bakker WH, et al: *Eur J Nucl Med* 20:716–731, 1993.)

Imaging Methods.—Both planar and SPECT images are acquired using a large-field-of-view gamma camera and a medium-energy parallel-hole collimator. Imaging is best accomplished 24 hours after injection of the radiopharmaceutical. Planar studies can be repeated at 48 hours and are especially useful when the 24-hour study shows activity accumulating in the abdomen.

Scintigraphic Findings.—The frequency of somatostatin receptors in various types of tumor and nonmalignant processes is shown in Tables 1, 2, and 3. Normally, the pituitary and thyroid glands, liver, spleen, kid-

TABLE 3.—Incidence of Somatostatin Receptors in Granulomatous
and Autoimmune Diseases

	In vivo scintigraphy		In vitro receptor status	
Non-Hodgkin's lymphoma	59/74	80%	26/30	87%
Hodgkin's disease	23/24	96%	2/2	100%
Sarcoidosis	23/23	100%	3/3	100%
Wegener's granulomatosis	4/4	100%	–	
Tuberculosis	6/6	100%	2/2	100%
Graves' disease: thyroid	9	*	1	
Graves' ophthalmopathy	25	†	–	

Note: Results of [^{111}In-DTPA-D-Phe^1]-octreotide scintigraphy as compared with in vitro somatostatin receptor autoradiography. In vivo and in vitro data are from different patient groups.

*Increased accumulation of radioactivity in the thyroid gland in untreated hyperthyroidism.

†Correlation with clinical activity score of orbital inflammation.

(Courtesy of Krenning EP, Kwekkeboom DJ, Bakker WH, et al: *Eur J Nucl Med* 20:716–731, 1993.)

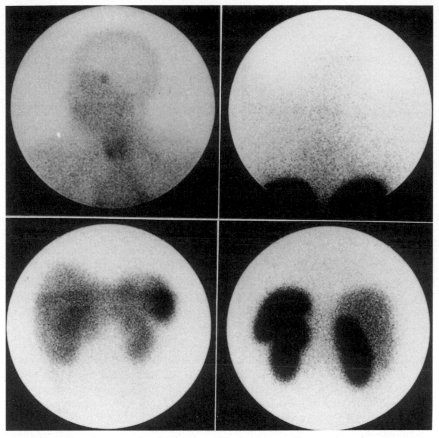

Fig 12–2.—Normal scintigraphic distribution of [¹¹¹In-DTPA-D-Phe¹]-octreotide in a man 24 hours after IV injection. Usually the pituitary, thyroid gland, liver, spleen, kidneys, and urinary bladder are visualized. Visualization of intestinal radioactivity depends on the time of scintigraphy and the use of laxatives. **Top left,** left lateral part of the head; **top right,** anterior chest; **lower left,** anterior abdomen; **lower right,** posterior abdomen. (Courtesy of Krenning EP, Kwekkeboom DJ, Bakker WH, et al: *Eur J Nucl Med* 20:716–731, 1993.)

neys, and bladder are visualized (Fig 12–2). Pituitary tumors producing growth hormone or thyrotropin and clinically nonfunctioning adenomas can be visualized by octreotide scintigraphy. Most endocrine pancreatic tumors are visualized, as are many paragangliomas, neuroblastomas, pheochromocytomas, medullary thyroid carcinomas, and carcinoid tumors. Octreotide scintigraphy can be used to select patients with carcinoid syndrome who may respond well to octreotide therapy. In addition to endocrine tumors, many astrocytomas, Merkel's cell tumors, breast cancers, and small-cell lung cancers are demonstrated by octreotide scintigraphy. The presence of somatostatin receptors on white blood cells enables the detection of malignant lymphomas and granulomatous diseases.

TABLE 4.—Comparison of [^{111} In-DTPA-D-Phe^1]-Octreotide Scintigraphy (OC) and ^{123}I-MIBG Scintigraphy Performed in the Same (27) Patients

Tumour type (number)	Number of lesions visualized		
	OC>MIBG	Equal	MIBG>OC
Phaeochromocytoma (8)	2	4	2
Neuroblastoma (5)	0	4	1
Paraganglioma (4)	3	1	0
Carcinoid (1)	0	1	0
Unclassified APUDoma (1)	1	0	0
Medullary thyroid carcinoma (1)	1	0	0
Adenocarcinoma (primary unknown) (1)	1	0	0

Note: No uptake in either investigation: carcinoid (1), non-Hodgkin's lymphoma (2), adrenal hematoma (1), liposarcoma (1), plasma cell granuloma of lung (1). In all patients, histologic proof of the tumor was obtained.
(Courtesy of Krenning EP, Kwekkeboom DJ, Bakker WH, et al: *Eur J Nucl Med* 20:716–731, 1993.)

Comparison to Meta-iodobenzylguanidine (MIBG) Scintigraphy.— Octreotide scintigraphy has proved to be equal to or occasionally better than MIBG scintigraphy in evaluating patients with pheochromocytoma or neuroblastoma (Table 4). An example is shown in Figure 12–3.

▶ Among the extensive publications on indium-111 octreotide analogue, if you have time to read only 1 article, this is the best. Because the Food and Drug Administration finally approved this agent earlier this year, we can now play catch-up with our European colleagues. Many centers now like to do planar and SPECT imaging at both 4 and 24 hours and total body scans after 4 hours—following 6 mCi of the indium-111 compound. The highest activity can be expected in the spleen, with activity in the kidneys, liver, gallbladder, intestinal contents, bladder, thyroid, and pituitary as well. The intestinal activity is less at 4 hours and often shows abdominal tumors better than at 24 hours. Breast activity is often seen in females at 24 hours. Nasopharyngeal or lung hilar activity may be seen with colds or other respiratory infections. Increased lung uptake occurs with bleomycin or radiation therapy. Recent surgical sites also show uptake.

This agent not only demonstrates many types of tumor well, but it predicts which ones will respond to octreotide therapy. The neuroendocrine tumors are derived from the amine precursor uptake and decarboxylation system. The mechanism of localization in nonendocrine neoplasms, granulomas, and other diseases is not clear.—J.G. McAfee, M.D.

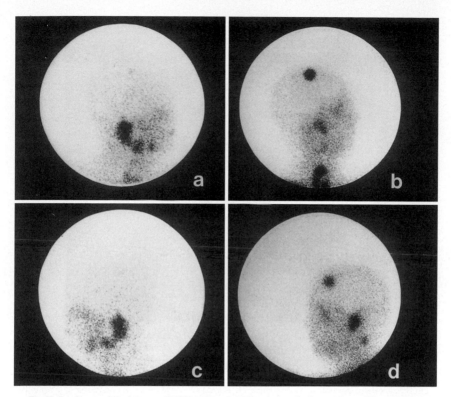

Fig 12–3.—Comparison between MIBG and octreotide scintigraphy in a patient with multiple paragangliomas. Right (**a, b**) and left (**c, d**) lateral image of the head and neck. **a, c,** after ^{123}I-MIBG; **b, d** after [^{111} In-DTPA-D-Phe^1]-octreotide. On the right lateral image, abnormal uptake of labeled octreotide is seen in the parietal region and above the thyroid, as well as the contralateral temporal paraganglioma (**b**). With ^{123} I-MIBG, only the parietal lesion is faintly visualized (**a**). On the left lateral image, increased uptake of labeled octreotide is present in a temporal and vagal paraganglioma, and the contralateral parietal metastasis of the paraganglioma is also seen (**d**). On the MIBG scintigram, only the parotid and submandibular salivary glands are visualized (**c**). Note that uptake of ^{123} I-MIBG in the parotid and submandibular salivary glands can hamper the recognition of paragangliomas. (Courtesy of Krenning EP, Kwekkeboom DJ, Bakker WH, et al: *Eur J Nucl Med* 20:716–731, 1993.)

---

^{111}In-Octreotide Scintigraphy in Oncology

Krenning EP, Kwekkeboom DJ, Reubi JC, van Hagen PM, van Eijck CHJ, Oei HY, Lamberts SWJ (Univ Hosp Dijkzigt, Rotterdam, The Netherlands; Sandoz Research Inst, Berne, Switzerland)
Digestion 54:84S–87S, 1993   1 24-95-1 2–2

Introduction.—Scintigraphy with indium-111 (^{111}In) octreotide is a simple and sensitive technique for demonstrating tumor localization in most patients with amine precursor and decarboxylation (APUD) cell tumors and in those with lymphomas or granulomas. In addition, in vivo somatostatin receptor imaging may be used to select patients with

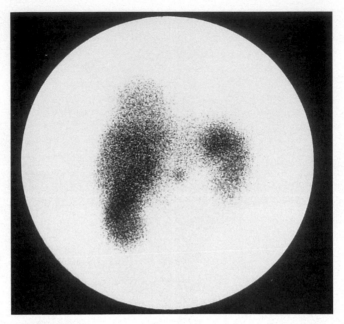

Fig 12-4.—Abdominal image in patient with multiple endocrine neoplasia syndrome. Anterior abdominal planar image 24 hours after injection of ^{111}In-octreotide. There is normal uptake of radioactivity in kidneys and liver. The unusual distribution of liver radioactivity is the result of several operations in the past. There is no uptake of radioactivity at the site of the spleen, which has been removed. There is abnormal accumulation of radioactivity medial to the right kidney and possibly a spot of radioactivity overprojecting the upper pole of the left kidney. (Courtesy of Krenning EP, Kwekkeboom DJ, Reubi JC, et al: *Digestion* 54:84S-87S, 1993.)

APUD cell tumors who are likely to respond to octreotide treatment. An overview of the results of using ^{111}In-octreotide scintigraphy for imaging various tumors was presented.

Somatostatin and Somatostatin Receptor Imaging.—Somatostatin is a small peptide that consists of 14 amino acids. The somatostatin analogue, octreotide, which is 8 amino acids long, binds to somatostatin receptors on both tumorous and nontumorous tissues. Octreotide is effective in the medical treatment of pituitary acromegaly. In addition, ^{111}In-octreotide, a radionuclide-coupled somatostatin analogue, can be used to visualize somatostatin receptor–bearing tumors after 24 hours. Static images were obtained 24 and 48 hours after patients were injected with the ^{111}In-coupled somatostatin analogue. The results were compared with those obtained using in vivo somatostatin receptor autoradiography.

Results.—The results of imaging in vivo corresponded with the somatostatin receptor status of the tumors in vitro. Imaging was successful in all 7 patients with gastrinoma (Fig 12-4), 1 of whom also had a glucagonoma. Other types of tumors for which imaging was 100% successful included small-cell lung cancer, sarcoidosis, paraganglioma, and carcinoids. In addition, ^{111}In-octreotide scintigraphy was better than conventional imaging techniques in demonstrating multicentricity of tumors.

Conclusion.—In most patients with APUD cell tumors, lymphomas, or granulomas, ^{111}In-octreotide scintigraphy successfully demonstrated tumor localization. With its ability to visualize somatostatin receptor-positive tumors in vivo, it can be used to predict which patients are likely to benefit from octreotide therapy. Because multicentricity is common in paragangliomas, somatostatin receptor imaging should be the method of choice in establishing the number and localizations of these tumors.

▶ This is a brief, general review of the virtues of somatostatin receptor imaging of various tumors and a few granulomas. Subsequent publications from these and other authors tend to emphasize images at 4 and 24 hours, rather than the 24- and 48-hour images in this article.—J.G. McAfee, M.D.

Octreotide and Related Somatostatin Analogs in the Diagnosis and Treatment of Pituitary Disease and Somatostatin Receptor Scintigraphy
Lamberts SWJ, Hofland LJ, de Herder WW, Kwekkeboom DJ, Reubi J-C, Krenning EP (Erasmus Univ, Rotterdam, The Netherlands; Univ of Berne, Switzerland)
Front Neuroendocrinol 14:27–55, 1993   124-95-12–3

Introduction.—Octreotide, a somatostatin analogue is effective in treating patients with pituitary tumors that secrete growth hormone (GH). However, its efficacy in controlling the pituitary secretion of thyroid-stimulating hormone, adrenocorticotrophic hormone (ACTH), and prolactin has not been adequately investigated. It should be possible to visualize most endocrine tumors with somatostatin receptors in high density in vivo through injection of a radionuclide-labeled somatostatin analogue.

Methods.—Scintigraphic visualization using ^{123}I-coupled [3]Tyr-octreotide was effective in localizing several endocrine tumors, including GH-secreting pituitary adenomas. This radionuclide, however, is difficult to obtain, store, and use, and it is prohibitively expensive. An alternative compound, which contains DTPA for binding ^{111}In, was even more effective in visualizing tumors with somatostatin receptors. It also was easier to use and more cost-effective.

Results.—Visualization of both a normal pituitary gland and a GH-secreting pituitary tumor in a patient with acromegaly was achieved using ^{111}In-DTPA-octreotide scintigraphy. When a GH-secreting tumor could not be visualized, the abnormally high GH levels could not be controlled by octreotide. Whole body scans localized rare ectopic tumors that were secreting GH-releasing hormone (GHRH). The [123]I-[3]Tyr-octreotide imaging clearly visualized uncommon pituitary adenomas that secreted thyroid-stimulating hormone in hyperthyroid patients who responded to octreotide therapy. Prolactin-secreting pituitary tumors could not be visualized, and they were not affected by octreotide therapy. Although ACTH-secreting pituitary tumors could not be visualized, ectopic sources of ACTH secretion in Cushing's syndrome could be localized, and octreotide therapy in these patients was successful.

Conclusion.—Good visualization with somatostatin receptor scintigraphy predicts the efficacy of octreotide therapy in treating patients with pituitary tumors that are secreting inappropriate amounts of GH or thyroid-stimulating hormone and in patients with ectopic ACTH-secreting tumors. Somatostatin receptor scintigraphy can also be used effectively to differentiate between GH- and ACTH-secreting pituitary tumors and ectopic GHRH- and ACTH-secreting tumors.

▶ The management of patients with the drug octreotide is presented in detail for pituitary tumors using high-density somatostatin receptors demonstrated by imaging. For example, octreotide therapy shrinks the tumor in about half the patients with acromegaly. This makes the tumor softer, so that it is easier to remove surgically. It is surprising that about 75% of clinically nonfunctioning adenomas can be visualized in images and that octreotide therapy may relieve chiasmal compression and improve visual acuity. These tumors compose about one third of all pituitary adenomas.—J.G. McAfee, M.D.

Use of Isotope-Labeled Somatostatin Analogs for Visualization of Islet Cell Tumors

van Eyck CHJ, Bruining HA, Reubi J-C, Bakker WH, Oei HY, Krenning EP, Lamberts SWJ (Erasmus Univ, Rotterdam, The Netherlands)
World J Surg 17:444–447, 1993   124-95-12-4

Objective.—In vitro autoradiographic studies demonstrate that most endocrine tumors show a high concentration of somatostatin receptors, in contrast to the virtual absence of binding sites in surrounding normal tissue. These findings agree with the clinical observation that tumor hormone secretion is suppressed after octreotide administration. The feasibility of in vivo detection of somatostatin receptor–positive tumors after administration of a radioactive iodine-labeled analogue was examined.

Methods.—Two isotope-labeled somatostatin analogues were injected intravenously into 25 patients with suspected somatostatin receptor-positive islet cell tumors. The analogues used were iodine-123 Tyr^3-octreotide in 9 patients and indium-111 octreotide in the remaining 16 patients. A gamma camera was used to make planar or SPECT images.

Results.—The imaging studies demonstrated the primary tumor—as well as distant metastases that were previously unrecognized in some cases—in 20 of 25 patients. Somatostatin receptors were also detected in vitro in these tumors, suggesting that the in vivo ligand binding to the tumor reflected binding to specific somatostatin receptors. In tumors with somatostatin receptors that were detected in vivo, octreotide had a good suppressive effect on hormonal hypersecretion.

Discussion.—Somatostatin receptor scintigraphy is a simple, painless, noninvasive technique for the diagnosis of islet cell tumors and carcinoids. It may be of considerable value in localizing primary tumors and metastases. Prospective studies are needed to compare this new method with other techniques and to establish its sensitivity and specificity.

▶ These authors concluded that the indium-111 (^{111}In)–labeled peptide is better than the iodine-123 peptide, because the liver, biliary excretion, gut, and thyroid activity is less with the former. Nonetheless, thyroid, gut, liver, spleen, and kidney activity is usually seen in 24-hour images with the ^{111}In peptide.

Of the 25 pancreatic endocrine tumors in this study, the sensitivity of detection of insulinomas (5 of 8) was not as high as in gastrinomas (10 of 11). Although SPECT imaging may be helpful, most tumors are well demonstrated on planar images, because the target-nontarget concentration ratios are so high. Unlike most published images of radiolabeled monoclonal antibodies, arrows are not needed here!—J.G. McAfee, M.D.

Octreotide Scintigraphy for the Detection of Paragangliomas
Kwekkeboom DJ, van Urk H, Pauw BKH, Lamberts SWJ, Kooij PPM, Hoogma RPLM, Krenning EP (Univ Hosp Dijkzigt, Rotterdam, The Netherlands)
J Nucl Med 34:873–878, 1993   124-95-12-5

Background.—Previous studies have accomplished the successful in vivo visualization of tumors of neuroendocrine origin, such as paragangliomas (formerly called glomus tumors) after injection of the radiolabeled somatostatin analogue octreotide. The results of in vivo indium-111 (^{111}In) octreotide scintigraphy were compared with the results of other techniques in 34 patients who were referred for known or suspected paragangliomas.

Method.—Thirty-four patients who received ^{111}In-octreotide scintigraphy were investigated. Participation in the study required either histologic or radiologic confirmation of a paraganglioma of a present or previously operated-on lesion or a history of paraganglioma-related signs and symptoms. The results of octreotide scintigraphy were compared with the outcomes of other imaging techniques used in the diagnosis or follow-up of these patients.

Results.—Fifty of 53 known localizations in 25 patients with paragangliomas were visualized by octreotide scintigraphy. The paragangliomas were identified in the carotid body, jugulotympanic parasympathetic paraganglia (Fig 12–5), and other sites. Three localizations were missed in 2 patients, probably because the tumors were too small or they had an ex-

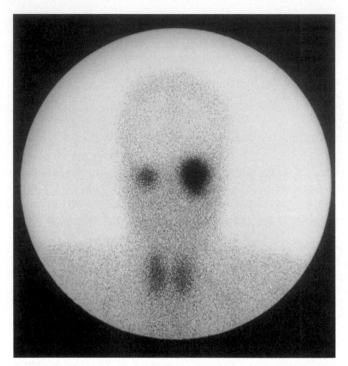

Fig 12–5.—Anterior image of the head and neck 24 hours after injection of ^{111}In-octreotide. There is normal accumulation of radioactivity in the thyroid and accumulation of radioactivity at the site of bilateral jugulotympanic paragangliomas. (Courtesy of Kwekkeboom DJ, van Urk H, Pauw BKH, et al: *J Nucl Med* 34:873–878, 1993.)

tremely low density of somatostatin receptors. Unexpected additional paraganglioma sites that had not been previously detected through conventional techniques were found in 9 of 25 patients. In 8 of 9 patients with suspected paragangliomas that had not shown up with routine screening, octreotide scintigraphy was also negative. Three patients showed signs of other diseases, indicating that octreotide scintigraphy can help distinguish paraganglioma from other lesions.

Conclusion.—Almost all paragangliomas can be visualized using in vivo ^{111}In-octreotide scintigraphy. Moreover, unlike conventional imaging, which is usually limited to the suspected site of the paraganglioma, octreotide scintigraphy provides information on potential tumor sites in the whole body; therefore, it has potential for detecting multicentricity or metastases in patients with paraganglioma.

▶ Indium-111 octreotide imaging is an important added diagnostic modality for these tumors, not only for the primary lesions, but for recurrences, metastases, and unsuspected multiple lesions. About 9% of these tumors are familial, 10% are multicentric, and about 10% are malignant. Postoperatively, recurrences or residual tumor are seen in about 10% of carotid body tumors and in 29% to 50% of jugulotympanic paragangliomas.

In 5 patients in this series who had known paragangliomas, meta-iodobenzylguanidine (MIBG) images were compared with the ^{111}In-octreotide images. In 1 of these patients, some lesions were not apparent in the MIBG study, and other lesions were faint. In keeping with the experience of others, labeled octreotide will probably prove superior to MIBG in demonstrating these tumors.—J.G. McAfee, M.D.

Somatostatin-Receptor Scintigraphy in Primary Breast Cancer
van Eijck CHJ, Krenning EP, Bootsma A, Oei HY, van Pel R, Lindemans J, Jeekel J, Reubi JC, Lamberts SWJ (Erasmus Univ, Rotterdam, The Netherlands; Univ of Berne, Switzerland)
Lancet 343:640–643, 1994   124-95-12–6

Background.—Primary cancers and metastases can be demonstrated by somatostatin-receptor (SS-R) scintigraphy in most patients with neuroendocrine tumors such as carcinoids, islet cell tumors, and paragangliomas. Somatostatin receptors have also been seen in human breast cancers, according to previous in vitro studies. The use of SS-R scintigraphy in 50 patients with breast cancer was assessed.

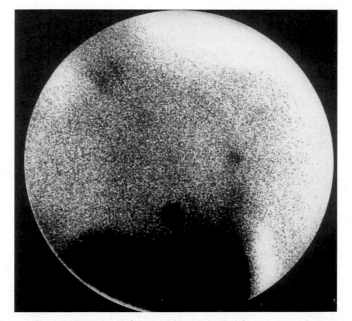

Fig 12–6.—Indium-111 DTPA-D-Phe[1])-octreotide scintigraphy of a patient, aged 39 years, showing breast cancer on the left side and axillary-node metastases. (Courtesy of van Eijck CHJ, Krenning EP, Bootsma A, et al: *Lancet* 343:640–643, 1994.)

Methods.—The patients were all cytologically confirmed as having breast cancer. All underwent scintigraphy using the somatostatin analogue [DTPA-D-Phe¹]-octreotide, in doses ranging from 200 to 272 MBq (5.4–7.3 mCi) of ultrapure indium-111. The value of this study in the detection of recurrent disease was compared with that of the serum markers carcinoembryonic antigen and CA15-3.

Results.—Scintigraphy was positive in 39 of 52 (75%) primary cancers. Eighty-five percent of the invasive ductal cancers were demonstrated compared with 56% of the invasive lobular carcinomas. Nonpalpable cancer-containing axillary lymph nodes were detected in 4 of the 13 patients with subsequently histologically proven metastases (Fig 12–6). In vivo positivity of the cancers was unrelated to patient age. Six of 28 patients with SS-R–positive primary cancers had recurrent disseminated breast cancer on SS-R scintigraphy; only 3 of these patients had abnormal serum cancer markers.

Conclusion.—Somatostatin-receptor scintigraphy appears to be effective in the early detection of SS-R–positive breast cancer recurrence. It may prove useful in the selection of patients for somatostatin analogue treatment and other forms of treatment. For patients with SS-R–positive breast cancers, it appears to be more sensitive than the usual serum cancer markers in detecting recurrences.

▶ This article did not discuss somatostatin receptors in benign breast lesions. With a detection sensitivity of 75% for primary breast carcinomas, ¹¹¹In-octreotide may not be useful in differentiating malignant from benign breast lesions. Although van Eijck et al. believe that octreotide will be of minor value in detecting axillary node involvement, this study indicated that images made with octreotide can detect unsuspected, symptom-free metastases.—J.G. McAfee, M.D.

The Role of Iodine-123-Tyr-3-Octreotide Scintigraphy in the Staging of Small-Cell Lung Cancer

Leitha T, Meghdadi S, Studnicka M, Wolzt M, Marosi C, Angelberger P, Neumann M, Schlick W, Kletter K, Dudczak R (Univ Clinics of Nuclear Medicine and Internal Medicine, Vienna; Austrian Research Ctr Seibersdorf, Austria; Ctr for Pulmonary Diseases, Vienna; et al)

J Nucl Med 34:1397–1402, 1993   124-95-12–7

Introduction.—The major prognostic factors in small-cell lung cancer (SCLC) are clinical performance status and the extent of tumor dissemination. Rapid identification of extensive disease in the staging workup would save further time-consuming examinations. The role of iodine-123 (¹²³I) Tyr-3-octreotide scintigraphy in staging SCLC, its ability to discriminate between limited and extensive disease stages, and its regional sensitivity for different metastatic locations were investigated.

Patients and Methods.—Twenty patients with histologically confirmed SCLC took part in the study. The diagnostic workup included chest films taken in 2 planes, bronchoscopy, thoracic CT scan, abdominal sonography, bone scanning within 4 weeks, and ^{123}I-Tyr-3-octreotide scintigraphy. The imaging protocol included dynamic (0–30 minutes post injection), static (30 minutes, 90 minutes, 4 hours, and 24 hours post injection), and SPECT (90 minutes post injection) studies.

Results.—Metastases were found in the lymph nodes in 15 patients, in bone in 4, in the liver in 2, and in the brain in 2; 5 patients had pleuropulmonal metastases. Clinical and radiologic staging classified 9 patients as having extensive disease and 11 as having limited disease. The primary tumor site was imaged best in the early planar images (15–30 minutes post injection) and by SPECT. Both methods were comparable in the number of scintigraphically positive results. However, the optimal imaging time and study type varied with each primary tumor, and 16 of 19 tumors were positive in at least 1 study. Although lymph node metastases were noted in 75% of patients, anatomical localization required the use of SPECT. Sequential planar images identified all 3 adrenal metastases. The sensitivity for bone metastases was 50%, and the sensitivity for pleuropulmonal metastases was 40%. Previous radiation therapy or chemotherapy appeared to have no effect on imaging results.

Conclusion.—The primary tumor was detected by ^{123}I-Tyr-3-octreotide scintigraphy in 84% of patients. Scintigraphy alone identified 7 of the 9 patients (78%) with extensive disease. When it is performed as the initial step in a staging workup, extensive disease can be quickly confirmed, further examinations foregone, and chemotherapy started without delay. However, this imaging method cannot substitute for liver sonography or conventional bone scanning in patients without scintigraphic evidence of distant tumor spread.

Somatostatin Receptor Imaging in Small Cell Lung Cancer Using ^{111}In-DTPA-Octreotide: A Preliminary Study

Maini CL, Tofani A, Venturo I, Pigorini F, Sciuto R, Semprebene A, Boni S, Giunta S, Lopez M ('Regina Elena' Natl Cancer Inst, Rome; 'C Forlanini' Hosp, Rome)
Nucl Med Commun 14:962–968, 1993   124-95-12–8

Introduction.—Small-cell lung cancer (SCLC) has a mortality of 87% and a median survival of 40 weeks for patients with disseminated disease. Prognostic factors previously identified include disease extent, sex, performance status, age, and tumor markers. Somatostatin (SS) receptors that are detected on biopsy specimens from patients with SCLC may be associated with less aggressive evolution. The results of SCLC scanning using indium-111 (^{111}In) octreotide were presented.

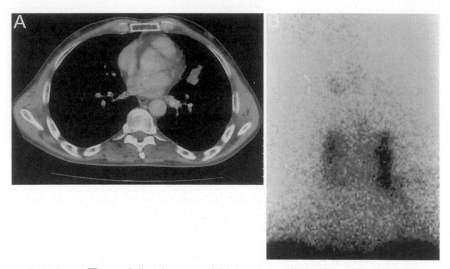

Fig 12–7.—A, CT scan of chest showing a solid 2.5-cm mass with irregular margins in the superior segment of the lingular lobe. **B,** ^{111}In-octreotide scan at 24 hours. Posterior view of thorax shows intense tracer uptake in both lungs, suggesting more extensive disease than did the CT scan. (Courtesy of Maini CL, Tofani A, Venturo I, et al: *Nucl Med Commun* 14:962–968, 1993.)

Patients and Methods.—Fifteen patients who ranged in age from 49 to 69 years underwent SS receptor imaging; all had histologically confirmed SCLC. Nine had undergone at least 1 cycle of chemotherapy, and 6 were studied before chemotherapy. The ^{111}In-DTPA-D-Phe-1-octreotide was injected as an IV bolus with an activity of 5 mCi (185 MBq). Acquisition was performed at 4 and 24 hours. Two independent observers rated uptake as absent, faint, moderate, or intense. Thirteen of the 15 patients had positive scans.

Results.—Two patients who had undergone chemotherapy showed no uptake on early or late scans. The tumor was visualized at 4 hours in all patients with a positive scan. The 24-hour scan yielded better images in 2 cases and worse images in 3. In general, the octreotide uptake was more extensive in these scans than was apparent at CT (Fig 12–7). None of the patients experienced side effects after injection of the radiopharmaceutical.

Conclusion.—Preliminary observations suggest that a more extensive disease and a worse evolution seem to be associated with the absence of SS receptors in patients with SCLC. Therefore, evaluation of SS receptor status may offer prognostic information in this aggressive tumor. Indium-111 octreotide can assess the SS receptor status of SCLC. Previous chemotherapy generally did not affect tumor visualization.

▶ This is a horrible disease because dissemination occurs so early, resulting in a 2-year survival of about 15% and a 5-year survival of about 2%. This type of lung cancer is almost unknown in nonsmokers. Unfortunately, most of the smoking public does not know this.

In the preceding article (Abstract 124-95-12-7), the greater gallbladder and bowel concentrations with the ^{123}I-octreotide analogue made detection of abdominal lesions more difficult than with ^{111}In-octreotide. Certainly, the ^{111}In compound is more practical. The advantage of this SS imaging for this neoplasm is the rapid detection of sites of dissemination by the total body imaging. As the authors point out, this imaging does not eliminate the need for bone or liver imaging, and it does not replace chest radiographs and CT studies.—J.G. McAfee, M.D.

Somatostatin Receptors in Meningiomas: A Scintigraphic Study Using ^{111}In-DTPA-D-Phe-1-Octreotide

Maini CL, Tofani A, Sciuto R, Carapella C, Cioffi R, Crecco M ('Regina Elena' Natl Cancer Inst, Rome)

Nucl Med Commun 14:550–558, 1993   124-95-12-9

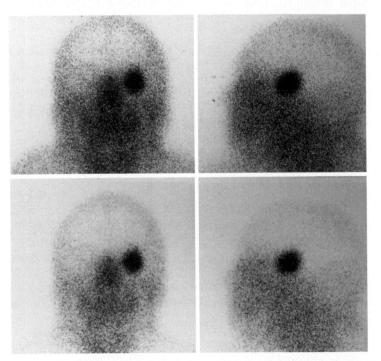

Fig 12–8.—Scintigraphic images recorded at 2 hours (**top**) and at 24 hours (**bottom**). Anterior (**left**) and left lateral (**right**) views are shown. The intense ^{111}In-octreotide uptake by the sphenoidal-ridge meningioma is clearly evident in the early scans, whereas the late scans do not add any new information. (Courtesy of Maini CL, Tofani A, Sciuto R, et al: *Nucl Med Commun* 14:550–558, 1993.)

Objective.—The somatostatin derivate DTPA-D-Phe-1-octreotide (Octreoscan), radiolabeled with indium-111 (^{111}In) chloride, was used to evaluate 12 patients with suspected meningioma, a tumor with high-affinity receptors for somatostatin. No previous study has reported meningioma scintigraphy using ^{111}In-labeled octreotide.

Patients and Methods.—The patients were 12 to 60 years of age. Eleven underwent surgery, and a histologic diagnosis was obtained. One patient had a very small tumor and was treated conservatively with 12-month follow-up. The tracer was injected as an IV bolus with an activity of 185 MBq. Planar images were obtained in 4 projections; acquisition was performed at 2 and 24 hours, with a preset time of 10 minutes and a matrix resolution of 512 × 512.

Results.—The ^{111}In-octreotide scans were positive in all 9 patients with histologic confirmation of meningioma. In all patients, the tumor was apparent at 2 hours, and 24-hour scans did not add information or increase the diagnostic quality (Fig 12–8). Scintigraphy also detected the small meningioma in the patient who did not undergo surgery. The ^{111}In-octreotide scintigraphy was negative in 2 patients, who were referred for differential diagnosis between acoustic neurinoma and meningioma. None of the patients experienced side effects after IV injection of the tracer.

Conclusion.—The high uptake of ^{111}In-octreotide demonstrated the suitability of this imaging method for in vivo visualization of somatostatin receptors. In 1 patient with meningioma, a marked thickening of the frontal theca prevented CT and MRI from visualizing the underlying tumor. Indium-111 octreotide scintigraphy is a safe, fast test that increases the diagnostic specificity of traditional neuroimaging.

▶ That meningiomas have a very high expression of somatostatin receptors came as a complete surprise to me and perhaps to others. Indium-111 octreotide imaging may not be indicated for uncomplicated meningiomas but to differentiate them from other intracranial tumors. Therapy of unresectable meningiomas may be attempted with the drug octreotide or with a radioisotopic analogue such as yttrium-90 octreotide.—J.G. McAfee, M.D.

A Ticket to Ride: Peptide Radiopharmaceuticals
Fischman AJ, Babich JW, Strauss HW (Massachusetts Gen Hosp, Boston; Harvard Med School, Boston)
J Nucl Med 34:2253–2263, 1993   124-95-12–10

Introduction.—Within recent decades, attempts to image patients using biospecific agents have progressed from large proteins and antibody fragments to smaller "molecular recognition units," including antigen-binding domain fragments and small, biologically active peptides. The use of smaller molecules provides higher target-to-background activity ratios and more rapid blood clearance.

Technical Aspects.—Modern molecular engineering methods make it possible for the peptide to carry the radionuclide-binding group in its structure while at the same time maintaining high-affinity binding to the receptor site. In addition to single-chain antigen-binding proteins, hypervariable-region peptide analogues and natural biologically active peptides have been used. Natural peptides of low and intermediate molecular weight may be more suitable for use as radiopharmaceuticals than antibodies. Short-lived nuclides such as technetium-99m are preferred.

Current Peptide Radiopharmaceuticals.—The somatostatin analogue octreotide has been used to image pancreatic and gastrointestinal tract endocrine tumors, which express somatostatin receptors. Chemotactic peptides may prove useful in detecting sites of focal infection. Technetium-labeled peptides of this type have proven to be excellent agents for use in imaging infection in a number of species.

Other Applications.—Growth factors, which are highly expressed in tumors and after injury, may prove to be useful imaging agents. It may be possible to design radiopharmaceuticals by independently manipulating segments of the reagent that regulate binding, radiolabeling, and biodistribution. The use of multiple binding determinants might enhance affinity.

▶ This is an excellent review article on the present and future applications of peptides and their analogues for radionuclide imaging. Because of the outstanding success of octreotide analogues for imaging neuroendocrine and other tumors, many believe that peptides will be more successful than radiolabeled monoclonal antibodies. More than 800 bioactive peptides are available commercially. The challenge is to select those that are capable of targeting specific receptors in vivo.—J.G. McAfee, M.D.

Phase II Scintigraphic Clinical Trial of Malignant Melanoma and Metastases With Iodine-123-N-(2-Diethylaminoethyl 4-Iodobenzamide)
Michelot JM, Moreau MFC, Veyre AJ, Bonafous JF, Bacin FJ, Madelmont JC, Bussiere F, Souteyrand PA, Mauclaire LP, Chossat FM, Papon JM, Labarre PG, Kauffmann P, Plagne RJ (INSERM U 71, Clermont-Ferrand, France; CHU Gabriel Montpied, Clermont-Ferrand, France; Centre Antoine Lacassagne, Nice, France; et al)
J Nucl Med 34:1260–1266, 1993   124-95-12–11

Background.—Preclinical studies have shown that [^{125}I]-N-(2-diethylaminoethyl) 4-iodobenzamide (BZA) may be a useful radiopharmaceutical in the management of patients with malignant melanoma. In a phase II clinical trial, iodine-123 (^{123}I) BZA was assessed as an imaging agent of primary melanomas and metastases.

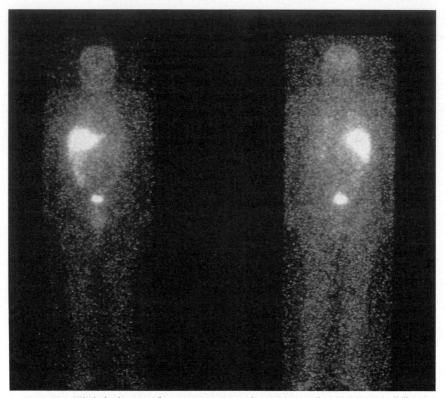

Fig 12–9.—Whole body scan of a group 3 patient taken 24 hours after IV injection of ¹²³I-BZA shows normal uptake in the liver and kidneys (**left,** anterior; **right,** posterior). (Courtesy of Michelot JM, Moreau MFC, Veyre AJ, et al: *J Nucl Med* 34:1260–1266, 1993.)

Patients and Methods.—One hundred ten patients aged 16–89 years with a history of melanoma were included. Investigations were conducted in 2 nuclear medicine departments. Patients were imaged 20–24 hours after the IV injection of 3.5 mCi (130 MBq) of ¹²³I-BZA.

Results.—No short- or long-term side effects were noted after injection. At 24 hours post injection, a considerable clearance of radioactivity from the blood pool was seen (Fig 12–9). Homogenous distribution of radioactivity was noted in the lung, liver, and intestinal tract, with occasional concentration in the gallbladder. The uptake in normal eyes was symmetric and weak. In 18 of 19 patients examined for suspected ocular melanoma, clear, intense, homogenous concentration in the pathologic eye was noted (Fig 12–10). In a patient who was treated for a primary ocular melanoma by surgery 6 years earlier, in situ orbital recurrence, multiple liver metastases, and diffuse bone infiltration were observed. The melanomatous nature of previously occult lesions was verified by clinical and/or laboratory findings in follow-up studies (Fig 12–11). In 44 patients who experienced clinical remission after treatment of malig-

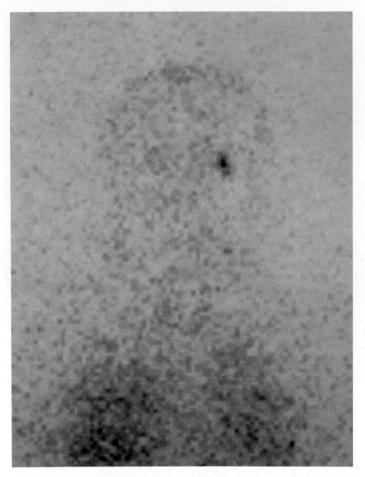

Fig 12–10.—Scan of the head (anterior) 24 hours after injection. Increased uptake is visible on the left eye. (Courtesy of Michelot JM, Moreau MFC, Veyre AJ, et al: *J Nucl Med* 34:1260–1266, 1993.)

nant melanoma and in 7 patients with nonmelanomatous disease, the scintigraphic results were normal. No false positive results were noted. Diagnostic sensitivity, accuracy, and specificity, which were calculated on a lesion-site basis, were 81%, 87%, and 100%, respectively.

Conclusion.—In patients with malignant melanoma, ^{123}I-BZA scintigraphy seems to be a safe and useful agent for detection and follow-up purposes.

▶ This agent appears to be very promising for detecting malignant melanoma. It is unfortunate that it concentrates mainly in the normal liver, a common site for metastases. Many stable drugs, particularly antipsychotics, are

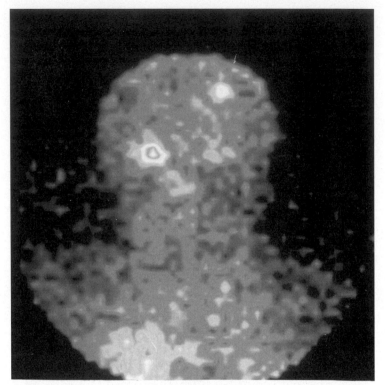

Fig 12–11.—Anterior scan of the head taken 22 hours after injection. Two lesions that could be brain metastases are visible. (Courtesy of Michelot JM, Moreau MFC, Veyre AJ, et al: *J Nucl Med* 34:1260–1266, 1993.)

iodobenzamides. The rationale for this imaging success is explained in the next article (Abstract 124-95-12–12).—J.G. McAfee, M.D.

A Malignant Melanoma Imaging Agent: Synthesis, Characterization, In Vitro Binding and Biodistribution of Iodine-125-(2-Piperidinylamino-ethyl)4-Iodobenzamide

John CS, Bowen WD, Saga T, Kinuya S, Vilner BJ, Baumgold J, Paik CH, Reba RC, Neumann RD, Varma VM, McAfee JG (George Washington Univ, Washington, DC; Natl Inst of Diabetes and Digestive and Kidney Diseases and Nuclear Medicine, Bethesda, Md)
J Nucl Med 34:2169–2175, 1993   124-95-12–12

Objective.—To develop improved radiopharmaceuticals with which to image malignant melanoma, both iodine-125 (^{125}I) and ^{131}I-labeled forms of 2-piperidinylaminoethyl)4-iodobenzamide (PAB) were developed. In vitro binding profiles were recorded for iodine-labeled PAB (IPAB) and for a structurally related analogue, N-(2-diethylaminoethyl)4-iodobenzamide (IDAB). In addition, biodistribution studies were performed in mice, and imaging studies were performed in nude mice bearing xenografts of human melanoma.

Results.—The in vitro binding profiles of IPAB and IDAB, which were determined using a variety of neurotransmitter receptors, indicated that both radiopharmaceuticals have high sigma-1 affinity and low affinity for sigma-2 sites. Competition binding studies of ^{125}I-PAB using a human malignant melanoma cell line showed the tracer to be bound to the cells with high affinity; the binding was saturable. Biodistribution studies in mice bearing xenografts of human malignant melanoma indicated good tumor uptake of ^{125}I-PAB. High tumor-to–nontarget organ ratios were recorded 24 hours after nuclide injection. Tumor images acquired at 24 hours clearly delineated the tumor; there was very little activity at other sites.

Conclusion.—Sigma-1 receptors may be used as external markers when using SPECT to image tumors (e.g., malignant melanoma) and characterize their molecular composition.

▶ This group discovered that certain radioiodinated iodobenzamides localize in sigma-1 and sigma-2 receptors that are normally present, particularly in normal brain, breast, liver, and kidney, as well as in high density in a variety of tumors including malignant melanomas. Their first compound (IDAB) is the same as I-BZA in the preceding article (Abstract 124-95-12–11), with a higher specific activity. In both melanotic and amelanotic melanoma xenografts in nude mice, another iodobenzamide (IPAB) achieved a higher tumor concentration than IDAP. The race is now on for synthetic chemists to develop even better agents of this class for localizing various neoplasms.

Another iodobenzamide, I-BZM, which was developed for brain imaging of dopamine receptors, is available commercially in Europe, but it has a low sensitivity for detecting melanomas such as meta-iodobenzylguanide (1). —J.G. McAfee, M.D.

Reference

1.   Hoefnagel CA, et al: *Eur J Nucl Med* 21:587, 1994.

Imaging Tumor Hypoxia and Tumor Perfusion

Groshar D, McEwan AJB, Parliament MB, Urtasun RC, Golberg LE, Hoskinson M, Mercer JR, Mannan RH, Wiege LI, Chapman JD (Cross Cancer Inst, Edmonton, Alta, Canada; Rebecca Sief Government Hosp, Safed, Israel; Univ of Alberta, Edmonton, Canada; et al)
J Nucl Med 34:885–888, 1993   1 2 4-95-1 2–1 3

Background.—It long has been recognized that inadequately oxygenated cells within some tumors may contribute to their resistance to irradiation and chemotherapy. Studies have shown that the binding of a

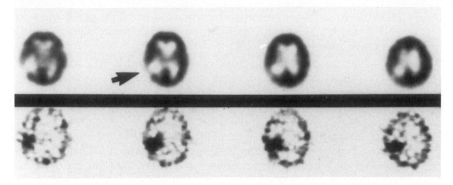

Fig 12–12.—Axial SPECT images of a patient with small-cell lung cancer brain metastasis. The HMPAO study (**top row**) shows decreased perfusion at the tumor site (**arrow**) with increased IAZA uptake (**bottom row**). (Courtesy of Groshar D, McEwan AJB, Parliament MB, et al: *J Nucl Med* 34:885–888, 1993.)

novel nitromisonidazole analogue, iodoazomycin arabinoside (IAZA), to EMT-6 cells is strongly dependent on the degree of hypoxia. Iodoazomycin arabinoside may be labeled with iodine-123 (^{123}I) and nuclide activity may be detected by planar scintigraphy or SPECT. Regional tissue perfusion, which can be assessed by technetium-labeled hexamethylpropyleneamine oxime (HMPAO), may also be an indicator of tissue viability.

Methods.—The distribution of HMPAO and IAZA was examined in 22 patients with a variety of tumors, including small-cell lung cancer, glioblastoma multiforme, squamous cell cancer of the head and neck, soft tissue sarcoma, and prostatic cancer. Twenty-seven tumors were examined using ^{123}I-IAZA and technetium-99m HMPAO as probes.

Findings.—Thirteen tumors (48%) exhibited increased uptake in IAZA images, and 1 had reduced uptake. In HMPAO images, 48% of tumors had decreased uptake and 26% showed increased uptake. The tumors with decreased HMPAO uptake tended to be IAZA-avid (Fig 12–12). None of the 4 glioblastomas were IAZA-avid, although all exhibited marked perfusion defects. Excluding these tumors, 89% of lesions with decreased HMPAO uptake exhibited increased IAZA uptake. Thirty-six percent of those with normal or increased HMPAO uptake were IAZA-avid.

Conclusion.—Measuring both HMPAO and IAZA in tumors may help in prescribing effective treatment.

▶ Radiolabeled misonidazole analogues have been studied since the mid-1970s to confirm the presence of hypoxic cells in tumors or ischemic myocardium. Their uptake probably reflects nitroreductase activity. Assessing the oxygenation status of tumors is of great interest in radiotherapy. Perfusion agents, such as technetium-99m HMPAO, cannot differentiate ischemic from necrotic areas in the brain, whereas IAZA localizes only in necrotic areas.

Iodoazomycin has successfully demonstrated thoracic and thigh malignancies as well (1). Images using SPECT are done 18–24 hours after 6 mCi of ^{123}I-IAZA. Nonetheless, there are practical disadvantages, including significant deiodination, and visualization of the thyroid, liver, and gut. Iodination at hospital sites for any ^{123}I radiopharmaceutical for imaging requires a shipment of 30 mCi at a cost of $100/mCi plus shipping and handling. At only 1 patient per shipment, that is a major expense.—J.G. McAfee, M.D.

Reference

1. Parliament MB, et al: *Br J Cancer* 65:90, 1992.

Selective Localization of a Radioiodinated Phospholipid Ether Analog in Human Tumor Xenografts
Plotzke KP, Fisher SJ, Wahl RL, Olken NM, Skinner S, Gross MD, Counsell RE
(Univ of Michigan, Ann Arbor; VA Med Ctr, Ann Arbor, MI)
J Nucl Med 34:787–792, 1993   124-95-12–14

Background.—Radioiodinated analogues of phospholipid ethers have been synthesized to assess their potential as noninvasive tumor-imaging agents. The capacity of $[^{125}I]$-*rac*-1-0-[12-(*m*-iodophenyl)dodecyl-2-0-methylglycero-3-phosphocholine (NM-294) to accumulate in various human tumor xenografts in athymic nude mice was investigated.

Methods and Findings.—Athymic mice that were implanted with human tumors of several histologies, including adenocarcinoma of the ovary and colon and melanoma and small-cell carcinoma of the lung, were given NM-294. Excellent tumor images were obtained using gamma camera scintigraphy. Tumor images were obtained at 5 days or more after injection when almost all background activity had cleared from the liver and gastrointestinal tract. At this time, tumor-blood ratios were very high, about 8:1, 17:1, and 30:1 in melanoma colon, and ovarian cancer, respectively. This is consistent with the scintigraphic images obtained in all human tumor models. Lipid extraction of the liver and tumor at 13 days after injection showed that most radioactivity in these tissues remained associated with the parent compound, with only a small amount retained by the liver.

Conclusion.—In athymic mice with human tumors, NM-294 was rapidly eliminated from the blood into the liver and then apparently redistributed into the kidney and intestine. In addition, NM-294 accumulated and was retained in various human tumors. Further research with NM-294 for eventual clinical evaluation is warranted.

▶ This is one of a series of papers on the development of these compounds for tumor imaging. Activity in the blood and viscera falls slowly, but the tumor-blood ratios are impressively high at 5 days. If these agents were used in humans, there would probably be an even longer wait for optimal tumor imaging.—J.G. McAfee, M.D.

Technetium-99m-Tetrofosmin as a New Radiopharmaceutical for Myocardial Perfusion Imaging
Kelly JD, Forster AM, Higley B, Archer CM, Booker FS, Canning LR, Chiu KW, Edwards B, Gill HK, McPartlin M, Nagle KR, Latham IA, Pickett RD, Storey AE, Webbon PM (Amersham Internatl plc, Buckinghamshire, England; Univ of North London; Royal Veterinary College, Hatfield, England)
J Nucl Med 34:222–227, 1993   124-95-12–15

Introduction.—The identification of superior technetium-99m (^{99m}Tc) cations for myocardial perfusion imaging has been the focus of many recent studies. It is possible that the introduction of heteroatomic functions may decrease the nontarget uptake of these compounds. Preclinical development of $[^{99m}Tc(tetrofosmin)_2O_2]^+$ (Fig 12–13) was reported.

Results.—Biodistribution was examined in rats and guinea pigs and revealed good uptake by the heart, with rapid clearance from blood and liver and no significant uptake by the lung. In the pig, the compound was excreted primarily through the hepatobiliary system. Acute toxicity studies in the rat demonstrated no toxicity at a dose equivalent to 400 times a single human dose or after 14 days at 100 times the human dose. No significant mutagenic potential was detected.

Conclusion.—This compound has been developed to provide excellent myocardial uptake with rapid background clearance. A lyophilized preparation provides the convenience of room-temperature reconstitution with 8 hours of stability. Clinical trials with this compound are now being performed.

▶ This new myocardial ^{99m}Tc complex is a diphosphinoethane compound and a close relative of an older agent known as DMPE. With alkyl phosphine complexes like DMPE, the blood clearance was slow, and the liver uptake was too high.

In this new complex, the dimethyl groups of DMPE were replaced by ether functional groups (ethoxyethane), resulting in faster blood clearance, lower

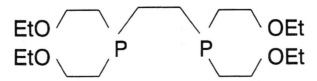

Fig 12–13.—Structure of the phosphine ligand tetrofosmin: 1,2-bis[bis(2-ethoxyethyl)phosphino]-ethane. (Courtesy of Kelly JD, Forster AM, Higley B, et al: *J Nucl Med* 34:222–227, 1993.)

liver and gastrointestinal concentrations, and higher cardiac uptake. Why didn't they call it EDEPE instead of tetrofosmin?—J.G. McAfee, M.D.

Biokinetics of Technetium-99m-Tetrofosmin: Myocardial Perfusion Imaging Agent: Implications for a One-Day Imaging Protocol

Jain D, Wackers FJT, Mattera J, McMahon M, Sinusas AJ, Zaret BL (Yale Univ, New Haven, Conn)
J Nucl Med 34:1254–1259, 1993   124-95-12–16

Purpose.—Stress radionuclide myocardial perfusion imaging is an integral part of the clinical evaluation of suspected or known coronary artery disease. The biokinetics of a new labeled myocardial perfusion imaging agent were evaluated after administration during exercise and at rest.

Methods.—The symptom-limited treadmill exercise was performed by 20 patients with suspected coronary artery disease. At peak exercise, 6–8 mCi of technetium-99m (^{99m}Tc) tetrofosmin was injected. After 4 hours of rest, 22–24 mCi was injected. Serial 5-minute planar images were obtained in the left anterior oblique view at 5, 10, 15, 30, 60, 120, and 180 minutes after injection. The average decay-corrected counts per pixel in the heart and other organs were plotted against time, and the heart-to–adjacent organ ratios were determined.

Results.—During stress imaging, the heart had the highest activity at all times, with the exception of the gallbladder, which had high activity for the first 15 minutes. During imaging at rest, the gallbladder, liver, and gastrointestinal tract initially had higher activity than the heart, but the activity in these nontarget organs cleared within the course of the subsequent 30–60 minutes (Fig 12–14). The heart-to–adjacent organ ratios were always greater than 1 during the stress images, and the heart-to–

SERIAL TETROFOSMIN IMAGES IN LAO VIEW

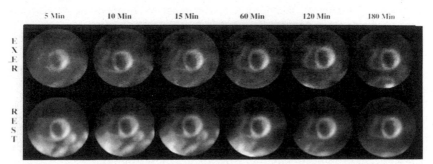

Fig 12–14.—Serial images in the left anterior oblique view after exercise and rest injections of ^{99m}Tc-tetrofosmin in patient with partially reversible septal and apical perfusion abnormality. Each image was obtained for 5 minutes. There is low subdiaphragmatic activity as early as 5 minutes after exercise injection. After rest injection, the first image shows significant hepatic activity, which rapidly clears and concentrates in the gallbladder. By 30 minutes, most subdiaphragmatic activity has cleared. (Courtesy of Jain D, Wackers FJT, Mattera J, et al: *J Nucl Med* 34:1254–1259, 1993.)

adjacent organ ratios were greater than 1 after the first 30 minutes during the rest images.

Conclusion.—Tetrofosmin images were of good to excellent quality, with good myocardial delineation and adequate contrast between the heart and background. Imaging can be initiated within 5 minutes after injection during exercise and within 30 minutes after injection during rest. Therefore, ^{99m}Tc-tetrofosmin may represent a significant advance in myocardial perfusion imaging.

▶ This is one of several ^{99m}Tc myocardial agents that theoretically should produce better images than thallium-201, but so far none has a normal myocardial clearance rate comparable to that of thallium. Teboroxime clears too quickly and the others clear too slowly, imposing time delays between studies and immediately after injection, waiting for hepatobiliary activity to clear.

Tetrofosmin is more convenient to prepare than sestamibi (no boiling required). In this article, good images were obtained after a 30- to 45-minute wait after stress injection but only 5 minutes after the injection during exercise.

More comparative studies of the new ^{99m}Tc agents are needed to test their efficacy in distinguishing reversible ischemic areas from irreversible, nonviable defects. In 1 study (1), sestamibi incorrectly identified 36% of myocardial defects as irreversible. They were subsequently found to be reversible by thallium redistribution/reinjection and by PET.—J.G. McAfee, M.D.

Reference

1. Dilsizian V, et al: *Circulation* 89:578, 1994.

Investigations of Ascorbate for Direct Labeling of Antibodies With Technetium-99m

Hnatowich DJ, Virzi F, Winnard P Jr, Fogarasi M, Rusckowski M (Univ of Massachusetts, Worcester)
J Nucl Med 35:127–134, 1994   124-95-12–17

Background.—In a recently described technique for directly labeling antibodies with technetium-99m (^{99m}Tc), sulfhydryls were generated by reduction of antibody disulfides with ascorbic acid. These proteins can then be labeled at high efficiency with ^{99m}Tc after reduction of pertechnetate with dithionite. The mechanism of the increased stability toward cysteine challenge reported for the label was assessed, and the role of ascorbate in the labeling process was determined.

Methods and Findings.—The reported high labeling efficiencies were reproduced by increasing the dithionite concentration fivefold, probably because of variations among lots of commercial sodium dithionite. Despite this success, antibody reduction after ascorbate treatment could not be confirmed. Using both Ellman's reagent and 2,2' dithiodipyridine as indicators, sulfhydryls could not be detected on 1 IgG antibody treated at 10 times the suggested ascorbate-to-antibody molar ratio. The number of sulfhydryls generated could not have been more than 1% or 2%. Also, radiolabeling efficiencies for 2 IgG antibodies and stabilities of the label to cysteine challenge did not change when the ascorbate was eliminated. The approximate number of sulfhydryls generated by antibody treatment with dithionite at 1 to 2 times the concentration needed for adequate labeling was 1% to 5%.

Conclusion.—Ascorbate played at best a minor role in the labeling process. Any antibody reduction was probably a result of residual dithionite presented to the protein along with the reduced ^{99m}Tc.

▶ There is still no universally accepted method for ^{99m}Tc labeling of monoclonal antibodies or other proteins with high stability, using either bifunctional chelates or "direct" labeling.

This is an excellent review of the direct approach, particularly the reduction methods for liberating endogenous sulfhydryl groups of protein molecules for chelation. These researchers successfully labeled a monoclonal antibody and polyclonal IgG with ^{99m}Tc and found dithionite to be important and ascorbate unimportant in the reduction step. However, their preparation is significantly different from the method of Thakur and colleagues, in which ascorbic acid is a major factor in the reduction (1–3).—J.G. McAfee, M.D.

References

1. Thakur ML, et al: *Nucl Med Biol* 18:227, 1991.
2. Thakur ML, et al: *J Immunol Methods* 137:217, 1991.
3. Thakur ML: Letter to the Editor. *J Nucl Med* (To be published).

Evidence for the Long-Term Biological Distribution of Technegas Particles

Burch WM (Australian Natl Univ, Canberra)
Nucl Med Commun 14:559–561, 1993   124-95-12–18

Background.—Technegas is a suspension of structured graphite ellipsoids labeled with technetium-99m in a carrier gas or argon. Its clinical use as a unique, dry, insoluble microaerosol for diagnostic lung imaging has expanded rapidly. The experimental evidence for predicting the fate of Technegas particles was reviewed.

Model.—A model that was originally developed for the kinetics of alveolobronchiolar transport of particles was validated experimentally. The 4 transport compartments identified were the mucociliary escalator, which showed clearance half-times to as long as a few hours; a surfactant-mediated movement along the lumen of the proximal respiratory bronchioles to the ciliated bronchi, resulting in a biphasic short-term clearance; centrilobular and peribronchial lymphatic drainage to the bronchial surface, for which a clearance half-time of at least 1 to 14 days would be needed; and trapping by subpleural, paraseptal, and perivascular lymphatics, from which clearance would be measured in months. These compartments are based on particles that do not swamp and occlude their respective conduits. Therefore, stated clearance times that are measured with large doses of insoluble aerosols should not be used.

Conclusion.—Although no exact parallel for Technegas exists, there is an extensive literature on associated aerosol behavior. Inhalation insults to the lung that deliver a mass of material many times greater than Technegas to the alveoli were well tolerated in human volunteers.

▶ As was lamented in last year's YEAR BOOK OF NUCLEAR MEDICINE (1), little progress has been made in obtaining Food and Drug Administration approval of Technegas either as a device or a radiopharmaceutical, despite its demonstrated safety and efficacy in improving the diagnosis of pulmonary embolism in more than 100,000 patient studies in other countries without a single adverse reaction. The regulatory concern is apparently based on the absence of metabolic breakdown of totally inert elemental carbon.

This article points out that some of the 50-μg dose of carbon inhaled during a Technegas diagnostic study is lost by bronchial drainage. This "dose" of elemental carbon is less than the amount of soot inhaled in a few hours in any industrialized city. Anyone who has attended an autopsy knows that human lungs are black from inhaled carbon and that the cut surfaces of draining lymph nodes exude black grit.

Regulatory policies in the United States are inconsistent. Sestamibi, which was only recently approved, is inert and is not metabolized but excreted. Elemental sulfur, which is administered intravenously in milligram quantities as technetium-99m sulfur colloid, is neither metabolized nor excreted.—J.G. McAfee, M.D.

Reference

1. 1994 YEAR BOOK OF NUCLEAR MEDICINE, p 108.

Synthesis and Labelling Characteristics of ^{99m}**Tc-Mercaptoacetyltripeptides**
Bormans G, Cleynhens B, Adriaens P, De Roo M, Verbruggen A (Inst of Pharmaceutical Sciences, KU Leuven, Belgium; Univ Hosp Gasthuisberg, Leuven, Belgium)
J Label Compound Radiopharmaceuticals 33:1065–1078, 1993
124-95-12-19

Introduction.—An intensive search for a technetium-99m (^{99m}Tc)–labeled alternative to radioiodinated Hippuran led to the development of some mercaptoacetyltriglycine derivatives in which 1 or more of the 3

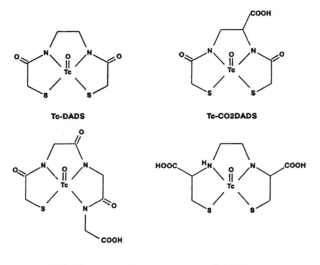

Fig 12–15.—Structure of 99mTc-N,N'-bis-(mercaptoacetamido)-ethylene diamine (*Tc-DADS*), 99mTc-N,N'-bis-(mercaptoacetyl)-2,3-diaminopropanoate (*Tc-CO2DADS*), 99mTc-mercaptoacetyltriglycine (*Tc-MAG₃*), and 99mTc-L,L-ethylene dicysteine (*Tc-L,L-EC*). (Courtesy of Bormans G, Cleynhens B, Adriaens P, et al: *J Label Compound Radiopharmaceuticals* 33:1065–1078, 1993.)

glycyl moieties are replaced by other amino acids (Fig 12–15). Mercaptoacetyltriglycine (99mTc-MAG₃) is now generally accepted as the best agent to use for routine renal imaging, to get relative renal function and transit time studies, and to estimate renal plasma flow.

Objective and Methods.—Fifteen derivatives of MAG₃ were synthesized in which 1, 2, or 3 glycyl groups were substituted by other amino acids including D- or L-alanine, D-serine, D-2-aminobutyric acid, D-valine, and D-phenylglycine. Because of the presence of a chiral carbon atom in the mercaptoacetyltripeptides, 99mTc labeling produced for each ligand a pair of diastereomers that were separable by reversed-phase high-pressure liquid chromatography.

Results.—Except for a serine derivative, all the 99mTc-labeled derivatives had longer retention times than the parent compound 99mTc-MAG₃. The relative amounts of the 2 diastereomers formed during labeling depended in part on the nature of the ligand, but they were influenced to a limited degree by the pH of the exchange labeling mixture.

▶ This group completed the monumental task of synthesizing and testing 15 analogues of MAG₃, which were different from the 12 analogues previously evaluated by Eshima, Taylor, and Fritsberg. It appears that none of these is superior to MAG₃. The separation of the diastereomers of these compounds for routine renal diagnostic studies is impractical.

This group has developed 99mTc–1,1-ethylene dicysteine (the diacid form of the brain agent ECD) as a renal imaging agent that has a faster clearance than MAG$_3$ (1). Although it will be marketed in Europe, unfortunately there are no plans to market it in the United States.—J.G. McAfee, M.D.

Reference

1. Van Nerom CG, et al: *Eur J Nucl Med* 20:738, 1993.

Chemistry and Biological Behavior of Samarium-153 and Rhenium-186–Labeled Hydroxyapatite Particles: Potential Radiopharmaceuticals for Radiation Synovectomy
Chinol M, Vallabhajosula S, Goldsmith SJ, Klein MJ, Deutsch KF, Chinen LK, Brodack JW, Deutsch EA, Watson BA, Tofe AJ (Long Island Jewish Med Ctr, New Hyde Park, NY; Mount Sinai Med Ctr, New York; Mallinckrodt Med Inc, St Louis, Mo; et al)
J Nucl Med 34:1536–1542, 1993   124-95-12–20

Background.—Although radiation synovectomy is effective, its safety has not been established definitively. The challenge remains to find an appropriate radiopharmaceutical. A new class of agents for radiation synovectomy that uses particles made from hydroxyapatite, a natural constituent of bone that is biologically compatible, has been developed. The safety of samarium-153 (^{153}Sm) and rhenium-186 (^{186}Re)–labeled hydroxyapatite particles in normal rabbits and rabbits with antigen-induced arthritis (AIA) was investigated.

Methods.—Particles were radiolabeled with ^{153}Sm or ^{186}Re. Their in vivo safety was assessed after intra-articular injection into the knees of normal rabbits and those with AIA.

Findings.—Radiolabeling efficiency exceeded 95%. In vitro studies showed a minimal loss of activity from particles over 6 days with ^{153}Sm-labeled hydroxyapatite and approximately 5% loss of activity over 5 days with ^{186}Re-labeled hydroxyapatite. The total cumulative extra-articular ^{153}Sm leakage over 6 days was .28% in normal rabbits and .09% in rabbits with AIA. Rhenium-186 leakage from the joint was 3.05% over 4 days, with 80% of extra-articular activity detected in the urine. Histopathologic assessment showed that hydroxyapatite particles were distributed throughout the synovium, where they were embedded in the synovial fat pad.

Conclusion.—This hydroxyapatite carrier is labeled easily and efficiently with ^{153}Sm and has a very low leakage rate from the joint. As a result, radiolabeled hydroxyapatite particles are an attractive candidate as a radiation synovectomy agent for intractable joint pain in patients with rheumatoid arthritis.

▶ These hydroxyapatite (HA) particles of controlled size (15–40 μm) seem ideal for radiation synovectomy, because HA is an endogenous substance that is capable of retaining ^{153}Sm until decay, but it is totally biodegraded by

6 weeks. Samarium-153 has a half-life of 1.95 days, a rather weak β-emission (β-max, .80 MeV), and a principal gamma emission of 103 KeV that is suitable for imaging. Would a stronger β-emitter, such as 2.7-day yttrium-90, be better (β-max, 2.27 MeV)?—J.G. McAfee, M.D.

Call Mosby Document Express at **1 (800) 55-MOSBY** to obtain copies of the original source documents of articles featured or referenced in the YEAR BOOK series.

13 Physics and Dosimetry

Introduction

As you can see, there have been some administrative changes under the new editorship of the YEAR BOOK OF NUCLEAR MEDICINE. The 2 chapters of Physics and Instrumentation and Health Physics have been combined into this 1 chapter entitled Physics and Dosimetry. Indeed, several times in the past, I found myself referencing back and forth between the 2 separate chapters (sometimes it is difficult to decide where to put an article). In this combined chapter, we strive to present technical issues that are closely associated with physics and instrumentation. Hopefully, the newest developments in reconstruction theory, instrument design, and associated health physics have been concisely reviewed here.

This year, the chapter has been loosely divided into 5 subsections. After a very interesting historic overview of instrument development in nuclear medicine, 3 articles deal with the ever-present problem of correcting for scatter in SPECT imaging. This reminds us that tomographic imaging in nuclear medicine continues to become more quantitative.

In the second subsection, 4 articles give highlights of new collimator geometries that are being developed, highlighting the impressive improvements in spatial resolution that SPECT has enjoyed. Reconstruction theory remains one of the most interesting fields of new development, as can be seen in the 4 articles included in the following group.

The dosimetry subsection of this chapter is further divided into 3 articles on specific radionuclides and their internal dose evaluations and 4 articles on general dosimetry updates.

Finally, it is a standing tradition to conclude this chapter with a report on unexpectedly interesting material used for dosimetry studies. In the past, we have found reports on sugar and tooth enamel, which were used to estimate exposure or dose. This tradition continues.

I. George Zubal, Ph.D.

Historic Perspective
Croll MN (Hahnemann Univ, Philadelphia)
Semin Nucl Med 24:3–10, 1994   124-95-13–1

Objective.—Because of the multidisciplinary nature of the specialty, it is difficult to write about the history of the instruments used in nuclear medicine. The sequence of events leading to the development of current nuclear medical instrumentation was reviewed.

History.—In the 1930s, John Lawrence was already treating patients with leukemia with phosphorus-32 at Berkeley, California. Not long after that came Fermi's achievement of a sustained nuclear reaction. This led to the Manhattan Project, which developed the bombs that were dropped at Hiroshima and Nagasaki. The Atomic Energy Commission was created in 1946. The same year, a New York internist named Sam Seidlin described the successful treatment of thyroid metastases using iodine-131. The Atomic Energy Commission's goals became twofold: to build bombs under utmost secrecy and to provide radioisotopes for cancer treatment with the greatest possible publicity.

The rectilinear scanner developed by Benedict Cassen at the University of California at Los Angeles was followed shortly by the development of the gamma scintillation camera by Hal O. Anger. The Anger camera soon became the primary instrument for nuclear medicine imaging. Additional cameras with different methods of operation began to appear, including Bender's digital autofluoroscope, Kuhl's efforts in tomographic imaging, and the development of SPECT. Anger first proposed and developed the idea of a positron camera, with PET eventually becoming commercially available in 1985.

Summary.—A review of the history of nuclear medical instrumentation—from the first sustained nuclear reaction to the development of PET—demonstrates that the development of this sophisticated technology owes a great deal to the work of pioneers in a number of related fields.

▶ The lead article in volume XXIV of *Seminars in Nuclear Medicine* gives a historic perspective on the development of nuclear medicine camera systems. The complete volume contains so many excellent individual articles that it is difficult to extract any one of them for review in the YEAR BOOK OF NUCLEAR MEDICINE. Therefore, I extracted the lead article and urge you to read the other 7 articles in this issue. They cover topics from planar imaging to convergent-beam collimation, to quantitative tomography, to networks and use of personal computers, with 2 articles devoted to the new cardiac procedures. This issue is a handy combination of overviews on both historical evolution and more recent developments in nuclear imaging techniques. It's worth putting on the shelf next to your textbooks.—I.G. Zubal, Ph.D.

Comparison of Four Scatter Correction Methods Using Monte Carlo Simulated Source Distributions

Ljungberg M, King MA, Hademenos GJ, Strand S-E (Univ of Lund, Sweden;

Univ of Massachusetts, Worcester)
J Nucl Med 35:143–151, 1994   124-95-13-2

Background.—In SPECT, scatter correction is important to improve image quality, boundary detection, and quantification of activity in different areas. Four scatter correction techniques were compared.

Methods.—Three methods using more than 1 energy window and 1 convolution-subtraction correction technique with spatial variant scatter line-spread functions were compared. Monte Carlo simulated data for point sources on- and off-axis, hot and cold spheres of different diameters, and a realistic source distribution that simulated brain imaging were used.

Findings.—Image quality and quantification were significantly improved by all correction methods compared with uncorrected images. No single technique was quantitatively better than the others when it was judged by all criteria for all source distribution. Three methods performed best when judged by at least 1 criterion for 1 of the source distributions. The differences among methods in brain imaging were much smaller than the difference between correction and no correction.

Conclusion.—Scatter correction is essential for accurate quantification of SPECT images. All 4 methods tested resulted in a good, although imperfect, scatter correction. Perhaps the choice of method should be based on its ease of use.

▶ There are at least 2 good reasons for selecting this article. First, it demonstrates the power of Monte Carlo simulations, which enable us to conduct measurements while easily accessing important experimental parameters. Such Monte Carlo calculations are coming into wider use because of the incredible speed and easy access to fast number-crunching computers. Second, the simulations presented here allow for a "fair" comparison of 4 different scatter correction techniques. Understanding the differences in the images caused by scatter subtraction corrections is important when implementing these techniques on clinical data; here is the "purest" form of that comparison.—I.G. Zubal, Ph.D.

Compton Scatter Compensation Using the Triple-Energy Window Method for Single- and Dual-Isotope SPECT

Ichihara T, Ogawa K, Motomura N, Kubo A, Hashimoto S (Toshiba Nasu Works, Tochigi-ken, Japan; Hosei Univ, Tokyo; Keio Univ, Tokyo)
J Nucl Med 34:2216–2221, 1993   124-95-13-3

Background.—Quantitative gamma camera–based SPECT studies may be complicated by Compton-scattered photons mixing into the preset energy window as well as by attenuation of photons within the body. Most of the scattered photons in the main window are single-scatter

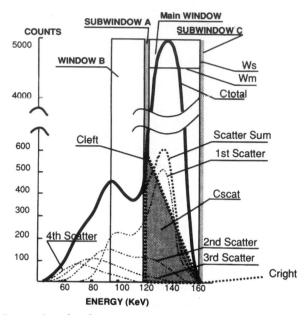

Fig 13–1.—Position-dependent Compton-scatter compensation method (TEW method) and a simulated energy spectrum of ⁹⁹ᵐTc using Monte Carlo modeling. Shown are the total energy spectrum (*total*), the first- to fourth-order scattering (*1st Scatter, . . ., 4th Scatter*), and sum of all orders of scattering (*Scatter Sum*). Most of the scattered photons in the main window are first-order scattered photons. To reduce scattered photons accurately, it is necessary to estimate the scatter sum in the main window, which is shown as a *shaded triangle,* using the counts in narrow scatter rejection windows A and C, adjacent to the main window. (Courtesy of Ichihara T, Ogawa K, Motomura N, et al: *J Nucl Med* 34:2216–2221, 1993.)

photons, making it necessary to estimate single-scatter intensity for each pixel. A Monte Carlo modeling method sometimes has been used to determine the distribution of scattered photons.

Objective and Method.—A triple-energy window (TEW) method was developed to determine position-dependent Compton scatter. Spatially dependent energy spectra were acquired and scattered photon components estimated for each region. The total values for 3 energy windows of the spectra were used rather than obtaining full-energy spectra. The count of primary photons at each pixel in the acquired image was estimated with the 24% main window centered at the photopeak energy and 3-keV scatter rejection windows on both sides of the main window.

Evaluation.—Energy spectra of primary and Compton-scattered photons were determined for a technetium-99m (⁹⁹ᵐTc) line source at the center of a 20-cm-diameter water-filled cylindrical vessel (Fig 13–1). In a preliminary clinical trial in which scatter compensation was examined for myocardial imaging using ⁹⁹ᵐTc-labeled tetrofosmin, the TEW method accurately compensated for Compton scatter.

Conclusion.—The TEW method is a relatively simple means of compensating for Compton scatter in quantitative isotope studies.

▶ Building on the knowledge contained in the previous article (Abstract 124-95-13-2), the data presented here include clinical results and may be considered the scatter subtraction technique that works best in the real world. It allows for imperfect energy resolution of the camera, septal penetration through collimators, and downscatter from higher-energy emissions. The figure included is a handy reference that reminds us of the contribution of higher-order scatters into typical energy windows.—I.G. Zubal, Ph.D.

A Transmission-Dependent Method for Scatter Correction in SPECT

Meikle SR, Hutton BF, Bailey DL (Royal Prince Alfred Hosp, Sydney, Australia)
J Nucl Med 35:360–367, 1994   124-95-13-4

Purpose.—The main factors that limit accuracy in SPECT are attenuation and Compton scattering. Transmission measurements, which are used along with iterative correction techniques, can sufficiently overcome the problem of attenuation. A number of different methods of compensating for scatter have been described, but they have been for dealing with complex scattering in objects of heterogenous density such as the chest. A scatter compensation technique that incorporates planar

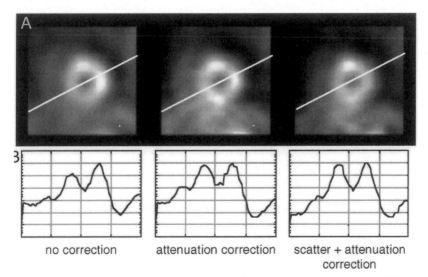

no correction   attenuation correction   scatter + attenuation
                                                    correction

Fig 13-2.—A, short-axis reconstructions of a clinical ²⁰¹Tl myocardial perfusion study and (**B**) corresponding count profiles along the line indicated through the myocardium. The images were processed using no scatter or attenuation correction (*left*), attenuation correction only (*middle*), and scatter correction followed by attenuation correction (*right*). Both scatter and attenuation correction methods incorporated transmission data that were acquired simultaneously with the emission data using a scanning collimated line source. (Courtesy of Meikle SR, Hutton BF, Bailey DL: *J Nucl Med* 35:360–367, 1994.)

transmission measurements in the estimation of photopeak scatter in SPECT was described.

Methods.—The new technique starts by estimating scatter distribution by convolving the planar projections with a monoexponential scatter function. Scatter fraction, which is defined as the number of scattered events that reach the detector as a proportion of total events, is determined for each point in the projections on the basis of narrow-beam transmission values that are obtained using an external source. To test the assumptions of the method, technetium-99m (^{99m}Tc) and thallium-201 (^{201}Tl) point and line sources were used. Realistic phantom experiments—simulating blood pool, lung, and myocardial perfusion studies—were performed to examine the quantitative and qualitative impact of transmission-dependent scatter correction.

Results.—In a variable-density phantom, the new technique accurately predicted scatter distribution from both ^{99m}Tc and ^{201}Tl line sources. Failure to remove scattered events from the projections before attenuation correction resulted in artificially enhanced reconstructed counts in area of high tissue density. Scatter was quantified with 95% or better accuracy in the heart and lungs using transmission-dependent scatter correction (Fig 13-2); by contrast, use of convolution-subtraction with a constant scatter fraction underestimated scatter in the heart and overestimated it in the lungs.

Conclusion.—With this new method, incorporating transmission data permits accurate scatter compensation in SPECT studies of objects of nonuniform density. So far, the method has been developed for use with ^{99m}Tc and ^{201}Tl sources, and it could be extended to other radionuclides as well.

▶ Here is a most intriguing new combination: the use of transmission images and applying scatter correction for SPECT. Transmission data have conventionally been applied for improved attenuation corrections. Of course, it is obvious that heterogenous densities within the object require heterogenous attenuation corrections. However, a more subtle realization is that heterogenous densities also influence the scatter correction techniques currently applied for SPECT. To my knowledge, that insight, together with a clinical example, is shown for the first time in this article. We see that heterogenous attenuation corrections (based on transmission images) are slowly becoming an accepted routine in SPECT tomography of the thorax.—I.G. Zubal, Ph.D.

Pinhole Collimation for Ultra-High-Resolution, Small-Field-of-View SPECT

Jaszczak RJ, Li J, Wang H, Zalutsky MR, Coleman RE (Duke Univ, Durham, NC)

Phys Med Biol 39:425–437, 1994   124-95-13–5

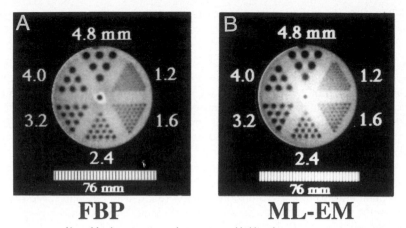

FBP   ML-EM

Fig 13–3.—**A,** filtered back-projection and **B** maximum likelihood–expectation maximization reconstructed transaxial images of the micro-cold-rod phantom. (Courtesy of Jaszczak RJ, Li J, Wang H, et al: *Phys Med Biol* 39:425–437, 1994.)

Background.—When imaging small objects such as animals in a laboratory, pinhole collimation may be preferable to conventional parallel-hole collimation. Geometric sensitivity increases for points close to the pinhole, making small-diameter and high-magnification pinhole geometries useful when using a large-field-of-view scintillation camera. Large magnification minimizes the loss of system resolution that is inherent in use of a scintillation camera.

Objective.—The concept of small-field-of-view, ultra-high-resolution pinhole collimation was applied to a rotating-camera SPECT system used to image small animals in the laboratory.

Method.—A pinhole collimator was designed to be mounted on 1 scintillation camera of a triple-headed SPECT system. Three pinhole inserts that had aperture diameters of approximately .6, 1.2, and 2 mm could be individually mounted on the collimator housing. A ramp filter was used with a 3-dimensional cone-beam filtered back-projection algorithm.

Results.—All the pinhole apertures improved spatial resolution compared with a parallel-hole collimator. Reconstructed SPECT resolutions for the .6-, 1.2-, and 2-mm pinhole apertures were 1.5, 1.9, and 2.8 mm, respectively. The 1.6-mm-diameter rods of a micro-cold-rod phantom were clearly visualized (Fig 13–3). Pinhole SPECT bone scans of rats demonstrated the skull bones and mandible. The anatomy of the liver was well visualized; areas that lacked activity represented vascular structures.

Conclusion.—Pinhole SPECT using ultra-high-resolution equipment is a simple and inexpensive means of imaging small animals in the laboratory that may be applied to existing rotating-camera SPECT systems. This method may prove especially useful for imaging nuclides such as iodine-131 that emit high-energy photons, because it minimizes septal penetration.

▶ Advances in SPECT imaging have prompted developments in design and application of nonparallel collimation geometries. Of particular interest is the pinhole collimator, which when used for SPECT imaging, gives incredibly high spatial resolution. Note that the resolution in the images shown in Figure 13–3 is better than the physical limitation of PET imaging. This is exciting proof that SPECT imaging can do better than PET in regard to spatial resolution.

This article also leads me to recommend an article in the March 1994 issue of *Physics in Medicine and Biology*. It is among many in this special edition dedicated to fully 3-dimensional image reconstruction, and it represents a concise accumulation of the newest techniques in volumetric imaging in nuclear medicine.—I.G. Zubal, Ph.D.

Fan-Beam Reconstruction Algorithm for a Spatially Varying Focal Length Collimator
Zeng GL, Gullberg GT, Jaszczak RJ, Li J (Univ of Utah, Salt Lake City; Duke Univ, Durham, NC)
IEEE Trans Med Imaging 12:575–582, 1993   124-95-13–6

Background.—The fan-beam collimator is used in SPECT studies to enhance sensitivity when imaging small organs, but projection data surrounding the site of interest are truncated. One possible solution to this problem is to use a spatially varying focal-length fan-beam collimator, which is designed so that the shortest focal lengths are at the center of the collimator and the longest one is at the periphery.

A New Approach.—A convolution back-projection algorithm was developed for a spatially varying focal-length fan-beam collimator, assuming that the focal length increases monotonically toward the edge of the collimator (Fig 13–4). The reconstruction algorithm is expressed as an infinite series of convolutions followed by a single back-projection. After the weighting and convolution are performed N times, N convolved projections are summed and 1 back-projection is performed, yielding the final reconstructed image.

Results.—Simulation studies showed that only a small number of N terms are needed to obtain high-quality reconstructions. When testing the algorithm for 2 spatially varying focal-length formulations, a singular artifact was apparent when the focal-length function was not smooth. For smooth functions, however, the reconstructions were free of artifact.

▶ The advantages of high sensitivity for fan-beam collimators is counterbalanced by their small field of view, which can lead to truncation artifacts. Lower-sensitivity, parallel-hole collimators have the advantage of larger fields

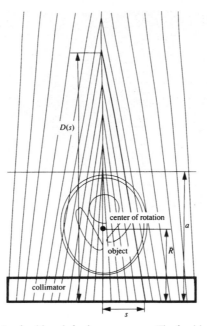

Fig 13–4.—Spatially varying focal-length fan-beam geometry. The focal length $D(s)$ increases as (s) increases. The distance from any part of the object to the collimator is always less than a for each projection angle and $D(s)$ is not less than a. (Courtesy of Zeng GL, Gullberg GT, Jaszczak RJ, et al: *IEEE Trans Med Imaging* 12:575–582, 1993.)

of view. This collimator is in effect a hybrid of these 2 geometries and represents, in my view, the most intriguing new development in collimator design associated with SPECT imaging.—I.G. Zubal, Ph.D.

A Cone Beam SPECT Reconstruction Algorithm With a Displaced Center of Rotation

Li J, Jaszczak RJ, Wang H, Gullberg GT, Greer KL, Coleman RE (Duke Univ, Durham, NC; Univ of Utah, Salt Lake City)
Med Phys 21:145–152, 1994   124-95-13–7

Objective.—Two major types of misalignments can lead to image artifacts in cone-beam SPECT: mechanical shift, which is the displacement of the midplane of the cone-beam geometry off the mechanical center of rotation, and electronic shift, which is the electronic centering misalignment. The 2 orthogonal components of mechanical shift are the shift of the midplane of the cone-beam collimator along the axis of rotation and the distance between the midline of the cone-beam collimator and the axis of rotation. A reconstruction algorithm for a cone-beam geometry with a displaced center of rotation has been developed.

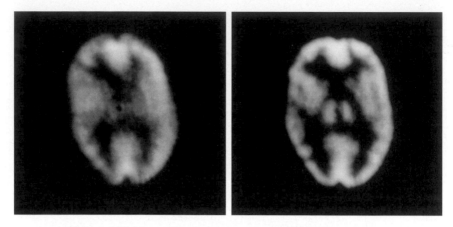

Without MS correction   With MS correction

Fig 13–5.—Transverse sectional images of the experimentally acquired Hoffman brain phantom. The image on the **left** is obtained without mechanical shift (MS) correction and the image on the **right** was obtained with MS correction. (Courtesy of Li J, Jaszczak RJ, Wang H, et al: *Med Phys* 21:145–152, 1994.)

Findings.—The algorithm directly corrects for mechanical shift by incorporating it into the algorithm. Both Monte Carlo simulations and experimental data indicated that the algorithm improved the distortions and artifacts caused by mechanical shift and improved image resolution (Fig 13–5). It also corrects for the blurring and "doughnut"-type artifacts caused by system mechanical shift. It cannot, however, correct for the insufficient sampling of planar-orbit cone-beam tomography.

Conclusion.—A cone-beam SPECT reconstruction algorithm that corrects directly for mechanical shift was described and evaluated. The shift for which the algorithm is designed is angular-independent; it is not applicable to angular-dependent cases.

▶ We have followed cone-beam SPECT reconstruction algorithm development over the past few years. Until now, the mathematics of fully 3-dimensional reconstructions have been outlined and grappled with. A sign of maturity is to see that center of rotation artifacts are currently being investigated for cone-beam geometries.

However well developed the reconstruction mathematics has become, the clinical use of cone-beam collimators has not yet made a strong impact in clinical nuclear medicine. Perhaps 1 reason for this is that cone-beam collimation was first developed, in part, to increase the sensitivity of single-headed SPECT cameras. I cannot help but observe that sensitivity improvements have been accomplished by the most straightforward method: tripling the number of cameras on the gantry. Because cone-beam collimation methods seem to have matured, it will be interesting to see whether they find routine application in clinical nuclear medicine.—I.G. Zubal, Ph.D.

A Scanning Line Source for Simultaneous Emission and Transmission Measurements in SPECT

Tan P, Bailey DL, Meikle SR, Eberl S, Fulton RR, Hutton BF (Royal Prince Alfred Hosp, Sydney, Australia; Univ of New South Wales, Sydney, Australia)
J Nucl Med 34:1752–1760, 1993   124-95-13–8

Background.—Incorrect compensation for photon attenuation is a major source of qualitative and quantitative inaccuracy in SPECT. A number of algorithms can achieve qualitative accuracy when they are combined with transmission measurements; however, clinical application of transmission-based quantitative SPECT requires the ability to acquire both emission and transmission data within a reasonable time. A scanning collimated line source for simultaneous acquisition of emission and transmission data has been developed.

Findings.—The microprocessor-controlled line source includes hardware that electronically windows the spatial gamma camera signal (Fig 13–6), separating the emission signals of the patient from the transmission signals of the line source. The advantages of the line source vs. previously described techniques using a flood source are that the transmission radionuclide need not have a lower energy than the emission radionuclide; narrow-beam, scatter-free attenuation measurements can be made; and the radiation exposure to staff is reduced. Measured attenuation coefficients for an elliptical water-filled phantom were $\mu = .15$ cm^{-1}. The technique was validated in both phantom and human studies using various radionuclide combinations and imaging geometries. The results were comparable using separate and simultaneous acquisitions.

Discussion.—The collimated scanning transmission line source permits accurate measurements of a narrow-beam attenuation coefficient of the object being studied, with simultaneous measurement of emission photons. The combination of emission and electronic collimation to separate the emission and transmission data permits much greater flexibility in the combinations of transmission and emission nuclides that can be used. Finally, transmission measurements can be acquired in a practi-

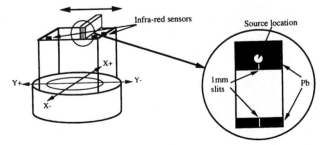

Fig 13–6.—Detail of the line-source collimation. The minimum thickness of lead is equivalent to 3 tenth-value layers for technetium-99m photons. (Courtesy of Tan P, Bailey DL, Meikle SR, et al: *J Nucl Med* 34:1752–1760, 1993.)

cal time frame, which is essential for the quantitative clinical use of SPECT.

▶ Today, a commercial 3-headed SPECT camera can be purchased with the option of using 1 head for transmission scanning. The geometry on these commercially available units uses a stationary rod source in conjunction with a fan-beam collimator whose line of focus corresponds to the position of the rod source.

An alternative to buying multiheaded SPECT cameras mounted with non-parallel collimators was demonstrated in this article. The ingenious method of electronic collimation that separates the emission from transmission gammas is noteworthy. Because cost reduction continues to be an ever more prevalent force in health care, such developments hold a real potential for use in smaller departments.—I.G. Zubal, Ph.D.

Rapidly Converging Iterative Reconstruction Algorithms in Single-Photon Emission Computed Tomography
Wallis JW, Miller TR (Washington Univ, St Louis, Mo)
J Nucl Med 34:1793–1800, 1993   124-95-13–9

Introduction.—A number of iterative reconstruction methods have been described to reduce noise, enhance resolution, and improve attenuation compensation, thereby improving image quality in SPECT. However, many of these algorithms are very time-consuming, which limits their clinical application. A number of new iterative reconstruction methods were described and evaluated.

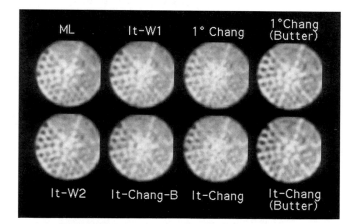

Fig 13–7.—Images of the Jaszczak phantom, presented after regularization to equivalent noise levels. Images marked *Butter* were smoothed with a fifth-order Butterworth filter; all other images were regularized with a gaussian filter (slight truncation at the image edge results from the FIR filter used). Note the similarity of the ML and iterative W2 (It-W2) images, despite the markedly fewer iterations required by It-W2. (Courtesy of Wallis JW, Miller TR: *J Nucl Med* 34:1793–1800, 1993.)

Methods.—Many of the iterative algorithms represented feedback loops, in which projections were generated from the current estimate and compared with measured projections. Some of the methods used a ramp filter during back-projection; the type of back-projection weighting varied, and sometimes camera and collimator blur were used in the projection step. The properties of convergence and resolution in reconstructions performed by maximum likelihood (ML), iterative Chang, and the newly proposed iterative algorithms were compared using simulated and real cylindrical phantoms with rod inserts. Kernel-sieve regularization was used to standardize the signal-to-noise ratio.

Results.—Techniques using a ramp demonstrated much faster conversion than ML reconstruction. One ramp method yielded images with the same resolution and noise as ML, which allowed the reconstruction to be terminated at 14 iterations compared with 1,000 with ML (Fig 13–7). An accurate model of the gamma camera imaging process in the projection step and the inclusion of attenuation weighting and depth-dependent blur in the back-projection step were the main determinants of resolution.

Conclusion.—A new iterative reconstruction method was described that achieved results comparable to those of ML reconstruction about 80 times faster. The new method incorporates attenuation and blur and uses a ramp filter. Visually and quantitatively, the results are nearly identical to those of the ML technique.

▶ Three recent developments in nuclear medicine have bootstrapped each other's progress in the last few years: faster computers, heterogenous attenuation correction, and iterative reconstruction algorithms. A new development in 1 aspect of this trio is caused by (and enhances) improvements in the remaining 2. Speeding up the convergence of iterative reconstruction algorithms is an important contribution to these recent developments. An additional insight was the comparison of image quality that was noted in some of the current iterative methods.—I.G. Zubal, Ph.D.

Artificial Neural Networks for Single Photon Emission Computed Tomography: A Study of Cold Lesion Detection and Localization
Tourassi GD, Floyd CE Jr (Duke Univ, Durham, NC)
Invest Radiol 28:671–677, 1993   124-95-13–10

Background.—The use of artificial neural networks in diagnosis in medical imaging has received much attention recently. An artificial neural network for cold lesion detection and localization in SPECT images was developed.

Methods and Findings.—The network was trained for several noise levels and lesion sizes to identify lesions in the middle of small-image neighborhoods. The network could identify cold abnormalities when it was scrolled across an image. Diagnostic performance was assessed at 2 noise levels and 2 lesion sizes using the free-response operating characteristic (FROC) analysis. The network was also tested in a situation for which it was not trained. A high sensitivity and low false positive rate per image were associated with the neural network for all test situations.

Conclusion.—Neural networks are promising for computer-aided clinical diagnosis in SPECT. This network was associated with a high sensitivity and low false positive rate per image in all test situations.

▶ Within the past several years, we have noticed an increased interest in iterative reconstruction methods over filtered back-projection algorithms. I believe we're seeing a third technique evolving for reconstructing images from projections: artificial neural networks. The use of neural networks as a reconstruction scheme is in its fledgling state, but it is a very exciting application for this still-evolving field. In the future, I think we can expect to see more development in neural networks for image reconstruction; I believe these are the first results of very interesting things to come.—I.G. Zubal, Ph.D.

Effect of Motion on Thallium-201 SPECT Studies: A Simulation and Clinical Study
Prigent FM, Hyun M, Berman DS, Rozanski A (Cedars-Sinai Med Ctr, Los Angeles; Univ of California, Los Angeles)
J Nucl Med 34:1845–1850, 1993   124-95-13–11

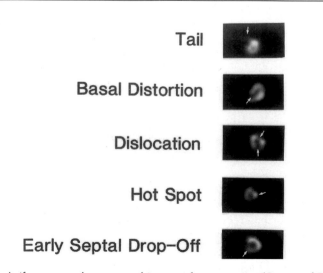

Tail

Basal Distortion

Dislocation

Hot Spot

Early Septal Drop–Off

Fig 13–8.—Artifacts commonly encountered in cases of severe motion. (Courtesy of Prigent FM, Hyun M, Berman DS, et al: *J Nucl Med* 34:1845–1850, 1993.)

Introduction.—Patient motion during acquisition of thallium-201 (^{201}Tl) SPECT studies is a potential source of artifacts and can produce false positive results. However, the effects of patient motion on test specificity are unknown. A simulation study was conducted to determine the effects of different motion patterns and the resultant artifacts.

Methods.—Seventy-four different motion patterns were simulated on a representative normal stress-redistribution ^{201}Tl SPECT study by moving 1 or more multiples of the original projections for a varying number of integral pixels. The simulations mimicked the common motion patterns in the laboratory, including bounce, shift, complex motion, and lateral motion. Data from recent studies of 164 normal patients were also reviewed.

Results.—The motion pixel "area index" of the simulations ranged from 1 to 83. Defects were present in 87% of simulations with an index of 21 or more; by contrast, 86% of simulations with an index less than 21 were normal. On review of normal studies, motion was found in 26%. However, motion-related defects were present in only 4% of cases.

Conclusion.—Mild motion appears to be unlikely to produce significant defects on ^{201}Tl-SPECT studies. When motion is severe, it produces recognizable patterns, depending on its direction, magnitude, and timing (Fig 13–8). Motion is now an unusual source of artifacts in this laboratory.

▶ Many clinicians have speculated on the artifacts created in tomographic images by patient motion. Many times we see artifacts that indicate the patient must have moved in a certain direction during acquisition. This type of inverse logic can certainly be frustrating.

The elegance of this article rests with taking the approach of creating known motion and looking at the resultant artifacts. Having done that, we now have powerful knowledge that can be applied to interpreting the clinical results; this is good science.—I.G. Zubal, Ph.D.

Results of a Clinical Receiver Operating Characteristic Study Comparing Filtered Backprojection and Maximum Likelihood Estimator Images in FDG PET Studies
Llacer J, Veklerov E, Baxter LR, Grafton ST, Griffeth LK, Hawkins RA, Hoh CK, Mazziotta JC, Hoffman EJ, Metz CE (Univ of California, Berkeley; Univ of California, Los Angeles; Univ of Southern California, Los Angeles; et al)
J Nucl Med 34:1198–1203, 1993   124-95-13–12

Introduction.—In image reconstruction for emission tomography, the maximum likelihood estimator (MLE) method has been investigated for its potential of lessening noise and producing higher effective sensitivity than is realized with standard filtered background projection (FBP) techniques. Reducing noise in low-uptake regions is expected to enhance the

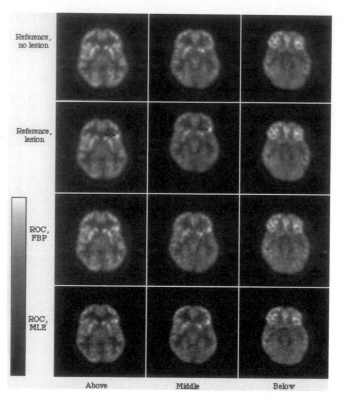

Fig 13–9.—High-count (reference) images reconstructed by FBP before adding a lesion (**top row**), after placing an additive lesion in grey matter indicated by an *arrow* (**second row**), FBP reconstruction of a 1.4-M data set corresponding to the second-row images (**third row**), and MLE reconstruction of the same 1.4-M data set. The images on the **left** and **right columns** are submitted together with the center image to provide anatomical information to the physician who has to rate the center image. The added lesion was extended to the plane above the center. (Courtesy of Llacer J, Veklerov E, Baxter LR, et al: *J Nucl Med* 34:1198–1203, 1993.)

detectability of small lesions more with the MLE method than with FBP reconstructions.

Methods.—The receiver operating characteristic (ROC) method was used to compare MLE reconstructions of human fluorodeoxyglucose (FDG) PET scan data to FBP reconstructions of the same data. The analysis focused on gray and white matter lesions whose nature and contrast level make them borderline-detectable. Ninety data sets were used; 42 were left in their original condition and 48 were modified by the addition of lesions. Each data set was reconstructed using both the MLE and FBP methods and evaluated by 5 physician observers.

Results.—The area under the ROC curve increased significantly with MLE reconstructions vs. FBP reconstructions—from .65 to .71—for 4 of the 5 observers. On high-count images, even subtle lesions were judged to be detectable; when transferred to low-count images, the lesions became more difficult to detect (Fig 13–9). Both methods of reconstruction gave nearly identical results for additive lesions in gray matter and in normal images.

Conclusion.—The MLE method of image reconstruction is superior to the FBP method for detecting small focal lesions at the threshold of detectability in human FDG PET studies. In some of the cases, the MLE technique may offer clinically significant advantages. The MLE reconstructions performed took about 10 minutes per plane, and faster ones will soon be widely available.

▶ Sometimes we make the mistake of preferring a certain reconstruction technique (or filter) based on the fact that the images look better. This holds the danger of delivering good-looking images with poor clinical information. As the investigators point out, it is more important and reasonable to prefer a reconstruction method because clinically relevant objects are more easily perceived in the images (after all, that is why we create the images in the first place isn't it?).

This well-constructed analysis reminds us that we should look at the most informative image, not necessarily the nicest or most convenient. We should remember this when we transfer tomographic slice information from the computer screen onto x-ray film, which some people prefer to view on light boxes.—I.G. Zubal, Ph.D.

Comparison of Personnel Radiation Dosimetry From Myocardial Perfusion Scintigraphy: Technetium-99m-Sestamibi Versus Thallium-201
Culver CM, Dworkin HJ (William Beaumont Hosp, Royal Oak, Mich)
J Nucl Med 34:1210–1213, 1993   124-95-13–13

Background.—Myocardial perfusion scintigraphy can be performed using technetium-99m (^{99m}Tc) sestamibi or thallium-201 (^{201}Tl) as the imaging agent. In selecting an imaging agent, the external radiation exposure to the technical staff is one of the factors to be considered. These 2 agents were compared in a retrospective radiation dosimetry study.

Methods.—Technical personnel were monitored using film badges for whole body and thermoluminescent dosimeters (TLDs) for hand/finger dose equivalents. Badge reports were reviewed for 3 periods of 4 months: 1 in which ^{201}Tl was used exclusively for stress myocardial perfusion imaging and 2 in which ^{99m}Tc-sestamibi was used exclusively, before and after implementation of a radiation reduction policy. Staff members studied included 10 nuclear medicine technologists and 2 radiopharmacy technologists.

Results.—When ^{99m}Tc-sestamibi replaced ^{201}Tl, the mean whole body film badge readings increased from 100 to 450 μSv/month. Corresponding values for the radiopharmacy technologists were from 240 to 560 μSv/month. Hand TLD readings increased as well, although the differ-

Monthly Dose Equivalent to Nuclear Medicine Technologists

Time period	Dosimetry reports	Whole body (μSv)	Hand/Finger (μSv)
I, ^{201}Tl	14	100 ± 100 (0–300)	750 ± 550 (300–1900)
II, ^{99m}Tc	16	450 ± 210 (200–1000)	1390 ± 790 (400–2700)
III*, ^{99m}Tc	15	310 ± 80 (200–500)	1030 ± 620 (200–2100)

Whole body: $p < 0.001$ (I vs II); ns (II vs III). Hand/Finger: ns (I vs II); ns (II vs III).

Abbreviation: ns, not significant.
Note: Results are expressed as means ± 1 SD. Values in parentheses indicate the range.
* Radiation reduction policy was introduced before period III.
(Courtesy of Culver CM, Dworkin HJ: *J Nucl Med* 34:1210–1213, 1993.)

ence was not significant for the nuclear medicine technologists (table). The mean whole-body dose equivalent for 8 staff members of a noninvasive cardiology unit after implementation of the radiation reduction policy was 360 μSv/month. The most effective radiation reduction methods were the use of a lead face shield and lead-lined storage container in the noninvasive imaging area, handling spills by shielding rather than decontamination, and reducing the time spent in close proximity to the patient.

Conclusion.—An increase in the radiation dose after changing imaging agents from ^{201}Tl to ^{99m}Tc-sestamibi was documented. Although radiation reduction measures have reduced mean whole body and hand dose equivalents, current levels are still higher than when ^{201}Tl was used as the imaging agent for myocardial perfusion studies.

▶ There is consolation in knowing that although 10 times the activity is injected for sestamibi studies compared with thallium, the dose levels experienced by the technologists are less.—I.G. Zubal, Ph.D.

Cellular Dosimetry: Absorbed Fractions for Monoenergetic Electron and Alpha Particle Sources and S-Values for Radionuclides Uniformly Distributed in Different Cell Compartments
Goddu SM, Howell RW, Rao DV (Univ of Medicine and Dentistry of New Jersey, Newark)
J Nucl Med 35:303–316, 1994   124-95-13–14

Introduction.—The standard dosimetric approach when using incorporated radionuclides to combat cancer is to calculate the mean absorbed doses to bulk tumor and normal organs using data from the medical internal radiation dose (MIRD) publications. Sometimes, it is more appropriate to determine the absorbed dose to individual cells, especially when nuclides concentrate in cells or emit radiation whose range is comparable to the cell dimensions.

Objective and Methods.—Cellular absorbed fractions were calculated for a number of sources of monoenergetic electrons and alpha-particles that were assumed to be uniformly distributed in various cell compartments. Cells were assumed to be spherically symmetric; cell and nuclear radii ranged from 2 to 10 μm. Absorbed fractions were estimated for electron sources that had energies of .1 keV to 1 MeV, and for monoenergetic alpha-particle sources having energies of 3 MeV to 10 MeV.

Results.—Both absorbed fractions and cellular S-values were obtained for a number of different-sized cells and cellular nuclei. S-values for intracellular technetium-99m are shown in the table.

Conclusion.—Using data on absorbed fractions and S-values as well as experimental data on radionuclide biokinetics and subcellular distribution makes it possible to conveniently calculate cellular self-absorbed radiation doses.

▶ Out of the several isotopes presented in this report, technetium-99m is the most interesting to us and is extracted as a table. From left to right, the columns represent the cell radius and cell nucleus radius, and then 5 col-

S-Values for Intracellular Technetium-99m

R_C (μm)	R_N (μm)	C←C (Gy/Bq·s)	C←CS (Gy/Bq·s)	N←N (Gy/Bq·s)	N←Cy (Gy/Bq·s)	N←CS (Gy/Bq·s)
3	2	3.58E-03	1.85E-03	1.17E-02	3.33E-04	1.19E-04
3	1	3.58E-03	1.85E-03	8.85E-02	4.56E-04	1.10E-04
4	3	1.55E-03	8.05E-04	3.58E-03	1.54E-04	7.47E-05
4	2	1.55E-03	8.05E-04	1.17E-02	1.72E-04	7.23E-05
5	4	8.16E-04	4.23E-04	1.55E-03	8.68E-05	4.76E-05
5	3	8.16E-04	4.23E-04	3.58E-03	9.44E-05	4.63E-05
5	2	8.16E-04	4.23E-04	1.17E-02	1.13E-04	4.76E-05
6	5	4.82E-04	2.50E-04	8.16E-04	5.38E-05	3.17E-05
6	4	4.82E-04	2.50E-04	1.55E-03	5.72E-05	3.00E-05
6	3	4.82E-04	2.50E-04	3.58E-03	6.67E-05	2.96E-05
7	6	3.09E-04	1.61E-04	4.82E-04	3.60E-05	2.23E-05
7	5	3.09E-04	1.61E-04	8.16E-04	3.72E-05	2.06E-05
7	4	3.09E-04	1.61E-04	1.55E-03	4.21E-05	1.95E-05
8	7	2.11E-04	1.10E-04	3.09E-04	2.55E-05	1.64E-05
8	6	2.11E-04	1.10E-04	4.82E-04	2.58E-05	1.50E-05
8	5	2.11E-04	1.10E-04	8.16E-04	2.83E-05	1.38E-05
9	8	1.50E-04	7.83E-05	2.11E-04	1.89E-05	1.26E-05
9	7	1.50E-04	7.83E-05	3.09E-04	1.88E-05	1.13E-05
9	6	1.50E-04	7.83E-05	4.82E-04	2.01E-05	1.03E-05
10	9	1.11E-04	5.80E-05	1 50E-04	1.45E-05	9.93E-06
10	8	1.11E-04	5.80E-05	2.11E-04	1.42E-05	8.90E-06
10	7	1.11E-04	5.80E-05	3.09E-04	1.50E-05	8.05E-06

(Courtesy of Goddu SM, Howell RW, Rao DV: *J Nucl Med* 35:303–316, 1994.)

umns list the source and target doses for combinations of the following: C = entire cell, Cy = cytoplasm, CS = cell surface, and N = cell nucleus.—I.G. Zubal, Ph.D.

MIRD Dose Estimate Report No. 17: Radiation Absorbed Dose Estimates From Inhaled Krypton-81m Gas in Lung Imaging

Atkins HL, Robertson JS, Akabani G (Brookhaven Natl Lab, Upton, NY; State Univ of New York, Stony Brook; Battelle-Pacific Northwest Labs, Richland, Wash)
J Nucl Med 34:1382–1384, 1993   124-95-13–15

Background.—Krypton-81m (^{81m}Kr) is a daughter product of the radioactive decay of ribidium-81 used for ventilation lung imaging. It is mainly used to help diagnose pulmonary embolism. Estimated absorbed doses from ^{81m}Kr gas that was administered by inhalation were reported.

Radiation Absorbed Dose.—Krypton-81m has an extremely short physical half-life, which precludes obtaining biological data directly for

Estimated Absorbed Dose From Inhaled [81m]Kr Gas

Target organ	rad/mCi-min in lungs	mGy/MBq-min in lungs
Tracheal mucosa (surface)	4.6×10^{-1}	1.2×10^{-1}
Tracheal mucosa (mean)	2.1×10^{-3}	5.7×10^{-4}
Lungs	2.5×10^{-3}	6.7×10^{-4}
Liver	5.2×10^{-5}	1.4×10^{-5}
Spleen	4.9×10^{-5}	1.8×10^{-5}
Red marrow	3.9×10^{-5}	1.0×10^{-5}
Muscle	3.5×10^{-5}	9.3×10^{-6}
Kidneys	2.7×10^{-5}	7.2×10^{-6}
Ovaries	1.6×10^{-5}	4.2×10^{-6}
Testes	1.1×10^{-5}	2.9×10^{-6}
Total body	6.7×10^{-5}	1.8×10^{-5}

Note: Assumes equilibrium in the lung is attained, which requires inhalation of the gas for at least 2 minutes.
(Courtesy of Atkins HL, Robertson JS, Akabani G: *J Nucl Med* 34:1382-1384, 1993.)

an absorbed-dose estimate. In determining absorbed dose, it is assumed that the patient inhales [81m]Kr at a constant delivery rate and that at equilibrium, 37 MBq of the gas is in the lung spaces. Delivery of radioactivity is stopped abruptly after the image is obtained, and the [81m]Kr washes out of the lungs. The trachea was modeled as a right circular cylinder with a 1.1-cm inside diameter and a .2-cm mucosal thickness. It was assumed that the radionuclide would mix uniformly with air at a pressure of 1 atm and fill the inner cylinder at the same concentration as in the lung. Residence times for the various components of the washout were determined from the ratio of body content to lung content. Estimated absorbed doses are shown in the table.

▶ Although krypton ventilation lung studies are probably not as widespread as xenon or aerosols, a substantial number of departments use krypton and avoid some of the problems associated with trapping xenon and delivering the aerosol.—I.G. Zubal, Ph.D.

Dosimetry and Toxicity of Samarium-153-EDTMP Administered for Bone Pain Due to Skeletal Metastases

Bayouth JE, Macey DJ, Kasi LP, Fossella FV (Univ of Texas, Houston)
J Nucl Med 35:63–69, 1994   124-95-13–16

Introduction.—The bone-seeking phosphonate ethylenediaminetetramethylenephosphonic acid (EDTMP), chelated with the β-emitter samarium-153 ([153]Sm), is undergoing a trial at cancer centers for relieving

Estimates of Radiation Dose to Several Organs After the First Administration of ^{153}SM-EDTMP to 16 Patients

Patient number*	%ID in skeleton	Injected activity (GBq)	Bladder wall† (cGy/GBq)	Stomach (cGy/GBq)	Small intestine (cGy/GBq)	Large intestine (cGy/GBq)	Kidneys (cGy/GBq)	Liver (cGy/GBq)	Red marrow‡ (cGy/GBq)
11	82.9	3.12	5.5	2.0	2.4	3.2	5.4	2.5	108.2
1	65.6	1.11	9.1	2.3	2.7	4.3	9.2	3.2	85.5
15	57.8	2.39	10.7	2.5	2.8	4.8	10.9	3.6	75.3
4	57.3	0.84	10.8	2.5	2.8	4.9	11.0	3.6	74.7
16	55.5	2.85	11.2	2.5	2.8	5.0	11.4	3.7	72.3
5	51.7	1.20	12.0	2.6	2.9	5.2	12.2	3.8	67.4
9	50.8	1.19	12.2	2.6	2.9	5.3	12.4	3.9	66.3
17	49.8	2.26	12.4	2.6	2.9	5.3	12.7	3.9	65.0
19	49.6	3.50	12.4	2.6	2.9	5.4	12.7	3.9	64.7
10	48.7	2.27	12.6	2.6	2.9	5.4	12.9	4.0	63.5
14	46.5	4.16	13.1	2.6	3.0	5.6	13.4	4.1	60.6
18	42.1	3.51	14.0	2.7	3.0	5.8	14.3	4.3	54.8
8	41.6	1.66	14.1	2.7	3.0	5.9	14.4	4.3	54.3
13	37.7	3.09	14.9	2.8	3.1	6.1	15.3	4.5	49.2
7	35.3	1.06	15.4	2.8	3.1	6.3	15.8	4.6	46.0
6	13.8	1.52	19.9	3.2	3.5	7.6	20.5	5.5	17.9
Average values	49.18 ± 14.35		12.5 ± 3.0	2.6 ± 0.2	2.9 ± 0.2	5.4 ± 0.9	12.8 ± 3.1	4.0 ± 0.6	64.1 ± 18.7

Note: Doses are listed per mCi of ^{153}Sm administered. The cumulated activity in each organ was calculated from biodistribution data obtained from a rat model and weighted according to the percentage of the injected dose available, i.e., not taken up by the skeleton. The marrow doses are the exceptions.

* Urine samples were not available for patients 2, 3, and 12.

† The mean residence time in the bladder was determined from estimates of urinary clearance assuming 75% voiding every 30 minutes.

‡ Estimated dose to the marrow assumes that skeletal activity was uniformly distributed in the bones in accordance with the medical internal radiation dose approach. No specific uptake in the marrow itself was observed.

(Courtesy of Bayouth JE, Macey DJ, Kasi LP, et al: *J Nucl Med* 35:63–69, 1994.)

bone pain caused by metastatic cancer. The phase I/II clinical trial defined the pharmacokinetics of repeated injections of ¹⁵³Sm-EDTMP and its skeletal uptake and determined radiation doses to various organs.

Methods.—Nineteen patients received as many as 4 injections of ¹⁵³Sm-EDTMP in a dose of either .5 or 1 mCi/kg of body weight. The radiopharmaceutical was injected intravenously over 1 minute in a volume that did not exceed 1 mL. Skeletal retention of radioactivity was estimated from urinary excretion.

Findings.—The mean biological half-life of skeletal activity was 520 hours or infinite for purposes of dosimetry because the biological half-life of the nuclide is 10-fold greater than its physical half-life. Blood activity declined rapidly to about 20% of the injected dose in the first 30 minutes and then more slowly. Skeletal uptake varied widely, but it averaged 50% of the injected dose. Radiation dose estimates are shown in the table. Bone marrow toxicity, as reflected by changes in platelet counts, was dose-related. Thirteen of the 19 patients (68%) reported significant relief of bone pain.

Conclusion.—Bone pain from metastatic cancer may be relieved by injecting ¹⁵³Sm-EDTMP, which results in a limited dose to the red marrow and has no toxic effects on other organs.

▶ This presentation of the data is interesting because the error with which doses are calculated can be appreciated. Not only are the standard deviations given, but some of the extreme high or low doses are shown. Such considerations are important, because we obviously rarely treat an "average" patient; every patient has some degree of individual conditions that must be taken into consideration.—I.G. Zubal, Ph.D.

The Influence of Tracer Localization on the Electron Dose Rate Delivered to the Cell Nucleus
Faraggi M, Gardin I, de Labriolle-Vaylet C, Moretti J-L, Bok BD (Bichat Hosp, Paris; Beaujon Hosp, Clichy, France; Saint Antoine Hosp, Paris; et al)
J Nucl Med 35:113–119, 1994   124-95-13–17

Background.—Both photons and electrons are emitted by most of the photon emitters used in diagnostic nuclear medical procedures. If cellular uptake of radionuclides remains stable over time, the absorbed dose at the cellular level may be great. Dose calculation at the cellular level is more accurate than that of conventional dosimetry.

Methods.—The radiation dose rate delivered by electron emissions of technetium-99m (⁹⁹ᵐTc), indium-123 (¹²³In), gallium-67 (⁶⁷Ga), and thallium-201 (²⁰¹Tl) at the subcellular level was calculated using spherical models to simulate various cellular localizations of radionuclides. The models were applied to large lymphocytes, and uniform distributions of radioactivity throughout the nucleus, cytoplasm, or cell membrane surface were assumed.

Ratio Between the Dose Rate $\dot{D}$ (0) to the Nucleus Center for
Nucleus, Cytoplasm, and Cell Membrane Localizations vs.
Homogenous Distribution Over the Entire Cell

	^{99m}Tc	^{123}I	^{111}In	^{67}Ga	^{201}Tl
$\dfrac{D\,(0)\text{nucleus}}{D\,(0)\text{cell}}$	3.2	3.0	2.8	3.2	3.1
$\dfrac{D\,(0)\text{cytopla.}}{D\,(0)\text{cell}}$	0.068	0.17	0.23	0.056	0.10
$\dfrac{D\,(0)\text{memb.}}{D\,(0)\text{cell}}$	0.034	0.14	0.16	0.043	0.041

Note: Total activity is the same for all the localizations.
(Courtesy of Faraggi M, Gardin I, de Labriolle-Vaylet C, et al: *J Nucl Med* 35:113–119, 1994.)

Findings.—The dose rate strongly depended on the subcellular distribution of the radioisotope. When the radioactivity was localized in the cell nucleus rather than on the cell membrane only, the absorbed dose rate $\dot{D}(0)$ at the center of the cell delivered by a constant cellular radioactivity of ^{99m}Tc, ^{123}I, ^{111}In, ^{67}Ga, and ^{201}Tl was, respectively, 94, 21, 18, 74, and 76 times greater. Assuming that radioactivity is distributed uniformly throughout the cell may result in underestimation of the dose rate from 2.8- to 3.2-fold if the tracer is localized only in the nucleus or an overestimation from 4.3- to 30-fold if the tracer is localized in the cytoplasm or on the cell membrane, depending on the radionuclide (table).

Conclusion.—Failure to consider subcellular localization of a radiopharmaceutical may result in an underestimation or overestimation of the dose rate and therefore the dose to the nucleus. Even if dosimetry alone is inadequate for predicting radiobiological effects, it may be very important in accurately determining dose estimates at the subcellular level in the study of cell survival of Auger emitters as a function of absorbed dose.

▶ This article nicely complements the previous one (Abstract 124-95-13–16), and both remind us that we are enhancing our understanding of doses to living tissue by more closely examining where the dose is delivered within the cell. The table enables us to compare the cellular dose for several commonly used isotopes.—I.G. Zubal, Ph.D.

Radon Update: Facts Concerning Environmental Radon: Levels, Mitigation Strategies, Dosimetry, Effects and Guidelines

Brill AB, for the SNM Committee on Radiobiological Effects of Ionizing Radiation (Univ of Massachusetts, Worcester)
J Nucl Med 35:368–385, 1994   124-95-13-18

Introduction.—The potential danger from naturally occurring radon gas and its daughters has become a matter of public concern. Evidence of the nature and severity of this problem was reviewed, and the abatement procedures and related costs were described.

Discussion.—Although the radiation dose from external radon is very low, inhaled radon can deliver a high-energy dose to the tracheobronchial epithelium. The primary source of the radon in the home is the soil. Levels in the home are usually highest in the winter, when the house is closed up. Radon levels are highest in home levels that make contact with the ground. There is a large geographic variation in the distribution of radon. High levels of radon are associated with granite igneous rocks, shale, dirty quartz sedimentary rocks, phosphate deposits, and some beach sands. Fractured bedrock and porous home foundations can also increase exposure to radon. Radon can also outgas from contaminated water supplies, with deep well aquifers being particularly vulnerable to contamination. Abatement involves water purification and aeration, if contaminated water is the source. Ventilation can be used to lower high radon gas levels in the home. Sealing cracks and openings in the foundation and covering exposed earth can reduce the home's intake of radon. Studies of miners have demonstrated that the major health risk from radon exposure is bronchogenic carcinoma. Smoking is a very important co-factor. The effect of the natural background of radon on cancer is too small to be detected in epidemiologic studies.

Conclusion.—Radon is a naturally occurring gas that can cause lung cancer at high doses. Individuals who live in areas with a high natural radon background should test their home. This can be done simply and inexpensively. Based on the results, a risk-benefit analysis must be used to determine what action, if any, should be taken. The costs of remediation appear to exceed the potential benefits for radon levels of less than 8 pCi/L.

▶ Over the years, we have presented updates on radon levels in various areas of the country. This article does more than that; it gives us an excellent overview of the physics of decay, instrumentation, measurement, health effects, and regulations. All aspects are insightfully covered, which makes this an excellent reference article.—I.G. Zubal, Ph.D.

Determining Person-Years of Life Lost Using the Beir V Method
Maillie HD, Simon W, Watts RJ, Quinn BR (Univ of Rochester, NY; Rochester Gas and Electric Corp, NY)
Health Phys 64:461–466, 1993   124-95-13-19

Objective.—Several studies have presented estimates of the risks of exposure to ionizing radiation, including many on the production of fatal cancers. However, it is believed that risk is better expressed as person-years of life lost. The BEIR V report provides data on years of life lost for only 3 sets of circumstances; here, a technique for making risk estimates under a variety of conditions was presented.

Findings.—Estimated person-years of life lost were calculated when groups of males or females were exposed to low linear energy transfer (LET) ionizing radiation. For example, for each 1 million females receiving an acute dose of 10 mSv, the total number of radiation-induced fatal cancers was 835. Although the total number of person-years of life lost is low—1.4×10^4, or an average of about 5 days—the 22 women who die of leukemia will suffer for about 34 years. Women who die of other forms of cancer lose an average of about 16 years. These estimates agree well with some previous examples reported by the United States National Academy of Sciences. For 1 million males exposed to 1 mSv y^{-1}, a total of 8.7×10^4 person-years would be lost. The result is 7% higher than that reported in BEIR V, whereas the result of a similar calculation for females was 3% higher.

Discussion.—This method allows calculation of the risk of radiation injury to groups that are exposed to whole body low LET ionizing radiation. Loss of life because of such exposure is low compared with normally occurring deaths for dose equivalents of less than 4 Sv, so the estimates presented are conservative. The methods described can be used to make similar calculations to apply to other scenarios.

▶ This article serves as a very good tutorial, which teaches some of the parameters and mathematics involved in making these difficult estimations. The definition of terms and graph of parameters over population lifetimes are very helpful in understanding the process of calculating risk associated with radiation dose.—I.G. Zubal, Ph.D.

Long-Term Radon Concentrations Estimated From ^{210}Po Embedded in Glass

Lively RS, Steck DJ (Minnesota Geological Survey, St Paul; St John's Univ, Collegeville, Minn)
Health Phys 64:485–490, 1993   124-95-13–20

Objective.—Measured alpha-activity on glass surfaces is positively correlated with radon exposure. However, the general application of this technique has been limited by uncertainties regarding glass exposure in the home and the fate of radon progeny deposited on glass. A model for estimating the fraction of embedded radon progeny that permits more accurate estimation of average radon concentrations from alpha-activity on glass was developed.

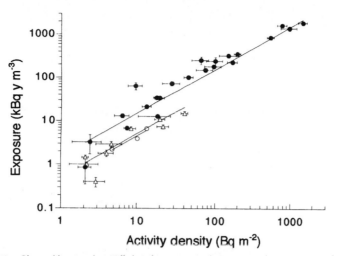

Fig 13–10.—Glass calibration data. *Filled circles* represent the Revigator data; *open triangles* indicate the mixed-air data; *open circles* indicate the EPALV data. Regression lines have been separately calculated for each data set. *Error bars* on the *vertical axis* indicate uncertainty in the concentration of radon in the chambers. *Horizontal error bars* are uncertainties associated with counting statistics and the standard deviation of activity from multiple glass samples of a given exposure. (Courtesy of Lively RS, Steck DJ: *Health Phys* 64:485–490, 1993.)

Methods.—Surface alpha-activity was measured on glass samples that were exposed in radon chambers and interior and exterior glass samples from 6 houses. Radon concentrations ranged between 100 Bq m^{-3} and 9 MBq m^{-3}, with durations of a few days to several years. The new model was designed to calculate the fractions of attached and unattached progeny deposited on the surface, the adsorbed fraction, and the fraction embedded into the glass by alpha-recoil.

Results.—There was a linear relationship between the product of the average radon concentration and the integrated exposure time with the activity of polonium-210 (^{210}Po) embedded in the glass surfaces across the range of exposures. The theoretical calculations of exposure vs. activity agreed with both the radon chamber and household glass measurements (Fig 13–10). Household cleaning or thin films did not significantly affect the embedded fraction of ^{210}Po. Adsorbed activity varied widely, however.

Conclusion.—Measurement of ^{210}Po embedded in glass provides a better means of estimating long-term radon exposure than short-term radon measurements do. A regression model reflecting the deposition model of the glass will improve the effectiveness and general applicability of this method.

▶ It appears that the number of intriguing new methods for estimating the dose may well be endless. Every year, new methods are investigated, and an interesting example is presented here. This year, we learn that by estimating the number of embedded radon progeny in glass, we can estimate the concentrations of radon-222 levels.—I.G. Zubal, Ph.D.

Subject Index*

A

Abdomen
infections and inflammations,
technetium-99m-HMPAO
leukocytes in, 93: 168
Abscess
brain, discordance between fluorine-18
fluorodeoxyglucose uptake and
contrast enhancement in, 95: 74
Absorptiometry
dual photon, for bone mineral
measurements with gamma camera,
95: 158
Abuse
cocaine, brain perfusion SPECT in,
94: 304
Acalculous
biliary colic, hepatobiliary scintigraphy
in, 94: 239
gallbladder disease, gallbladder ejection
fraction predicting, 94: 238
Acetate
carbon-11-, for myocardial perfusion
evaluation, 93: 54
Acetazolamide
effect on vascular responses in
diaschisis, 94: 299
N-Acetylaspartate
in brain after stroke, 94: 91
Acquired immunodeficiency syndrome (see
AIDS)
Adenocarcinoma
papillary, in thyroid hemiagenesis,
94: 191
Adenoma
liver, or follicular nodular hyperplasia,
94: 359
parathyroid, with thyroid hemiagenesis,
94: 194
Adenomyosis
bone scintigraphy of, blood flow and
blood pool, 95: 249
Adenosine
coronary hyperemia
with technetium-99m-teboroxime in
tomographic myocardial perfusion
imaging, 93: 35
with thallium-201 SPECT in coronary
artery disease, 93: 12
tomography in, 94: 17
for coronary vasodilatation with
thallium-201 scintigraphy in
coronary artery disease, 93: 10
myocardial thallium-201 tomography,
94: 25

SPECT thallium-201 for high-risk left
main and three-vessel coronary
artery disease, 94: 7
thallium-201, superior to exercise
thallium-201 in coronary artery
disease in left bundle branch block,
94: 4
vs. exercise thallium-201 SPECT for
myocardial perfusion imaging,
93: 11
Adolescence
spinal disorders during, scintigraphy of,
95: 136
Adrenal
cortex masses, benign, chemical shift
MRI of, 94: 378
masses
chemical shift, fast low-angle shot
MRI of, 94: 380
lipid in, 94: 380
Adrenergic
tumors, iodine-131
metaiodobenzylguanidine for,
95: xxiv
Adrenocorticotropin
secreting bronchial carcinoid,
somatostatin analogs in, 95: 160
Adriamycin
cardiomyopathy, myocardial substrate
utilization and left ventricular
function in, 95: 337
Aerosol
inhaled, three different sized aerosols,
differences in deposition patterns in
lungs, 94: 111
phytate, in ventilation studies, vs.
technetium-99m C, 94: 110
scintigraphy in cystic fibrosis therapy
assessment, 93: 138
technetium-99m DTPA, radiation
absorbed dose from, 94: 341
ultrafine, in infant with bronchial
stenosis, inhalation scintigraphy of,
94: 113
Aged
coronary artery bypass, risk stratification
in, cineangiography of, 95: 327
dipyridamole thallium-201 imaging in,
prognostic value, 94: 29
AIDS
cholangitis
sclerosing, hepatobiliary imaging in,
95: 214
sclerosing, hepatobiliary scintigraphy
in, 93: 249

---

*All entries refer to the year and page number(s) for data appearing in this and the
previous edition of the YEAR BOOK.*

technetium-99m DISIDA
hepatobiliary scintigraphy in,
95: 85
dementia complex, brain perfusion
SPECT in, 94: 304
gastric uptake of gallium-67 in, 93: 172
lung clearance of technetium-99m
diethylene triamine penta-acetate
in, 93: 134
nuclear medicine and, 95: 82
Pneumocystis carinii pneumonia in,
gallium-67 scintigraphy and CT of,
94: 162
(*See also* HIV)
Albumin
macroaggregates, technetium-99m
for lung imaging, arterial oxygen
saturation in, 93: 126
for perfusion scintigraphy, hypoxia
associated with, 94: 106
sonicated, in myocardial contrast
echocardiography, 94: 16
Alcoholic
liver disease assessment with SPECT,
94: 256
Algorithm
cone beam SPECT reconstruction, with
displaced center of rotation,
95: 429
fan beam reconstruction, for spatially
varying focal length collimator,
95: 428
rapidly converging iterative
reconstruction, in SPECT, 95: 432
Alimentation
enteral, percutaneous, gastrostomy vs.
gastrojejunostomy in, 94: 258
Alkali
milk alkali syndrome, technetium-99m
methylene diphosphonate increased
skeletal uptake in, 95: 127
Alveolitis
fibrosing, inhaled technetium-99m
DTPA clearance predicting clinical
course of, 95: 36
Alzheimer dementia
energy metabolism and mobile
phosphoesters quantification by
phosphorus-31 magnetic resonance
spectroscopy in, 94: 93
Alzheimer's disease
cerebrospinal fluid volumes in, 95: 370
PET and MRI in, brain metabolism as
reliable discriminator in, 95: 265
probable, PET in, 93: 287
probable, technetium-99m HMPAO
SPECT vs. fluorine-18 FDG PET in,
95: 268

temporal lobe blood flow reduction in,
94: 295
AMI-227
for magnetic resonance lymphography
of filariasis (in ferret), 94: 371
L-Amino acid
natural, brain uptake of, 93: 329
p-Aminohippurate
clearance, in renal artery blood flow, vs.
MRI, 95: 180
Ammonia, nitrogen-13 (*see* Nitrogen-13
ammonia)
Amobarbital
injection, intracarotid, for anatomic
correlates of memory, with
technetium-99m HMPAO SPECT,
95: 278
Aneurysm
intracranial, surgery, temporary clipping
in, cerebral blood flow variations
during, 95: 261
popliteal vein, pulmonary embolism
from, 94: 104
pulmonary artery, thrombosed, causing
high-probability lung imaging,
94: 105
Angelman syndrome
cerebral blood flow in, regional,
95: 280
Angina
pectoris
effort, myocardial scintigraphy with
technetium-99m-sestamibi and
dipyridamole in, 93: 26
with left ventricular dysfunction
during exercise, and normal
coronary arteries, 95: 328
thallium perfusion imaging
abnormality in, with low myocardial
and skeletal muscle energy charge,
94: 20
unstable, myocardial perfusion imaging
in, thallium-201, prognostic value,
93: 4
Angiography
with blood pool imaging for hand
radiation injury assessment, 94: 345
in chest pain, spontaneous, 93: 28
cineangiography after coronary artery
bypass in aged, for risk
stratification, 95: 327
coronary, vs. planar myocardial
perfusion imaging, 94: 42
in gastrointestinal bleeding, vs.
technetium-99m red blood cell
scintigraphy, 94: 244
gated radionuclide, in left ventricular
ejection fraction assessment, 93: 39

in Klippel-Trenaunay syndrome,
radionuclide total body, 94: 272
magnetic resonance (*see* Magnetic
resonance angiography)
pulmonary
with MRI, experience, 95: 38
for suspected pulmonary embolism,
quantitative plasma D-dimer levels
in, 95: 2
radionuclide, in dobutamine stress test,
with thallium-201 SPECT, after
infarction, 95: 301
Angioplasty
balloon, of coronary artery, left
ventricular function, monitoring for
myocardial ischemia during, 93: 45
cerebral, in delayed ischemia due to
vasospasm, 94: 282
coronary
percutaneous transluminal, early
thallium imaging after, 94: 17
with positive exercise test, restenosis
in, exercise thallium scintigraphy vs.
dipyridamole echocardiography in,
94: 15
in myocardial infarction, exercise
thallium-201 scintigraphy after,
94: 12
percutaneous transluminal, vascular
injury imaging with technetium-99m
monoclonal antiplatelet antibody
S12 in, 94: 72
Angiotensin
converting enzyme inhibitor in
renovascular hypertension, causing
transplant artery thrombosis,
95: 200
Anisotropy
in MRI
diffusion-weighted, 93: 64
with simultaneous spin and stimulated
echoes, 94: 73
Anorexia
nervosa, with osteomalacia, 95: 128
Antenatal
diagnosis of pelvic hydronephrosis,
93: 233
Anthracycline
myocardial damage assessment by
indium-111 myosin monoclonal
antibodies, 93: 49
Anti-CD4
monoclonal antibodies, technetium-99m
specific murine, in imaging of
inflamed joints in rheumatoid
arthritis, 95: 105
Anti-CEA monoclonal antibody
indium-111

in thyroid medullary carcinoma
imaging, 93: 159
ZCE 025 in colorectal carcinoma
follow-up, 93: 160
Anti-fibrin
monoclonal antibody fab fragment,
technetium-99m DD-3B6/22, in
deep venous thrombosis and
pulmonary embolism detection,
95: 245
Anti-thyroglobulin antibodies
circulating, in thyroid cancer, meaning
of, 94: 189
Antianginal
drugs, in exercise myocardial perfusion
imaging, 95: 298
Antibodies
anti-thyroglobulin, circulating, in thyroid
cancer, meaning of, 94: 189
antimyosin
indium-111, for visualization of
myocardial infarction, 94: 71
uptake of, and myocardial infarction
age, 93: 48
ascorbate for direct labeling, with
technetium-99m, 95: 414
fab fragment, technetium-99m
radiolabeling of, 93: 335
granulocyte antibody, technetium-99m,
in inflammatory disease, 93: 170
guiding scintigraphy in uveal melanoma,
93: 117
monoclonal antiplatelet, S12,
monoclonal, technetium-99m, for
vascular injury imaging, 94: 72
monoclonal (*see* Monoclonal antibody)
for MRI imaging, 93: 76
Anticoagulation
ventilation perfusion lung scintigraphy
reporting and, 95: 15
Antifibrin
monoclonal antibody, indium-111, in
venous thrombosis, 93: 268
Antigen
carcinoembryonic, monoclonal antibody
fragments, iodine-123, for
colorectal cancer imaging, 94: 136
MHC complex class II antigen
induction by rejecting heart, 93: 51
prostate specific (*see* Prostate specific
antigen)
Antimyosin
antibody
indium-111, for visualization of
myocardial infarction, 94: 71
uptake, indium-111, and myocardial
infarction age, 93: 48

fab, indium-111 monoclonal,
    myocardial uptake in doxorubicin
    cardiotoxicity detection (in rat),
    94: 70
Antiplatelet
    antibody S12, monoclonal,
    technetium-99m, for vascular injury
    imaging, 94: 72
Aortic
    dissection, ascending, causing unilateral
        absence of perfusion on lung
        imaging, 95: 24
    graft
        early postoperative, technetium-99m
            leukocytes in, 93: 270
        infection detection with
            technetium-99m hexametazime
            leukocytes in, 94: 158
Aortofemoral
    Dacron prosthesis, knitted vs. woven,
        94: 265
Aortoiliac
    Dacron prosthesis, knitted vs. woven,
        94: 265
Appendicitis
    detection, with technetium-99m
        monoclonal antibodies against
        granulocytes, 95: 104
Arrhythmogenic
    foci in Wolff-Parkinson-White syndrome
        and ventricular tachycardia, 94: 51
    right ventricular disease, impairment of
        sympathetic innervation of left
        ventricle in, 94: 68
Arteries
    carotid (see Carotid artery)
    cerebral, obstruction, consecutive
        technetium-99m HMPAO SPECT
        in, for carbon dioxide reactivity,
        95: 257
    coronary (see Coronary artery)
    infarct related, totally occluded, in acute
        myocardial infarction, thallium-201
        imaging of viability in, 95: 294
    intracerebral, temporary balloon
        occlusion of, brain blood flow
        SPECT in, 95: 259
    oxygen saturation in lung imaging,
        93: 126
    peripheral, disease, leg muscle
        scintigraphy with technetium-99m
        MIBI in, 94: 271
    pulmonary, aneurysm, thrombosed,
        causing high-probability lung
        imaging, 94: 105
    renal (see Renal artery)
    thrombosis, platelet-specific
        monoclonal antibody in, 93: 265

vertebral, stenosis, causing
    vertebrobasilar insufficiency,
    93: 293
Arteriography
    contrast, in peripheral vascular disease,
        94: 269
    coronary, in coronary artery disease,
        93: 105
Arteriovenous fistula
    pulmonary, scintigraphy in, 93: 129
Arteriovenous malformation
    cerebral, resection, intracranial
        hypertension after, 95: 368
Arthritis
    inflammatory activity of, indium-111
        leukocytes in, 93: 174
    osteoarthritis of knee, MRI, radiography
        and scintigraphy in, 93: 113
    rheumatoid (see Rheumatoid arthritis)
Arthrography
    combined contrast and radionuclide, in
        hip prosthesis suspected loosening,
        95: 356
Artifact
    correction, two-D translational motion,
        improved algorithm for, 93: 85
    phase-encode order effects on, in
        single-shot RARE sequences,
        93: 81
Ascorbate
    for antibody direct labeling with
        technetium-99m, 95: 414
Aspiration
    biopsy, fine-needle
        effect on thyroid imaging, 95: 174
        in kidney transplant acute
            dysfunction, 94: 232
Aspirin
    renography, for renovascular
        hypertension detection, 95: 194
Astrocytoma
    pilocytic, juvenile, neuroimaging of,
        95: 366
Asynergic regions
    severe, rest-injected thallium-201 for
        viability assessment, 93: 22
Athlete
    endurance, iliotibial band injury in,
        scintigraphy of, 93: 199

B

Back
    pain, low, SPECT, radiography and CT
        in, 93: 194
Backprojection

filtered, clinical receiver operating
characteristic study, in
fluorodeoxyglucose PET, 95: 435

Bacterial
infection, imaging focal sites of, with
technetium-99m hydrazino
nicotinamide derivatized
chemotactic peptide analogs,
95: 106

Ballet
overuse injury, of second metatarsal
base, as diagnostic problem,
95: 147

Balloon
angioplasty in coronary artery, left
ventricular function monitoring for
myocardial ischemia during, 93: 45
occlusion
of coronary artery, sequential
teboroxime imaging of, 95: 319
temporary, of carotid and
intracerebral arteries, 95: 259
temporary, of carotid artery to predict
tolerance before carotid sacrifice,
94: 280
test occlusion
of carotid artery, 93: 295
in carotid occlusion, permanent,
sequelae prediction, 94: 358

Basketball
professional players, tibiofibular
synostosis in, 95: 146

Beam
combined cone beam and parallel beam
data reconstructed by
three-dimensional SPECT, 93: 303
cone beam transmission CT with
gamma camera for torso imaging,
93: 304

Behavioral
factors, in mental stress induced silent
left ventricular dysfunction in
coronary artery disease, 95: 330
sequelae of severe closed head injury,
SPECT in, 94: 286

Beir V method
determining person years of life lost
using, 95: 445

Benzamides
iodinated, brain distribution of (in rat),
93: 321

Benzodiazepine
receptor
and binding sites, radioligands for
PET of, 94: 331
central and peripheral, and
epileptogenic tissue, 93: 283
ligand, iomazenil as, 93: 323

radioligand, SPECT, iodine-123
iomazenil, pharmacokinetics of,
94: 329
SPECT of, 93: 319

Beta-adrenergic
receptors in idiopathic dilated
cardiomyopathy, PET for, 94: 64

Beta adrenoceptors
myocardial, reduction in hypertrophic
cardiomyopathy, PET of, 95: 346

Beta-methyl fatty acid
in CT in hypertrophic cardiomyopathy,
93: 46

Beta oxidation
of 1-[carbon-14]-17-[iodine-131]-
iodoheptadecanoic acid after
intracoronary injection, 94: 66

Beta receptors
in heart, scintigraphy of, 93: 47

Bicycle
stress echocardiography vs. exercise
thallium-201 tomography for
coronary artery disease detection,
94: 13

Bile
duct
leakage, after laparoscopic
cholecystectomy, imaging of,
95: 215
obstruction in cystic fibrosis,
hepatobiliary scintigraphy of,
93: 256
leak
after falciform ligament tear,
hepatobiliary imaging of, 93: 254
after laparoscopic cholecystectomy,
scintigraphy of, 94: 258
secretion, effect of somatostatin analog
and octreotide on,
cholescintigraphy in, 95: 235

Biliary
colic, acalculous, hepatobiliary
scintigraphy in, 94: 239
dyskinesia, cholecystectomy in,
abnormal gallbladder nuclear
ejection fraction predicting success,
95: 210
fistula, traumatic, nonsurgical
management, 95: 218

Biopsy
aspiration, fine-needle
effect on thyroid imaging, 95: 174
in kidney transplant acute
dysfunction, 94: 232
marrow, iliac crest, vs. imaging for bone
metastases in lung cancer, 95: 131

Biotin
for infection localization, 94: 163

1,2-Bis[bis(2-ethoxyethyl)phosphino]ethane
technetium-99m, as new myocardial
perfusion imaging agent, 94: 46
Bis(dithiocarbamato) nitrido
technetium-99m neutral myocardial
imaging agents (in animals),
95: 324
Bladder
renography radiation dose to, 95: 185
variants on bone and kidney imaging,
94: 227
Blastomycosis
pulmonary, North American, gallium-67
imaging in, 95: 89
Block, bundle branch (see Bundle branch
block)
Blood
absorbed dose calculation to, of
radionuclides, 93: 350
flow
bone scintigraphy, of adenomyosis,
95: 249
brain, imaging to predict tolerance
before carotid sacrifice, 94: 280
cerebral, abnormalities,
technetium-99m ECD vs.
xenon-133 SPECT in, 94: 304
cerebral, changes in depression,
technetium-99m HMPAO SPECT
in, 94: 302
cerebral, in dementia, degenerative,
with iodine-123 IMP, 93: 286
cerebral, rCBF SPECT in ischemic
stroke thrombolysis, 93: 296
cerebral, regional, improvement with
cocaine polydrug users treatment,
95: 251
cerebral, regional, in Angelman
syndrome, 95: 280
cerebral, regional, measurement with
N-isopropyl-p-iodine 123
iodoamphetamine, redistribution in
ischemic cerebrovascular disease,
95: 253
cerebral, regional, variations during
temporary clipping in intracranial
aneurysm surgery, 95: 261
cerebral, SPECT for dementia
evaluation, interobserver agreement
in, 95: 262
cerebral, SPECT study, 94: 286
cerebral, technetium-99m HMPAO
SPECT of, 94: 278
cerebral, tomography in frontal brain
lesion volume measurement,
93: 299
concurrent quantification with tissue
metabolism with

hydrogen-2/phosphorus-31
magnetic resonance imaging, 89,
94: 88
leg, by plethysmography, vs. regional
distribution of thallium-201 during
lone leg exercise, 95: 239
limb, radionuclide measurements in
diagnostic problems in vascular
surgery, 95: 240
measurement with oxygen-17 MRI (in
rat), 93: 89
myocardial, and myocardial retention
of technetium-99m teboroxime,
94: 43
myocardial, assessment, new strategy,
94: 56
myocardial, assessment with
technetium-99m tetrofosmin, in
ischemia model (in dog), 95: 322
myocardial, glucose uptake and, in
ischemic myocardium (in dog),
94: 58
myocardial, noninvasive quantification
in coronary artery disease, 93: 53
myocardial, PET of, identifies
nonviable myocardium in chronic
myocardial infarction, 95: 334
myocardial, PET polar map displays
in, 94: 59
myocardial, quantification with
nitrogen-13 ammonia and dynamic
PET, 94: 62
myocardial, quantification with
nitrogen-13 ammonia and
reoriented dynamic PET, 94: 60
penis, in impotence, with papaverine
test, 94: 230
prostate, measurements by PET,
94: 229
renal artery, cine phase-contrast MRI
vs. p-aminohippurate clearance in,
95: 180
SPECT, brain, in temporary balloon
occlusion of carotid and
intracerebral arteries, 95: 259
temporal lobe, reduction in
Alzheimer's disease, 94: 295
penile flow during tumescence
dual-radioisotope technique in,
93: 230
pool
imaging, in bone scintigraphy of
adenomyosis, 95: 249
imaging with angiography for hand
radiation injury assessment, 94: 345
scintigraphy, false-positive hepatic, in
metastatic colon carcinoma,
93: 242

subtraction technique for indium-111 antimyosin antibodies in myocardial infarction visualization, 94: 71

pooling, in ventriculography in Kawasaki disease in children, with ventricular dysfunction and carditis, 95: 90

radioactivity concentration of technetium-99m, factors influencing, 94: 47

vessels, absorbed dose calculations to, of radionuclides, 93: 350

volume of prostate, measurements by PET, 94: 229

Bone, 94: 167

cancer, metastatic, pain palliation, 95: xxii

heterotopic new, accumulation of indium-111 leukocytes, 94: 158

imaging

bladder variants on, 94: 227

bony lesions in, 24 hour/3 hour radio-uptake technique for, 95: 133

correlation with prostate specific antigen in prostate cancer staging and monitoring, 94: 172

in gangrene, peripheral, due to fulminant meningococcemia, 95: 99

in hip fracture, occult, vs. MRI, 94: 377

of joint inflammation in rheumatoid arthritis, 94: 178

of limping toddlers, occult, 94: 170

of lung cancer, non-small cell, 93: 205

in non-united fracture management, 94: 177

in osteoma, osteoid, of femoral neck, 94: 376

in osteomyelitis in children, 94: 154

of pleural effusion, pleural fluid cytopathology in, 95: 76

SPECT, of kidney transplant with subclinical hip abnormality, 94: 176

technetium, negative, in histologically proven pressure sore related osteomyelitis, 95: 112

three-phase, of hypervascular brown tumors, 95: 122

triple phase, prognostic value for reflex sympathetic dystrophy in hemiplegia, 95: 281

vs. MRI for spinal metastases detection, 95: 355

infections, indium-111 IgG scintigraphy in, 93: 189

involvement in sarcoidosis, multiple atypical, 95: 118

lesions, in bone imaging, 24 hour/3 hour radio-uptake technique for, 95: 133

metastases

in breast cancer, CA 15-3 indicating, 94: 144

in small cell lung cancer, iliac crest marrow biopsy vs. imaging for, 95: 131

mineral measurements, with dual photon absorptiometry, and gamma camera, 95: 158

Paget disease, sarcoma in, features and radiography of, 93: 206

pain, skeletal metastases causing, samarium-153 EDTMP in, 95: 441

periarticular sites in trauma, false positives with indium-111 leukocytes and technetium-99m methylene diphosphonate scintigraphy, 94: 180

scintigraphy (*see* Scintigraphy, bone)

Bowel

inflammatory disease

indium-111 whole body retention in, 93: 175

simultaneous technetium-99m HMPAO and indium-111 oxine leukocytes for imaging of, 94: 248

technetium-99m and indium-111 leukocyte scintigraphy in, 94: 148

technetium-99m IgG imaging not predicting intestinal inflammation in, 94: 147

technetium-99m white blood cells vs. indium-111 granulocytes in, 95: 225

Brain

abscess, discordance between fluorine-18 fluorodeoxyglucose uptake and contrast enhancement in, 95: 74

after stroke, acute, N-acetylaspartate, creatine, phosphocreatine and choline compounds in, proton magnetic resonance spectroscopy of, 94: 91

anatomy, normal, fluorine-18 FDG PET and MRI, 95: 365

blood flow imaging to predict tolerance before carotid sacrifice, 94: 280

concentrations of putative radioligands, *ex vivo* binding to measure, 94: 334

death, magnetic resonance in, 94: 351

distribution of iodinated benzamides (in rat), 93: 321

fluoxetine and trifluoperazine in,
fluorine-19 magnetic resonance
spectroscopy of, 94: 352
frontal brain lesions, chronic traumatic,
volume measurement with MRI and
CBF tomography, 93: 299
function regional, neuroleptic effects
on, technetium-99m HMPAO
SPECT in, 93: 282
glucose metabolism changes in cocaine
dependence and withdrawal,
93: 290
imaging
functional, at 1.5 T with gradient echo
MRI techniques, 94: 350
three-dimensional, SPECT imager for,
stationary hemispherical, 94: 311
magnetic resonance and,
computer-assisted superimposition,
93: 279
magnetic resonance imaging, negative,
with stroke, 94: 354
magnetic resonance spectroscopy of,
proton, 94: 90
mapping, functional, with MRI, 94: 349
metabolism, as reliable discriminator in
Alzheimer's disease, PET and MRI
in, 95: 265
model, three-dimensional SPECT
simulations of, 93: 305
monoamine reuptake sites in, SPECT of,
93: 317
myo-inositol in, carbon-13 magnetic
resonance spectroscopy of, 94: 87
neurons in, cholinergic, mapping with
SPECT and iodine-123 IBVM,
95: 275
PET, fluorine-18 substituted
corticosteroids for, 94: 337
phantom physical, three-dimensional
SPECT simulations of, 93: 305
reorganization, functional, in
striatocapsular infarction recovery,
94: 305
SPECT (see SPECT, brain)
structures, and cognitive functions,
cerebrospinal fluid volumes in
Alzheimer's disease, 95: 370
technetium-99m HMPAO uptake,
quantification of, 95: 273
tumors
in children, thallium-201 vs.
technetium-99m MIBI SPECT of,
95: 44
thallium-201 SPECT of, 95: 45
uptake of
L-3-[iodine-123]iodo-α-methyl
tyrosine, 93: 329

Breast
cancer
bone metastases in, CA 15-3
indicating, 94: 144
detection and staging with
indium-111 B72.3 monoclonal
antibody, 93: 155
somatostatin receptor scintigraphy in,
95: 399
thallium-201 scintigraphy with
mammography for diagnosis,
95: 52
vertebral metastases of, MRI of,
94: 378
carcinoma
PET with fluorodeoxyglucose in,
94: 128
suspicion, prone scintimammography
in, 95: 376
disease, PET with fluorodeoxyglucose,
94: 128
mass abnormalities, thallium-201
scintigraphy of, 94: 138
milk, excretion of gallium-67 in, and
ingestion by infant, 93: 349
MRI of, 94: 78
Bronchi
stenosis, in infant, inhalation
scintigraphy in, 94: 113
stump postpneumonectomy, open,
xenon-133 ventilation imaging in,
94: 116
Bronchial
carcinoid,
adrenocorticotropin-secreting,
somatostatin analogs in, 95: 160
Bronchoalveolar
lavage
causing ventilation perfusion lung
imaging abnormalities, 95: 34
in lung disposition of gallium-67 in
Pneumocystis pneumonia, 93: 171
Bronchogenic
carcinoma, post-irradiation lung
function in, perfusion lung imaging
of, 94: 124
Bronchopleural
fistula, xenon-133 ventilation imaging
of, 94: 117
Brown
tumors, hypervascular, three-phase bone
imaging of, 95: 122
Brucellosis
musculoskeletal, imaging features,
95: 114
skeletal, bone scintigraphy in, 93: 190
Budd-Chiari syndrome

liver necrosis of, technetium-99m medronate uptake in, *94:* 254
Buerger's disease
microcirculatory characteristics in, *94:* 268
Bundle branch block
left
with coronary artery disease, adenosine superior to exercise thallium-201 in, *94:* 4
myocardial scintigraphy with thallium-201 and technetium-99m hexakis-methoxyisobutylisonitrile, *94:* 33
Burn
ossification after, heterotopic, causing vocal cord dysfunction, *95:* 150
Bypass
coronary artery, in aged, risk stratification in, cineangiography for, *95:* 327

C

CA 15-3
indicating metastatic bone in breast cancer, *94:* 144
Calcification
in tendinitis in proximal thigh, *95:* 359
Calcium
overload of myocardial cells and mitochondria causing myocardial ischemia, *94:* 31
Calibration
survey instrument, technetium-99m wipe standard for, *94:* 343
Camera
gamma (*see* Gamma camera)
in nuclear medicine, historic perspective, *95:* 421
SPECT, multi-head, sensitivity, resolution and image quality, *94:* 308
Cancer
bone, metastatic, pain palliation, *95:* xxii
breast (*see* Breast cancer)
cells, proliferative activity measurement by FDG uptake, *94:* 130
with central venous catheter, upper extremity radionuclide venography in, *94:* 266
in children, glomerular filtration rate estimation with technetium-99m DTPA clearance, *95:* 201
colorectal (*see* Colorectal cancer)

detection in solitary lung nodules with PET with 2-[fluorine-18]-fluoro-2-deoxy-D-glucose, *94:* 127
fluorodeoxyglucose uptake in, and blood glucose concentration, PET in, *94:* 131
head and neck, imaging with carbon-11-methionine and PET, *93:* 158
liver, metastatic, treatment, *95:* xxv
lung (*see* Lung cancer)
ovaries (*see* Ovaries, cancer)
prostate (*see* Prostate cancer)
rectum, and scar, differentiation with PET and MRI, *93:* 116
soft tissue, detection with gallium scintigraphy, *93:* 150
therapy assessment with fluorine-18 fluorodeoxyglucose and PET, *93:* 153
thyroid (*see* Thyroid cancer)
Capillary
network, link between IVIM and classical perfusion, *94:* 74
Captopril
during diuretics, renal functional response to, *93:* 235
renography
in renal artery stenosis, *93:* 237
technetium-99m DTPA, in renal artery stenosis, *95:* 199
renoscintigraphy with technetium-99m DTPA in suspected renovascular hypertension, *95:* 191
scintigraphy, renal
in hypertension and chronic renal failure, *95:* 198
in renovascular hypertension, and prognosis, *94:* 221
Carbon-11
acetate
in myocardial perfusion evaluation, *93:* 54
vs. fluorine-18-fluorodeoxyglucose, for myocardium viability delineation, by PET, *95:* 338
CGP-12177 for PET of beta-adrenergic receptors in idiopathic dilated cardiomyopathy, *94:* 64
hydroxyephedrine
for cardiac diabetic neuropathy assessment, *95:* 342
with PET for assessment of cardiac adrenergic neuronal function after acute myocardial infarction, *95:* 343

McN-5652Z, as PET radiotracer for serotonin uptake sites, 94: 333
methionine in head and neck cancer imaging, 93: 158
tropanyl benzilate, study of, 93: 325
Carbon-13
magnetic resonance spectroscopy of *myo*-inositol in brain, 94: 87
1-[Carbon-14]-17-[iodine-131]-iodoheptadecanoic acid
beta oxidation after intracoronary injection, 94: 66
Carbon dioxide
inhalation, oxygen-15-, for myocardial blood flow quantification in coronary artery disease, 93: 53
reactivity by consecutive technetium-99m HMPAO SPECT, in cerebral artery obstruction, 95: 257
Carcinoembryonic antigen
monoclonal antibody fragments, iodine-123, for colorectal cancer imaging, 94: 136
Carcinoid
bronchial, adrenocorticotropin-secreting, somatostatin analogs in, 95: 160
metastatic, scintigraphy with iodine-123 metaiodobenzylguanidine vs. iodine-123 Tyr-3-octreotide in, 94: 204
octreotide in, iodine-123, 94: 203
treatment with iodine-131 metaiodobenzylguanidine, 95: 56
Carcinoma
breast
PET with fluorodeoxyglucose in, 94: 128
suspicion, prone scintimammography in, 95: 376
bronchogenic, post-irradiation lung function in, perfusion lung imaging of, 94: 124
colon, metastatic, false-positive hepatic blood pool scintigraphy in, 93: 242
colorectal, follow-up, indium-111-anti-CEA monoclonal antibody ZCE 025 in, 93: 160
lung, squamous cell, radioiodine uptake by, 95: 31
thyroid (see Thyroid carcinoma)
Cardiac (see Heart)
Cardiomegaly
lower lobe ventilation impairment in, left, 94: 115
Cardiomyopathy

adriamycin, myocardial substrate utilization and left ventricular function in, 95: 337
dilated
distinction of ischemic from idiopathic, with thallium-201, 94: 8
idiopathic, beta-adrenergic receptors in, PET of, 94: 64
hypertrophic
cardiac arrest and syncope in, with myocardial ischemia, 95: 299
myocardial beta adrenoceptors reduction in, PET of, 95: 346
myocardial emission CT in, 93: 46
right ventricular, arrhythmogenic, regional myocardial sympathetic dysinnervation in, iodine-123 metaiodobenzylquanidine scintigraphy in, 95: 326
Cardiopulmonary
disease, prior, and strengthening diagnostic value of ventilation perfusion lung imaging in acute pulmonary embolism, 95: 10
Cardiotoxicity
doxorubicin, detection by myocardial uptake of indium-111 monoclonal antimyosin fab (in rat), 94: 70
Cardiovascular, 94: 1, 95: 283
Carditis
in Kawasaki disease in children, ventriculography and heart imaging in, 95: 90
Carotid
artery
balloon test occlusion of, 93: 295
temporary balloon occlusion of, brain blood flow SPECT in, 95: 259
temporary balloon occlusion of, to predict tolerance before carotid sacrifice, 94: 280
occlusion, permanent, sequelae prediction with MRI, technetium-99m HMPAO scintigraphy and balloon test occlusion, 94: 358
sacrifice, permanent, temporary balloon occlusion of carotid artery and brain blood flow imaging to predict tolerance before, 94: 280
Carpal
instability, missed diagnosis in suspected scaphoid fracture, 95: 141
Catecholamine
elevation, influencing heart volumes serial measurements by count-based methods, 94: 47

uptake and storage site in transplanted heart, PET in, 93: 59

Catheter
central venous, in cancer, upper extremity venography in, 94: 266

Catheterization
unnecessary, false positive thallium-01 imaging leading to, 94: 1

CBF (*see* Cerebral blood flow)

CCK
cholescintigraphy in differentiation of choledochal cyst and gallbladder, 93: 255

CEA
monoclonal antibody fragments, iodine-123, for imaging in colorectal cancer, 94: 136

Cells
cancer, proliferative activity measurement by FDG uptake, 94: 130
nucleus of, tracer localization in electron dose rate delivery to, 95: 443

Cellular
dosimetry, absorbed fractions for monoenergetic electron and alpha particle sources and S values for radionuclides, 95: 439

Central nervous system, 94: 277, 95: 251

Central venous catheter
in cancer, upper extremity venography in, 94: 266

Cerebellar diaschisis (*see* Diaschisis, cerebellar)

Cerebral
angioplasty in delayed ischemia due to vasospasm, 94: 282
arteriovenous malformation resection, intracranial hypertension after, 95: 368
artery, obstruction, consecutive technetium-99m HMPAO SPECT, for carbon dioxide reactivity, 95: 257
blood flow (*see* Blood flow, cerebral)
cortical activity, technetium-99m HMPAO of, 93: 291
glucose metabolism in Parkinson's disease, and dementia, 94: 292
infarction
chronic, proton magnetic resonance spectroscopy of, 94: 90
leukocyte infiltration in, 93: 300
ischemia, MRI of
contrast-enhanced, 93: 96
diffusion/perfusion, 93: 99
findings in first 24 hours, 93: 97

oxygen consumption measurement with oxygen-17 MRI (in rat), 93: 89

Cerebrospinal fluid
leak, pleural, indium-111 DTPA myelography of, 94: 123
suppressed quantitative single-shot diffusion imaging, 93: 62
volumes, in Alzheimer's disease, 95: 370

Cerebrovascular
disease, ischemic, redistribution in cerebral blood flow measurement with N-isopropyl-*p*-iodine-123 iodoamphetamine, 95: 253

Chelates
Dy, for T2 contrast-enhanced imaging, 93: 71
gadolinium (*see* Gadolinium chelates)
paramagnetic, metal ion release from, 93: 73
ribonucleoside-technetium, water-stable, for ribonuclease inhibition, 94: 323

Chelating agent
diamide dimercaptide, in technetium-99m radiolabeling of antibody fab fragment, 93: 335

Chemotactic
peptide analogs, technetium-99m hydrazino nicotinamide derivatized, for imaging focal sites of bacterial infection, 95: 106

Chemotherapy
in Hodgkin's disease, thymic rebound after, gallium in, 95: 60
response, phosphorus-31 magnetic resonance spectroscopy of, 94: 368

Chest pain (*see* Pain, chest)

Children
brain tumor evaluation, thallium-201 vs. technetium-99m MIBI SPECT of, 95: 44
cancer, glomerular filtration rate estimation in, with technetium-99m DTPA clearance, 95: 201
gastrointestinal bleeding, obscure, repeated technetium-99m pertechnetate in, 95: 233
Hodgkin's disease, residual mediastinal mass assessment with gallium-67 and CT, 93: 143
hydronephrosis, unilateral, ultrasound and renal scintigraphy in, 95: 187
Kawasaki disease, ventricular dysfunction and carditis in, ventriculography and heart imaging in, 95: 90
kidney scanning, dynamic, what proportion of isotope injected does child receive, 94: 220

kidney tract disease, technetium-99m
     mercapto acetyl triglycine in,
     93: 237
kidney washout during technetium-99m
     DTPA diuresis renography, ureteral
     status in, 93: 239
osteoma, osteoid, diagnosis, 95: 134
ostcomyclitis, multifocal, bone imaging
     in, 94: 154
pilocytic astrocytoma, juvenile,
     neuroimaging of, 95: 366
pneumonia, simple focal, uneventful
     recovery from, pulmonary
     scintigraphic defects after, 95: 32
pyelonephritis, reflux and nonreflux,
     kidney scarring after,
     technetium-99m DMSA
     scintigraphy of, 94: 226
sacrum fracture, fatigue, 95: 144
technetium-99m investigations, radiation
     dose from, 93: 342
Cholangitis
  AIDS
     sclerosing, hepatobiliary imaging in,
        95: 214
     sclerosing, hepatobiliary scintigraphy
        in, 93: 249
     technetium-99m DISIDA
        hepatobiliary scintigraphy in,
        95: 85
Cholecystectomy
  in biliary dyskinesia, abnormal
     gallbladder nuclear ejection fraction
     predicting success, 95: 210
  laparoscopic
     bile duct leakage after, imaging of,
        95: 215
     bile leakage after, scintigraphy of,
        94: 258
Cholecystitis
  acute
     cholescintigraphy in, with morphine
        augmentation, 95: 209
     morphine-augmented
        cholescintigraphy in, 93: 246
     rim sign portending, 94: 240
     scintigraphy with technetium-99m
        HMPAO leukocytes in, 93: 258
     suspected, hepatobiliary scintigraphy
        in, morphine-augmented, 94: 237
  acute or subacute, gallbladder with rim
     sign in, 95: 216
Cholecystokinin
  cholescintigraphy to differentiate
     choledochal cyst from gallbladder,
     93: 255
  second dose during imaging, gallbladder
     response to, 94: 236

Choledochal
  cyst differentiated from gallbladder by
     CCK cholescintigraphy, 93: 255
Cholescintigraphy
  CCK, to differentiate choledochal cyst
     from gallbladder, 93: 255
  of cholecystitis, acute, morphine
     augmentation in, 95: 209
  morphine-augmented
     in cholecystitis, acute, 93: 246
     false-negative, in gallbladder
        perforation, 93: 248
  results in VA hospital, 94: 235
  rim sign in, and grading hyperperfusion
     diagnostic value, 95: 212
  of somatostatin analog and octreotide,
     effect on bile secretion and
     gallbladder emptying, 95: 235
Choline
  compounds containing, in brain after
     stroke, proton magnetic resonance
     spectroscopy of, 94: 91
Chondrolysis
  bone scintigraphy of, 94: 169
Chromatography
  to identify radioiodinated thyroid
     hormones after iodine-131
     scintigraphy in thyroid carcinoma
     follow-up, 95: 162
Chromic
  phosphate therapy, in ovarian cancer,
     intraperitoneal distribution imaging
     before, 95: 172
Cigarette smoking (see Smoking)
Cimetidine
  enhancing technetium-99m
     pertechnetate in Meckel's
     diverticulum visualization, 93: 262
Cine
  MRI of global left ventricular perfusion,
     93: 106
Cineangiography
  for risk stratification after coronary
     artery bypass in aged, 95: 327
Circuitry
  fast photon-counting, for germanium
     detector system, 93: 315
Circulation
  collateral, adequacy during balloon test
     occlusion of carotid artery, 93: 295
  magnetic resonance in brain death and,
     94: 351
  microcirculatory characteristics in
     Buerger's disease, 94: 268
Cirrhosis
  with portal hypertension, liver
     hemangioma in, technetium-99m
     red blood cell SPECT of, 95: 221

spleen infarction in, liver spleen
scintigraphy in, 95: 373
thallium-201 scintigraphy by rectum in,
95: 238
CIT
iodine-123, in SPECT of monoamine
reuptake sites in brain, 93: 317
Cocaine
abuse, brain perfusion SPECT in,
94: 304
crack cocaine use and pulmonary
infarction, 93: 125
dependence and withdrawal, brain
glucose metabolism changes in,
93: 290
polydrug users, chronic, treatment of,
improving regional cerebral blood
flow, 95: 251
Cognitive
activation, monitoring, with dual isotope
brain SPECT, 95: 276
functions, and brain structures,
cerebrospinal fluid volumes in
Alzheimer's disease, 95: 370
Colic
biliary, acalculous, hepatobiliary
scintigraphy in, 94: 239
kidney (*see* Kidney, colic)
Colitis
ulcerative, technetium-99m HMPAO
leukocyte scintigraphy in, 95: 93
Collimation
pinhole, for SPECT, ultra high
resolution, small field of view,
95: 426
Collimator
511-keV, for positron emitters with
gamma camera, 94: 321
higher-resolution, for SPECT, 94: 309
spatially varying focal length, fan beam
reconstruction algorithm for,
95: 428
Colon
carcinoma, metastatic, false-positive
hepatic blood pool scintigraphy in,
93: 242
regional transit, in constipation,
radioisotope determination vs.
radioopaque markers, 95: 237
Color
Doppler ultrasound in liver hyperplasia,
focal nodular, 94: 360
Colorectal
cancer
iodine-123 CEA monoclonal antibody
fragment imaging in, 94: 136

technetium-99m IMMU-4
monoclonal antibody imaging in,
94: 135
carcinoma follow-up
indium-111-anti-CEA monoclonal
antibody ZCE 025 in, 93: 160
Compton scatter compensation
with triple-energy window method for
SPECT, 95: 423
Computed tomography
cone-beam transmission, with gamma
camera for torso imaging, 93: 304
in epilepsy, partial, 94: 355
of femoral neck osteoma, osteoid,
94: 376
with gallium-67 imaging in Hodgkin's
disease in children, 93: 143
in head injury, closed, comparison with
SPECT and MRI, 93: 100
of hepatomegaly, congestive, 93: 260
for kidney depth measurement, vs.
technetium-99m DMSA, 94: 224
of liver hemangioma, 93: 119
in low back pain, chronic, 93: 194
myocardial emission, in hypertrophic
cardiomyopathy, 93: 46
of paraganglioma, for preoperative and
postoperative evaluation, vs.
iodine-131
metaiodobenzylguanidine
scintigraphy, 95: 55
of *Pneumocystis carinii* pneumonia in
AIDS, 94: 162
single photon emission (*see* SPECT)
in sternocostoclavicular hyperostosis,
95: 358
of stress fracture, bilateral pedicle,
93: 201
Computer
assisted superimposition of magnetic
resonance for brain images,
93: 279
generated marrow subtraction image, in
musculoskeletal infection, 95: 113
Cone
beam SPECT reconstruction algorithm,
with displaced center of rotation,
95: 429
Constipation
rectal emptying in, scintigraphy of,
94: 262
severe, regional colonic transit in,
radioisotope determination vs.
radioopaque markers, 95: 237
Contrast
magnetization transfer, in fat-suppressed
steady-state three-dimensional
MRI, 94: 77

material iodides, effects on radioactive
    iodine thyroid uptake, 93: 219
media for MRI (*see* Magnetic resonance
    imaging, contrast media)
in MRI, fast spin-echo, factors
    influencing, 94: 75
phase-encode order effects, in
    single-shot RARE sequences,
    93: 81
Copper
    binding sites in immunoglobulin G,
        94: 328
Coronary
    angiography
        magnetic resonance, vs. conventional
            angiography, 94: 364
        vs. myocardial perfusion imaging,
            planar, 94: 42
    angioplasty (*see* Angioplasty, coronary)
    arteriography in coronary artery disease,
        93: 105
    artery
        angioplasty, left ventricular function
            monitoring for myocardial ischemia
            during, 93: 45
        balloon occlusion, sequential
            teboroxime imaging of, 95: 319
        bypass, in aged, risk stratification in,
            cineangiography in, 95: 327
        disease (*see* /ibelow/I)
        occlusion, teboroxime imaging to
            detect, sequential, 95: 317
        occlusion, total, myocardial perfusion
            and ventricular function
            measurements during, 95: 311
        occlusion and reperfusion, extent of
            jeopardized myocardium during,
            93: 31
        reperfusion, teboroxime imaging,
            sequential, to detect, 95: 317
    artery disease
        advanced, outcome after viability
            studies with PET, 94: 52
        after heart transplant, exercise
            thallium scintigraphy of, 94: 19
        angiographically significant,
            prognostic value of exercise
            myocardial perfusion imaging in,
            94: 11
        chronic, left ventricular wall
            thickening in, 94: 57
        chronic, myocardial viability
            assessment in, 95: 315
        chronic, myocardial viability
            assessment in, with thallium-201
            SPECT vs. fluorodeoxyglucose
            PET, 95: 293

chronic, viable myocardium
    identification in, 93: 26
detection, accuracy of dipyridamole
    thallium-201 myocardial perfusion
    imaging, 94: 30
detection, bicycle stress
    echocardiography vs. exercise
    thallium-201 tomography for,
    94: 13
detection, with technetium-99m Q3
    and thallium-201, 95: 323
dipyridamole-MRI and coronary
    arteriography in, 93: 105
evaluation with technetium-99m
    tetrofosmin myocardial
    tomography, 95: 321
exercise SPECT thallium in, 95: 286
high risk, dipyridamole thallium
    imaging safety in, 93: 7
hypoperfused myocardium secondary
    to, stress redistribution
    thallium-201 SPECT indexes in,
    94: 22
identification in women by exercise
    SPECT thallium-201, 94: 2
with left bundle branch block,
    adenosine superior to exercise
    thallium-201 in, 94: 4
left main and three-vessel high-risk,
    adenosine SPECT thallium-201 in,
    94: 7
low C/M ratio identifying left
    ventricular dysfunction at rest,
    94: 22
management, nuclear exercise testing
    in, 93: 16
mental stress inducing silent left
    ventricular dysfunction in, 95: 330
myocardial blood flow noninvasive
    quantification in, 93: 53
myocardial perfusion imaging in,
    planar, 94: 41
myocardial scintigraphy with
    thallium-201 and technetium-99m
    hexakis-methoxyisobutylisonitrile,
    94: 33
myocardial viability in perfusion
    defects, 94: 55
one-vessel, stress thallium-201
    myocardial perfusion SPECT
    defects in, 95: 287
PET in, metabolic imaging value for
    prognosis, 95: 332
scintigraphy in, exercise thallium,
    prognostic value of, 93: 2
severe, exercise thallium-201
    tomography in, 94: 9

stable, iodine-123 IPPA metabolic and thallium-201 perfusion imaging in, 95: 300

suspected, dobutamine thallium-201 tomography in, 94: 5

suspected, exercise thallium test in, qualitatively normal planar, follow-up, 95: 283

thallium-201 scintigraphy with adenosine coronary vasodilatation in, 93: 10

thallium-201 SPECT during adenosine coronary hyperemia, 93: 12

thallium-201 SPECT vs. exercise echocardiography in, 93: 14

thallium-201 SPECT vs. rubidium-82 PET in, 93: 24

thallium-201 testing in, exercise, over 70, prognostic significance, 93: 5

in young men, exercise thallium-201 scintigraphy with false-positives, 94: 4

hyperemia (*see* Hyperemia, coronary)

patency after myocardial infarction, reverse redistribution on exercise thallium scintigraphy in, 94: 23

reserve, assessment with PET with oxygen-15 water vs. intracoronary Doppler technique, 95: 340

stenosis severity, and perfusion defects with myocardial contrast echocardiography, thallium-201 SPECT in, 94: 16

vasodilation with adenosine and thallium-201 scintigraphy in coronary artery disease, 93: 10

venous outflow phase velocity mapping of left ventricular perfusion, 93: 106

Correlative imaging, 95: 349

Corticosteroids
fluorine-18 substituted, for brain PET, 94: 337

Cost
analysis of kidney transplant acute dysfunction, biopsy, ultrasound and scintigraphy in, 94: 232

Count
based methods for heart volumes serial measurements, 94: 47

Counters
in vivo, potential contaminants from radionuclides, 93: 355

Creatine
in brain after stroke, proton magnetic resonance spectroscopy of, 94: 91

Crohn's disease

acute, indium-111 imaging in, and mucosal damage severity, 95: 228

with fistula and sinus tract, indium-111 white blood cell scintigraphy in, 95: 227

scintigraphy with indium-111 leukocytes and ultrasound in, 94: 250

technetium-99m HMPAO leukocyte scintigraphy in, 95: 93

Curettage
intraoperative, probe-guided, of osteoid osteoma, 95: 364

Cutaneous (see Skin)

Cyst
choledochal, differentiated from gallbladder by CCK cholescintigraphy, 93: 255

Cystic fibrosis
bile duct obstruction in, hepatobiliary scintigraphy in, 93: 256

therapy assessment with aerosol scintigraphy, 93: 138

Cytometry
DNA flow, to measure cancer cell proliferative activity, 94: 130

Cytopathology
pleural fluid, in bone imaging of pleural effusion, 95: 76

D

D-dimer
levels, quantitative plasma, in pulmonary angiography for suspected pulmonary embolism, 95: 2

plasma measurement in pulmonary embolism diagnosis, 95: 4

D2 receptors
decrease in neurologic deficit in treated Wilson's disease, 94: 294

Dacron
prosthesis, aortoiliac and aortofemoral, knitted vs. woven, 94: 265

Death
brain, magnetic resonance in, 94: 351

Defecatory
difficulty, rectal emptying in, scintigraphy of, 94: 262

Deferoxamine
gallium-67, 93: 341

Dementia
AIDS dementia complex, brain perfusion SPECT in, 94: 304

Alzheimer, energy metabolism and mobile phosphoesters quantification with phosphorus-31 magnetic resonance spectroscopy, 94: 93

degenerative, cerebral blood flow in, with iodine-123 IMP, 93: 286

evaluation, interobserver agreement with cerebral blood flow SPECT, technetium-99m exametazime and HMPAO, 95: 262

in Parkinson's disease, and cerebral glucose metabolism, 94: 292

SPECT in, technetium-99m HMPAO, 93: 284

Deoxyglucose, fluorine-18 (see Fluorine-18 deoxyglucose)

Deoxyhemoglobin
susceptibility effect in magnetic resonance venography, 94: 79

Depression
major, cerebral blood flow changes in, technetium-99m HMPAO SPECT in, 94: 302

Deuterium
magnetic resonance washout method, validation for organ perfusion measurement, 94: 89

Diabetes mellitus
cardiac neuropathy, assessment with carbon-11 hydroxyephedrine and PET, 95: 342

foot complications in, infectious, indium-111 immunoglobulin G imaging in, 94: 149

with foot ulcer, osteomyelitis in, MRI of, 95: 353

insulin-dependent, myocardial glucose uptake in, dynamic PET in, 95: 336

osteomyelitis of foot in, indium-111 leukocyte scintigraphy in, 93: 183

Diagnosis
images of gas-forming infections, 95: 100

Dialdehyde starch
gallium-67, 93: 341

Diamide dimercaptide
chelating agent in technetium-99m radiolabeling of antibody fab fragment, 93: 335

Diaschisis
cerebellar, crossed
hemispheric flow reduction in, SPECT of, 94: 296

reverse in partial complex seizures in herpes simplex encephalitis, 94: 297

vascular response in, and acetazolamide, 94: 299

Diethylene

triamine penta-acetate, technetium-99m, lung clearance in AIDS, 93: 134

Diffusion
mediated susceptibility losses in tissues, and paramagnetic relaxation, 93: 71

MRI (see Magnetic resonance imaging, diffusion)

Dimercaptosuccinic acid, technetium-99m (see Technetium-99m DMSA)

Dipyridamole
echocardiography vs. exercise thallium scintigraphy for restenosis with positive exercise test after coronary angioplasty, 94: 15

induced technetium-99m MIBI perfusion abnormality on SPECT, 94: 39

MRI in coronary artery disease detection, 93: 105

in myocardial perfusion imaging
for cardiac risk stratification before vascular surgery, 94: 28

thallium-201, with low-level exercise unmasking ischemia, 93: 8

for myocardial scintigraphy with technetium-99m-sestamibi in effort angina, 93: 26

stress, thallium-201 myocardial imaging of perioperative cardiac events in major nonvascular surgery, 95: 288

technetium-99m sestamibi myocardial tomography, in stable chest pain, 95: 303

thallium-201
imaging, in aged, prognostic value, 94: 29

myocardial perfusion imaging for coronary artery disease detection and side-effect profile, 94: 30

scintigraphy, as preoperative screening test, 93: 9

scintigraphy, in stable chest pain, prognostic value, 93: 6

thallium imaging
negative, prognostic implications, 94: 29

for preoperative cardiac risk in nonvascular surgery, 94: 26

safety in high risk coronary artery disease, 93: 7

thallium scintigraphy predicting survival after major vascular surgery, 94: 27

DISIDA
technetium-99m, in hepatobiliary scintigraphy in AIDS cholangitis, 95: 85

Diuresis

renography, technetium-99m DTPA, kidney washout during, in children, ureteral status in, 93: 239

Diuretic renography (*see* Renography, diuretic)

Diuretics
captopril during, renal functional response to, 93: 235

Diverticulum
Meckel's
"fading," scintigraphy of, 94: 253
false-positive imaging, 95: 232
visualization with cimetidine-enhanced technetium-99m pertechnetate, 93: 262

DMSA, technetium-99m (*see* Technetium-99m DMSA)

DNA
flow cytometry to measure cancer cell proliferative activity, 94: 130

Dobutamine
infusion, myocardial oxidative metabolism during, 94: 60
stress
in quantitative technetium-99m sestamibi defect size, 95: 313
scintigraphy, 94: 5
test with thallium-201 SPECT, and radionuclide angiography, after infarction, 95: 301
thallium-201 tomography for suspected coronary artery disease, 94: 5
thallium myocardial perfusion tomography, 93: 13

L-Dopa
production and metabolism, 93: 327

Dopamine
cells, fetal implanted, survival in transplant for Parkinson's disease, 94: 290
D2 receptor-radioligands, 93: 321
D1 receptors in Parkinson's disease and striatonigral degeneration, PET of, 95: 270
receptor
D₂, in Parkinson's disease, SPECT with iodine-123 iodobenzamide in, 94: 293
SPECT in Parkinson's disease, 95: 271
uptake inhibitor binding (in mice), 93: 318

Doppler
color ultrasound in liver hyperplasia, focal nodular, 94: 360
intracoronary technique, in coronary reserve assessment, 95: 340

ultrasound, in kidney transplant acute dysfunction, 94: 232

Dosimetry, 95: 421
for adult female and fetus from iodine-131 in hyperthyroidism, 93: 214
cellular absorbed fractions for monoenergetic electron and alpha particle sources and S values for radionuclides, 95: 439
personnel dosimetry systems, determining lower limit of detection for, 93: 351
radiation (*see* Radiation dosimetry)
of radon, 95: 444
of samarium-153 EDTMP for bone pain due to skeletal metastases, 95: 441
thermoluminescence, detection and determination limits for, 93: 352

DOTA
Gd-, renal tolerance evaluation in chronic renal failure, 93: 74

Doxorubicin
cardiotoxicity detection by myocardial uptake of indium-111 monoclonal antimyosin fab (in rat), 94: 70

Drugs
antianginal, in exercise myocardial perfusion imaging, 95: 298
inducing pneumonitis, indium-111 leukocyte pulmonary uptake in, 94: 121

DTPA
D-Phe-1
indium-111, for somatostatin receptor scintigraphy, Rotterdam experience, 95: 388
octreotide, indium-111, for somatostatin receptor scintigraphy, 93: 147
octreotide, indium-111, for somatostatin receptor scintigraphy, of meningioma, 95: 403
gadolinium (*see* Gadolinium DTPA)
indium-111
for myelography of pleural cerebrospinal fluid leak, 94: 123
octreotide, for somatostatin receptor imaging of small cell lung cancer, 95: 401
technetium-99m (*see* Technetium-99m DTPA)

Duodenum
ileal duplication of, technetium-99m pertechnetate scintigraphy in, 94: 251

Dy

chelates for T2 contrast-enhanced
imaging, 93: 71
Dysinnervation
myocardial sympathetic, regional, in
arrhythmogenic right ventricular
cardiomyopathy, iodine-123
metaiodobenzylguanidine
scintigraphy in, 95: 326
Dyskinesia
biliary, cholecystectomy in, abnormal
gallbladder nuclear ejection fraction
predicting success in, 95: 210
Dystrophy, reflex sympathetic (see Reflex
sympathetic dystrophy)

E

Echocardiography
bicycle stress, vs. exercise thallium-201
tomography in coronary artery
disease detection, 94: 13
dipyridamole, vs. exercise thallium
scintigraphy for restenosis with
positive exercise test after coronary
angioplasty, 94: 15
exercise, vs. thallium-201 SPECT in
coronary artery disease, 93: 14
myocardial contrast, of perfusion
defects, and coronary stenosis
severity, thallium-201 SPECT in,
94: 16
resting two-dimensional, of
perioperative cardiac events in
major nonvascular surgery, 95: 288
in stress myocardial perfusion,
postexercise regional ventricular
function and myocardial
assessment, 95: 305
Ectopic
thyroid, intracardiac, conservative
surgery, 95: 379
EDTMP
samarium-153, dosimetry and toxicity in
bone pain due to skeletal
metastases, 95: 441
Elderly (see Aged)
Electrocardiography
in chest pain, spontaneous, 93: 28
exercise, in coronary artery disease,
93: 2
monitoring, ambulatory, before vascular
surgery, 94: 28
in myocardial infarction, recent, for
residual tissue viability assessment,
93: 20

nondiagnostic, noninvasive
identification of myocardium at risk
in, 93: 30
Electrocorticography
in epilepsy, partial, ictal and interictal
activity, 94: 357
Electroencephalography
in epilepsy, partial, 94: 355
ictal and interictal activity, 94: 357
Electron
dose rate delivery to cell nucleus, tracer
localization in, 95: 443
Embolism
pulmonary
acute, artificial neural network
approach, 95: 18
acute, ventilation/perfusion lung
imaging in, 93: 124
acute, ventilation perfusion lung
imaging in, strengthening the
diagnostic value of, 95: 10
D-dimer plasma measurement and
lower extremity venous ultrasound
in, 95: 4
fibrin-specific monoclonal antibody
localizing and visualizing, 93: 128
frequent asymptomatic, with deep
vein thrombosis, 95: 1
in Klippel-Trenaunay syndrome,
94: 274
during lower extremity compression
ultrasound, 94: 103
lung imaging in, 94: 98
massive, false-positive V/Q imaging
mimicking, 93: 127
from popliteal vein aneurysm,
94: 104
posterior view ventilation imaging in,
limitations of, 95: 21
Prospective Investigation of Diagnosis
Study, ventilation perfusion
scintigraphy in, 95: 8
scintigraphy, Technegas vs.
krypton-81m for, 94: 108
scintigraphy, technetium-99m
technegas ventilation, 93: 131
suspected, intermediate probability
lung imaging in, 93: 123
suspected, pulmonary angiography
for, quantitative plasma D-dimer
levels in, 95: 2
suspected, ventilation imaging of,
technetium-99m micro aerosol
pertechnegas for, 95: 22
suspected, when can treatment be
withheld, 95: 6

technetium-99m DD-3B6/22
anti-fibrin monoclonal antibody fab
fragment in, 95: 245
ventilation perfusion lung imaging,
mismatched vascular defects in,
95: 13
Encephalitis
herpes simplex
partial complex seizures in, reverse
crossed cerebellar diaschisis in,
94: 297
SPECT and MRI in, 93: 101
Encephalography
HIV, SPECT in, 93: 288
Endocrine, 94: 185, 95: 153
tumors, gastrointestinal, preoperative
localization, with somatostatin
receptor scintigraphy, 95: 381
Endoprosthesis
infected, monoclonal antibody
leukocyte scintigraphy of, 94: 161
Energy
charge, low of myocardial and skeletal
muscle, in angina pectoris with
thallium perfusion imaging
abnormality, 94: 20
metabolism, quantification in Alzheimer
dementia with phosphorus-31
magnetic resonance spectroscopy,
94: 93
Enteral
alimentation, percutaneous, gastrostomy
vs. gastrojejunostomy in, 94: 258
Epilepsy
partial
comparison of SPECT, EEG, CT and
MRI in, 94: 355
ictal and interictal activity recorded
with
magnetoelectroencephalography,
94: 357
temporal lobe
neuroimaging in, 94: 354
phosphorus-32 magnetic resonance
spectroscopy of, 94: 92
Epileptogenic tissue
benzodiazepine receptors and, 93: 283
Epiphysis
femoral, slipped capital, and bone
scintigraphy of chondrolysis,
94: 169
Erythrocyte (*see* Red blood cell)
Esophagus
dysmotility on ventilation perfusion lung
imaging, 94: 122
retained radioactivity, giving
false-positive thyroid cancer

metastases on radioiodine imaging,
95: 166
Estrogen
receptor imaging with MIVE$_2$, 93: 337
Ether
radioiodinated phospholipid ether
analog, localization in tumor
xenografts, 95: 411
Ethyl cysteinate dimer
technetium-99m, in SPECT of stroke,
95: 252
L,L-Ethylenedicysteine
technetium-99m, as new kidney imaging
agent, 95: 177
Exametazime
multidose, for leukocyte labeling, with
tin enhancement, 95: 103
reconstituted, long-term stability,
93: 330
Exercise
capacity improvement after
revascularization, PET in, 93: 58
ECG in coronary artery disease, 93: 2
echocardiography vs. thallium-201
SPECT in coronary artery disease,
93: 14
inadequate, leading to suboptimal
imaging, 93: 8
induced ischemia, reinjection as
alternative to rest imaging, in
thallium-201 emission tomography,
94: 6
influencing technetium-99m blood
radioactivity concentration, 94: 47
intramyocardial distribution during,
technetium-99m sestamibi
myocardial SPECT for, 95: 310
left ventricular dysfunction during, in
angina pectoris with normal
coronary arteries, 95: 328
in left ventricular performance
assessment after thrombolytics in
acute myocardial infarction, 93: 37
in myocardial perfusion and ventricular
function measurements during total
coronary artery occlusion, 95: 311
myocardial perfusion imaging,
antianginal drugs, peak heart rate
and stress level in, 95: 298
one leg, thallium-201 during, regional
distribution, vs. leg blood flow by
plethysmography, 95: 239
technetium-99m sestamibi myocardial
tomography, of right ventricular
perfusion defects after inferior
myocardial infarction, 95: 308

technetium-99m sestamibi tomography,
for cardiac risk stratification in
stable chest pain, 95: 304

test, positive, after coronary angioplasty,
restenosis in, exercise thallium
scintigraphy vs. dipyridamole
echocardiography for, 94: 15

testing
in myocardial infarction, recent,
residual tissue viability assessment
by, 93: 20
nuclear, in coronary artery disease
management, 93: 16

thallium
scintigraphy in coronary artery
disease, prognostic value, 93: 2
SPECT, in coronary artery disease,
95: 286
test, qualitatively normal planar, in
suspected coronary artery disease,
follow-up, 95: 283

thallium-201
SPECT vs. adenosine for myocardial
perfusion imaging, 93: 11
test, ischemic, poor prognosis in,
94: 10
testing in coronary artery disease over
70, prognostic significance, 93: 5

Extremities
blood flow radionuclide measurements,
for vascular surgery diagnostic
problems, 95: 240
lower
compression ultrasound of,
pulmonary embolism during,
94: 103
pain, in preschool children, bone
scintigraphy of, 93: 196
venous ultrasound in pulmonary
embolism diagnosis for, 95: 4
reflex sympathetic dystrophy of, MRI
failure in, 93: 110
upper, venography in cancer with
central venous catheter, 94: 266

Eye
MRI of, high resolution, with short TR,
short TE and partial-echo
acquisition, 93: 82
vitrectomized, partial oxygen pressure
in, with fluorine-19 MRI (in rabbit),
93: 87

F

Fab fragment
anti-fibrin monoclonal antibody,
technetium-99m DD-3B6/22, in

deep venous thrombosis and
pulmonary embolism detection,
95: 245

Face
nerve palsy, peripheral, after radioiodine
therapy of papillary thyroid
carcinoma, 95: 170

Falciform
ligament tear, bile leak after,
hepatobiliary imaging of, 93: 254

Fallopian tube
passive transport processes, serial
scintigraphy in, 93: 236

Fan beam
reconstruction algorithm for spatially
varying focal length collimator,
95: 428

Fat
necrosis, intraosseous, with pancreatitis,
95: 130
suppressed MRI, magnetization transfer
contrast in, 94: 77

Fatty
acid
analog, iodinated branched, for
SPECT in myocardial infarction
regional metabolic abnormality,
94: 67
in CT in hypertrophic
cardiomyopathy, 93: 46
uptake, differentiation from regional
perfusion in myocardial injury
zones, 93: 46
liver causing liver spleen imaging defect,
93: 154

FDG (*see* Fluorodeoxyglucose)

Feet (*see* Foot)

Felodipine
oral, kidney effects of, scintigraphy with
technetium-99m mercaptoacetyl
triglycine, 95: 189

Femur
epiphysis, slipped capital, and bone
scintigraphy of chondrolysis,
94: 169
fracture, occult proximal, MRI of,
95: 349
head ischemia, early traumatic, MRI vs.
bone scintigraphy in, 94: 374
neck
fracture, gadopentetate dimeglumine
MRI in, 94: 375
osteoma, osteoid, bone imaging, CT
and MRI in, 94: 376

Fetus
dopamine cells, implanted, survival in
transplant for Parkinson's disease,
94: 290

mesencephalic graft in Parkinson's disease due to MPTP, 94: 291

radiation dosimetry from iodine-131 in maternal hyperthyroidism, 93: 214

Fever

of unknown origin, immunoscintigraphy in diagnosis of, 95: 80

Fibrin

specific monoclonal antibody localizing and visualizing pulmonary embolism, 93: 128

Fibrosing

alveolitis, inhaled technetium-99m DTPA clearance predicting clinical course of, 95: 36

mediastinitis, superior vena cava obstruction in, 93: 271

Fibrosis, cystic (*see* Cystic fibrosis)

Filariasis

magnetic resonance lymphography of, with AMI-227 (in ferret), 94: 371

Fistula

biliary, traumatic, nonsurgical management, 95: 218

bronchopleural, xenon-133 ventilation imaging of, 94: 117

in Crohn's disease, with sinus tract, indium-111 white blood cell scintigraphy in, 95: 227

pulmonary arteriovenous, scintigraphy in, 93: 129

subarachnoid pleural, indium-111 DTPA myelography of, 94: 123

Flow

cytometry, DNA, to measure cancer cell proliferative activity, 94: 130

rate effect on adherence of leukocytes, 93: 330

Fluoride ion

fluorine-18, for whole body skeletal imaging, 94: 181

Fluorine-18

2-fluoro-2-deoxy-D-glucose, myocardial uptake in PET, 95: 335

6-fluorodopa PET in Parkinson's disease after nitecapone inhibition, 94: 335

deoxyglucose

in ischemic myocardium, myocardial blood flow and glucose uptake in (in dog), 94: 58

PET, in myocardial viability in perfusion defects, 94: 55

PET, of exercise capacity improvement after revascularization, 93: 58

PET, of heart, effect of metabolic milieu on, 93: 55

PET, vs. thallium-201 reinjection, 93: 21

uptake in left ventricular wall thickening, 94: 57

fluoride ion, for whole body skeletal imaging, 94: 181

fluoro-2-deoxy-D-glucose

for PET in solitary lung nodule cancer detection, 94: 127

for PET of soft tissue masses, 93: 151

fluorodeoxyglucose (*see* Fluorodeoxyglucose, fluorine-18)

fluoromisonidazole for hypoxic myocardium detection, 94: 65

L-DOPA production and metabolism, 93: 327

substituted corticosteroids for PET of brain, 94: 337

Fluorine-19

magnetic resonance spectroscopy

of 5-fluorouracil metabolism in liver (in mice), 94: 369

of fluoxetine and trifluoperazine in brain, 94: 352

of myocardial oxygen tension, 94: 86

MRI of partial oxygen pressure in vitrectomized eye (in rabbit), 93: 87

U-FLARE for fast perfluorocarbon imaging, 94: 85

Fluoro-2-deoxy-D-glucose

fluorine-18, for PET

of soft tissue masses, 93: 151

in solitary lung nodule cancer detection, 94: 127

uptake to measure cancer cell proliferative activity, 94: 130

2-[F-18]-Fluoro-2-deoxy-D-glucose

myocardial uptake in PET, 95: 335

for PET of solitary pulmonary nodule, 95: 26

Fluorodeoxyglucose

fluorine-18

for cancer therapy assessment, with PET, 93: 153

in cancer therapy assessment, with PET, 93: 153

discordance between uptake and contrast enhancement in brain abscess, 95: 74

intratumoral distribution (in mice), 94: 130

myocardial uptake of, regional, with SPECT, 95: 331

in myocardial viability in chronic coronary artery disease, 95: 315

PET, in probable Alzheimer's disease, vs. technetium-99m HMPAO SPECT, 95: 268

PET, of normal brain anatomy,
95: 365
of residual tissue viability after
myocardial infarction, time
dependence of, 95: 339
vs. carbon-11 acetate, for myocardium
viability delineation by PET,
95. 338
PET
in breast disease, 94: 128
clinical receiver operating
characteristic study of filtered
backprojection vs. maximum
likelihood estimator images in,
95: 435
vs. thallium-201 SPECT, for
myocardial viability assessment in
chronic coronary artery disease,
95: 293
uptake in cancer, and blood glucose
concentrations, PET in, 94: 131
6-Fluorodopa
fluorine-18, for PET in Parkinson's
disease after nitecapone inhibition,
94: 335
Fluoromisonidazole
fluorine-18, for hypoxic myocardium
detection, 94: 65
5-Fluorouracil
liver metabolism, thymidine-modulated,
fluorine-19 magnetic resonance
spectroscopy of (in mice), 94: 369
Fluoxetine
in brain, fluorine-19 magnetic resonance
spectroscopy of, 94: 352
Foot
diabetic complications, infectious,
indium-111 immunoglobulin G
imaging in, 94: 149
osteomyelitis in diabetes, indium-111
leukocyte scintigraphy in, 93: 183
reflex sympathetic dystrophy,
scintigraphy of, 94: 174
ulcer, in diabetes, osteomyelitis in, MRI
of, 95: 353
Fracture
femur
neck, gadopentetate dimeglumine
MRI in, 94: 375
occult proximal, MRI of, 95: 349
hip, occult, MRI vs. bone imaging in,
94: 377
pelvis, radiation-induced scintigraphy,
technetium-99m MDP scintigraphy
in, 93: 198
sacrum, fatigue, in children, 95: 144
scaphoid, suspected

carpal instability as missed diagnosis
in, 95: 141
radiography and bone scintigraphy in,
95: 353
radiography and scintigraphy of,
94: 167
spine, in multiple injury, negative
scintigraphy in, 95. 351
stress, bilateral pedicle, SPECT and CT
of, 93: 201
talar dome, bone scintigraphy of,
93: 204
tibia, insufficiency, after kidney
transplant, 95: 125
ununited
infection diagnosis in, imaging with
indium-111 leukocytes and
technetium-99m methylene
diphosphonate, 95: 97
management, bone imaging in,
94: 177

G

Gadolinium
chelates
dissociation, relationship to chemical
characteristics (in mice), 94: 94
high-dose in MRI, 93: 75
reaction with endogenously available
ions, 93: 73
for T2 contrast-enhanced imaging,
93: 71
DOTA, renal tolerance evaluation in
chronic renal failure, 93: 74
DTPA
for synergistic enhancement of MRI,
93: 79
for ultrafast MRI in myocardial
perfusion imaging, 93: 104
Gadopentetate
dimeglumine for MRI in femoral neck
fracture, 94: 375
Gallbladder
abnormal nuclear ejection fraction
predicting success of
cholecystectomy in biliary
dyskinesia, 95: 210
activity after IV technetium-99m
mercaptoacetyltriglycine, simulating
obstructive uropathy, 94: 211
differentiated from choledochal cyst by
CCK cholescintigraphy, 93: 255
disease, acalculous, gallbladder ejection
fraction predicting, 94: 238
ejection fraction

calculation, sincalide infusion and
    three-minute infusion in, 93: 245
predicting acalculous gallbladder
    disease, 94: 238
emptying, effect of somatostatin analog
    and octreotide on,
    cholescintigraphy in, 95: 235
perforation
    false-negative morphine-augmented
        cholescintigraphy in, 93: 248
    malrotation simulating,
        technetium-99m IDA scintigraphy
        in, 93: 251
response to cholecystokinin second
    dose during imaging, 94: 236
visualization
    early, during technetium-99m red
        blood cell scintigraphy, 94: 241
    prompt, with rim sign, as acute or
        subacute cholecystitis, 95: 216
Gallium
scintigraphy in soft tissue cancer
    detection, 93: 150
in thymic rebound after chemotherapy
    for Hodgkin's disease, 95: 60
Gallium-67
avid mediastinal mass after Hodgkin's
    disease treatment, thallium-201
    scintigraphy of, 95: 63
citrate
    for imaging in lung disease, and
        transferrin receptor expression,
        94: 164
    imaging in tuberculosis, acute
        disseminated, vs. chest radiography,
        95: 88
    imaging of salivary gland disease in
        HIV infection, 94: 197
    SPECT in Hodgkin's disease in
        mediastinum, 93: 145
deferoxamine-dialdehyde starch-IgG,
    93: 341
excretion in breast milk and ingestion by
    infant, 93: 349
gastric uptake in AIDS, 93: 172
IgG polyclonal, in inflammatory lesions,
    acute focal, 93: 163
imaging
    of blastomycosis, North American
        pulmonary, 95: 89
    with CT in Hodgkin's disease in
        children, 93: 143
lung disposition in *Pneumocystis*
    pneumonia, 93: 171
scintigraphy
    after treatment of lymphoma, 93: 144
    in leprosy, borderline lepromatous,
        95: 90

in lymphoma, small, non-cleaved cell,
    94: 137
in otitis, differentiating necrotizing
    from severe, 93: 176
of *Pneumocystis carinii* pneumonia in
    AIDS, 94: 162
uptake, in benign transformation mass
    mimicking Hodgkin's disease
    recurrence, 95: 61
whole-body, in sarcoidosis diagnosis,
    93: 178
Gamma camera
for 511-keV collimator for positron
    emitters, 94: 321
for bone mineral measurements, using
    dual photon absorptiometry,
    95: 158
in cone-beam transmission CT for torso
    imaging, 93: 304
in imaging therapeutic dose of
    iodine-131, 93: 156
renography, standardization of, 94: 222
Ganglia
lunate, communicating intraosseous,
    95: 362
Gangrene
peripheral, due to fulminant
    meningococcemia, bone imaging in,
    95: 99
Gas
forming infection, diagnostic images of,
    95: 100
pulmonary gas volume, regional
    ventilation, measurement of, and
    PET, 93: 140
Gastric
emptying
    measurement by MRI, 94: 362
    rate of solids, menstrual cycle and
        menopause in, 95: 236
uptake of gallium-67 in AIDS, 93: 172
(*See also* Stomach)
Gastrointestinal, 94: 235, 95: 205
bleeding
    localization with technetium-99m red
        blood cell scintigraphy, 95: 223
    obscure, in children, repeated
        technetium-99m pertechnetate in,
        95: 233
    studies with technetium-99m
        erythrocytes, 93: 241
    study, technetium-99m red blood cell,
        spleen rupture incidental detection
        during, 94: 243
    technetium-99m red blood cell
        scintigraphy vs. angiography in,
        94: 244

true positive imaging of, and
false-positive Meckel's diverticulum
imaging, 95: 232
endocrine tumors, preoperative
localization, with somatostatin
receptor scintigraphy, 95: 381
Gastrojejunostomy
in enteral alimentation, percutaneous,
vs. gastrostomy, 94: 258
Gastrostomy
in enteral alimentation, percutaneous,
vs. gastrojejunostomy, 94: 258
Gd (see Gadolinium)
Genitourinary, 94: 207
Geometry
ventricular, in quantitative
technetium-99m sestamibi defect
size, 95: 313
Germanium
detector system with fast
photon-counting circuitry for
imaging, 93: 315
Glass
household, for indoor radon estimation
of past exposure, 94: 347
^{210}Po embedded in, for long-term radon
concentrations estimation, 95: 446
Glioma
recurrent, vs. radiation necrosis, 94: 288
supratentorial, thallium-201 SPECT of,
95: 48
Glomerular
filtration rate, in cancer in children,
technetium-99m DTPA clearance to
estimate, 95: 201
Glucose
blood concentration, and
fluorodeoxyglucose uptake in
cancer, PET of, 94: 131
cerebral metabolism in Parkinson's
disease, and dementia, 94: 292
metabolism
changes, of brain, in cocaine
dependence and withdrawal,
93: 290
in uveal melanoma, 93: 117
myocardial uptake in insulin-dependent
diabetes, dynamic PET of, 95: 336
uptake and myocardial blood flow in
ischemic myocardium (in dog),
94: 58
Glycolipopeptide
J001 macrophage targeting, for
scintigraphy in sarcoidosis, 94: 165
P-Glycoprotein
multidrug-resistant, imaging with
organotechnetium complex,
94: 327

Graft
aortic
early postoperative technetium-99m
leukocytes in, 93: 270
infection detection with
technetium-99m hexametazime
leukocytes, 94: 158
mesencephalic, fetal, in Parkinson's
disease due to MPTP, 94: 291
Granulation
tissue, fluorine-18 fluorodeoxyglucose
distribution in (in mice), 94: 130
Granulocyte
antibody, technetium-99m, in
inflammatory diseases, 93: 170
indium-111, vs. technetium-99m white
blood cells in inflammatory bowel
disease, 95: 225
technetium-99m monoclonal antibodies
against, in appendicitis detection,
95: 104
Granulocytopenia
febrile patients, infection of, indium-111
IgG in, 93: 179
Graves' disease
euthyroid, with thyroid carcinoma,
94: 192

H

Hamartoma
pulmonary, technetium-99m methylene
diphosphonate uptake by, 94: 118
Hand
radiation dose to, in nuclear medicine,
93: 353
radiation injuries, assessment with
angiography and blood pool
imaging, 94: 345
Head
injury, closed, comparison of SPECT,
CT and MRI in, 93: 100
and neck cancer imaging,
carbon-11-methionine and PET in,
93: 158
region, indium-111 leukocyte
accumulation in, 93: 166
Health
physics, 94: 339
Heart
adrenergic neuronal function assessment
after acute myocardial function,
with carbon-11 hydroxyephedrine
and PET, 95: 343
arrest, in hypertrophic cardiomyopathy,
myocardial ischemia in, 95: 299

beta receptors in, scintigraphy of,
93: 47
diabetic neuropathy, assessment with
carbon-11 hydroxyephedrine and
PET, 95: 342
disease not diminishing lung imaging in
acute pulmonary embolism,
93: 124
failure
congestive, with intact systolic left
ventricular performance, outcome,
93: 41
iodine-123 metaiodobenzylguanidine
scintigraphy in, 94: 69
hypertrophy, iodine-123
metaiodobenzylguanidine
scintigraphy in, 94: 69
imaging
SPECT for, attenuation and scatter
correction method, 94: 312
technetium-99m HMPAO white
blood cell, in Kawasaki disease in
children, with ventricular
dysfunction and carditis, 95: 90
with technetium-99m sestamibi,
normal, prognostic value of,
95: 302
metabolism, regional substrate,
evaluation with PET, 93: 56
patient outcome, and rubidium-82 PET
myocardial perfusion imaging,
94: 61
perioperative events in major
nonvascular surgery, risk indexes,
echocardiography and myocardial
imaging of, 95: 288
PET
attenuation imaging,
three-dimensional registration,
94: 64
effect of metabolic milieu on, 93: 55
polar map displays for myocardial
blood flow and viability assessment,
94: 59
rate, peak, in exercise myocardial
perfusion imaging, 95: 298
rejecting, MHC class II antigen
induction by, 93: 51
risk
in nonvascular surgery, preoperative,
dipyridamole thallium imaging in,
94: 26
stratification, in stable chest pain,
exercise technetium-99m sestamibi
tomography for, 95: 304
stratification, with dipyridamole
myocardial perfusion imaging and

ECG monitoring before vascular
surgery, 94: 28
shape deformity measurement, model in
measurement of, 93: 43
sympathetic neuronal dysfunction,
regional, and ventricular
refractoriness, 95: 343
transplant (*see* Transplantation, heart)
volume assessment by gated
angiography, 93: 39
volumes serial measurements by
count-based methods, 94: 47
Hemangioma
differentiated from liver metastases with
ultrafast MRI, 93: 115
in Kasabach-Merritt syndrome,
technetium-99m red blood cell
imaging in, 94: 274
liver
cavernous, lack of enlargement over
time, 95: 372
in cirrhosis with portal hypertension,
technetium-99m red blood cell
SPECT in, 95: 221
metastatic malignancy masquerading
as, on red blood cell scintigraphy,
95: 68
MRI, CT and SPECT of, 93: 119
small cavernous, SPECT in, 93: 244
technetium-99m red blood cell
SPECT in, 94: 246
Hematology, 95: 41
Hemiagenesis, thyroid (*see* Thyroid
hemiagenesis)
Hemiplegia
reflex sympathetic dystrophy in, triple
phase bone imaging for, 95: 281
Hemispheric
flow reduction, SPECT of, in crossed
cerebellar diaschisis, 94: 296
Hemoglobin
sickle cell disease, splenic infarction and
sequestration in, 93: 274
Hemorrhage
gastrointestinal (*see* Gastrointestinal
bleeding)
intraperitoneal bleeding,
technetium-99m red blood cell
scintigraphy in, 94: 247
Hepatic (*see* Liver)
Hepatitis
radiation, magnetic resonance
appearance of, 94: 361
Hepatobiliary
excretion of MAG3, as urinary leak
simulation, 95: 220
imaging

in AIDS related sclerosing cholangitis,
95: 214
of bile leak after falciform ligament
tear, 93: 254
hot spot in focal nodular hyperplasia,
95: 205
scintigraphy (see Scintigraphy,
hepatobiliary)
Hepatomegaly
congestive, CT, ultrasound and nuclear
medicine in, 93: 260
Hernia
hiatal, on whole body radioiodine
imaging, mimicking metastatic
thyroid cancer, 95: 378
Herpes
simplex encephalitis
partial complex seizures in, reverse
crossed cerebellar diaschisis in,
94: 297
SPECT and MRI in, 93: 101
Heterogenous
systems, water-photon magnetic
relaxation in, 93: 69
Heterotopic
liver transplant for liver failure, liver
regeneration after, 94: 261
new bone, accumulation of indium-111
leukocytes by, 94: 158
Hexakis-methoxyisobutylisonitrile
technetium-99m
after stress for SPECT of myocardial
perfusion defect size, 94: 40
for myocardial scintigraphy of left
bundle branch block and coronary
artery disease, 94: 33
Hexametazime
technetium-99m, with leukocytes, in
aortic graft infection detection,
94: 158
Hexamethylpropylene amine oxime,
technetium-99m (see
Technetium-99m
HMPAO)
Hiatal
hernia, on whole body radioiodine
imaging, mimicking metastatic
thyroid cancer, 95: 378
High field imaging
RF penetration effects reduction in,
93: 86
Hip
fracture, occult, MRI vs. bone imaging
in, 94: 377
osteoporosis (see Osteoporosis,
transient, of hip)
prosthesis, suspected loosening,
combined contrast and

radionuclide arthrography in,
95: 356
subclinical abnormality after kidney
transplant, MRI and SPECT bone
imaging in, 94: 176
Hippuran
iodine-131, for kidney transplant
evaluation, 94: 214
Histiocytosis
sinus, with lymphadenopathy, skeletal
involvement, 95: 57
HIV
encephalopathy, SPECT in, 93: 288
infection, salivary gland disease in,
gallium-67 citrate imaging of,
94: 197
(See also AIDS)
HMPAO
brain SPECT, abnormalities in,
assessment method, 95: 267
technetium-99m (see Technetium-99m
HMPAO)
Hodgkin's disease
chemotherapy, thymic rebound after,
gallium in, 95: 60
in children, residual mediastinal mass
assessment with gallium-67 and CT,
93: 143
in mediastinum, gallium-67-citrate
SPECT in, 93: 145
nodular lymphocytic recurrence,
gallium-67 uptake in benign
transformation mass mimicking,
95: 61
treatment, thallium-67 avid mediastinal
mass after, thallium-201
scintigraphy of, 95: 63
Hormone, thyroid (see Thyroid hormones)
HSA
technetium-99m, for vascular exam in
reflex sympathetic dystrophy,
93: 272
Hydrated
lysosome results in water-proton
magnetic relaxation, 93: 69
Hydration
relaxation in protein solutions and tissue
and, 94: 78
Hydrazino nicotinamide
derivatized chemotactic peptide analogs,
technetium-99m, for imaging focal
sites of bacterial infection, 95: 106
Hydrocephalus
normal pressure, SPECT with
technetium-99m d,l-HMPAO,
before and after shunt operation,
95: 279
Hydrogen-1

MRI, quantitation of metabolites by,
93: 90
Hydrogen-2
phosphorus-31 magnetic resonance
imaging for concurrent
quantification of tissue metabolism
and blood flow, 89, 94: 88
Hydronephrosis
pelvic, antenatal diagnosis, 93: 233
unilateral, in children, ultrasound and
kidney scintigraphy in, 95: 187
Hydroxyapatite
particles, samarium-153 and
rhenium-186, as
radiopharmaceuticals for radiation
synovectomy (in rabbit), 95: 418
Hydroxyephedrine
carbon-11 (*see* Carbon-11
hydroxyephedrine)
for PET in pheochromocytoma
localization, 94: 195
Hyperemia
coronary, adenosine
with thallium-201 SPECT in coronary
artery disease, 93: 12
in tomographic myocardial perfusion
imaging, 93: 35
tomography of, 94: 17
Hyperglycemia
reducing fluorodeoxyglucose uptake in
tumors, 94: 132
Hyperostosis
sternocostoclavicular, CT of, 95: 358
Hyperparathyroidism
10 MHz ultrasound vs. thallium-201
technetium-99m subtraction
imaging of, 95: 155
parathyroid abnormalities in,
technetium-99m iodine-123
imaging vs. ultrasound of, 95: 157
surgery, localization with
technetium-99m sestamibi, 95: 42
Hyperperfusion
grading, diagnostic value of, and rim
sign in cholescintigraphy, 95: 212
Hyperplasia
focal nodular
hot spot hepatobiliary imaging in,
95: 205
of liver (*see* Liver, hyperplasia, focal
nodular)
Hypertension
intracranial, after cerebral arteriovenous
malformation resection, 95: 368
kidney scintigraphy in, captopril,
95: 198

portal, in cirrhosis, with liver
hemangioma, technetium-99m red
blood cell SPECT in, 95: 221
pulmonary, perfusion lung scintigraphy
in, 95: 37
renovascular (*see* Renovascular
hypertension)
Hyperthyroidism
iodine-131 in, radiation dosimetry for
adult female and fetus from,
93: 214
iodine-induced, intrathyroid iodine store
measurement in, 93: 218
Hypertrophic cardiomyopathy (*see*
Cardiomyopathy, hypertrophic)
Hypertrophy
heart, iodine-123
metaiodobenzylguanidine
scintigraphy in, 94: 69
Hypoperfused
myocardium secondary to coronary
artery disease, stress redistribution
thallium-201 SPECT in, 94: 22
Hypoperfusion
of myocardium, contrast-enhanced MRI
of, 93: 102
Hypothesis
linear, nonthreshold, for low-dose
radiation, 93: 348
Hypothyroidism
permanent congenital, radionuclide
imaging in, 93: 218
Hypoxia
myocardial
with fluorine-18 fluoromisonidazole
and PET, 94: 65
marking with iodovinylmisonidazole,
95: 325
in technetium-99m Technegas
ventilation and technetium-99m
MAA perfusion scintigraphy,
94: 106
tissue, iodoazomycin arabinoside as
marker of, 93: 338
tumor, imaging of, 95: 409
Hysterosalpingography
radionuclide, simplified technique,
95: 203

I

IBVM
iodine-123, of neurons, cholinergic,
mapping in brain, 95: 275
IBZM

iodine-123, for dopamine receptor SPECT in Parkinson's disease, 95: 271

IDA
technetium-99m, for scintigraphy in malrotation simulating gallbladder perforation, 93: 251

Ig (*see* Immunoglobulin)

Ileal
duplication of stomach and duodenum, technetium-99m pertechnetate scintigraphy in, 94: 251

Iliac
crest marrow biopsy vs. imaging for bone metastases in lung cancer, 95: 131

Iliotibial band injury
in endurance athlete, scintigraphy of, 93: 199

Imager
SPECT, stationary hemispherical, for three-dimensional brain imaging, 94: 311

Images
diagnostic, of gas-forming infection, 95: 100

Imaging
correlative, 95: 349
high field, RF penetrating effects reduction in, 93: 86
iodine-131 dose with gamma camera, 93: 156
liver spleen, defect due to fatty liver, 93: 154
lung (*see* Lung imaging)
magnetic resonance (*see* Magnetic resonance)
MRI (*see* Magnetic resonance imaging)
myocardial perfusion (*see* Myocardial perfusion imaging)
neuroimaging (*see* Neuroimaging)
T2 contrast-enhanced, Gd- and Dy-chelates for, 93: 71
V/Q, false-positive, mimicking pulmonary embolism, 93: 127

Immunodiagnosis
of tumors, 95: 70

Immunoglobulin
G
copper and technetium-99m binding sites similarity in, 94: 328
gallium-67, 93: 341
gallium-67 polyclonal, in inflammatory lesions, acute focal, 93: 163
indium-111 (*see* Indium-111 IgG)

nonspecific, indium-111, in scintigraphy of inflammations and infections, 93: 174
polyclonal, labeled with polymeric iron oxide, 93: 76
polyclonal, technetium-99m, in purulent disease diagnosis, focal, 95: 101
polyclonal, technetium-99m, to detect joint inflammation in rheumatoid arthritis, 94: 178
technetium-99m, not predicting intestinal inflammation in inflammatory bowel disease, 94: 147
nonspecific human, for imaging of inflamed joints in rheumatoid arthritis, 95: 105
polyclonal, for infection localization, 94: 163

Immunoradiometric
assay with metallic radionuclides, 93: 341

Immunoscintigraphy
in fever of unknown origin diagnosis, 95: 80
indium-111 OC-125, in ovarian cancer recurrence diagnosis, 94: 134
in ovarian cancer management, 94: 143

IMP, iodine-123 (*see* Iodine-123 IMP)

Impotence
papaverine test with radionuclide penile blood flow in, 94: 230

In vivo counters
potential contaminants from radionuclides, 93: 355

Indium-111
anti-CEA monoclonal antibody
in thyroid medullary carcinoma imaging, 93: 159
ZCE 025 in colorectal carcinoma follow-up, 93: 160
antifibrin monoclonal antibody in venous thrombosis, 93: 268
antimyosin antibodies
for myocardial infarction visualization, 94: 71
uptake and myocardial infarction age, 93: 48
B72.3 monoclonal antibody in breast cancer detection and staging, 93: 155

DTPA
myelography of pleural cerebrospinal fluid leak, 94: 123
octreotide, for somatostatin receptor imaging of small cell lung cancer, 95: 401

DTPA-D-Phe-1
octreotide, for scintigraphy,
  somatostatin receptor, of
  meningioma, 95: 403
octreotide, for somatostatin receptor
  scintigraphy, 93: 147
for somatostatin receptor
  scintigraphy, 95: 388
granulocyte, vs. technetium-99m white
  blood cells, in inflammatory bowel
  disease, 95: 225
IgG
in granulocytopenia, febrile infection
  in, 93: 179
imaging of infectious diabetic foot
  complications, 94: 149
nonspecific, in scintigraphy of
  inflammations and infections,
  93: 174
nonspecific, in subacute infections
  foci detection, 93: 164
scintigraphy in bone, joint and joint
  prosthesis infections, 93: 189
imaging, in Crohn's disease, acute,
  mucosal damage severity in,
  95: 228
leukocytes
accumulation in head and neck
  region, 93: 166
accumulation in heterotopic new
  bone, 94: 158
in arthritis, of inflammatory activity,
  93: 174
autologous, in subacute infectious foci
  detection, 93: 164
in deep venous thrombosis, 93: 269
imaging, in mesenteric lymphadenitis,
  95: 95
imaging, of infected knee prosthesis,
  93: 184
imaging, of ununited fracture
  infection, 95: 97
in inflammatory lesions, acute focal,
  93: 163
oxine, flow rate effect on adherence
  of, 93: 330
in polycystic liver disease with normal
  tissue remnants, 95: 229
pulmonary uptake in drug-induced
  pneumonitis, 94: 121
scintigraphy, false positives in
  periarticular bone sites in trauma,
  94: 180
scintigraphy, in Crohn's disease,
  94: 250
scintigraphy, in Crohn's disease with
  fistula and sinus tract, 95: 227

scintigraphy, in inflammatory bowel
  disease, 94: 148
scintigraphy, in osteomyelitis of foot
  in diabetes, 93: 183
scintigraphy, of cutaneous sarcoidosis,
  94: 118
scintigraphy, of marrow alterations in
  osteomyelitis, 93: 186
scintigraphy, of marrow-containing
  skeleton, photopenic defects,
  94: 155
in sulfur colloid scintigraphy of
  musculoskeletal infection, 95: 113
monoclonal antibody against tissue
  plasminogen activator in deep
  venous thrombosis, 93: 267
monoclonal antimyosin fab, myocardial
  uptake in doxorubicin
  cardiotoxicity detection (in rat),
  94: 70
myosin-specific monoclonal antibodies
  in myocardial damage due to
  anthracycline, 93: 49
OC-125 immunoscintigraphy in ovarian
  cancer recurrence diagnosis,
  94: 134
octreotide scintigraphy, in oncology,
  95: 393
oxine leukocytes, for imaging in
  inflammatory bowel disease,
  94: 248
whole body retention in inflammatory
  bowel disease, 93: 175
Infant
bronchial stenosis, inhalation
  scintigraphy in, 94: 113
ingestion of breast milk with gallium-67,
  93: 349
limping toddlers, occult, bone imaging
  in, 94: 170
Infarction
cerebral, leukocyte infiltration in,
  93: 300
chronic, proton magnetic resonance
  spectroscopy of, 94: 90
dobutamine stress test with thallium-201
  SPECT and radionuclide
  angiography after, 95: 301
myocardial (*see* Myocardial infarction)
pancreatitis and, 95: 130
pulmonary, in crack cocaine use,
  93: 125
related artery, totally occluded, in acute
  myocardial infarction, thallium-201
  imaging of viability in, 95: 294
spleen
in cirrhosis, liver spleen scintigraphy
  in, 95: 373

in hemoglobin sickle cell disease,
93: 274
striatocapsular, recovery from, brain
functional reorganization in,
94: 305
Infection, 94: 147, 95: 79
aortic graft, detection with
technetium-99m hexametazime
leukocytes, 94: 158
bacterial, imaging focal sites, with
technetium-99m hydrazino
nicotinamide derivatized
chemotactic peptide analogs,
95: 106
diseases in competitive sports, 95: 86
of endoprosthesis, monoclonal antibody
leukocyte scintigraphy of, 94: 161
focal, imaging with technetium-99m
liposomes (in rat), 95: 107
foci, subacute, detection with
indium-111 leukocytes and
immunoglobulin G, 93: 164
gas-forming, diagnostic images of,
95: 100
localization with streptavidin, biotin and
polyclonal immunoglobulin,
94: 163
musculoskeletal, marrow subtraction
image and sulfur colloid
scintigraphy in, 95: 113
phantom, in asymptomatic vessels,
95: 247
scintigraphy of, indium-111 nonspecific
IgG in, 93: 174
in ununited fractures, imaging with
indium-111 leukocytes and
technetium-99m methylene
diphosphonate, 95: 97
Inflammation, 95: 79
foci, technetium-99m proteins in
imaging of, 93: 332
of joints in rheumatoid arthritis, imaging
with technetium-99m monoclonal
antibodies and immunoglobulin,
95: 105
scintigraphy of, indium-111 nonspecific
IgG in, 93: 174
Inflammatory
bowel disease (see Bowel, inflammatory
disease), 95: 225
diseases, technetium-99m granulocyte
antibody in, 93: 170
lesions, acute focal, radioactive agents
including indium-111 leukocytes
and gallium-67 polyclonal IgG,
93: 163
Innervation

sympathetic, of left ventricle,
impairment in arrhythmogenic right
ventricular disease, 94: 68
Instrumentation, 94: 307
Insulin
dependent diabetes, myocardial glucose
uptake in, dynamic PET of, 95: 336
low-dose, before fluorodeoxyglucose
uptake in cancer studies, 94: 132
Intestine, 94: 235
inflammation in inflammatory bowel
disease, technetium-99m IgG
imaging not predicting, 94: 147
Intracardiac
ectopic thyroid, conservative surgery,
95: 379
Intracerebral
artery, temporary balloon occlusion of,
brain blood flow SPECT in,
95: 259
Intracoronary Doppler technique
in coronary reserve assessment, 95: 340
Intracranial
aneurysm surgery, temporary clipping in,
regional cerebral blood flow
variations during, 95: 261
hypertension, after cerebral
arteriovenous malformation
resection, 95: 368
Intramyocardial
distribution during exercise,
technetium-99m sestamibi
myocardial SPECT for, 95: 310
Intraperitoneal
bleeding, technetium-99m red blood
cell scintigraphy in, 94: 247
distribution imaging before chromic
phosphate therapy in ovarian
cancer, 95: 172
Iodide
contrast material iodides effects on
radioactive iodine thyroid uptake,
93: 219
hyperthyroidism due to, intrathyroidal
iodine store measurement in,
93: 218
iodine-131, thyroid carcinoma
concentrating, 93: 216
Iodinated
benzamides, brain distribution of (in
rat), 93: 321
Iodine
radioactive, thyroid uptake, effects of
contrast material iodides on,
93: 219
radioiodine uptake by pelvis in rectal
wall teratoma after thyroidectomy
for carcinoma, 94: 190

stores, intrathyroid, measurement in
iodide-induced hyperthyroidism,
93: 218
uptake, thyrotropin stimulating (in
monkey), 94: 185
Iodine-123
for brain SPECT, 94: 277
CEA monoclonal antibody fragment
imaging in colorectal cancer,
94: 136
CIT in monoamine reuptake sites in
brain, 93: 317
fatty acid for CT in hypertrophic
cardiomyopathy, 93: 46
IBVM, of neurons, cholinergic, mapping
in brain, 95: 275
IBZM, for dopamine receptor SPECT in
Parkinson's disease, 95: 271
imaging, in hyperparathyroidism, with
parathyroid abnormalities, 95: 157
IMP
for cerebral blood flow in
degenerative dementia, 93: 286
for lung imaging, abnormal
accumulation mechanism, 93: 137
iodoamphetamine
N-isopropyl-*p*-, for cerebral blood
flow measurement, redistribution in
ischemic cerebrovascular disease,
95: 253
in SPECT of stroke, 95: 252
iodobenzamide
for SPECT of D$_2$ dopamine receptors
in Parkinson's disease, 94: 293
for SPECT of D2 receptor decrease in
neurologic deficit in treated
Wilson's disease, 94: 294
iomazenil, pharmacokinetics of, 94: 329
metaiodobenzylguanidine
in metastatic carcinoid, 94: 204
scintigraphy, in heart hypertrophy and
failure, 94: 69
scintigraphy, of regional myocardial
sympathetic dysinnervation in
arrhythmogenic right ventricular
cardiomyopathy, 95: 326
scintigraphy, with thallium-201 for
neuroendocrine tumor detection,
95: 53
SPECT of denervated but viable
myocardium (in dog), 93: 50
N-(2-diethylaminoethyl
4-iodobenzamide), for scintigraphy
of malignant melanoma and
metastases, 95: 405
N-isopropyl-p-iodoamphetamine lung
clearance and smoking, 93: 136

octreotide in carcinoid and islet cell
tumors, 94: 203
phenylpentadecanoic acid metabolic, in
stable coronary artery disease,
95: 300
for SPECT, recent developments,
93: 333
Tyr-3-octreotide
in metastatic carcinoid, 94: 204
scintigraphy, in lung cancer staging,
small cell, 95: 400
for somatostatin receptor
scintigraphy, 93: 147, 95: 388
Iodine-125
(2-piperidinylaminoethyl)
4-iodobenzamide, as malignant
melanoma imaging agent, 95: 408
metaiodobenzylguanidine
intraoperative, of metastatic
pheochromocytoma, 94: 196
for pheochromocytoma intraoperative
detection, 95: 171
Iodine-131
contamination from thyroid cancer,
94: 188
hippuran for kidney transplant
evaluation, 94: 214
in hyperthyroidism, radiation dosimetry
to adult female and fetus in,
93: 214
imaging
therapeutic dose with gamma camera,
93: 156
whole body, in thyroid carcinoma,
metastatic differentiated, diagnosis
and treatment assessment, 95: 164
iodide, thyroid carcinoma
concentrating, 93: 216
localization in thyroid carcinoma,
insular, 93: 220
metaiodobenzylguanidine
for adrenergic tumors, 95: xxiv
for bone scintigraphy of
neuroblastoma, 94: 141
for malignant pheochromocytoma,
paraganglioma and carcinoid
treatment, 95: 56
scintigraphy, for paraganglioma
preoperative and postoperative
evaluation, vs. CT and MRI, 95: 55
scintigraphy, in suspected
pheochromocytoma, 93: 227
scintigraphy, whole body,
radioiodinated thyroid hormones
after, in thyroid carcinoma
follow-up, 95: 162

therapy for thyroid carcinoma, complications, sequelae and dosimetry, 94: 187

thyroid ablation, efficacy assessment, 95: 169

Iodoamphetamine
iodine-123
N-isopropyl-p-, for cerebral blood flow measurement, redistribution in ischemic cerebrovascular disease, 95: 253
in SPECT of stroke, 95: 252

Iodoazomycin arabinoside
as tissue hypoxia marker, 93: 338

Iodobenzamide
iodine-123
N-(2-diethylaminoethyl 4-), for scintigraphy of malignant melanoma and metastases, 95: 405
for SPECT, of D$_2$ dopamine receptors in Parkinson's disease, 94: 293
for SPECT, of D2 receptor decrease in neurologic deficit in treated Wilson's disease, 94: 294
iodine-125 (2-piperidinylaminoethyl) 4-, as malignant melanoma imaging agent, 95: 408

1-[carbon-14]-17-[iodine-131]-Iodoheptade-canoic acid
beta oxidation after intracoronary injection, 94: 66

Iodovinylmisonidazole
for myocardial hypoxia marker, 95: 325

Iomazenil
as benzodiazepine receptor ligand, 93: 323
iodine-123, pharmacokinetics of, 94: 329

IPPA
metabolic, iodine-123, in stable coronary artery disease, 95: 300

Iron
oxide
compound AMI-227, for magnetic resonance lymphography if filariasis (in ferret), 94: 371
nanoparticles for MRI contrast media, 93: 76
polymeric, polyclonal immunoglobulin G labeled with, 93: 76

Irradiation (see Radiation)

Ischemia
cerebral (see Cerebral ischemia)
exercise-induced, reinjection as alternative to rest imaging with thallium-201 emission tomography, 94: 6

femoral head, traumatic, MRI vs. bone scintigraphy in, 94: 374
model, of myocardial blood flow, technetium-99m tetrofosmin to assess (in dog), 95: 322
myocardium (see Myocardium, ischemia)
thallium-201 myocardial perfusion imaging with dipyridamole and low-level exercise unmasking ischemia, 93: 8
vasospasm causing, delayed, brain SPECT and cerebral angioplasty in, 94: 282

Ischemic
but viable myocardium, nitrates improving detection of, by thallium-201 reinjection SPECT, 95: 291
cardiomyopathy, dilated, thallium-201 in, 94: 8
cerebrovascular disease, redistribution in cerebral blood flow measurement with N-isopropyl-p-iodine-123 iodoamphetamine, 95: 253
stroke, thrombolysis with recombinant tissue plasminogen activator in, 93: 296
thallium-201 exercise test, poor prognosis in, 94: 10

Islet cell tumors
octreotide in, iodine-123, 94: 203
visualization with somatostatin analogs, 95: 396

n-Isopropyl-p-iodoamphetamine
SPECT in complex partial seizure disorders, 93: 280

J

Joint, 94: 167
infections and joint prosthesis infections, indium-111 IgG scintigraphy in, 93: 189
inflammation
active, in rheumatoid arthritis, technetium-99m polyclonal IgG and bone imaging in, 94: 178
in rheumatoid arthritis, imaging with technetium-99m monoclonal antibodies and immunoglobulin, 95: 105

K

Kasabach-Merritt syndrome
familial cases, 94: 274

hemangioma in, technetium-99m red
blood cell imaging in, 94: 274
Kawasaki disease
in children, with ventricular dysfunction
and carditis, ventriculography and
heart imaging in, 95: 90
Kidney, 95: 177
colic, scintigraphy in initial evaluation,
renal, 94: 219
depth
improved formula for estimation in
adult, 95: 183
measurement with technetium-99m
DMSA vs. CT, 94: 224
effects of oral felodipine, scintigraphy
with technetium-99m
mercaptoacetyl triglycine, 95: 189
excretion characteristics of
technetium-99m
mercaptoacetylglycyl-D-
alanylglycine, 94: 213
failure, chronic
kidney scintigraphy in, captopril,
95: 198
renal tolerance evaluation of
Gd-DOTA in, 93: 74
function
and drainage in management of pelvic
hydronephrosis, antenatal
diagnosis, 93: 233
monitor of, ambulatory, 94: 208
pyeloplasty, early, does it really avert
loss of function, 95: 186
functional response to captopril during
diuretics, 93: 235
imaging
bladder variants on, 94: 227
dynamic, in children, what proportion
of isotope injected does child
receive, 94: 220
in kidney donor preoperative
evaluation, 95: 190
new agent, technetium-99m
L,L-ethylenedicysteine as, 95: 177
technetium-99m
mercaptoacetyltriglycine replacing
technetium-99m DMSA, 94: 212
renography radiation dose to, 95: 185
scarring
after reflux and nonreflux
pyelonephritis in children,
technetium-99m DMSA
scintigraphy of, 94: 226
after vesicoureteral reflux, 94: 227
scintigraphy (*see* Scintigraphy, kidney)
tract disease, in children,
technetium-99m mercapto acetyl
triglycine in, 93: 237

transplant (*see* Transplantation, kidney)
uropathy, obstructive, gallbladder
activity after IV technetium-99m
mercaptoacetyltriglycine simulating,
94: 211
washout, during technetium-99m DTPA
diuresis renography in children,
ureteral status in, 93: 239
(*See also* Renal)
Klippel-Trenaunay syndrome
angiography of, radionuclide total body,
94: 272
pulmonary embolism in, 94: 274
Knee
osteoarthritis, MRI, radiography and
scintigraphy in, 93: 113
prosthesis, infected, indium-111
leukocyte, technetium-99m sulfur
colloid and MDP imaging in,
93: 184
Krypton-81m
inhaled gas, radiation absorbed dose
estimates from, in lung imaging,
95: 440
for ventilation scintigraphy of
respiratory disease, 94: 109
vs. Technegas in scintigraphy of
pulmonary embolism, 94: 108

L

L-DOPA
production and metabolism, 93: 327
Laparoscopic
cholecystectomy
bile duct leakage after, imaging of,
95: 215
bile leakage after, scintigraphy of,
94: 258
Lavage
bronchoalveolar
causing ventilation perfusion lung
imaging abnormalities, 95: 34
in lung disposition of gallium-67 in
Pneumocystis pneumonia, 93: 171
Leg
blood flow, by plethysmography, vs.
regional distribution of
thallium-201 during one leg
exercise, 95: 239
muscle scintigraphy with
technetium-99m MIBI in peripheral
vascular disease, 94: 271
Leprosy
borderline lepromatous, gallium-67
scintigraphy in, 95: 90
Leukemia

lymphoma, T cell, in adult, radiographic
features, 95: 374
Leukocyte
exametazime, multidose, for labeling of,
with tin enhancement, 95: 103
flow rate effect on adherence of,
93: 330
heart imaging, technetium-99m
HMPAO, in Kawasaki disease in
children, with ventricular
dysfunction and carditis, 95: 90
indium-111 (see Indium-111 leukocytes)
infiltration in cerebral infarct, 93: 300
monoclonal antibody scintigraphy of
infected endoprosthesis, 94: 161
scintigraphy (see Scintigraphy, leukocyte)
technetium-99m
hexametazime, for aortic graft
infection detection, 94: 158
HMPAO, for scintigraphy in
cholecystitis, 93: 258
HMPAO, imaging, in suspected
orthopedic infection, 94: 152
HMPAO, in abdominal infections and
inflammations, 93: 168
HMPAO, in purulent disease
diagnosis, focal, 95: 101
vs. indium-111 granulocytes in
inflammatory bowel disease,
95: 225
(See also Technetium-99m leukocytes)
Ligament
falciform, tear, bile leak after,
hepatobiliary imaging, 93: 254
Limb (see Extremities)
Limping toddlers
occult, bone imaging of, 94: 170
Linear
nonthreshold hypothesis for low-dose
radiation, 93: 348
Lipid
in adrenal masses, 94: 380
Liposome
nitroxide system for oximetry, 93: 88
technetium-99m, for imaging focal
infection (in rat), 95: 107
Liver
alcoholic disease, assessment with
SPECT, 94: 256
blood pool scintigraphy, false-positive,
in metastatic colon carcinoma,
93: 242
cancer, metastatic, treatment, 95: xxv
failure, fulminant, heterotopic liver
transplant for, liver regeneration
after, 94: 261
fatty, causing liver spleen imaging
defect, 93: 154

5-fluorouracil metabolism in,
thymidine-modulated, fluorine-19
magnetic resonance spectroscopy
of (in mice), 94: 369
hemangioma (see Hemangioma, liver)
hyperplasia, focal nodular
color Doppler ultrasound and MRI
in, 94: 360
MRI and pathologic correlation,
94: 360
resection of liver tumors, 94: 358
masses, solitary solid, scintigraphy of,
94: 139
metastases
differentiated from hemangioma with
ultrafast MRI, 93: 115
technetium-99m MAA intraarterial
infusion targeting, 95: 66
necrosis of Budd-Chiari syndrome,
technetium-99m medronate uptake
in, 94: 254
polycystic disease, normal tissue
remnants in, indium-111 white
blood cells in, 95: 229
regeneration after heterotopic liver
transplant for liver failure, 94: 261
spleen
imaging, defect due to fatty liver,
93: 154
scintigraphy, of splenic infarction in
cirrhosis, 95: 373
transplant, heterotopic, for liver failure,
liver regeneration after, 94: 261
tumors, benign, resection, 94: 358
uptake of technetium-99m PYP, 93: 259
L,L-ethylenedicysteine
technetium-99m, as new kidney imaging
agent, 95: 177
Low back pain
SPECT, radiography and CT in, 93: 194
Lunate
ganglion, communicating intraosseous,
95: 362
Lung, 94: 97, 95: 1
aerosol deposition pattern differences,
inhaled, due to three different sized
aerosols, 94: 111
cancer
non-small cell, bone imaging of,
93: 205
PET and, satellite, in surgical patients,
95: 71
small cell, bone metastases in, iliac
crest marrow biopsy vs. imaging for,
95: 131
small cell, somatostatin receptor
imaging, with indium-111 DTPA
octreotide, 95: 401

small cell, staging, with iodine-123
Tyr^3 octreotide scintigraphy,
95: 400
carcinoma, squamous cell, radioiodine
uptake by, 95: 31
clearance
of iodine-123
N-isopropyl-p-iodoamphetamine,
and smoking, 93: 136
of technetium-99m diethylene
triamine penta-acetate, in AIDS,
93: 134
disease
not diminishing lung imaging in acute
pulmonary embolism, 93: 124
transferrin receptor expression in, and
gallium-67 citrate imaging, 94: 164
disposition of gallium-67 in
Pneumocystis pneumonia, 93: 171
function, post-irradiation, in
bronchogenic carcinoma, perfusion
lung imaging in, 94: 124
imaging
high-probability, pulmonary artery
aneurysm causing, thrombosed,
94: 105
inhaled krypton-81m gas in, radiation
absorbed dose estimates from,
95: 440
intermediate probability, in suspected
pulmonary embolism, 93: 123
interpretation, do diagnostic
algorithms always produce uniform,
94: 100
with iodine-123-IMP, abnormal
accumulation mechanism, 93: 137
perfusion, arterial oxygen saturation
in, 93: 126
perfusion, of post-irradiation lung
function in bronchogenic
carcinoma, 94: 124
in pulmonary embolism, 94: 98
reports, interpretation by clinicians,
95: 16
segmental defect size underestimation
in, 94: 97
unilateral absence of perfusion on,
ascending aortic dissection causing,
95: 24
ventilation perfusion, abnormalities
due to bronchoalveolar lavage,
95: 34
ventilation perfusion, esophageal
dysmotility on, 94: 122
ventilation perfusion, in pulmonary
embolism, acute, 93: 124

ventilation perfusion, in pulmonary
embolism, acute, strengthening the
diagnostic value of, 95: 10
ventilation perfusion, in pulmonary
embolism, mismatched vascular
defects in, 95: 13
ventilation perfusion, neural network
analysis in, 94: 102
left lower lobe ventilation impairment in
cardiomegaly, 94: 115
MRI, contrast-enhanced, ventilation
perfusion assessments, 94: 366
nodules, solitary, malignancy detection
with PET with
2-[fluorine-18]-fluoro-2-deoxy-D-
glucose, 94: 127
scintigraphy
perfusion in pulmonary hypertension,
95: 37
ventilation perfusion, reporting, and
anticoagulation, 95: 15
uptake of indium-111 leukocytes in
drug-induced pneumonitis, 94: 121
(*See also* Pulmonary)
Lying
pathological, in thalamic dysfunction,
technetium-99m HMPAO SPECT
in, 94: 300
Lymph
node metastases, magnetic resonance
lymphography of (in rabbit),
94: 370
Lymphadenitis
mesenteric, indium-111 white blood cell
imaging in, 95: 95
Lymphadenopathy
massive, with sinus histiocytosis, skeletal
involvement, 95: 57
Lymphangioscintigraphy
of lymphedema, vs. MRI, 94: 371
Lymphedema
lymphoscintigraphy in, as reliable test,
95: 246
MRI vs. lymphangioscintigraphy in,
94: 371
Lymphocytosis
syndrome, diffuse infiltrative, salivary
gland radiotracer activity in,
94: 197
Lymphography, magnetic resonance (*see*
Magnetic resonance lymphography)
Lymphoma
gallium-67 scintigraphy after treatment,
93: 144
leukemia, T cell, in adult, radiographic
features, 95: 374
non-Hodgkin's, residual masses after
treatment, MRI of, 94: 367

small, non-cleaved cell, gallium-67
scintigraphy in, 94: 137
Lymphoscintigraphy
of lymphedema, as reliable test, 95: 246
in melanoma of trunk, high-risk, 95: 75
Lysozyme
results, hydrated, in water-proton
magnetic relaxation, 93: 69

M

Macrophages
fluorine-18 fluorodeoxyglucose
distribution in (in mice), 94: 130
targeting glycolipopeptide, J001, for
scintigraphy in sarcoidosis, 94: 165
MAG3
hepatobiliary excretion of, as urinary
leak simulation, 95: 220
technetium-99m (see Technetium-99m
mercaptoacetyltriglycine)
Magnet
magnetic resonance, high-field
superferric, 94: 85
Magnetic
relaxation, water-proton, in
heterogenous systems, hydrated
lysozyme results, 93: 69
resonance (see below)
Magnetic fields
4.0-tesla, human exposure in
whole-body scanner, 94: 95
dependence of proton spin relaxation in
tissues, 93: 68
static, in radiation survey instruments
response, 94: 344
Magnetic resonance
angiography
coronary, vs. conventional
angiography, 94: 364
magnetization transfer time-of-flight
in, 94: 76
with quasi-half-echo scanning, 93: 80
of renal arteries, 93: 120
susceptibility-based, 94: 80
appearance of radiation hepatitis,
94: 361
in brain death, 94: 351
computer-assisted superimposition, for
brain images, 93: 279
deuterium washout method, validation
for organ perfusion measurement,
94: 89
imaging (see below)
lymphography
of filariasis, with AMI-227 (in ferret),
94: 371

of lymph node metastases (in rabbit),
94: 370
magnet, high-field superferric, 94: 85
microscopy, high-temperature
superconducting receiver for,
94: 84
spectroscopy
carbon-13, of myo-inositol in brain,
94: 87
fluorine-19, of 5-fluorouracil
metabolism in liver (in mice),
94: 369
fluorine-19, of fluoxetine and
trifluoperazine in brain, 94: 352
fluorine-19, of myocardial oxygen
tension, 94: 86
generalized series approach to, 93: 91
phosphorus-31, in Alzheimer
dementia for quantification of
energy metabolism and mobile
phosphoesters, 94: 93
phosphorus-31, in temporal lobe
epilepsy, 94: 92
phosphorus-31, of chemotherapy
response, 94: 368
proton, in stroke, acute, 94: 353
proton, of brain, 94: 90
proton, of N-acetylaspartate, creatine,
phosphocreatine and choline
compounds in brain after acute
stroke, 94: 91
studies and nuclear medicine, 94: 349
tagged image sequences, motion
estimation from, 94: 81
venography with deoxyhemoglobin
susceptibility effect, 94: 79
Magnetic resonance imaging
of adrenal masses, chemical shift, fast
low-angle shot, 94: 380
in Alzheimer's disease, brain metabolism
as reliable discriminator of, 95: 265
of anisotropic and restricted diffusion
by simultaneous spin and stimulated
echoes, 94: 73
antibody, 93: 76
brain, negative, in stroke, 94: 354
of brain anatomy, normal, 95: 365
for brain mapping, functional, 94: 349
of breast, 94: 78
in carotid occlusion, permanent,
sequelae prediction, 94: 358
of cerebral ischemia
contrast-enhanced MRI, 93: 96
findings in first 24 hours, 93: 97
chemical shift, of benign adrenal cortex
masses, 94: 378
cine

of global left ventricular perfusion, 93: 106

phase-contrast, of renal artery blood flow, vs. p-aminohippurate clearance, 95: 180

contrast media

development of, new directions in, 93: 70

iron oxide nanoparticles for, 93: 76

superparamagnetic, target-specific, 93: 77

diffusion, 93: 61

of cerebral ischemia, 93: 99

CSF-suppressed quantitative single-shot, 93: 62

weighted, anisotropy in, 93: 64

dipyridamole, for coronary artery disease detection, 93: 105

in epilepsy, partial, 94: 355

ictal and interictal activity, 94: 357

in extremity reflex sympathetic dystrophy, failure of, 93: 110

of eye, high-resolution with short TR, short TE and partial-echo acquisition, 93: 82

fast gradient-recalled technique with dynamic susceptibility effects sensitivity, 94: 80

fast spin-echo, contrast in, factors influencing, 94: 75

fat-suppressed steady-state three-dimensional, magnetization transfer contrast in, 94: 77

of femur

fracture, occult proximal, 95: 349

head ischemia, vs. bone scintigraphy, 94: 374

neck osteoma, osteoid, 94: 376

flash, MTC in, 93: 67

fluorine-19, of partial oxygen pressure in vitrectomized eye (in rabbit), 93: 87

of frontal brain lesions, chronic traumatic, volume measurement, 93: 299

gadolinium chelates in, high-dose, 93: 75

with gadopentetate dimeglumine, in femoral neck fracture, 94: 375

for gastric emptying measurement, 94: 362

gradient echo, functional brain imaging at 1.5 T, 94: 350

in head injury, closed, comparison with SPECT and CT, 93: 100

hemangioma differentiated from liver metastases by, ultrafast MRI, 93: 115

in herpes simplex encephalitis, 93: 101

of hip

fracture, occult, vs. bone imaging, 94: 377

transient osteoporosis, 94: 372

hydrogen-1, for quantitation of metabolites, 93: 90

hydrogen2/phosphorus-31, for concurrent quantification of tissue metabolism and blood flow, 89, 94: 88

of kidney transplant hip abnormality, subclinical, 94: 176

of liver

hemangioma, 93: 119

hyperplasia, focal nodular, 94: 360

hyperplasia, focal nodular, with color Doppler ultrasound, 94: 360

of lung, contrast-enhanced, ventilation perfusion assessments, 94: 366

in lymphedema, vs. lymphangioscintigraphy, 94: 371

of lymphoma, non-Hodgkin's, of residual masses after treatment, 94: 367

magnetization transfer contrast in in flash MRI, 93: 67

with periodic pulsed saturation, 93: 65

magnetization transfer pulsed sequences in, design and implementation, 93: 66

marrow, in osteoporosis, 93: 114

motion effects in, reduction with projection reconstruction techniques, 94: 82

of myocardium

contrast-enhancement for, 93: 103

hypoperfused, contrast-enhanced MRI, 93: 102

perfusion imaging with Gd-DTPA, 93: 104

in osteoarthritis of knee, correlation with radiography and scintigraphy, 93: 113

in osteomyelitis (*see* Osteomyelitis, MRI in)

osteonecrosis misdiagnosed in hip transient osteoporosis, 94: 373

oxygen-17, to measure cerebral oxygen consumption and blood flow (in rat), 93: 89

of paraganglioma, for preoperative and postoperative evaluation, vs. iodine-131 metaiodobenzylguanidine scintigraphy, 95: 55

in parathyroid disease, for preoperative localization, vs. imaging and ultrasound, 95: 155

perfusion, 63, 93: 61

of cerebral ischemia, 93: 99

phosphorus-31, in human body, 93: 90

projection reconstruction techniques for, consistent, 94: 83

with pulmonary angiography, experience, 95: 38

of pulmonary vessels, single breath-hold MRI, 94: 366

in rectal cancer and scar differentiation, 93: 116

in sacroiliitis, septic, 93: 109

shimming, rapid, fully automatic, arbitrary volume, 93: 92

of spine in metastases, correlation with scintigraphy, 93: 112

in stroke, acute, 94: 353

synergistic enhancement with Gd-DTPA and magnetization transfer, 93: 79

three D

acquisition and visualization in, improvement of, 93: 83

of pulmonary vasculature, 93: 118

three-DFT, low-field aspects of, 93: 84

two-D translational motion artifact correction, improved algorithm for, 93: 85

in uveal melanoma, 93: 117

of vertebral metastases of breast cancer, 94: 378

of visual cortex, for functional mapping, 93: 95

vs. bone imaging, for spinal metastases detection, 95: 355

wavelet-encoded, 93: 86

of wrist, high-resolution, with short TR, short TE and partial-echo acquisition, 93: 82

Magnetization transfer

contrast

in fat-suppressed steady-state three-dimensional MRI, 94: 77

in MRI (see Magnetic resonance imaging magnetization transfer contrast in)

in multisection fast spin echo imaging, 94: 76

relaxation in protein solutions and tissue and, 94: 78

for synergistic enhancement of MRI, 93: 79

time-of-flight magnetic resonance angiography, 94: 76

Magnetoelectroencephalography

in epilepsy, partial, of ictal and interictal activity, 94: 357

Major histocompatibility complex

class II antigen induction by rejecting heart, 93: 51

Malformation

cerebral arteriovenous, resection, intracranial hypertension after, 95: 368

Malignancy (see Cancer)

Malrotation

simulating gallbladder perforation, technetium-99m IDA scintigraphy in, 93: 251

Mammography

scintimammography, prone, in breast carcinoma suspicion, 95: 376

with thallium-201 scintigraphy in breast cancer diagnosis, 95: 52

Marrow

alterations in osteomyelitis, indium-111 leukocyte scintigraphy in, 93: 186

biopsy, iliac crest, vs. imaging for bone metastases in lung cancer, 95: 131

containing skeleton, photopenic defects on indium-111 leukocyte scintigraphy, 94: 155

scintigraphy and MRI in osteopetrosis, 93: 114

subtraction image, computer generated, in musculoskeletal infection, 95: 113

Maximum

likelihood-expectation maximization reconstruction by ROC analysis, 93: 307

McN-5652Z

carbon-11, as PET radiotracer for serotonin uptake sites, 94: 333

MDP, technetium-99m (see Technetium-99m, MDP)

Meckel's diverticulum

"fading" scintigraphy of, 94: 253

false-positive imaging, 95: 232

visualization with cimetidine-enhanced technetium-99m pertechnetate, 93: 262

Mediastinal

Hodgkin's disease, gallium-67-citrate SPECT of, 93: 145

mass

gallium-67 avid, after Hodgkin's disease treatment, thallium-201 scintigraphy of, 95: 63

residual, in Hodgkin's disease in children, 93: 143

Mediastinitis

fibrosing, superior vena cava obstruction in, 93: 271
Medications (see Drugs)
Medicine, nuclear (see Nuclear medicine)
Medronate
technetium-99m, uptake in liver necrosis of Budd-Chiari syndrome, 94: 254
Melanoma
malignant
imaging agent, iodine-125 (2-piperidinylaminoethyl) 4-iodobenzamide, 95: 408
scintigraphy of, with iodine-123 N-(2-diethylaminoethyl 4-iodobenzamide), 95: 405
of trunk, high-risk, lymphoscintigraphy of, 95: 75
uveal, MRI, scintigraphy and glucose metabolism in, 93: 117
Mcmory
anatomic correlates of, from intracarotid amobarbital injection with technetium-99m HMPAO SPECT, 95: 278
Meningioma
scintigraphy of, somatostatin receptor, with indium-111 DTPA-D-Phe[1] octreotide, 95: 403
Meningococcemia
fulminant, peripheral gangrene in, bone imaging of, 95: 99
Menopause
in gastric emptying rate of solids, 95: 236
Menstrual
cycle, in gastric emptying rate of solids, 95: 236
Mental
stress inducing silent left ventricular dysfunction in coronary artery disease, 95: 330
Mercaptoacetylglycyl-D-alanylglycine
technetium-99m, kidney excretion characteristics of, 94: 213
Mercaptoacetyltriglycine, technetium-99m (see Technetium-99m mercaptoacetyltriglycine)
Mercaptoacetyltripeptides
technetium-99m, synthesis and labeling characteristics of, 95: 416
Mesencephalic
graft, fetal, in Parkinson's disease due to MPTP, 94: 291
Mesenchymoma
pulmonary, technetium-99m methylene diphosphonate uptake by, 94: 118
Mesenteric

lymphadenitis, indium-111 white blood cell imaging in, 95: 95
Metaiodobenzylguanidine
iodine-123
in metastatic carcinoid, 94: 204
scintigraphy, in heart hypertrophy and failure, 94: 69
scintigraphy, in regional myocardial sympathetic dysinnervation in arrhythmogenic right ventricular cardiomyopathy, 95: 326
scintigraphy, with thallium-201 for neuroendocrine tumor detection, 95: 53
for SPECT of denervated but viable myocardium (in dog), 93: 50
iodine-125
intraoperative, of metastatic pheochromocytoma, 94: 196
for pheochromocytoma intraoperative detection, 95: 171
iodine-131 (see Iodine-131 metaiodobenzylguanidine)
Metal
ion release from paramagnetic chelates, 93: 73
Metallic
radionuclides, immunoradiometric assay with, 93: 341
Metastases
bone
in breast cancer, CA 15-3 indicating, 94: 144
in small cell lung cancer, iliac crest marrow biopsy vs. imaging for, 95: 131
of bone cancer, pain palliation, 95: xxii
of carcinoid, scintigraphy with iodine-123 metaiodobenzylguanidine vs. iodine-123 Tyr-3-octreotide in, 94: 204
of colon carcinoma, false-positive hepatic blood pool scintigraphy in, 93: 242
of liver
cancer, treatment, 95: xxv
differentiated from hemangioma with ultrafast MRI, 93: 115
technetium-99m MAA intraarterial infusion targeting, 95: 66
lymph node, magnetic resonance lymphography of (in rabbit), 94: 370
masquerading as liver hemangioma on red blood cell scintigraphy, 95: 68
of pheochromocytoma, intraoperative iodine-125

metaiodobenzylguanidine imaging
of, 94: 196
prostate cancer, follow-up, prostate
specific antigen replacing bone
scintigraphy in, 94: 172
scintigraphy of, with iodine-123
N-(2-diethylaminoethyl
4-iodobenzamide), 95: 405
skeletal, bone pain due to,
samarium-153 EDTMP in, 95: 441
spine, detection, bone imaging vs. MRI
in, 95: 355
suspected, spinal MRI in, correlation
with scintigraphy, 93: 112
of thyroid
cancer, false-positive, on radioiodine
imaging due to esophageal retained
radioactivity, 95: 166
cancer, hiatal hernia on whole body
radioiodine imaging mimicking,
95: 378
carcinoma, differentiated,
thyroglobulin and iodine-131
imaging in diagnosis and treatment
assessment, 95: 164
vertebral, of breast cancer, MRI of,
94: 378
Metatarsal
second, base, overuse ballet injury of, as
diagnostic problem, 95: 147
Methionine
carbon-11, in head and neck cancer
imaging, 93: 158
Methotrexate
infiltration, extraskeletal localization of
MDP in soft tissue secondary to,
95: 150
Methoxyestradiol
in estrogen receptor imaging, 93: 337
Methyl tyrosine
L-3-[iodine-123]iodo-α-, brain uptake
of, 93: 329
Methylene diphosphonate (see MDP)
MIBI, technetium-99m (see
Technetium-99m
methoxyisobutylisonitrile)
Microautoradiography
of fluorine-18 fluorodeoxyglucose
intratumoral distribution (in mice),
94: 130
Microcirculation
characteristics in Buerger's disease,
94: 268
Microscopy
magnetic resonance, high-temperature
superconducting receiver for,
94: 84
Milk

alkali syndrome, technetium-99m
methylene diphosphonate increased
skeletal uptake in, 95: 127
breast, excretion of gallium-67 and
ingestion by infant, 93: 349
Mineral
bone, measurement with dual photon
absorptiometry, with gamma
camera, 95: 158
Mitochondria
viability and metabolism effect on
technetium-99m sestamibi
myocardial retention, 94: 31
MIVE$_2$
in estrogen receptor imaging, 93: 337
Model
brain, three-dimensional SPECT
simulations of, 93: 305
in cardiac shape deformity
measurement, 93: 43
ischemia, of myocardial blood flow
assessment with technetium-99m
tetrofosmin (in dog), 95: 322
of lymph node metastases, magnetic
resonance lymphography of (in
rabbit), 94: 370
Monitor
ambulatory, radionuclide
of left ventricular systolic and diastolic
function, 95: 329
for left ventricular systolic and
diastolic function measurements,
94: 48
of function in left ventricular ejection
fraction measurements, 93: 44
of kidney function, ambulatory, 94: 208
Monitoring
cognitive activation, dual isotope brain
SPECT for, 95: 276
ECG, ambulatory, before vascular
surgery, 94: 28
of kidney function, ambulatory monitor,
94: 208
left ventricular function, for myocardial
ischemia during coronary artery
angioplasty, 93: 45
prostate cancer, prostate specific
antigen and bone imaging in,
94: 172
of reflex sympathetic dystrophy therapy,
93: 272
Monoamine
reuptake sites in brain, SPECT of,
93: 317
Monoclonal antibody
to activated platelets, in thrombus
imaging with technetium-99m
synthetic peptides, 95: 244

CEA fragments, iodine-123, for imaging in colorectal cancer, 94: 136

fab fragment, technetium-99m DD-3B6/22 anti-fibrin, in deep venous thrombosis and pulmonary embolism detection, 95: 245

fibrin-specific, localizing and visualizing pulmonary embolism, 93: 128

IMMU-4, technetium-99m, for imaging in colorectal cancer, 94: 135

indium-111
anti-CEA, in thyroid medullary carcinoma imaging, 93: 159
anti-CEA, ZCE 025 in colorectal carcinoma follow-up, 93: 160
antifibrin, in venous thrombosis, 93: 268
B72.3 in breast cancer detection and staging, 93: 155
myosin-specific, in myocardial damage due to anthracycline, 93: 49
against tissue plasminogen activator in deep venous thrombosis, 93: 267
leukocyte scintigraphy of infected endoprosthesis, 94: 161
platelet-specific, in arterial thrombosis, 93: 265
research on ligands, nuclides and labeling techniques, 93: 332
technetium-99m (see Technetium-99m monoclonal antibodies)

Monoclonal antimyosin fab
indium-111, myocardial uptake in doxorubicin cardiotoxicity detection (in rat), 94: 70

Monoclonal antiplatelet antibody
S12, technetium-99m, for vascular injury imaging, 94: 72

Morphine
augmented
cholescintigraphy (see Cholescintigraphy, morphine augmented)
hepatobiliary scintigraphy in cholecystitis, 94: 237

Mortality
with revascularization, in myocardial infarction size and myocardial viability, 95: 333

Motion
effects
in MRI, reduction with projection reconstruction techniques, 94: 82
on thallium-201 SPECT, 95: 434
estimation from tagged magnetic resonance image sequences, 94: 81

intravoxel incoherent, link with classical perfusion in capillary network, 94: 74
of patient, effect on myocardial perfusion SPECT, 94: 24

Motor
recovery after stroke, PET in, 93: 277
stroke recovery, stroke due to striatocapsular infarction, 94: 306

MPTP
Parkinson's disease due to, fetal mesencephalic graft in, 94: 291

MTC (see Magnetic resonance imaging, magnetization transfer contrast in)

Mucosal
damage severity in acute Crohn's disease, indium-111 imaging in, 95: 228

Muscarinic receptors
central, imaging agent, 93: 325
myocardial, quantificaation by PET, 95: 344
subtype selectivity of QNB analogues, 93: 324

Muscle, 94: 167
leg, scintigraphy with technetium-99m MIBI in peripheral vascular disease, 94: 271
myocardial and skeletal, low energy charge, in angina pectoris with thallium perfusion imaging abnormality, 94: 20
skeletal, in sarcoidosis, imaging of, 95: 120

Musculoskeletal, 95: 109
brucellosis, imaging features, 95: 114
infection, marrow subtraction image and sulfur colloid scintigraphy in, 95: 113

Myelography
indium-111 DTPA, of pleural cerebrospinal fluid leak, 94: 123

myo-inositol
in brain, carbon-13 magnetic resonance spectroscopy of, 94: 87

Myocardial infarction
acute
cardiac adrenergic neuronal function assessment after, with carbon-11 hydroxyephedrine and PET, 95: 343
clinical, radionuclide and hemodynamic data in, incremental prognostic accuracy of, 93: 15
denervated but viable myocardial assessment after (in dog), 93: 50
noninvasive identification of myocardium at risk in, 93: 30

streptokinase in, left ventricular function assessment after, 93: 38

thrombolytics and angioplasty in, exercise thallium-201 scintigraphy after, 94: 12

thrombolytics in, evaluation with technetium-99m-sestamibi myocardial scintigraphy, 93: 33

thrombolytics in, left ventricular performance assessment after, 93: 37

with totally occluded infarct-related artery, thallium-201 imaging of viability in, 95: 294

age and indium-111 antimyosin antibody uptake, 93: 48

assessment with technetium-99m-sestamibi myocardial imaging, 93: 32

chronic, nonviable myocardium in, PET of myocardial blood flow identifies, 95: 334

coronary artery occlusion and reperfusion in, sequential teboroxime imaging to detect, 95: 317

coronary patency and ventricular function after, reverse redistribution on exercise thallium scintigraphy in, 94: 23

inferior, right ventricular perfusion defects after, assessment by exercise with technetium-99m sestamibi myocardial tomography, 95: 308

inferior wall left ventricular, right ventricular dysfunction during, thrombolytics in, 94: 49

metabolism after, oxidative, 93: 56

myocardial viability detection after, rest sestamibi vs. rest redistribution thallium-201 SPECT in, 94: 38

regional metabolic abnormality in relation to perfusion and wall motion, SPECT in, 94: 67

residual tissue viability after, time dependence of, fluorine-18 fluorodeoxyglucose and PET in, 95: 339

size

estimation from nitrogen-13 ammonia PET, 94: 63

and myocardial viability, PET of, 95: 333

visualization after indium-111 antimyosin antibodies, 94: 71

Myocardial perfusion

abnormalities, gated SPECT with technetium-99m sestamibi in, 94: 34

defect size after SPECT with technetium-99m hexakis-methoxyisobutylisonitrile after stress, 94: 40

defects, reversibility of, quantitative criteria for, 93: 1

dipyridamole, for cardiac risk stratification before vascular surgery, 94: 28

evaluation with carbon-11-acetate, 93: 54

imaging

agent, technetium-99m tetrofosmin as, 95: 412, 413

exercise, antianginal drugs, peak heart rate and stress level in, 95: 298

exercise, prognostic value in angiographically significant coronary artery disease, 94: 11

new agent, technetium-99m 1,2-bis[bis(2-ethoxyethyl) phosphino]ethane, 94: 46

with PET and SPECT, disparate results, 93: 25

planar, in coronary artery disease, 94: 41

rubidium-82 PET, and heart patient outcome, 94: 61

SPECT, exercise-thallium-201, vs. adenosine for, 93: 11

technetium-99m methoxyisobutylisonitrile, stress only vs. stress rest, 94: 32

with technetium-99m teboroxime, 94: 42

thallium-201, dipyridamole, for coronary artery disease detection accuracy and side-effect profile, 94: 30

thallium-201, dipyridamole, with low-level exercise unmasking ischemia, 93: 8

thallium-201, in unstable angina, prognostic value, 93: 4

thallium-201, SPECT, of myocardial defect, according to extent, 95: 284

tomographic, with technetium-99m-teboroxime during adenosine coronary hyperemia, 93: 35

with ultrafast MRI with Gd-DTPA, 93: 104

measurements during total coronary artery occlusion, 95: 311

quantification of PET after heart
transplant, 93: 52
scintigraphy
in myocardial infarction, recent, for
residual tissue assessment, 93: 20
personnel radiation dosimetry from,
95: 437
SPECT
effect of motion of patient on, 94: 24
rest thallium-201/stress
technetium-99m sestamibi
dual-isotope, validation of, 95: 289
stress thallium-201, defects in
one-vessel coronary artery disease,
95: 287
with thallium-201 and
technetium-99m sestamibi (in dog),
94: 36
stress, gated technetium-99m sestamibi
to assess, 95: 305
technetium-99m sestamibi, gated planar,
for validation of global and
segmental left ventricular
contractile function, 95: 312
tomography, dobutamine thallium,
93: 13
Myocardium
beta adrenoceptors reduction in
hypertrophic cardiomyopathy, PET
of, 95: 346
blood flow (*see* Blood flow, myocardial)
clearance kinetics of technetium-99m
teboroxime differentiate normal
and flow-restricted myocardium (in
dog), 94: 45
damage due to anthracycline,
indium-111 myosin monoclonal
antibodies in, 93: 49
defect, thallium-201 SPECT myocardial
perfusion imaging of, according to
extent, 95: 284
denervated by viable, assessment after
acute myocardial infarction (in
dog), 93: 50
echocardiography, contrast, of perfusion
defects, and coronary stenosis
severity, thallium-201 SPECT in,
94: 16
emission CT in hypertrophic
cardiomyopathy, 93: 46
flow-restricted at rest, and myocardial
clearance kinetics of
technetium-99m teboroxime (in
dog), 94: 45
hypoperfused
contrast-enhanced MRI of, 93: 102

secondary to coronary artery disease,
stress redistribution thallium-201
SPECT indexes in, 94: 22
hypoxia
detection with fluorine-18
fluoromisonidazole and PET,
94: 65
marking with iodovinylmisonidazole,
95: 325
imaging
dipyridamole stress thallium-201, of
perioperative cardiac events in
major nonvascular surgery, 95: 288
dual-isotope, feasibility, advantages
and limitations, 95: 291
at rest with technetium-99m-sestamibi
in myocardial infarction assessment
and first-pass ejection fraction,
93: 32
in SPECT, technetium-99m-SQ30217
in, 93: 34
with technetium-99m-sestamibi,
comparison of same-day protocols,
93: 33
infarction (*see* Myocardial infarction)
injury zones, differentiation of regional
perfusion and fatty acid uptake in,
93: 46
intramyocardial distribution during
exercise, technetium-99m sestamibi
myocardial SPECT for, 95: 310
ischemia
in calcium overload of myocardial
cells and mitochondria, 94: 31
detected by thallium scintigraphy,
related to cardiac arrest and
syncope in hypertrophic
cardiomyopathy, 95: 299
myocardial blood flow and glucose
uptake in (in dog), 94: 58
silent, during coronary artery
angioplasty, left ventricular function
monitoring for, 93: 45
teboroxime to detect, sequential,
coronary artery occlusion and
reperfusion in, 95: 317
technetium-99m sestamibi uptake and
retention during, 95: 314
ischemic but viable, nitrates improving
detection of, by thallium-201
reinjection SPECT, 95: 291
jeopardized, extent assessment during
coronary artery occlusion and
reperfusion, 93: 31
MRI of, contrast-enhancement for,
93: 103
muscarinic receptor quantification, by
PET, 95: 344

muscle energy charge, low, in angina
    pectoris with thallium perfusion
    imaging abnormality, 94: 20
neutral imaging agents,
    bis(dithiocarbamato) nitrido
    technetium-99m (in animals),
    95: 324
oxidative metabolism during
    dobutamine infusion, 94: 60
oxygen tension, fluorine-19 magnetic
    resonance spectroscopy of, 94: 86
perfusion (*see* Myocardial perfusion)
reperfusion
    prolonged metabolic abnormalities in
        (in dog), 93: 57
    technetium-99m sestamibi uptake and
        retention during, 95: 314
retention
    of technetium-99m sestamibi, effect
        of mitochondrial viability and
        metabolism on, 94: 31
    of technetium-99m teboroxime, and
        myocardial blood flow, 94: 43
    at risk, noninvasive identification in
        acute myocardial infarction and
        nondiagnostic ECG, 93: 30
scintigraphy
    exercise thallium-201, accuracy in
        asymptomatic young men, 94: 3
    with technetium-99m-sestamibi and
        dipyridamole in effort angina,
        93: 26
    with technetium-99m-sestamibi in
        evaluation of thrombolytics in
        myocardial infarction, 93: 33
    with thallium-201 and
        technetium-99m
        hexakis-methoxyisobutylisonitrile in
        left bundle branch block and
        coronary artery disease, 94: 33
SPECT
    stress-rest, with technetium-99m
        tetrofosmin, 95: 320
    technetium-99m sestamibi, for
        intramyocardial distribution during
        exercise, 95: 310
    thallium-201 chloride, of denervated
        but viable myocardium (in dog),
        93: 50
substrate utilization in adriamycin
    cardiomyopathy, 95: 337
sympathetic dysinnervation, regional, in
    arrhythmogenic right ventricular
    cardiomyopathy, iodine-123
    metaiodobenzylguanidine
    scintigraphy in, 95: 326

technetium-99m sestamibi and
    thallium-201 retention
    characteristics in (in dog), 94: 35
thallium-201 tomography, equivalence
    between adenosine and exercise,
    94: 25
to-left ventricular cavity count ratio in
    left ventricular dysfunction from
    thallium perfusion tomographic
    scintigraphy, 94: 21
tomography
    dipyridamole technetium-99m
        sestamibi, in stable chest pain,
        95: 303
    technetium-99m sestamibi, rest-stress,
        95: 306
    technetium-99m sestamibi, with
        exercise, to assess right ventricular
        perfusion defects after inferior
        myocardial infarction, 95: 308
    with technetium-99m tetrofosmin, in
        coronary artery disease evaluation,
        95: 321
uptake
    of 2-[fluorine-18]fluoro-2-deoxy-D-
        glucose, in PET, 95: 335
    of fluorine-18 fluorodeoxyglucose,
        with SPECT, 95: 331
    of glucose, in insulin-dependent
        diabetes, dynamic PET in, 95: 336
    of indium-111 monoclonal antimyosin
        fab in doxorubicin cardiotoxicity
        detection (in rat), 94: 70
viability
    assessment, in chronic coronary
        disease with thallium-201 SPECT
        vs. fluorodeoxyglucose PET,
        95: 293
    assessment, new strategy, 94: 56
    assessment,
        stress-redistribution-reinjection vs.
        rest-redistribution thallium imaging
        for, vs. metabolic activity by PET,
        95: 296
    assessment, with sestamibi
        scintigraphy, 94: 36
    in coronary artery disease, chronic,
        95: 315
    delineation with carbon-11 acetate vs.
        fluorine-18-fluorodeoxyglucose, by
        PET, 95: 338
    detection after infarction, rest
        sestamibi vs. rest-redistribution
        thallium-201 SPECT in, 94: 38
    gated technetium-99m sestamibi to
        assess, 95: 305
    metabolic, PET of, 94: 53

myocardial infarction size and, PET of, 95: 333

in perfusion defects, fluorine-18 deoxyglucose PET in, 94: 55

PET polar map displays in, 94: 59

thallium-201 immediate reinjection after stress imaging of, 95: 292

thallium reinjection demonstrating, in regions with reverse redistribution, 95: 297

viable, identification in chronic coronary artery disease, 93: 26

viable and nonviable, thallium activity after reinjection distinguishing, 93: 18

Myosin

specific monoclonal antibodies, indium-111, in myocardial damage due to anthracycline, 93: 49

N

N-acetylaspartate

in brain after stroke, proton magnetic resonance spectroscopy of, 94: 91

N-isopropyl-*p*-iodine 123 iodoamphetamine, for cerebral blood flow

measurement, redistribution in ischemic cerebrovascular disease, 95: 253

N-isopropyl-p-iodoamphetamine lung clearance, iodine-123, and smoking, 93: 136

Neck

cancer imaging, carbon-11-methionine and PET in, 93: 158

region, indium-111 leukocyte accumulation in, 93: 166

Necrosis

fat, intraosseous, with pancreatitis, 95: 130

liver, of Budd-Chiari syndrome, technetium-99m medronate uptake in, 94: 254

radiation, vs. recurrent glioma, 94: 288

Necrotizing

otitis, scintigraphy in, bone and gallium-67, 93: 176

Neoplasm (*see* Tumor)

Nephropathy

reflux, scintigraphy with ultrasound in, 95: 383

Nerve

facial, peripheral, palsy after radioiodine therapy of papillary thyroid carcinoma, 95: 170

sympathetic innervation of left ventricle, impairment in arrhythmogenic right ventricular disease, 94: 68

Neural

network

analysis of ventilation-perfusion lung imaging, 94: 102

artificial, approach for acute pulmonary embolism, 95: 18

artificial, for SPECT, 95: 433

Neuroblastoma

bone scintigraphy of, with iodine-131 metaiodobenzylguanidine, 94: 141

Neuroendocrine

tumor detection with thallium-201 and iodine-123 metaiodobenzylguanidine for scintigraphy of, 95: 53

Neuroimaging

of pilocytic astrocytoma, juvenile, 95: 366

in temporal lobe epilepsy, 94: 354

Neuroleptic

effects on regional brain function, technetium-99m HMPAO SPECT of, 93: 282

Neuron

cardiac adrenergic function assessment after acute myocardial infarction, with carbon-11 hydroxyephedrine and PET, 95: 343

cholinergic, mapping in brain with SPECT and iodine-123 IBVM, 95: 275

dysfunction, regional sympathetic, scintigraphy of, in heart, 95: 343

Neuropathy

cardiac diabetic, assessment with carbon-11 hydroxyephedrine and PET, 95: 342

Nitecapone

inhibition for fluorine-18-6-fluorodopa PET in Parkinson's disease, 94: 335

Nitrates

improving detection of ischemic but viable myocardium by thallium-201 reinjection SPECT, 95: 291

Nitrogen-13

ammonia PET

heart, effect of metabolic milieu on, 93: 55

for left ventricular mass and infarct size estimation, 94: 63

in myocardial blood flow, 94: 60

in myocardial blood flow quantification, 94: 62

Nitroglycerin

splanchnic vein volume-pressure relation
with radionuclide plethysmography
and, 94: 50
Nitroxide
liposome system for oximetry, 93: 88
Non-united fracture
management, bone imaging in, 94: 177
North American
pulmonary blastomycosis, gallium-67
imaging in, 95: 89
Nuclear
ejection fraction, abnormal gallbladder,
predicting success of
cholecystectomy in biliary
dyskinesia, 95: 210
magnetic resonance (see Magnetic
resonance)
medicine
AIDS and, 95: 82
camera systems, historic perspective,
95: 421
in hepatomegaly, congestive, 93: 260
information for patients and staff
about, 94: 339
investigations of radiation dose to
adults, 93: 344
radionuclides (see Radionuclide)
therapeutic, 95: xxi
therapeutic, future expectations,
95: xxx
Nucleus
cell, tracer localization in electron dose
rate delivery to, 95: 443

O

OC-125
indium-111, for immunoscintigraphy in
ovarian cancer recurrence
diagnosis, 94: 134
Octreotide
effect on bile secretion and gallbladder
emptying, cholescintigraphy in,
95: 235
indium-111
DTPA, for somatostatin receptor
imaging of small cell lung cancer,
95: 401
DTPA-D-Phe-1, for somatosatin
receptor scintigraphy, 93: 147
DTPA-D-Phe-1, for somatostatin
receptor scintigraphy of
meningioma, 95: 403
for scintigraphy in oncology, 95: 393
iodine-123
in carcinoid and islet cell tumors,
94: 203

Tyr-3, for somatostatin receptor
scintigraphy, 93: 147
Tyr-3, for somatostatin receptor
scintigraphy, Rotterdam experience,
95: 388
Tyr-3, in metastatic carcinoid,
94: 204
Tyr-3, scintigraphy, in lung cancer
staging, small cell, 95: 400
in pituitary disease, and somatostatin
receptor scintigraphy, 95: 395
scintigraphy, for paraganglioma
detection, 95: 397
Oncology, 94: 127, 95: 41
scintigraphy in, indium-111 octreotide,
95: 393
Ophthalmopathy
Graves', unilateral, with thyroid
carcinoma, 94: 192
OR-462
inhibition for fluorine-18-6-fluorodopa
PET in Parkinson's disease, 94: 335
Organotechnetium
complex, for imaging of
multidrug-resistant P glycoprotein,
94: 327
Orthopedic
infection, suspected, technetium-99m
HMPAO leukocyte imaging in,
94: 152
Ossification
heterotopic, after burns, causing vocal
cord dysfunction, 95: 150
Osteoarthritis
of knee, MRI, radiography and
scintigraphy in, 93: 113
Osteoarticular
tuberculosis, multifocal, case review,
95: 117
Osteoid osteoma (see Osteoma, osteoid)
Osteoma
osteoid
curettage of, intraoperative,
probe-guided, 95: 364
diagnosis in child, 95: 134
of femoral neck, bone imaging, CT
and MRI in, 94: 376
Osteomalacia
with anorexia nervosa, 95: 128
Osteomyelitis
bone imaging in, in children, 94: 154
in diabetes with foot ulcer, MRI in,
95: 353
of foot in diabetes, indium-111
leukocyte scintigraphy in, 93: 183
histologically proven pressure sore
related, with negative technetium
bone imaging, 95: 112

marrow alterations in, indium-111
leukocyte scintigraphy in, 93: 186
MRI in
comparison with skeletal scintigraphy,
93: 107
diagnostic pitfalls and characteristics,
93: 108
of pelvis, 95: 110
pubic, due to *Staphylococcus simulans*,
95: 111
of skull base, 93: 111
with soft-tissue infection and osseous
abnormalities, leukocyte
scintigraphy in, 93: 181
suspected, indium-111 leukocyte
scintigraphy of, 94: 155
Osteonecrosis
misdiagnosed, for hip transient
osteoporosis, on MRI, 94: 373
Osteopetrosis
marrow scintigraphy and MRI in,
93: 114
Osteoporosis
transient, of hip
misdiagnosed as osteonecrosis on
MRI, 94: 373
MRI in, 94: 372
Osteosarcoma
thallium-201 imaging of, 95: 50
Otitis
differentiating necrotizing from severe
with bone and gallium-67
scintigraphy, 93: 176
malignant external, scintigraphy of,
results, 95: 98
OV-TL 3 fab
technetium-99m, in suspected ovarian
cancer, 94: 132
Ovaries
cancer
chromic phosphate therapy,
intraperitoneal distribution imaging
before, 95: 172
management, immunoscintigraphy in,
94: 143
recurrences, diagnosis by correlative
imaging study, 94: 134
suspected, technetium-99m OV-TL 3
fab in, 94: 132
struma ovarii, 94: 191
Oxidation
beta, of
1-[carbon-14]-17-[iodine-131]-iodoh-
eptadecanoic acid after
intracoronary injection, 94: 66
Oxidative
metabolism
after myocardial infarction, 93: 56

in myocardium during dobutamine
infusion, 94: 60
Oxide
particles for magnetic resonance
lymphography of lymph node
metastases (in rabbit), 94: 370
Oximetry
with nitroxide-liposome system, 93: 88
Oxine
leukocytes, indium-111, for imaging in
inflammatory bowel disease,
94: 248
Oxygen
arterial oxygen saturation in lung
imaging, 93: 126
cerebral oxygen consumption
measurement with oxygen-17 MRI
(in rat), 93: 89
partial oxygen pressure in vitrectomized
eye with fluorine-19 MRI (in
rabbit), 93: 87
tension, myocardial, fluorine-19
magnetic resonance spectroscopy
of, 94: 86
Oxygen-15
carbon dioxide inhalation to quantify
myocardial blood flow in coronary
artery disease, 93: 53
water, for PET in coronary reserve
assessment, 95: 340
Oxygen-17
MRI to measure cerebral oxygen
consumption and blood flow (in
rat), 93: 89

P

P-32
therapy in ovarian cancer,
intraperitoneal distribution imaging
before, 95: 172
p-aminohippurate
clearance, for renal artery blood flow,
vs. MRI, 95: 180
P256 fab
in arterial thrombosis, 93: 265
P glycoprotein
multidrug-resistant, imaging with
organotechnetium complex,
94: 327
Pachydermoperiostosis
technetium-99m MDP scintigraphy of,
93: 208
Paget disease
of bone, sarcoma in, features and
radiography of, 93: 206
Pain

bone, skeletal metastases causing, samarium-153 EDTMP in, 95: 441
of bone cancer, metastatic, palliation, 95: xxii
chest (*see* Chest pain)
low back, SPECT, radiography and CT in, 93: 194
of lower extremity, in preschool children, bone scintigraphy of, 93: 196
Palsy
peripheral facial nerve, after radioiodine therapy of papillary thyroid carcinoma, 95: 170
Pancreatitis
fat necrosis, intraosseous, and infarction in, 95: 130
Papaverine
test in impotence, with radionuclide penile blood flow imaging, 94: 230
Paraganglioma
octreotide scintigraphy for detection, 95: 397
preoperative and postoperative evaluation with iodine-131 metaiodobenzylguanidine scintigraphy, vs. CT and MRI, 95: 55
treatment with iodine-131 metaiodobenzylguanidine, 95: 56
Paramagnetic
chelates, metal ion release from, 93: 73
relaxation
agents, magnetically coupled, 93: 79
with diffusion-mediated susceptibility losses in tissues, 93: 71
Parathyroid
abnormalities, in hyperparathyroidism, technetium-99m iodine-123 imaging vs. ultrasound of, 95: 157
adenoma, with thyroid hemiagenesis, 94: 194
disease, preoperative localization, MRI vs. imaging and ultrasound in, 95: 155
imaging with technetium-99m sestamibi, 93: 223
localization before exploration, 95: 153
pathology, dual isotope SPECT of, 93: 222
tumor localization, comparison of imaging methods, 94: 199
Parkinson's disease
cerebral glucose metabolism in, and dementia, 94: 292
D_2 dopamine receptors in SPECT with iodine-123 iodobenzamide in, 94: 293

dopamine D1 receptors in, PET of, 95: 270
dopamine receptor SPECT in, 95: 271
MPTP causing, fetal mesencephalic graft in, 94: 291
PET with fluorine-18-6-fluorodopa, after nitecapone inhibition, 94: 335
transplant for, fetal dopamine cell survival and neurologic improvement after, 94: 290
Pediatric (*see* Children)
Pedicle
stress fracture, bilateral, SPECT and CT of, 93: 201
Pelvic-uretero junction obstruction
postnatal suspected, diuretic renography in, 94: 216
Pelvis
fracture, radiation-induced insufficiency, technetium-99m MDP scintigraphy in, 93: 198
hydronephrosis, prenatal diagnosis, 93: 233
osteomyelitis of, 95: 110
radioiodine uptake in rectal wall teratoma after thyroidectomy for carcinoma, 94: 190
Penis
blood flow
in impotence, with papaverine test, 94: 230
during tumescence, dual-radioisotope technique for, 93: 230
corporal venous leak, technetium-99m erythrocytes in, 93: 229
Peptide
radiopharmaceuticals, as ticket to ride, 95: 404
receptor system, 95: xxix
Perfluorocarbon
emulsion, sequestered, for fluorine-19 magnetic resonance spectroscopy of myocardial oxygen tension, 94: 86
imaging, fast, with fluorine-19 U-FLARE, 94: 85
Perfusion
abnormality in dipyridamole-induced technetium-99m MIBI on SPECT, 94: 39
classical, link with IVIM in capillary network, 94: 74
defects
mismatched segmental equivalent, in strengthening diagnostic value of ventilation perfusion lung imaging in acute pulmonary embolism, 95: 10

mismatched segmental equivalent, in ventilation perfusion lung imaging in pulmonary embolism interpretation, 95: 13

myocardial contrast echocardiography of, and coronary stenosis severity, thallium-201 SPECT in, 94: 16

myocardial viability in, fluorine-18 deoxyglucose PET for, 94: 55

on thallium-201 scintigraphy, quantitative planar, outcome, 94: 1

left ventricular, global, measurement with cine MRI and coronary venous outflow phase velocity mapping, 93: 106

lung imaging
  arterial oxygen saturation in, 93: 126
  of post-irradiation lung function in bronchogenic carcinoma, 94: 124

MRI, 63, 93: 61
  of cerebral ischemia, 93: 99

myocardial (*see* Myocardial perfusion)

organ, measurement, deuterium magnetic resonance washout method validation for, 94: 89

quantification in gated SPECT, 93: 36

regional, differentiation from fatty acid uptake in myocardial injury zones, 93: 46

scintigraphy, technetium-99m MAA, hypoxia associated with, 94: 106

studies, interobserver variability in interpretation, 94: 19

in thallium imaging, abnormality in angina pectoris, with low myocardial and skeletal muscle energy charge, 94: 20

tumor, imaging of, 95: 409

unilateral absence of, on lung imaging, due to ascending aortic dissection, 95: 24

ventilation (*see* Ventilation perfusion)

Peripheral
  facial nerve palsy after radioiodine treatment of papillary thyroid carcinoma, 95: 170
  vessels, 94: 265
    disease, leg muscle scintigraphy with technetium-99m MIBI in, 94: 271
    disease, thallium perfusion imaging vs. arteriography in, 94: 269

Peritoneum
  bleeding, technetium-99m red blood cell scintigraphy in, 94: 247

Personnel
  dosimetry systems, determining the lower limit of detection for, 93: 351

radiation dosimetry from myocardial perfusion scintigraphy, 95: 437

Pertechnegas
  micro aerosol, technetium-99m, for ventilation imaging in suspected pulmonary embolism, 95: 22

Pertechnetate
  technetium-99m
    cimetidine-enhanced, in Meckel's diverticulum visualization, 93: 262
    for scintigraphy of ileal duplication of stomach and duodenum, 94: 251
    thyroid carcinoma concentrating, 93: 216

PET (*see* Positron emission tomography)

Pharmacokinetics
  of SPECT benzodiazepine receptor radioligand, iodine-123 iomazenil, 94: 329

Phase
  encode order, effect on contrast and artifact in single-shot RARE sequences, 93: 81

Phenylpentadecanoic acid
  metabolic, iodine-123, in stable coronary artery disease, 95: 300

Pheochromocytoma
  intraoperative detection with iodine-125 metaiodobenzylguanidine, 95: 171
  localization with PET hydroxyephedrine, 94: 195
  malignant, treatment with iodine-131 metaiodobenzylguanidine, 95: 56
  metastatic, intraoperative iodine-125 metaiodobenzylguanidine imaging of, 94: 196
  suspected, iodine-131 metaiodobenzylguanidine scintigraphy in, 93: 227

Phosphate
  radiolabeled, uptake by hepatic necrosis, 94: 256

Phosphocreatine
  in brain after stroke, proton magnetic resonance spectroscopy of, 94: 91

Phosphoesters
  mobile, quantification in Alzheimer dementia with phosphorus-31 magnetic resonance spectroscopy, 94: 93

Phospholipid
  ether analog, radioiodinated, localization in tumor xenografts, 95: 411

Phosphorus-31
  hydrogen-2 magnetic resonance imaging for concurrent quantification of

tissue metabolism and blood flow,
89, 94: 88

magnetic resonance spectroscopy (*see*
Magnetic resonance spectroscopy,
phosphorus-31)

MRI in human body, 93: 90

Photon

attenuation due to patient couches in
SPECT, correction method,
93: 309

fast photon-counting circuitry for
germanium detector system,
93: 315

Photopenic

defects in marrow-containing skeleton,
on indium-111 leukocyte
scintigraphy, 94: 155

Physics, 94: 307, 95: 421

health, 94: 339

Phytate

aerosol, in ventilation studies, vs.
technetium-99m C, 94: 110

Pilocytic

astrocytoma, juvenile, neuroimaging of,
95: 366

Pituitary

disease, octreotide and somatostatin
analogs in, and somatostatin
receptor scintigraphy, 95: 395

Plasminogen activator, tissue (*see* Tissue
plasminogen activator)

Platelet

activated, monoclonal antibody to, in
thrombus imaging with
technetium-99m synthetic peptides,
95: 244

specific monoclonal antibody in arterial
thrombosis, 93: 265

technetium-99m

HMPAO, for scintigraphy of venous
thrombosis, 93: 266

labeling of, 93: 339

Plethysmography

of leg blood flow, vs. regional
distribution of thallium-201 during
one leg exercise, 95: 239

radionuclide, of splanchnic vein
volume-pressure relation, and
nitroglycerin, 94: 50

Pleura

CSF leak, indium-111 DTPA
myelography of, 94: 123

effusion, bone imaging in, and pleural
fluid cytopathology, 95: 76

fluid cytopathology in bone imaging of
pleural effusion, 95: 76

Pneumocystis

carinii pneumonia, in AIDS, gallium-67
scintigraphy and CT of, 94: 162

pneumonia, lung disposition of
gallium-67 in, 93: 171

Pneumonectomy

open bronchial stump
post-pneumonectomy, xenon-133
ventilation imaging in, 94: 116

Pneumonia

Pneumocystis

carinii, in AIDS, gallium-67
scintigraphy and CT of, 94: 162

lung disposition of gallium-67 in,
93: 171

simple focal, uneventful recovery, in
children, pulmonary scintigraphic
defects after, 95: 32

Pneumonitis

drug-induced, indium-111 leukocyte
pulmonary uptake in, 94: 121

^{210}Po

embedded in glass, for long-term radon
concentrations estimation, 95: 446

Polar map

displays of cardiac PET, in myocardial
blood flow and viability assessment,
94: 59

Polycystic

liver disease, normal tissue remnants in,
indium-111 white blood cells in,
95: 229

Popliteal

pseudoaneurysm, radionuclide imaging
of, 94: 275

vein aneurysm, pulmonary embolism
from, 94: 104

Portal

hypertension, in cirrhosis, with liver
hemangioma, technetium-99m red
blood cell SPECT in, 95: 221

Positron emission tomography

in Alzheimer's disease

brain metabolism as reliable
discriminators in, 95: 265

probable, 93: 287

of brain, fluorine-18 substituted
corticosteroids for, 94: 337

in breast disease with
fluorodeoxyglucose, 94: 128

in cancer therapy assessment, with
fluorine-18 fluorodeoxyglucose,
93: 153

with carbon-11 CGP-12177 of
beta-adrenergic receptors in
idiopathic dilated cardiomyopathy,
94: 64

cardiac

Pneumocystis

attenuation imaging,
three-dimensional registration,
94: 64
effect of metabolic milieu on, 93: 55
polar map displays for myocardial
blood flow and viability assessment,
94: 59
for cardiac adrenergic neuronal function
assessment after acute myocardial
infarction, 95: 343
in cardiac diabetic neuropathy
assessment, 95: 342
in coronary artery disease
advanced, outcome after viability
studies, 94: 52
metabolic imaging value for
prognosis, 95: 332
in coronary reserve assessment, with
oxygen-15 water, 95: 340
detecting evidence of viability in rest
technetium-99m sestamibi defects,
95: 316
in dipyridamole induced
technetium-99m MIBI perfusion
abnormality on SPECT, 94: 39
dynamic
of myocardial glucose uptake in
insulin-dependent diabetes,
95: 336
in myocardial viability and myocardial
blood flow assessment, 94: 56
in epilepsy, partial, of ictal and interictal
activity, 94: 357
FDG imaging, of solitary pulmonary
nodule, 95: 26
fluorine-18 deoxyglucose
of exercise capacity improvement
after revascularization, 93: 58
in myocardial viability in perfusion
defects, 94: 55
vs. thallium-201 reinjection, 93: 21
fluorine-18 fluorodeoxyglucose
of normal brain anatomy, 95: 365
in probable Alzheimer's disease, vs.
technetium-99m HMPAO SPECT,
95: 268
fluorodeoxyglucose
clinical receiver operating
characteristic study of filtered
backprojection vs. maximum
likelihood estimator images in,
95: 435
uptake in cancer, and blood glucose
concentration, 94: 131
vs. thallium-201 SPECT, for
myocardial viability assessment in
chronic coronary artery disease,
95: 293

in head and neck cancer imaging,
93: 158
in heart metabolism evaluation, 93: 56
in heart transplant of catecholamine
uptake and storage sites, 93: 59
hydroxyephedrine, for
pheochromocytoma localization,
94: 195
for hypoxia in myocardium using
fluorine-18 fluoromisonidazole,
94: 65
imaging suite, radiation protection
design for, 94: 346
in left ventricular dysfunction, metabolic
imaging value for prognosis,
95: 332
of metabolic activity for myocardial
viability assessment, vs. thallium
imaging, 95: 296
of motor recovery after stroke, 93: 277
of myocardial beta adrenoceptors
reduction in hypertrophic
cardiomyopathy, 95: 346
of myocardial blood flow
identifies nonviable myocardium in
chronic myocardial infarction,
95: 334
quantification in coronary artery
disease, 93: 53
of myocardial infarction size and
myocardial viability, 95: 333
of myocardial metabolic viability, 94: 53
for myocardial muscarinic receptors
quantification, 95: 344
for myocardial perfusion quantification
after heart transplant, 93: 52
of myocardial uptake of
2-[fluorine-18]fluoro-2-deoxy-D-
glucose, 95: 335
in myocardial viability delineation, with
carbon-11 acetate vs.
fluorine-18-fluorodeoxyglucose,
95: 338
nitrogen-13 ammonia, for left
ventricular mass and infarct size
estimation, 94: 63
nitrogen-13 ammonia and dynamic, in
myocardial blood flow
quantification, 94: 62
nitrogen-13 ammonia and reoriented
dynamic, in myocardial blood flow
quantification, 94: 60
in Parkinson's disease
dopamine D1 receptors, 95: 270
with fluorine-18-6-fluorodopa, after
nitecapone inhibition, 94: 335

point source deconvolution in, cross-plane scattering correction, 93: 312

in prostatic blood flow and volume measurements, 94: 229

pulmonary gas volume measurements and, regional ventilation, 93: 140

radioligands of benzodiazepine receptors and binding sites, 94: 331

radiotracer for serotonin uptake sites, carbon-11 McN-5652Z, 94: 333

in rectal cancer and scar differentiation, 93: 116

of residual tissue viability after myocardial infarction, time dependence of, 95: 339

rubidium-82
for myocardial perfusion imaging, and heart patient outcome, 94: 61
vs. thallium-201 SPECT in coronary artery disease, 93: 24

satellite, and lung cancer, in surgical patients, 95: 71

of soft tissue masses with fluorine-18 fluoro-2-deoxy-D-glucose, 93: 151

of solitary lung nodules for cancer detection with 2-[fluorine-18]-fluoro-2-deoxy-D-glucose, 94: 127

with SPECT for myocardial perfusion imaging, disparate results, 93: 25

in striatonigral degeneration, of dopamine D1 receptors, 95: 270

three-dimensional
with conventional multislice tomograph without septa, 93: 311
scattered events in, with scanner with retractable septa, 94: 319

of thyroid masses, 95: 173

for whole body skeletal imaging, 94: 181

Positron emitters
511-keV collimator for, with gamma camera, 94: 321

Pregnancy
of nuclear medicine workers, ICRP recommendations for, 94: 340

Prenatal diagnosis
of pelvic hydronephrosis, 93: 233

Pressure sore
related osteomyelitis, histologically proven, with negative technetium bone imaging, 95: 112

Progestin
11beta-substituted, labeled with technetium-99m and rhenium-186, 94: 324

Prostate
blood flow and volume, measurements by PET, 94: 229

cancer
metastatic, follow-up, prostate specific antigen replacing bone scintigraphy in, 94: 172
newly diagnosed, prostate specific antigen in staging of, 94: 171
staging and monitoring, prostate specific antigen and bone imaging correlation in, 94: 172

specific antigen
bone scan correlation in prostate cancer staging and monitoring, 94: 172
in prostate cancer staging, newly diagnosed, 94: 171
replacing bone scintigraphy in metastatic prostate cancer follow-up, 94: 172

Prosthesis
aortoiliac and aortofemoral Dacron, knitted vs. woven, 94: 265

hip, suspected loosening, combined contrast and radionuclide arthrography in, 95: 356

infected endoprosthesis, monoclonal antibody leukocyte scintigraphy of, 94: 161

joint, infections, indium-111 IgG scintigraphy in, 93: 189

knee, infected, indium-111 leukocyte, technetium-99m sulfur colloid and MDP imaging in, 93: 184

Protein
solutions, relaxation in, including hydration and magnetization transfer, 94: 78

technetium-99m, in inflammatory foci imaging, 93: 332

Proton
magnetic resonance spectroscopy (see Magnetic resonance spectroscopy, proton)

spin relaxation in tissues, magnetic field dependence of, 93: 68

water magnetic relaxation in heterogenous systems, hydrated lysosome results, 93: 69

Pseudoaneurysm
popliteal, radionuclide imaging of, 94: 275

Psychological
factors, in mental stress induced silent left ventricular dysfunction in coronary artery disease, 95: 330

Psychosocial

sequelae of severe closed head injury, SPECT of, 94: 286
Pubic
osteomyelitis, due to *Staphylococcus simulans*, 95: 111
Pulmonary, 94: 97, 95: 1
angiography
with MRI, experience, 95: 38
for suspected pulmonary embolism, quantitative plasma D-dimer levels in, 95: 2
arteriovenous fistula, scintigraphy in, 93: 129
artery aneurysm, thrombosed, causing high-probability lung imaging, 94: 105
blastomycosis, North American, gallium-67 imaging in, 95: 89
embolism (*see* Embolism, pulmonary)
gas volume, regional ventilation, measurement of, and PET, 93: 140
hamartoma/mesenchymoma, technetium-99m methylene diphosphonate uptake by, 94: 118
hypertension, perfusion lung scintigraphy in, 95: 37
infarction with crack cocaine use, 93: 125
malignant lesions, suspected, thallium-201 SPECT of, 95: 28
nodule, solitary, PET-FDG imaging of, 95: 26
permeability alteration, detection with radionuclide technique, 93: 134
scintigraphy, defects after pneumonia recovery in children, 95: 32
vasculature, MRI of, three-dimensional, 93: 118
vessels, single breath-hold MRI of, 94: 366
(*See also* Lung)
Purulent disease
focal, technetium-99m HMPAO leukocytes and technetium-99m polyclonal immunoglobulin G in, 95: 101
Pyelonephritis
reflux and nonreflux, in children, kidney scarring after, technetium-99m DMSA scintigraphy of, 94: 226
Pyeloplasty
early, does it really avert loss of kidney function, 95: 186
PYP
technetium-99m, liver uptake of, 93: 259

Q

QNB
analogues, muscarinic receptor subtype selectivity of, 93: 324
Quality
control method for technetium-99m-sestamibi, 93: 27

R

Radiation
absorbed dose
estimated from inhaled krypton-81m gas in lung imaging, 95: 440
from technetium-99m DTPA aerosol, 94: 341
dose
to adults from nuclear medicine investigations, 93: 344
to children from technetium-99m investigations, 93: 342
to hands in nuclear medicine, 93: 353
during renography to kidney and bladder, 95: 185
doses from nuclear medicine patients to imaging technologist, 94: 340
dosimetry (*see* Dosimetry)
hand injuries due to, assessment with angiography and blood pool imaging, 94: 345
hepatitis, magnetic resonance appearance of, 94: 361
induced insufficiency fracture of pelvis, technetium-99m-MDP scintigraphy in, 93: 198
International Commission on Radiation Protection, recommendations for pregnant workers, 94: 340
low-dose, linear, nonthreshold hypothesis for, 93: 348
necrosis vs. recurrent glioma, 94: 288
protection design for PET imaging suite, 94: 346
risks, how real they are, 93: 347
survey instruments response, to static magnetic field, 94: 344
synovectomy, 95: xxv
samarium-153 and rhenium-186 hydroxyapatite particles as radiopharmaceuticals for (in rabbit), 95: 418
Radiochemistry, 94: 323
Radiofrequency
penetration effects in high field imaging, reduction of, 93: 86
Radiography

chest
  opacities, and matched ventilation
      perfusion defects, 95: 19
  in tuberculosis, acute disseminated, vs.
      gallium-67 citrate imaging in,
      95: 88
  of leukemia lymphoma, T cell, adult,
      95: 374
  in low back pain, chronic, 93: 194
  microautoradiography of fluorine-18
      fluorodeoxyglucose intratumoral
      distribution (in mice), 94: 130
  in osseous abnormalities in
      osteomyelitis, 93: 181
  in osteoarthritis of knee, 93: 113
  in Paget disease of bone with sarcoma,
      93: 206
  of scaphoid fracture, suspected, 94: 167
      with bone scintigraphy, 95: 353
Radioimmunodetection
  of solid tumors, 95: 69
Radioimmunotherapy, 95: xxvii
  future horizons and applications for,
      95: 69
Radioiodine
  imaging
      whole body, giving false-positive
          thyroid cancer metastases, due to
          esophageal retained radioactivity,
          95: 166
      whole body, hiatal hernia on,
          mimicking metastatic thyroid
          cancer, 95: 378
  therapy, in papillary thyroid carcinoma,
      peripheral facial nerve palsy after,
      95: 170
  in thyroid cancer, local reactions to,
      93: 211
  uptake, by lung carcinoma, squamous
      cell, 95: 31
Radiolabeled
  particles, 95: xxv
  small molecules, 95: xxii
Radioligands
  iodine-123 iomazenil, pharmacokinetics
      of, 94: 329
  for PET of benzodiazepine receptors
      and binding sites, 94: 331
  putative, brain concentrations of, *ex
      vivo* binding to measure, 94: 334
Radionuclide
  hysterosalpingography, simplified
      technique, 95: 203
  imaging in hypothyroidism, permanent
      congenital, 93: 218
  internally deposited, absorbed dose
      calculations to blood and blood
      vessels, 93: 350

list, 93: 355
  metallic, immunoradiometric assay with,
      93: 341
  monitor, ambulatory, for left ventricular
      systolic and diastolic function
      measurements, 94: 48
  plethysmography of splanchnic vein
      volume-pressure relation, and
      nitroglycerin, 94: 50
  potential contaminants for operators of
      in vivo counters, 93: 355
  uniformly distributed in different cell
      compartments, cellular dosimetry,
      95: 439
  ventriculography (*see* Ventriculography,
      radionuclide)
Radioopaque
  markers, vs. radioisotope determination
      of regional colonic transit in severe
      constipation, 95: 237
Radiopharmaceuticals, 95: 387
  peptide, as ticket to ride, 95: 404
  with rapid clearance for simulation of
      dynamic SPECT, 94: 309
Radiopharmacy, 94: 323
Radiotherapy
  of bronchogenic carcinoma, lung
      function after, perfusion lung
      imaging in, 94: 124
Radiotracer
  PET, for serotonin uptake sites,
      carbon-11 McN-5652Z, 94: 333
Radon
  concentrations, long-term, from ^{210}Po
      embedded in glass, 95: 446
  indoor, estimating past exposure from
      household glass, 94: 347
  levels, mitigation strategies, dosimetry,
      effects and guidelines, 95: 444
RARE sequences
  single-shot, phase-encode order effect
      on contrast and artifact in, 93: 81
RBC, technetium-99m (*see*
      Technetium-99m red blood cell)
Receiver
  high-temperature superconducting, for
      magnetic resonance microscopy,
      94: 84
  operating characteristics, clinical,
      filtered backprojection vs.
      maximum likelihood estimator
      images in fluorodeoxyglucose PET,
      95: 435
Reconstruction
  maximum-likelihood, clinically
      important characteristics of,
      94: 317

of SPECT images with generalized
matrix inverses, *94:* 318
Rectum
cancer and scar, differentiation with
PET and MRI, *93:* 116
colorectal carcinoma follow-up,
indium-111-anti-CEA monoclonal
antibody ZCE 025 in, *93:* 160
emptying in constipation and defecatory
difficulty, scintigraphy of, *94:* 262
scintigraphy by, thallium-201, in
cirrhosis, *95:* 238
wall teratoma after thyroidectomy for
carcinoma, pelvic radioiodine
uptake in, *94:* 190
Red blood cell
imaging, denatured, residual spleen
found with, *93:* 275
scintigraphy, of metastatic malignancy
masquerading as liver hemangioma,
95: 68
SPECT of liver hemangioma, *93:* 119
technetium-99m (*see* Technetium-99m
red blood cell)
Reflex
sympathetic dystrophy
of extremity, MRI failure in, *93:* 110
in foot, scintigraphy of, *94:* 174
in hemiplegia, triple phase bone
imaging in, *95:* 281
technetium-99m HSA vascular exam
in, *93:* 272
Reflux
nephropathy, scintigraphy with
ultrasound in, *95:* 383
pyelonephritis in children, kidney
scarring after, technetium-99m
DMSA scintigraphy of, *94:* 226
vesicoureteral, kidney scarring after,
94: 227
Reinjection
as alternative to rest imaging in
exercise-induced ischemia with
thallium-201 emission tomography,
94: 6
Relaxation
in protein solutions and tissue, including
hydration and magnetization
transfer, *94:* 78
Renal
artery
blood flow, cine phase-contrast MRI
of vs. p-aminohippurate clearance,
95: 180
magnetic resonance angiography of,
93: 120
stenosis, captopril renography in,
93: 237

stenosis, technetium-99m DTPA
captopril renography in, *95:* 199
(*See also* Kidney)
Renography
aspirin, in renovascular hypertension
detection, *95:* 194
captopril
in renal artery stenosis, *93:* 237
technetium-99m DTPA, in renal artery
stenosis, *95:* 199
diuretic
additional view after gravity assisted
drainage, *94:* 218
in postnatal suspected uretero-pelvic
junction obstruction, *94:* 216
gamma camera, standardization of,
94: 222
radiation dose to kidney and bladder
during, *95:* 185
technetium-99m DTPA
diuresis, kidney washout during,
ureteral status in, in children,
93: 239
processing variability of, interpolative
background subtraction in, *95:* 179
Renoscintigraphy
captopril, with technetium-99m DTPA,
in suspected renovascular
hypertension, *95:* 191
Renovascular
hypertension
angiotensin converting enzyme
inhibitor in, causing transplant
artery thrombosis, *95:* 200
captopril renal scintigraphy in, and
prognosis, *94:* 221
suspected, captopril renoscintigraphy
with technetium-99m DTPA in,
95: 191
unilateral, detection with aspirin
renography, *95:* 194
Reperfusion
coronary artery
extent of jeopardized myocardium
during, *93:* 31
teboroxime imaging to detect,
sequential, *95:* 317
myocardial
prolonged metabolic abnormalities in
(in dog), *93:* 57
technetium-99m sestamibi uptake and
retention during, *95:* 314
Respiratory
disease, scintigraphy of, technetium-99m
Technegas vs. krypton-81m
ventilation, *94:* 109
Restenosis

with positive exercise test after coronary angioplasty, exercise thallium scintigraphy vs. dipyridamole echocardiography in, 94: 15

Revascularization
exercise capacity improvement after, PET in, 93: 58
mortality, in myocardial infarction size and myocardial viability, 95: 333
in ventricular dysfunction, PET studies, 94: 53

Rhenium-186
hydroxyapatite particles, as radiopharmaceutical for radiation synovectomy (in rabbit), 95: 418
labeling progestin, 11beta-substituted, 94: 324

Rheumatoid arthritis
chronic, joint inflammation in, technetium-99m polyclonal Ig and bone imaging in, 94: 178
inflamed joints in, imaging with technetium-99m monoclonal antibodies and immunoglobulin, 95: 105

Ribonucleases
inhibition of, water-stable ribonucleoside-technetium chelate, 94: 323

Ribonucleoside
technetium chelate, water-stable, for ribonuclease inhibition, 94: 323

Ribose
infusion accelerating thallium redistribution, 93: 23

Rim sign
in cholescintigraphy, and grading hyperperfusion diagnostic value, 95: 212
gallbladder with, as acute or subacute cholecystitis, 95: 216
portending cholecystitis, 94: 240

ROC
analysis for maximum likelihood-expectation maximization reconstruction, 93: 307

Rubidium-82
PET myocardial perfusion imaging and heart patient outcome, 94: 61
PET vs. thallium-201 SPECT in coronary artery disease, 93: 24

Rupture
spleen, incidental detection during technetium-99m red blood cell gastrointestinal bleeding study, 94: 243

S

Sacroiliitis
septic, MRI in, 93: 109

Sacrum
fracture, fatigue, in children, 95: 144

Salivary gland
disease in HIV infection, gallium-67 citrate imaging of, 94: 197

Samarium-153
EDTMP, dosimetry and toxicity in bone pain due to skeletal metastases, 95: 441
hydroxyapatite particles, as radiopharmaceutical for radiation synovectomy (in rabbit), 95: 418

Sarcoidosis
bone involvement in, multiple atypical, 95: 118
cutaneous, indium-111 leukocyte scintigraphy of, 94: 118
gallium-67 imaging in, whole-body, 93: 178
scintigraphy with J001 macrophage targeting glycolipopeptide, 94: 165
skeletal muscle in, imaging of, 95: 120

Sarcoma
in Paget disease of bone, features and radiography of, 93: 206
soft tissue, thallium-201 imaging of, 95: 50

Scanner
with retractable septa for three-dimensional PET, scattered events in, 94: 319
whole-body, human exposure to 4.0-tesla magnetic fields in, 94: 95

Scanning (see Imaging)

Scaphoid
fracture, suspected
carpal instability as missed diagnosis in, 95: 141
radiography and bone scintigraphy in, 95: 353
radiography and scintigraphy of, 94: 167

Scar
differentiated from rectal cancer with PET and MRI, 93: 116

Scarring, kidney (see Kidney, scarring)

Scatter
Compton scatter compensation, with triple-energy window method for SPECT, 95: 423
correction
cross-plane, point source deconvolution in PET, 93: 312

in SPECT, transmission-dependent
method, 95: 425
window method for, dual-photopeak,
93: 308
four scatter correction methods using
Monte Carlo simulated source
distributions, 95: 422
Scintigraphy
aerosol, in cystic fibrosis therapy
assessment, 93: 138
of beta receptors in heart, 93: 47
of bile leakage after laparoscopic
cholecystectomy, 94: 258
bone
blood flow and blood pool, of
adenomyosis, 95: 249
in brucellosis, skeletal, 93: 190
of chondrolysis, 94: 169
in femoral head ischemia, vs. MRI,
94: 374
intraoperative, technique for, 93: 200
with iodine-131
metaiodobenzylguanidine of
neuroblastoma, 94: 141
in lower extremity pain in preschool
children, 93: 196
in otitis, differentiating necrotizing
from severe, 93: 176
prostate specific antigen replacing, in
metastatic prostate cancer
follow-up, 94: 172
in scaphoid fracture, suspected, with
radiography, 95: 353
of talar dome fracture, 93: 204
dobutamine stress, 94: 6
gallium-67
after treatment of lymphoma, 93: 144
in leprosy, borderline lepromatous,
95: 90
in lymphoma, small, non-cleaved cell,
94: 137
in otitis, differentiating necrotizing
from severe, 93: 176
in *Pneumocystis carinii* pneumonia in
AIDS, 94: 162
gallium, in soft tissue cancer detection,
93: 150
hepatic blood pool, false-positive, in
metastatic colon carcinoma,
93: 242
hepatobiliary
in biliary colic, acalculous, 94: 239
in cholangitis, AIDS-related
sclerosing, 93: 249
in cystic fibrosis of bile duct
obstruction, 93: 256
morphine-augmented, in cholecystitis,
94: 237

IgG, indium-111, in bone, joint and
joint prosthesis infections, 93: 189
of iliotibial band injury in endurance
athlete, 93: 199
immunoscintigraphy (*see*
Immunoscintigraphy)
indium-111
IgG, nonspecific, in diagnosis of
inflammations and infections,
93: 174
leukocyte, imaging in Crohn's disease,
94: 250
leukocyte, in Crohn's disease with
fistula and sinus tract, 95: 227
leukocyte, in cutaneous sarcoidosis,
94: 118
leukocyte, in osteomyelitis of foot in
diabetes, 93: 183
leukocyte, of marrow alterations in
osteomyelitis, 93: 186
leukocyte and technetium-99m
methylene diphosphonate, false
positives in periarticular bone sites
in trauma, 94: 180
octreotide, in oncology, 95: 393
inhalation, in bronchial stenosis in
infant, 94: 113
iodine-123 metaiodobenzylguanidine
in heart hypertrophy and failure,
94: 69
in regional myocardial sympathetic
dysinnervation in arrhythmogenic
right ventricular cardiomyopathy,
95: 326
vs. iodine Tyr-3-octreotide in
metastatic carcinoid, 94: 204
iodine-131 metaiodobenzylguanidine
for paraganglioma preoperative and
postoperative evaluation, vs. CT
and MRI, 95: 55
in suspected pheochromocytoma,
93: 227
iodine-123 Tyr^3 octreotide, in lung
cancer staging, small cell, 95: 400
kidney
captopril, in hypertension and chronic
renal failure, 95: 198
captopril, in renovascular
hypertension, and prognosis,
94: 221
in hydronephrosis in children, and
ultrasound, 95: 187
in kidney colic initial evaluation,
94: 219
of kidney effects of oral felodipine, with
technetium-99m mercaptoacetyl
triglycine, 95: 189

in kidney transplant acute dysfunction, 94: 232

leg muscle, with technetium-99m MIBI in peripheral vascular disease, 94: 271

leukocyte
monoclonal antibody, of infected endoprosthesis, 94: 161
in osteomyelitis with soft-tissue infection and osseous abnormalities, 93: 181
technetium-99m HMPAO, in ulcerative colitis and Crohn's disease, 95: 93

of liver masses, solitary solid, 94: 139

liver spleen, in splenic infarction in cirrhosis, 95: 373

lung
perfusion, in pulmonary hypertension, 95: 37
ventilation perfusion, reporting, and anticoagulation, 95: 15

lymphangioscintigraphy of lymphedema, vs. MRI, 94: 371

macrophage targeting glycolipopeptide, J001, in sarcoidosis, 94: 165

marrow, in osteopetrosis, 93: 114

of Meckel's diverticulum, "fading," 94: 253

of melanoma, malignant, and metastases, with iodine-123 N-(2-diethylaminoethyl 4-iodobenzamide), 95: 405

in metastases, correlation with spinal MRI, 93: 112

myocardial, with technetium-99m-sestamibi and dipyridamole in effort angina, 93: 26
in evaluation of thrombolytics in myocardial infarction, 93: 33

myocardial, with thallium-201 and technetium-99m hexakis-methoxyisobutylisonitrile in left bundle branch block and coronary artery disease, 94: 33

myocardial perfusion
in myocardial infarction, recent, for residual tissue viability assessment, 93: 20
personnel radiation dosimetry from, 95: 437

negative, despite spinal fractures in multiple injury, 95: 351

octreotide, for paraganglioma detection, 95: 397

in osteoarthritis of knee, 93: 113

of otitis, malignant external, results, 95: 98

in peripheral vascular disease, 94: 270

pharmacologic stress perfusion, superior to exercise, 94: 5

in pulmonary arteriovenous fistula, 93: 129

pulmonary defects after pneumonia recovery in children, 95: 32

of pulmonary embolism, Technegas vs. krypton-81m for, 94: 108

of rectal emptying in constipation and defecatory difficulty, 94: 262

red blood cell, of metastatic malignancy masquerading as liver hemangioma, 95: 68

of reflex sympathetic dystrophy in foot, 94: 174

in respiratory disease, technetium-99m Technegas vs. krypton-81m ventilation for, 94: 109

of scaphoid fracture, suspected, 94: 167

serial, in fallopian tube passive transport processes, 93: 236

sestamibi, for myocardial viability assessment, 94: 36

skeletal, in osteomyelitis, 93: 107

somatostatin receptor
in breast cancer, 95: 399
for gastrointestinal endocrine tumor preoperative localization, 95: 381
with indium-111-DTPA-D-Phe-1-octreotide, 93: 147
with indium-111 DTPA-D-Phe[1] and iodine-123 Tyr[3] octreotide, Rotterdam experience with, 95: 388
indium-111 DTPA-D-Phe[1] octreotide in meningioma, 95: 403
in pituitary disease, octreotide and somatostatin analogs in, 95: 395

SPECT, in alcoholic liver disease, 94: 257

of spine disorders during adolescence, 95: 136

sulfur colloid, in musculoskeletal infection, 95: 113

of sympathetic neuronal dysfunction, regional, in heart, 95: 343

technetium-99m
DISIDA, hepatobiliary, in AIDS cholangitis, 95: 85
DMSA, of kidney scarring after pyelonephritis in children, 94: 226
DSMA (V), for soft tissue tumor diagnosis, 95: 64

HMPAO, in carotid occlusion, permanent, sequelae prediction, 94: 358

HMPAO leukocytes in cholecystitis, 93: 258

HMPAO platelets in venous thrombosis, 93: 266

IDA in malrotation simulating gallbladder perforation, 93: 251

and indium-111 leukocyte, in inflammatory bowel disease, 94: 148

MDP in pachydermoperiostosis, 93: 208

MDP in pelvic fracture, radiation-induced insufficiency, 93: 198

pertechnetate, in ileal duplication of stomach and duodenum, 94: 251

red blood cell, in gallbladder visualization, early, 94: 241

red blood cell, in gastrointestinal bleeding, localization, 95: 223

red blood cell, in gastrointestinal bleeding, vs. angiography, 94: 244

red blood cell, in intraperitoneal bleeding, 94: 247

Technegas and technetium-99m MAA perfusion, hypoxia associated with, 94: 106

Technegas ventilation, in pulmonary embolism, 93: 131

thallium
   dipyridamole, predicting survival after major vascular surgery, 94: 27
   exercise, in coronary artery disease, prognostic value, 93: 2
   exercise, of coronary artery disease after heart transplant, 94: 19
   exercise, reverse redistribution, and coronary patency and ventricular function after myocardial infarction, 94: 23
   exercise, vs. dipyridamole echocardiography for restenosis in positive exercise test after coronary angioplasty, 94: 15
   in myocardial ischemia detection, related to cardiac arrest and syncope in hypertrophic cardiomyopathy, 95: 299
   tomographic perfusion, left ventricular cavity-to-myocardial count ratio in, in resting left ventricular dysfunction, 94: 21

thallium-201
   with adenosine coronary vasodilatation in coronary artery disease, 93: 10
   of breast mass abnormalities, 94: 138
   dipyridamole, as preoperative screening test, 93: 9
   dipyridamole, in stable chest pain, prognostic value, 93: 6
   exercise, after thrombolytics and angioplasty in myocardial infarction, 94: 12
   exercise, myocardial, accuracy in asymptomatic young men, 94: 3
   in Hodgkin's disease treatment assessment, with gallium-67 avid mediastinal mass after, 95: 63
   with iodine-123 metaiodobenzylguanidine, for neuroendocrine tumor detection, 95: 53
   with mammography in breast cancer diagnosis, 95: 52
   myocardial, in left bundle branch block and coronary artery disease, 94: 33
   quantitative planar, perfusion defects on, outcome, 94: 1
   quantitative planar, reproducibility of, 93: 1
   by rectum, in cirrhosis 95: 238
   with reinfarction for viable myocardium identification in chronic coronary artery disease, 93: 26
   rest, to assess stress myocardial perfusion, postexercise regional ventricular function and myocardial viability, 95: 305
   in thyroid cancer postoperative patients, 93: 217
   with ultrasound, in reflux nephropathy, 95: 383
   ventilation perfusion
      in Prospective Investigation of Pulmonary Embolism Diagnosis Study, 95: 8
      stripe sign validation in, 94: 99

Scintimammography
   prone, in breast carcinoma suspicion, 95: 376

Sclerosing cholangitis (*see* Cholangitis, sclerosing)

Seizure
   complex partial
      disorders, SPECT in, 93: 280
      in herpes simplex encephalitis, reverse crossed cerebellar diaschisis in, 94: 297

Sensory
  stimulation, intrinsic signal changes
    accompanying, 94: 349
Septic
  sacroiliitis, MRI in, 93: 109
Serotonin
  uptake sites, PET radiotracer for,
    carbon-11 McN-5652Z, 94: 333
Sestamibi
  rest, vs. rest redistribution thallium-201
    SPECT in myocardial viability
    detection after infarction, 94: 38
  scintigraphy for myocardial viability
    assessment, 94: 36
  technetium-99m (see Technetium-99m
    sestamibi)
Shimming
  rapid, fully automatic, arbitrary volume,
    93: 92
Shunt
  operation, in hydrocephalus, normal
    pressure, SPECT with
    technetium-99m d,l-HMPAO,
    95: 279
  right-to-left, in superior vena cava
    obstruction in fibrosing
    mediastinitis, 93: 271
Shunting
  technetium-99m MAA intraarterial
    infusion targeting, 95: 66
Sickle cell
  hemoglobin disease, splenic infarction
    and sequestration in, 93: 274
Sincalide
  infusion for gallbladder ejection fraction
    calculation, 93: 245
Sinus
  histiocytosis, with lymphadenopathy,
    skeletal involvement, 95: 57
  tract, in Crohn's disease, with fistula,
    indium-111 white blood cell
    scintigraphy in, 95: 227
Skeletal
  muscle
    energy charge, low, in angina pectoris
      with thallium perfusion imaging
      abnormality, 94: 20
    in sarcoidosis, imaging of, 95: 120
Skeleton
  brucellosis, bone scintigraphy of,
    93: 190
  involvement in sinus histiocytosis with
    lymphadenopathy, 95: 57
  marrow-containing, photopenic defects
    on indium-111 leukocyte
    scintigraphy, 94: 155
  metastases, causing bone pain,
    samarium-153 EDTMP in, 95: 441

whole body imaging with fluorine-18
    fluoride ion and PET, 94: 181
Skin
  sarcoidosis, indium-111 leukocyte
    scintigraphy of, 94: 118
Skull
  base osteomyelitis, 93: 111
Smoking
  lung clearance of iodine-123
    N-isopropyl-p-iodoamphetamine
    and, 93: 136
Soft tissue
  cancer, detection with gallium
    scintigraphy, 93: 150
  masses, PET of, with fluorine-18
    fluoro-2-deoxy-D-glucose, 93: 151
  MDP extraskeletal localization in,
    secondary to methotrexate
    infiltration, 95: 150
  sarcoma, thallium-201 imaging of,
    95: 50
  tumors, technetium-99m (V) DSMA
    scintigraphy of, 95: 64
Somatostatin
  analog
    in corticotropin-secreting bronchial
      carcinoid, 95: 160
    effect on bile secretion and
      gallbladder emptying,
      cholescintigraphy in, 95: 235
    iodine-123 octreotide, in carcinoid
      and islet cell tumors, 94: 203
    isotope labeled, for islet cell tumor
      visualization, 95: 396
    in pituitary disease, and somatostatin
      receptor scintigraphy, 95: 395
    Tyr-3-octreotide in metastatic
      carcinoid, 94: 204
  receptor
    imaging, in lung cancer, small cell,
      with indium-111 DTPA octreotide,
      95: 401
    scintigraphy (see Scintigraphy,
      somatostatin receptor)
SPECT
  in alcoholic liver disease assessment,
    94: 256
  algorithms in, rapidly converging
    iterative reconstruction, 95: 432
  of benzodiazepine receptor, 93: 319
    radioligand, iodine-123 iomazenil,
      pharmacokinetics of, 94: 329
  bone imaging of kidney transplant with
    subclinical hip abnormality, 94: 176
  brain
    blood flow, in temporary balloon
      occlusion of carotid and
      intracerebral arteries, 95: 259

dual isotope, for cognitive activation monitoring, 95: 276

HMPAO, abnormalities in, assessment method, 95: 267

in ischemia, delayed, due to vasospasm, 94: 282

perfusion, in cocaine abuse and AIDS dementia complex, 94: 304

technetium-99m and iodine-123, 94: 277

technetium-99m HMPAO, in acetazolamide effect on vascular response in diaschisis, 94: 299

camera, multi-head, sensitivity, resolution and image quality, 94: 308

cerebral blood flow

for dementia evaluation, interobserver agreement in, 95: 262

study, 94: 286

collimation for, pinhole, ultra high resolution, small field of view, 95: 426

collimators for, higher-resolution, 94: 309

for Compton scatter compensation, with triple-energy window method, 95: 423

cone beam reconstruction algorithm for, with displaced center of rotation, 95: 429

dipyridamole induced technetium-99m MIBI perfusion abnormality on, 94: 39

dopamine receptor, in Parkinson's disease, 95: 271

double-angulated integrated, for arrhythmogenic foci localization in Wolff-Parkinson-White syndrome and ventricular tachycardia, 94: 51

dual-isotope, of parathyroid pathology, 93: 222

dynamic, simulation with radiopharmaceuticals with rapid clearance, 94: 309

emission and transmission measurements in, simultaneous, scanning line source for, 95: 431

in epilepsy, partial, 94: 355

of ictal and interictal activity, 94: 357

exercise thallium imaging, in coronary artery disease, 95: 286

gallium-67-citrate, in Hodgkin's disease in mediastinum, 93: 145

gated

with technetium-99m sestamibi in myocardial perfusion abnormalities, 94: 34

three-dimensional motion and perfusion quantification in, 93: 36

in head injury

closed, comparison with CT and MRI, 93: 100

severe closed, with sequelae, 94: 286

for heart imaging, attenuation and scatter correction method, 94: 312

of hemispheric flow reduction in crossed cerebellar diaschisis, 94: 296

in herpes simplex encephalitis, 93: 101

high resolution

scatter, spatial resolution and quantitative recovery in, 94: 315

three-headed, in liver hemangioma, 93: 244

in HIV encephalopathy, 93: 288

imager, stationary hemispherical, for three-dimensional brain imaging, 94: 311

iodine-123

iodobenzamide, of D_2 dopamine receptors in Parkinson's disease, 94: 293

radiopharmaceuticals, recent developments, 93: 333

in low back pain, chronic, 93: 194

of monoamine reuptake sites in brain, 93: 317

myocardial, thallium-201 chloride, of denervated but viable myocardium (in dog), 93: 50

in myocardial infarction, of regional metabolic abnormality in relation to perfusion and wall motion, 94: 67

myocardial perfusion

dual-isotope, rest thallium-201/stress technetium-99m sestamibi, validation of, 95: 289

effect of patient motion on, 94: 24

imaging with thallium-201 and technetium-99m sestamibi (in dog), 94: 36

in myocardial uptake, regional, of fluorine-18 fluorodeoxyglucose, 95: 331

n-isopropyl-p-iodoamphetamine, in complex partial seizure disorders, 93: 280

neural networks for, artificial, 95: 433

of neurons, cholinergic, mapping in brain, 95: 275

patient couches causing photon attenuation, correction method, 93: 309

with PET for myocardial perfusion imaging, disparate results, 93: 25

rCBF, of thrombolysis in ischemic stroke, 93: 296

reconstruction of images with generalized matrix inverses, 94: 318

red blood cell, of liver hemangioma, 93: 119

scatter correction, transmission-dependent method, 95: 425

of spondylolysis, unilateral, 95: 139

of stress fracture, bilateral pedicle, 93: 201

of stroke
 acute, therapeutic trials, 95: 254
 with technetium-99m ethyl cysteinate dimer, iodine-123 iodoamphetamine and technetium-99m HMPAO, 95: 252

technetium-99m
 ECD, in cerebral blood flow abnormalities, vs. xenon-133 SPECT, 94: 304
 hexakis-methoxyisobutylisonitrile after stress for SPECT of myocardial perfusion defect size, 94: 40
 HMPAO, consecutive, for carbon dioxide reactivity, in cerebral artery obstruction, 95: 257
 HMPAO, d,l-, in hydrocephalus, normal pressure, before and after shunt operation, 95: 279
 HMPAO, d,l-, of regional cerebral blood flow variations during temporary clipping in intracranial aneurysm surgery, 95: 261
 HMPAO, erythrocytes, of brain in cerebral infarct, 93: 300
 HMPAO, for brain imaging, attenuation correction, 94: 314
 HMPAO, for memory anatomic correlates from intracarotid amobarbital injections, 95: 278
 HMPAO, in dementia, 93: 284
 HMPAO, in probable Alzheimer's disease, vs. fluorine-18 FDG PET, 95: 268
 HMPAO, in stroke, acute, 94: 285
 HMPAO, in thalamic dysfunction with pathological lying, 94: 300
 HMPAO, of brain, 93: 279
 HMPAO, of cerebral blood flow, 94: 278
 HMPAO, of cerebral flow changes in major depression, 94: 302
 HMPAO, of collateral circulation adequacy during balloon test occlusion of carotid artery, 93: 295

HMPAO, of neuroleptic effects on brain function, 93: 282

methoxyisobutylisonitrile, in myocardial viability in perfusion defects, 94: 55

recent developments in use, 93: 333

red blood cell, in liver hemangioma, 94: 246

red blood cell, in liver hemangioma in cirrhosis with portal hypertension, 95: 221

sestamibi, in right ventricular regional perfusion evaluation, 93: 29

sestamibi, myocardial, for intramyocardial distribution during exercise, 95: 310

sestamibi, rest-stress, of stress normal limits, 95: 309

thallium-201
 adenosine, for high-risk left main and three-vessel coronary artery disease, 94: 7
 during adenosine coronary hyperemia in coronary artery disease, 93: 12
 after rest injection, vs. fluorodeoxyglucose PET in myocardial viability assessment in chronic coronary artery disease, 95: 293
 of brain, 93: 279
 of brain tumors, 95: 45
 in coronary artery disease identification in women, 94: 2
 defects in detection of myocardial metabolic viability, 94: 53
 for dobutamine stress test, with radionuclide angiography, after infarction, 95: 301
 effect of motion on, 95: 434
 exercise, vs. adenosine for myocardial perfusion imaging, 93: 11
 myocardial perfusion, stress, defects in one-vessel coronary artery disease, 95: 287
 for myocardial perfusion imaging of myocardial defect, according to extent, 95: 284
 negative, with positive rubidium-82 PET myocardial perfusion imaging, and heart patient outcome, 94: 61
 perfusion defects with myocardial contrast echocardiography and coronary stenosis severity, 94: 16
 of pulmonary malignant lesions, suspected, 95: 28
 reinjection, of ischemic but viable myocardium, nitrates improving detection of, 95: 291

rest-redistribution vs. rest sestamibi in myocardial viability detection after infarction, 94: 38

stress redistribution indexes of hypoperfused myocardium secondary coronary artery disease, 94: 22

of supratentorial glioma, 95: 48

and technetium-99m HMPAO, in radiation necrosis vs. recurrent glioma, 94: 288

vs. exercise echocardiography in coronary artery disease, 93: 14

vs. rubidium-82 PET in coronary artery disease, 93: 24

three-dimensional

reconstruction of combined cone beam and parallel beam data, 93: 303

simulations of brain model and brain phantom, 93: 305

three-headed system, technetium-99m-SQ30217 myocardial imaging in, 93: 34

in vertebrobasilar insufficiency due to vertebral artery stenosis, 93: 293

volume quantitation in, image segmentation methods, 93: 314

xenon-133, in cerebral blood flow abnormalities, vs. technetium-99m ECD SPECT, 94: 304

Spectroscopy, magnetic resonance (*see* Magnetic resonance spectroscopy)

Spine

disorders during adolescence, scintigraphy of, 95: 136

fracture, in multiple injury, negative scintigraphy in, 95: 351

metastases

detection, bone imaging vs. MRI in, 95: 355

MRI and scintigraphy in, 93: 112

Splanchnic

vein volume-pressure relation during radionuclide plethysmography, and nitroglycerin, 94: 50

Spleen

infarction, in cirrhosis, liver spleen scintigraphy in, 95: 373

infarction and sequestration in hemoglobin sickle cell disease, 93: 274

liver

imaging, defect due to fatty liver, 93: 154

scintigraphy, of splenic infarction in cirrhosis, 95: 373

residual, on denatured erythrocyte imaging after negative colloid imaging, 93: 275

rupture, incidental detection during technetium-99m red blood cell gastrointestinal bleeding study, 94: 243

Spondylolysis

unilateral, SPECT of, 95: 139

Sports

competitive, infectious diseases in, 95: 86

SQ30217

technetium-99m-, for myocardial imaging in SPECT, 93: 34

Staphylococcus

simulans, causing pubic osteomyelitis, 95: 111

Stenosis

bronchial, in infant, inhalation scintigraphy in, 94: 113

coronary, severity, and perfusion defects with myocardial contrast echocardiography, and thallium-201 SPECT, 94: 16

renal artery

captopril renography in, 93: 237

technetium-99m DTPA captopril renography in, 95: 199

vertebral artery, causing vertebrobasilar insufficiency, 93: 293

Sternocostoclavicular

hyperostosis, CT of, 95: 358

Stomach

ileal duplication of, technetium-99m pertechnetate scintigraphy in, 94: 251

(*See also* Gastric)

Streptavidin

for infection localization, 94: 163

Streptokinase

in myocardial infarction, left ventricular function assessment after, 93: 38

Stress

bicycle stress echocardiography vs. exercise thallium-201 tomography in coronary artery disease detection, 94: 13

dipyridamole thallium-201 myocardial imaging of perioperative cardiac events in major nonvascular surgery, 95: 288

dobutamine (*see* Dobutamine stress)

fracture, bilateral pedicle, SPECT and CT of, 93: 201

imaging, thallium-201 immediate reinjection, in myocardial viability detection, 95: 292

level in exercise myocardial perfusion imaging, 95: 298

mental, inducing silent left ventricular dysfunction in coronary artery disease, 95: 330

myocardial perfusion

defect size with SPECT after, 94: 40

gated technetium-99m sestamibi to assess, 95: 305

normal limits, rest-stress technetium-99m sestamibi SPECT for, 95: 309

only vs. stress rest with technetium-99m methoxyisobutylisonitrile myocardial perfusion imaging, 94: 32

pharmacologic stress perfusion scintigraphy superior to exercise, 94: 5

redistribution thallium-201 SPECT indexes of hypoperfused myocardium secondary to coronary artery disease, 94: 22

test technetium-99m sestamibi myocardial tomography, validation, 95: 306

thallium-201

myocardial perfusion SPECT defects in one-vessel coronary artery disease, 95: 287

test, technetium-99m sestamibi myocardial perfusion SPECT, validation of, 95: 289

Striatocapsular

infarction recovery, brain functional reorganization in, 94: 305

Striatonigral

degeneration, dopamine D1 receptors in, PET of, 95: 270

Stripe sign

validation in ventilation-perfusion scintigraphy, 94: 99

Stroke

acute

MRI and proton magnetic resonance spectroscopy of, 94: 353

N-acetylaspartate, creatine, phosphocreatine and choline compounds in brain after, proton magnetic resonance spectroscopy of, 94: 91

technetium-99m HMPAO SPECT in, 94: 285

therapeutic trials, SPECT in, 95: 254

ischemia, thrombolysis with recombinant tissue plasminogen activator in, 93: 296

motor

recovery after, PET in, 93: 277

striatocapsular infarction causing, recovery from, 94: 306

with negative brain MRI, 94: 354

SPECT of, with technetium-99m ethyl cysteinate dimer, iodine-123 iodoamphetamine and technetium-99m HMPAO, 95: 252

Struma ovarii, 94: 191

Subarachnoid

pleural fistula, indium-111 DTPA myelography of, 94: 123

Suboptimal imaging

inadequate exercise leading to, 93: 8

Sulfur

colloid

scintigraphy of musculoskeletal infection, 95: 113

technetium-99m, imaging of infected knee prosthesis, 93: 184

Supratentorial

glioma, thallium-201 SPECT of, 95: 48

Surgery

major nonvascular, perioperative cardiac events in, risk indexes, echocardiography and myocardial imaging in, 95: 288

Sympathetic

dystrophy, reflex, in foot, scintigraphy of, 94: 174

innervation of left ventricle, impairment in arrhythmogenic right ventricular disease, 94: 68

Syncope

in hypertrophic cardiomyopathy, myocardial ischemia in, 95: 299

Syndome X

left ventricular dysfunction during exercise in angina pectoris with normal coronary arteries, 95: 328

Synostosis

tibiofibular, in professional basketball players, 95: 146

Synovectomy

radiation, 95: xxv

samarium-153 and rhenium-186 hydroxyapatite particles as radiopharmaceuticals for (in rabbit), 95: 418

T

T cell

leukemia lymphoma, in adult, radiographic features, 95: 374

T2 contrast-enhanced imaging

GD and Dy-chelates for, 93: 71

Tachycardia
ventricular, arrhythmogenic foci
localization by radionuclide
ventriculography, 94: 51
Talus
fracture, of dome, bone scintigraphy of,
93: 204
Teboroxime
imaging
sequential, in balloon occlusion of
coronary artery, 95: 319
sequential, to detect coronary artery
occlusion and reperfusion in
ischemic and infarcted
myocardium, 95: 317
rapid redistribution of, 94: 44
technetium-99m (*see* Technetium-99m
teboroxime)
Technegas
particles, biological distribution,
long-term, 95: 415
for scintigraphy, inhalation, in infant,
94: 113
technetium-99m (*see* Technetium-99m
Technegas)
ventilatory assistance device with,
93: 132
vs. krypton-81m in scintigraphy of
pulmonary embolism, 94: 108
Technetium
bone imaging, negative, in histologically
proven pressure sore related
osteomyelitis, 95: 112
ribonucleoside chelate, water-stable, for
ribonuclease inhibition, 94: 323
Technetium-99m
albumin macroaggregates for lung
imaging, arterial oxygen saturation
in, 93: 126
ascorbate for antibody direct labeling,
95: 414
binding sites in immunoglobulin G,
94: 328
1,2-bis[bis(2-ethoxyethyl)phosphino]-
ethane, as new myocardial
perfusion imaging agent, 94: 46
bis(dithiocarbamato) nitrido, for neutral
myocardial imaging agents (in
animals), 95: 324
blood radioactivity concentration,
factors influencing, 94: 47
for brain SPECT, 94: 277
C vs. phytate aerosol in ventilation
studies, 94: 110
DD-3B6/22 anti-fibrin monoclonal
antibody fab fragment, in deep
venous thrombosis and pulmonary
embolism detection, 95: 245

diethylene triamine penta-acetate lung
clearance in AIDS, 93: 134
dimercaptosuccinic acid (*see* DMSA
below)
DISIDA hepatobiliary scintigraphy in
AIDS cholangitis, 95: 85
DMSA
chemical identity of, 93: 336
kidney depth measurement by, vs. CT,
94: 224
for kidney imaging, technetium-99m
mercaptoacetyltriglycine replacing,
94: 212
scintigraphy, of kidney scarring after
pyelonephritis in children, 94: 226
(V), for scintigraphy of soft tissue
tumors, 95: 64
DTPA
aerosol, radiation absorbed dose
from, 94: 341
clearance, to estimate glomerular
filtration rate in cancer in children,
95: 201
diuresis renography, kidney washout
during, ureteral status in, in
children, 93: 239
inhaled, clearance predicting fibrosing
alveolitis clinical course, 95: 36
in kidney transplant evaluation,
94: 214
renography, captopril, in renal artery
stenosis, 95: 199
renography, processing variability,
interpolative background
subtraction in, 95: 179
for renoscintigraphy, captopril, in
suspected renovascular
hypertension, 95: 191
ECD SPECT in cerebral blood flow
abnormalities, vs. xenon-133
SPECT, 94: 304
erythrocyte (*see* red blood cell *below*)
ethyl cysteinate dimer, in SPECT of
stroke, 95: 252
exametazime, in cerebral blood flow
SPECT for dementia evaluation,
interobserver agreement in, 95: 262
granulocyte antibody in inflammatory
diseases, 93: 170
hexakis-methoxyisobutylisonitrile
after stress, for SPECT in myocardial
perfusion defect size, 94: 40
in left bundle branch block and
coronary artery disease, 94: 33
hexametazime leukocytes for aortic graft
infection detection, 94: 158
hexamethylpropylene amine oxime (*see*
HMPAO *below*)

HMPAO
  brain SPECT, of acetazolamide effect
    on vascular response in diaschisis,
    94: 299
  brain uptake, quantification of,
    95: 273
  for cerebral blood flow SPECT, in
    dementia evaluation, interobserver
    agreement in, 95: 262
  of cerebral cortical activity, reversible
    increased, 93: 291
  d,l-, for SPECT in hydrocephalus,
    normal pressure, before and after
    shunt operation, 95: 279
  d,l-, for SPECT of cerebral blood
    flow variations during temporary
    clipping in intracranial aneurysm
    surgery, 95: 261
  for dopamine receptor SPECT in
    Parkinson's disease, 95: 271
  for imaging in inflammatory bowel
    disease, 94: 248
  for leukocyte scintigraphy in ulcerative
    colitis and Crohn's disease, 95: 93
  leukocytes, imaging in suspected
    orthopedic infection, 94: 152
  leukocytes, in abdominal infections
    and inflammations, 93: 168
  leukocytes, in cholecystitis, 93: 258
  leukocytes, in purulent disease
    diagnosis, focal, 95: 101
  platelets for scintigraphy of venous
    thrombosis, 93: 266
  scintigraphy, in carotid occlusion,
    permanent, sequelae prediction,
    94: 358
  SPECT (see SPECT, technetium-99m
    HMPAO)
  white blood cell heart imaging in
    Kawasaki disease in children, with
    ventricular dysfunction and carditis,
    95: 90
HSA vascular exam in reflex sympathetic
    dystrophy, 93: 272
hydrazino nicotinamide derivatized
    chemotactic peptide analogs, for
    imaging focal sites of bacterial
    infection, 95: 106
IDA scintigraphy in malrotation
    simulating gallbladder perforation,
    93: 251
IMMU-4 monoclonal antibody imaging
    in colorectal cancer, 94: 135
immunoglobulin G
  imaging not predicting intestinal
    inflammation in inflammatory
    bowel disease, 94: 147

  polyclonal, in purulent disease
    diagnosis, focal, 95: 101
  polyclonal, to detect joint
    inflammation in rheumatoid
    arthritis, 94: 178
investigations, radiation dose to children
    from, 93: 342
labeling progestin, 11beta-substituted,
    94: 324
leukocytes
  in aortic graft, early postoperative,
    93: 270
  vs. indium-111 granulocytes in
    inflammatory bowel disease,
    95: 225
liposomes, for imaging focal infection
    (in rat), 95: 107
L,L-ethylenedicysteine, as new kidney
    imaging agent, 95: 177
MAA
  intraarterial infusion, in liver
    metastases and shunting, 95: 66
  perfusion scintigraphy, hypoxia
    associated with, 94: 106
MAG3 (see mercaptoacetyltriglycine
    below)
MDP
  imaging of infected knee prosthesis,
    93: 184
  for imaging of ununited fracture
    infection, 95: 97
  increased skeletal uptake in milk alkali
    syndrome, 95: 127
  scintigraphy (see Scintigraphy,
    technetium-99m MDP)
  in soft tissue secondary to
    methotrexate infiltration, 95: 150
  uptake by pulmonary
    hamartoma/mesenchymoma,
    94: 118
medronate uptake in liver necrosis of
    Budd-Chiari syndrome, 94: 254
mercaptoacetylglycyl-D-alanylglycine,
    kidney excretion characteristics of,
    94: 213
mercaptoacetyltriglycine
  clearance, validation of single sample
    technique, 94: 209
  IV, simulating obstructive uropathy,
    94: 211
  in kidney transplant evaluation,
    94: 214
  in renal tract disease, in children,
    93: 237
  for scintigraphy of kidney effects of
    oral felodipine, 95: 189
mercaptoacetyltripeptides, synthesis and
    labeling characteristics of, 95: 416

methoxyisobutylisonitrile (*see* sestamibi
below)
methylene diphosphonate (*see* MDP
above)
MIBI (*see* sestamibi *below*)
micro aerosol pertechnegas, for
ventilation imaging in suspected
pulmonary embolism, 95: 22
monoclonal antibodies
against granulocytes in appendicitis
detection, 95: 104
specific murine anti-CD4, for imaging
of inflamed joints in rheumatoid
arthritis, 95: 105
monoclonal antiplatelet antibody S12
for vascular injury imaging, 94: 72
organotechnetium complex for imaging
multidrug-resistant P glycoprotein,
94: 327
OV TL 3 fab in suspected ovarian
cancer, 94: 132
pertechnetate
cimetidine-enhanced, in Meckel's
diverticulum visualization, 93: 262
repeated, in children with obscure
gastrointestinal bleeding, 95: 233
scintigraphy in ileal duplication of
stomach and duodenum, 94: 251
thyroid carcinoma concentrating,
93: 216
platelets, labeling of, 93: 339
proteins in inflammatory foci imaging,
93: 332
PYP, liver uptake of, 93: 259
Q3, in coronary artery disease detection,
95: 323
radiolabeling of antibody fab fragment,
93: 335
RBC (*see* red blood cell *below*)
red blood cell
gastrointestinal bleeding studies,
93: 241
gastrointestinal bleeding study, spleen
rupture incidental detection during,
94: 243
of hemangioma in Kasabach-Merritt
syndrome, 94: 274
in penile corporal venous leak,
93: 229
scintigraphy (*see* Scintigraphy,
technetium-99m red blood cell)
SPECT, in liver hemangioma,
93: 119, 94: 246
SPECT, in liver hemangioma in
cirrhosis with portal hypertension,
95: 221
scintigraphy in inflammatory bowel
disease, 94: 148

sestamibi
cardiac imaging, normal, prognostic
value of, 95: 302
dipyridamole, myocardial tomography
in stable chest pain, 95: 303
exercise tomography, for cardiac risk
stratification in stable chest pain,
95: 304
gated, to assess stress myocardial
perfusion, ventricular function and
myocardial viability, 95: 305
for hyperparathyroidism imaging, with
parathyroid abnormalities, 95: 157
imaging of parathyroid, 93: 223
in jeopardized myocardium
assessment during coronary artery
occlusion and reperfusion, 93: 31
for leg muscle scintigraphy in
peripheral vascular disease, 94: 271
for localization in
hyperparathyroidism surgery,
95: 42
myocardial imaging, at rest in
myocardial infarction assessment
and first-pass ejection fraction,
93: 32
myocardial imaging, comparison of
same-day protocols for, 93: 33
myocardial perfusion, for validation
of global and segmental left
ventricular contractile function,
95: 312
myocardial perfusion, imaging, planar,
of coronary artery disease, 94: 41
myocardial perfusion, imaging, stress
only vs. stress rest, 94: 32
myocardial perfusion, SPECT, rest
thallium-201/stress, validation of,
95: 289
myocardial retention, effect of
mitochondrial viability and
metabolism on, 94: 31
myocardial scintigraphy, for
evaluation of thrombolytics in
myocardial infarction, 93: 33
myocardial scintigraphy, with
dipyridamole in effort angina,
93: 26
myocardial SPECT, intramyocardial
distribution during exercise,
95: 310
myocardial tomography, rest-stress,
validation, 95: 306
myocardial tomography, with
exercise, for right ventricular
perfusion defects after inferior
myocardial infarction, 95: 308

of myocardial viability in chronic coronary artery disease, 95: 315

in nondiagnostic ECG, 93: 30

perfusion abnormality, dipyridamole induced, on SPECT, 94: 39

quantitative, of defect size, regional ventricular function, geometry and dobutamine stress in, 95: 313

rapid preparation and quality control method for, 93: 27

rest, defects, PET detection of evidence of viability, 95: 316

SPECT, in myocardial viability in perfusion defects, 94: 55

SPECT, in right ventricular regional perfusion evaluation, 93: 29

SPECT, myocardial perfusion imaging, vs. thallium-201 (in dog), 94: 36

SPECT, rest-stress, of stress normal limits, 95: 309

SPECT, vs. thallium-201, for brain tumor evaluation in children, 95: 44

for tomography in spontaneous chest pain, 93: 28

uptake and retention during myocardial ischemia and reperfusion, 95: 314

in viable myocardium identification in chronic coronary artery disease, 93: 26

vs. thallium-201, in personnel radiation dosimetry from myocardial perfusion scintigraphy, 95: 437

vs. thallium-201, myocardial retention characteristics (in dog), 94: 35

SPECT, recent developments in, 93: 333

SQ30217 myocardial imaging in SPECT, 93: 34

subtraction, of hyperparathyroidism, 95: 155

sulfur colloid

imaging of infected knee prosthesis, 93: 184

scintigraphy of musculoskeletal infection, 95: 113

synthetic peptides, thrombus imaging with, monoclonal antibody to activated platelets in, 95: 244

teboroxime

during adenosine coronary hyperemia, 93: 35

myocardial clearance kinetics differentiating normal and

flow-restricted myocardium (in dog), 94: 45

myocardial perfusion imaging, planar, 94: 42

myocardial perfusion imaging, planar, in coronary artery disease, 94: 41

myocardial retention of, and myocardial blood flow, 94: 43

Technegas

for scintigraphy of respiratory disease, 94: 109

ventilation scintigraphy, hypoxia associated with, 94: 106

ventilation scintigraphy in pulmonary embolism, 93: 131

tetrofosmin, 94: 46

in myocardial blood flow assessment, in ischemia model (in dog), 95: 322

as myocardial perfusion imaging agent, 95: 412, 413

for myocardial SPECT, stress-rest, 95: 320

for myocardial tomography in coronary artery disease evaluation, 95: 321

wipe standard for survey instrument calibration, 94: 343

Technologist

imaging, radiation doses from nuclear medicine patients to, 94: 340

Temporal

lobe

blood flow reduction in Alzheimer's disease, 94: 295

epilepsy, neuroimaging in, 94: 354

epilepsy, phosphorus-31 magnetic resonance spectroscopy of, 94: 92

Tendinitis

calcific, in proximal thigh, 95: 359

Teratoma

rectal wall, after thyroidectomy for carcinoma, pelvic radioiodine uptake in, 94: 190

Tetrofosmin, technetium-99m (see Technetium-99m tetrofosmin)

Thalamus

dysfunction, pathological lying in, technetium-99m HMPAO SPECT of, 94: 300

Thallium

exercise

SPECT in coronary artery disease, 95: 286

test, qualitatively normal planar, in suspected coronary artery disease, follow-up, 95: 283

imaging

dipyridamole, for preoperative cardiac
risk in nonvascular surgery, 94: 26
dipyridamole, negative, prognostic
implications, 94: 29
dipyridamole, safety in high risk
coronary artery disease, 93: 7
early, after PTCA, 94: 17
perfusion, in angina pectoris with low
myocardial and skeletal muscle
energy charge, 94: 20
stress-redistribution-reinjection vs.
rest-redistribution, for myocardial
viability assessment, 95: 296
myocardial perfusion tomography, with
dobutamine, 93: 13
perfusion imaging, exercise whole-body,
in peripheral vascular disease,
94: 269
redistribution, ribose infusion
accelerating, 93: 23
reinjection
activity after, distinguishing viable and
nonviable myocardium, 93: 18
demonstrating viable myocardium in
regions with reverse redistribution,
95: 297
late redistribution imaging after,
93: 19
in myocardial viability in chronic
coronary artery disease, 95: 315
thallium uptake and washout after,
93: 19
scintigraphy (*see* Scintigraphy, thallium)
uptake, regional, in irreversible defects,
93: 18
Thallium-201
adenosine superior to exercise, in
coronary artery disease with left
bundle branch block, 94: 4
in cardiomyopathy, distinction of
ischemic from idiopathic dilated,
94: 8
in coronary artery disease detection,
95: 323
imaging
correlation with tomographic
myocardial perfusion imaging,
93: 35
dipyridamole, in aged, prognostic
value, 94: 29
false positive leading to unnecessary
catheterization, 94: 1
of osteosarcoma, 95: 50
planar, interpretation uniformity,
factors affecting, 94: 18
quantitative planar, for viability in
acute myocardial infarction with

totally occluded infarct-related
artery, 95: 294
of soft tissue sarcoma, 95: 50
subtraction, of hyperparathyroidism,
95: 155
ischemic exercise test, poor prognosis,
94: 10
myocardial imaging, dipyridamole stress,
of perioperative cardiac events in
major nonvascular surgery, 95: 288
myocardial perfusion, stress, SPECT
defects in one-vessel coronary
artery disease, 95: 287
myocardial perfusion imaging
in angina, unstable, prognostic value,
93: 4
dipyridamole, for coronary artery
disease detection accuracy and
side-effect profile, 94: 30
dipyridamole, with low-level exercise
unmasking ischemia, 93: 8
planar, 94: 42
planar, in coronary artery disease,
94: 41
myocardial SPECT of denervated but
viable myocardium (in dog), 93: 50
during one leg exercise, regional
distribution, vs. leg blood flow by
plethysmography, 95: 239
perfusion imaging, in stable coronary
artery disease, 95: 300
reinjection
immediate, after stress imaging, in
myocardial viability detection,
95: 292
metabolic activity in areas of new
fill-in after, 93: 21
rest-injected, in severe asynergic region
viability assessment, 93: 22
scintigraphy (*see* Scintigraphy,
thallium-201)
SPECT (*see* SPECT, thallium-201)
stress, rest, technetium-99m sestamibi
myocardial perfusion SPECT,
validation of, 95: 289
testing, exercise in coronary artery
disease over 70, prognostic
significance, 93: 5
thyroid imaging to differentiate benign
from malignant thyroid nodules,
93: 225
tomography
dobutamine, in suspected coronary
artery disease, 94: 5
emission, in exercise-induced
ischemia, reinjection as alternative
to rest imaging, 94: 6

exercise, in coronary artery disease, severe, 94: 9

exercise, vs. bicycle stress echocardiography in coronary artery disease detection, 94: 13

myocardial, equivalence between adenosine and exercise, 94: 25

uptake in left ventricular wall thickening, 94: 57

vs. technetium-99m sestamibi

myocardial retention characteristics (in dog), 94: 35

in personnel radiation dosimetry from myocardial perfusion scintigraphy, 95: 437

Thermoluminescence

dosimetry, detection and determination limits, 93: 352

Thigh

proximal, calcific tendinitis in, 95: 359

Thrombolysis

with recombinant tissue plasminogen activator in ischemic stroke, 93: 296

Thrombolytics

in myocardial infarction

evaluation with myocardial scintigraphy with technetium-99m-sestamibi, 93: 33

exercise thallium-201 scintigraphy after, 94: 12

inferior wall left ventricular, right ventricular dysfunction during, 94: 49

left ventricular performance assessment after, 93: 37

Thrombosed

pulmonary artery aneurysm causing high-probability lung imaging, 94: 105

Thrombosis

arterial, platelet-specific monoclonal antibody in, 93: 265

transplant artery, acute, due to angiotensin converting inhibitor in renovascular hypertension, 95: 200

venous

deep, indium-111 leukocytes in, 93: 269

deep, indium-111 monoclonal antibody against tissue plasminogen activator in, 93: 267

deep, proximal, venography of, 95: 243

deep, technetium-99m DD-3B6/22 anti-fibrin monoclonal antibody fab fragment in, 95: 245

deep, venography in diagnosis, radionuclide vs. contrast, 95: 241

deep, with pulmonary embolism, frequent asymptomatic, 95: 1

indium-111 antifibrin monoclonal antibody in, 93: 268

scintigraphy with technetium-99m HMPAO platelets vs. venography in, 93: 266

Thrombus

imaging with technetium-99m synthetic peptides, monoclonal antibody to activated platelets in, 95: 244

Thymidine

modulated 5-fluorouracil liver metabolism, fluorine-19 magnetic resonance spectroscopy of (in mice), 94: 369

uptake, tritiated, to measure cancer cell proliferative activity, 94: 130

Thymus

rebound after chemotherapy for Hodgkin's disease, gallium in, 95: 60

Thyroglobulin

measurement in thyroid cancer postoperative patients, 93: 217

in thyroid carcinoma, metastatic differentiated, for diagnosis and treatment assessment, 95: 164

Thyroid

ablation, iodine-131 for, efficacy assessment, 95: 169

cancer

differentiated, anti-thyroglobulin antibodies in, meaning of, 94: 189

differentiated, thyroid hormones in, 95: 161

iodine-131 contamination from, 94: 188

metastases, false-positive, on radioiodine imaging due to esophageal retained radioactivity, 95: 166

metastases, hiatal hernia on whole body radioiodine imaging mimicking, 95: 378

patients, cancer risks in, 93: 212

postoperative patients, thallium-201 scintigraphy and thyroglobulin measurement in, 93: 217

radioiodine in, local reactions to, 93: 211

carcinoma

autonomously functioning, with euthyroid Graves' disease, 94: 192

differentiated, chromatography of radioiodinated thyroid hormones after iodine-131 scintigraphy in follow-up of, 95: 162

differentiated, metastatic, thyroglobulin and iodine-131 imaging in diagnosis and treatment assessment, 95: 164

insular, iodine-131 localization in, 93: 220

iodine-131 therapy for, complications, sequelae and dosimetry, 94: 187

medullary, imaging with indium-111 anti-CEA monoclonal antibody fragments, 93: 159

papillary, concentrating technetium-99m sodium pertechnetate and iodine-131 iodide, 93: 216

papillary, radioiodine therapy of, peripheral facial nerve palsy after, 95: 170

thyroidectomy for, rectal wall teratoma after, pelvic radioiodine uptake in, 94: 190

thyrotropin for diagnosis, recombinant human, 95: 167

well differentiated, treatment modalities, results with, 94: 201

ectopic, intracardiac, conservative surgery, 95: 379

function, thyrotropin stimulating (in monkey), 94: 185

hemiagenesis
adenocarcinoma in, papillary, 94: 191
with parathyroid adenoma, 94: 194

hormones
radioiodinated, after iodine-131 scintigraphy in thyroid carcinoma follow-up, 95: 162
in thyroid cancer, 95: 161

imaging, effect of fine-needle aspiration biopsy on, 95: 174

masses, PET of, 95: 173

nodules, differentiating benign from malignant with thallium-201 thyroid imaging, 93: 225

uptake of radioactive iodine, effects of contrast material iodides on, 93: 219

Thyroidectomy
for thyroid carcinoma, rectal wall teratoma after, pelvic radioiodine uptake in, 94: 190

Thyrotropin
recombinant human
for diagnosis of thyroid carcinoma, 95: 167
stimulating thyroid function and iodine uptake (in monkey), 94: 185

Tibia
insufficiency fracture after kidney transplant, 95: 125

Tibiofibular
synostosis, in professional basketball players, 95: 146

Tin
enhancement in exametazime, multidose, for leukocyte labeling, 95: 103

Tissue
metabolism, concurrent quantification with blood flow with hydrogen-2/phosphorus-31 magnetic resonance imaging, 89, 94: 88

plasminogen activator
indium-111 monoclonal antibody against, in deep venous thrombosis, 93: 267
recombinant, for thrombolysis in ischemic stroke, 93: 296

relaxation in, including hydration and magnetization transfer, 94: 78

water, magnetic resonance behavior of, 94: 79

Toddlers
limping, occult, bone imaging in, 94: 170

Tomography
in adenosine-induced coronary hyperemia, 94: 17

CBF, in frontal brain lesion volume measurement, 93: 299

computed
single photon emission (see SPECT) (see Computed tomography)

exercise technetium-99m sestamibi, for cardiac risk stratification in stable chest pain, 95: 304

myocardial perfusion
with dobutamine thallium, 93: 13
with technetium-99m-teboroxime during adenosine coronary hyperemia, 93: 35

myocardium (see Myocardium, tomography)

positron emission (see Positron emission tomography)

technetium-99m-sestamibi, in spontaneous chest pain, 93: 28

thallium-201 (see Thallium-201 tomography)

Torso
imaging with cone-beam transmission CT with gamma camera, 93: 304

Toxicity

cardiotoxicity of doxorubicin detection
by myocardial uptake of indium-111
monoclonal antimyosin fab (in rat),
94: 70
of samarium-153 EDTMP in bone pain
due to skeletal metastases, 95: 441
Tracer
localization in electron dose rate
delivery to cell nucleus, 95: 443
Transferrin
receptor expression in lung disease and
gallium-67 citrate imaging, 94: 164
Transplantation
heart
catecholamine uptake and storage
sites after, PET in, 93: 59
coronary artery disease after, exercise
thallium scintigraphy in, 94: 19
myocardial perfusion, quantification
with PET after, 93: 52
orthotopic, left ventricular function
after, radionuclide ventriculography
of, 94: 48
kidney
acute dysfunction, biopsy, ultrasound
and scintigraphy in, 94: 232
artery thrombosis due to
angiotensin-converting inhibitor in
renovascular hypertension, 95: 200
donor preoperative evaluation with
kidney imaging, 95: 190
evaluation, technetium-99m MAG3 as
alternative to technetium-99m
DTPA and iodine-131 hippuran,
94: 214
with subclinical hip abnormality, MRI
and SPECT bone imaging in,
94: 176
tibial insufficiency fractures after,
95: 125
liver, heterotopic, for liver failure, liver
regeneration after, 94: 261
in Parkinson's disease, fetal dopamine
cell survival and neurologic
improvement after, 94: 290
Traumatic
biliary fistula, nonsurgical management,
95: 218
Trifluoperazine
in brain, fluorine-19 magnetic resonance
spectroscopy of, 94: 352
Tropanyl benzilate
carbon-11, study of, 93: 325
Trunk
melanoma, high-risk,
lymphoscintigraphy of, 95: 75
Tuberculosis

acute disseminated, gallium-67 citrate
imaging vs. chest radiography in,
95: 88
osteoarticular, multifocal, case review,
95: 117
Tumors
adrenergic, iodine-131
metaiodobenzylguanidine for,
95: xxiv
brain (see Brain tumors)
brown, hypervascular, three-phase bone
imaging of, 95: 122
carcinoid (see Carcinoid)
distribution of fluorine-18
fluorodeoxyglucose in (in mice),
94: 130
endocrine, gastrointestinal, preoperative
localization, with somatostatin
receptor scintigraphy, 95: 381
fatty liver masquerading as, 93: 154
hypoxia, imaging of, 95: 409
immunodiagnosis of, 95: 70
islet cell
octreotide in, iodine-123, 94: 203
visualization, with somatostatin
analogs, 95: 396
liver, benign, resection, 94: 358
neuroendocrine, detection with
thallium-201 and iodine-123
metaiodobenzylguanidine in
scintigraphy of, 95: 53
parathyroid, localization, comparison of
imaging methods, 94: 199
perfusion, imaging of, 95: 409
soft tissue, technetium-99m (V) DSMA
scintigraphy of, 95: 64
solid, radioimmunodetection of, 95: 69
xenografts, radioiodinated phospholipid
ether analog localization in,
95: 411

U

U-FLARE
fluorine-19, for fast perfluorocarbon
imaging, 94: 85
Ulcer
foot, in diabetes, with osteomyelitis,
MRI of, 95: 353
Ulcerative colitis
technetium-99m HMPAO leukocyte
scintigraphy in, 95: 93
Ultrasound
10 MHz, in hyperparathyroidism, vs.
thallium-201 technetium-99m
subtraction imaging, 95: 155

compression, of lower extremity, pulmonary embolism during, 94: 103

of Crohn's disease, 94: 250

Doppler

color, in liver hyperplasia, focal nodular, 94: 360

in kidney transplant acute dysfunction, 94: 232

of hepatomegaly, congestive, 93: 260

high-resolution, of hyperparathyroidism, with parathyroid abnormalities, 95: 157

of hydronephrosis in children, and renal scintigraphy, 95: 187

lower extremity venous, in pulmonary embolism, 95: 4

of parathyroid disease, vs. imaging and MRI, 95: 155

with scintigraphy, in reflux nephropathy, 95: 383

Ureteral

status in kidney washout during technetium-99m DTPA diuresis renography in children, 93: 239

Uretero-pelvic junction obstruction

postnatal suspected, diuretic renography in, 94: 216

Urinary

leak simulation, hepatobiliary excretion of MAG3 as, 95: 220

Uropathy

obstructive, gallbladder activity after IV technetium-99m mercaptoacetyltriglycine simulating, 94: 211

US (*see* Ultrasound)

Uvea

melanoma, MRI, scintigraphy and glucose metabolism in, 93: 117

V

V/Q

imaging, false-positive, mimicking pulmonary embolism, 93: 127

Vasodilation

adenosine coronary, with thallium-201 scintigraphy in coronary artery disease, 93: 10

Vasospasm

ischemia due to, delayed, brain SPECT and cerebral angioplasty in, 94: 282

Vein

central, catheter, in cancer, upper extremity venography in, 94: 266

collaterals in superior vena cava obstruction in fibrosing mediastinitis, 93: 271

coronary, outflow phase velocity mapping of left ventricular perfusion, 93: 106

lower extremity, ultrasound and pulmonary embolism diagnosis, 95: 4

popliteal, aneurysm, pulmonary embolism from, 94: 104

splanchnic, volume-pressure relation during radionuclide plethysmography, and nitroglycerin, 94: 50

thrombosis (*see* Thrombosis, venous)

Vena cava

obstruction, superior, in fibrosing mediastinitis, 93: 271

Venography

in deep vein thrombosis detection, proximal, 95: 243

magnetic resonance, with deoxyhemoglobin susceptibility effect, 94: 79

radionuclide

of upper extremity, in cancer with central venous catheter, 94: 266

vs. contrast, in deep venous thrombosis diagnosis, 95: 241

of venous thrombosis, 93: 266

Ventilation

imaging

posterior view, limitations in pulmonary embolism, 95: 21

in suspected pulmonary embolism, technetium-99m micro aerosol pertechnegas for, 95: 22

lower lobe impairment, left, in cardiomegaly, 94: 115

perfusion

assessments in contrast-enhanced lung MRI, 94: 366

defects, matched, and chest radiographic opacities, 95: 19

lung imaging, abnormalities due to bronchoalveolar lavage, 95: 34

lung imaging, esophageal dysmotility on, 94: 122

lung imaging, in pulmonary embolism, acute, 93: 124

lung imaging, in pulmonary embolism, acute, strengthening the diagnostic value of, 95: 10

lung imaging, in pulmonary embolism, mismatched vascular defects in, 95: 13

lung imaging, neural network analysis
in, 94: 102

lung scintigraphy, reporting, and
anticoagulation, 95: 15

scintigraphy, in Prospective
Investigation of Pulmonary
Embolism Diagnosis Study, 95: 8

scintigraphy, stripe sign validation in,
94: 99

pulmonary gas volume measurement,
and PET, 93: 140

scintigraphy
in pulmonary embolism, 93: 131
of respiratory disease, 94: 109
technetium-99m Technegas, hypoxia
associated with, 94: 106

studies, technetium-99m C vs. phytate
aerosol for, 94: 110

xenon-133 imaging of open bronchial
stump post-pneumonectomy,
94: 116

Ventilatory
assistance device with technegas,
93: 132

Ventricle
dysfunction
in Kawasaki disease in children,
ventriculography and heart imaging
in, 95: 90
suitable for revascularization, PET of,
94: 53
ejection fraction, first-pass, assessment
with technetium-99m-sestamibi
myocardial imaging, 93: 32
function
after myocardial infarction, reverse
redistribution on exercise thallium
scintigraphy in, 94: 23
measurements during total coronary
artery occlusion, 95: 311
postexercise regional, gated
technetium-99m sestamibi to assess,
95: 305
regional, in quantitative
technetium-99m sestamibi defect
size, 95: 313
geometry, in quantitative
technetium-99m sestamibi defect
size, 95: 313
left
cavity-to-myocardial count ratio in left
ventricular dysfunction, from
thallium perfusion tomographic
scintigraphy, 94: 21
diastolic filling in left ventricular
systolic function decrease, 93: 42

dysfunction, during exercise, in angina
pectoris with normal coronary
arteries, 95: 328

dysfunction, in left ventricular wall
thickening, 94: 57

dysfunction, PET of, metabolic
imaging value for prognosis,
95: 332

dysfunction, resting, left ventricular
cavity-to-myocardial count ratio in,
from thallium perfusion
tomographic scintigraphy, 94: 21

dysfunction, silent, mental stress
inducing, in coronary artery disease,
95: 330

ejection fraction, assessment by gated
angiography, 93: 39

ejection fraction, in PET of
myocardial infarction size and
myocardial viability, 95: 333

ejection fraction, measurements,
function monitor in, 93: 44

function, after heart transplant,
radionuclide ventriculography of,
94: 48

function, assessment after
streptokinase in myocardial
infarction, 93: 38

function, contractile, global and
segmental, validation with gated
planar technetium-99m sestamibi
myocardial perfusion, 95: 312

function, in adriamycin
cardiomyopathy, 95: 337

function, monitoring, continuous, for
myocardial ischemia during
coronary artery angioplasty, 93: 45

function, systolic and diastolic,
measurements with ambulatory
radionuclide monitor, 94: 48,
95: 329

mass estimation from nitrogen-13
ammonia PET, 94: 63

performance, assessment after
thrombolytics in myocardial
infarction, 93: 37

performance, intact systolic, in
congestive heart failure, outcome,
93: 41

perfusion, measurement with cine
MRI and coronary venous outflow
phase velocity mapping, 93: 106

systolic function decrease, left
ventricular diastolic filling in,
93: 42

volume determination, four
radionuclide methods, 93: 40

wall thickening, relation to fluorine-18 deoxyglucose and thallium-201 uptake, 94: 57
refractoriness in heart, 95: 343
right
arrhythmogenic disease, impairment of sympathetic innervation of left ventricle in, 94: 68
cardiomyopathy, arrhythmogenic, regional myocardial sympathetic dysinnervation in, iodine-123 metaiodobenzylquanidine scintigraphy in, 95: 326
dysfunction during inferior wall left ventricular myocardial infarction, thrombolytics in, 94: 49
perfusion defects after inferior myocardial infarction, assessment by exercise with technetium-99m sestamibi myocardial tomography, 95: 308
regional perfusion evaluation with technetium-99m-sestamibi SPECT, 93: 29
tachycardia, arrhythmogenic foci localization by radionuclide ventriculography, 94: 51
Ventriculography
equilibrium multigated blood pooling, in Kawasaki disease in children, with ventricular dysfunction and carditis, 95: 90
radionuclide
for arrhythmogenic foci localization in Wolff-Parkinson-White syndrome and ventricular tachycardia, 94: 51
of left ventricular function after heart transplant, 94: 48
for left ventricular function assessment after streptokinase in myocardial infarction, 93: 38
Vertebra
metastases of breast cancer, MRI of, 94: 378
Vertebral
artery stenosis causing vertebrobasilar insufficiency, 93: 293
Vertebrobasilar
insufficiency due to vertebral artery stenosis, 93: 293
Vesicoureteral
reflux, kidney scarring after, 94: 227
Vessels, 95: 239
asymptomatic, phantom infection in, 95: 247
blood, absorbed dose calculations to, of radionuclides, 93: 350

defects, mismatched, in ventilation perfusion lung imaging interpretation in pulmonary embolism, 95: 13
exam with technetium-99m HSA, in reflex sympathetic dystrophy, 93: 272
injury imaging with technetium-99m monoclonal antiplatelet antibody S12, 94: 72
peripheral (*see* Peripheral vessels)
pulmonary
MRI of, three-dimensional, 93: 118
single breath-hold MRI of, 94: 366
response in diaschisis to acetazolamide, 94: 299
surgery
diagnostic problems in, radionuclide limb blood flow measurements in, 95: 240
heart risk stratification with dipyridamole myocardial perfusion imaging and ambulatory ECG monitoring before, 94: 28
major, dipyridamole thallium scintigraphy predicting survival after, 94: 27
Visual
cortex, MRI for functional mapping, 93: 95
Vitrectomy
eye, partial oxygen pressure in, with fluorine-19 MRI (in rabbit), 93: 87
Vocal
cord dysfunction due to heterotopic ossification after burns, 95: 150

W

Water
labeled, in dipyridamole induced technetium-99m MIBI perfusion abnormality on SPECT, 94: 39
oxygen-15, for PET in coronary reserve assessment, 95: 340
proton magnetic relaxation in heterogenous systems, hydrated lysozyme results, 93: 69
tissue, magnetic resonance behavior of, 94: 79
Water-150
in myocardial viability and blood flow assessment, 94: 56
Wavelet
encodes MRI, 93: 86
White blood cell (*see* Leukocyte)
White matter

normal, proton magnetic resonance
spectroscopy of, 94: 90
signal hyperintensities in MRI, proton
magnetic resonance spectroscopy
of, 94: 90
Wilson's disease
treated, neurologic deficit in, D2
receptor decrease in, 94: 294
Window
method dual-photopeak, for scatter
correction, 93: 308
Wipe
technetium-99m wipe standard for
survey instrument calibration,
94: 343
Withdrawal
from cocaine, brain glucose metabolism
changes in, 93: 290
Wolff-Parkinson-White syndrome

arrhythmogenic foci localization by
radionuclide ventriculography,
94: 51
Wrist
MRI of, high-resolution, with short TR,
short TE and partial-echo
acquisition, 93: 82

X

Xenograft
tumor, radioiodinated phospholipid
ether analog localization in,
95: 411
Xenon-133
SPECT in cerebral blood flow
abnormalities, 94: 304
ventilation imaging of open bronchial
stump postpneumonectomy,
94: 116

Author Index

A

Aabed MY, 114
Abe H, 253
Abraham S, 334
Abrams MJ, 106
Aburano T, 28
Achong DM, 95, 113, 221
Ackermann RJ, 275
Adamopoulos G, 98
Adams JE, 358
Adamson DJA, 100
Adler LP, 173
Adriaens P, 416
Agress H Jr, 63
Akabani G, 440
Akkermans LMA, 237
Alavi A, 8, 19, 209, 246, 265, 355
Alavi K, 315
Alfano A, 281
Alle K, 376
Allen BC, 259
Allman K, 343
Allman KC, 316, 336, 342, 343
Almkvist O, 370
Alpert NM, 334
Al-Shahed MS, 114
Altehoefer C, 293
Altland E, 302
Alvarez VL, 244
Andersen AJ, 146
Andersen AR, 279
Anderson IF, 147
Andersson-Lundman G, 370
Andreasen NC, 276
Andrews J, 241
Andrich MP, 34
Angelberger P, 400
Angelides S, 245
Antico VF, 68
Antona C, 379
Aotsuka A, 270
Archer CM, 412
Areeda J, 306, 309
Arndt J-W, 225
Arnold R, 381
Arrighi JA, 296, 297, 315
Arsenault A, 310
Asahina M, 270
Ashburn WL, 22
Atkins HL, 440
Avraham A, 164
Awad IA, 368
Awender HM, 218

B

Babich JW, 106, 337, 404
Babyn PS, 99
Bacharach SL, 296, 297, 315
Bacin FJ, 405
Bailey DL, 425, 431
Bakheet S, 166
Bakker WH, 388, 396
Bakr MA, 190
Bandeen-Roche K, 278
Barax C, 349
Bardfeld P, 281
Barefield KP, 183
Barnes DC, 227, 229
Barnes PD, 44
Barron BJ, 254
Bar-Shalom R, 61
Bartenstein P, 326, 364
Bash J, 134
Basten A, 245
Basun H, 370
Bateman T, 306
Batjer H, 259
Battistin L, 271
Battle RW, 312
Baudouy M, 291
Baumgold J, 408
Bautovich G, 245
Bax JJ, 331
Baxter LR, 435
Bayer W, 174
Bayo F III, 130
Bayouth JE, 441
Beanlands RSB, 316
Beazley RM, 52
Becker E, 117
Becker W, 80, 105
Begley MG, 55
Beiras JMC, 301
Bekdik C, 189
Belezzuoli EV, 22
Bellande E, 324
Beller GA, 314
Bellina CR, 162
Bellotti C, 261
Ben-Arie Y, 61
Bendriem B, 340, 344
Bergmann SR, 338
Berland Y, 200
Berlangieri SU, 365
Berlin JA, 265
Berman D, 305
Berman DS, 287, 289, 306, 309, 434
Berná L, 236
Bernstein RM, 358
Bertagna X, 160
Bessent RG, 16
Besser GM, 56
Bevan DH, 374
Bhatnagar A, 133
Bianchi R, 162
Biersack HJ, 104
Biggs T, 21
Biglioli P, 379
Bijvoet OLM, 158
Biniakiewicz D, 323
Biskupiak JE, 325

Bizais Y, 131
Björkstén KS, 370
Björnebrink J, 351
Black CM, 36
Black HR, 199
Blacklow SC, 2
Blanchard RA, 52
Blend R, 155
Block J, 376
Blok D, 225
Blokland JAK, 158
Bloom AD, 173
Blumhardt R, 107
Bockisch A, 104
Bodenheimer MM, 283
Bohdiewicz PJ, 212
Bok BD, 443
Bolling S, 343
Bomanji J, 56
Bomanji JB, 198
Bombardieri E, 70
Bonafous JF, 405
Boni G, 162
Boni S, 401
Bonow RO, 296, 297, 299, 315
Bonte FJ, 259
Booker FS, 412
Bootsma A, 399
Borer JS, 327
Borges-Neto S, 311
Borggrefe M, 326
Borm JJJ, 353
Bormans G, 416
Bormans GM, 177
Borsato N, 271
Bos KE, 141
Boulahdour H, 205
Bounameaux H, 4
Bowen WD, 408
Boyd H, 346
Boyle IT, 155
Braat S, 320
Braverman LE, 167
Breeman WAP, 388
Breithardt G, 326
Bretagne J-F, 228
Brew B, 214
Briani C, 271
Briele B, 104
Brill AB, 444
Britton KE, 56, 198, 237
Broadwater JR, 210
Brodack JW, 418
Broekhuizen AH, 141, 353
Brooks MH, 174
Brown CV, 150
Brown EA, 198
Brown JW, 216
Brown KA, 298, 302, 312
Brucato V, 324
Bruining HA, 396
Brunden RC, 335
Brunet P, 200

525

Brunetti JC, 85
Brunken RC, 332
Bruyland M, 128
Buell U, 293
Buhe T, 131
Bundesen P, 245
Buraggi G, 70
Burch WM, 415
Burdge DR, 112
Burg MM, 330
Burke GJ, 42, 157
Burke K, 223
Burmester GR, 105
Burns DE, 60
Burroughs AK, 373
Buscombe JR, 15
Bussière F, 291, 405
Buxton DB, 335
Buyan N, 280
Byers SL, 288

C

Caillat-Vigneron N, 291
Calabuig R, 236
Caldwell JH, 325
Calkins H, 343
Callahan RJ, 337
Cameron K, 245
Camici PG, 346
Campbell SB, 127
Camps JAJ, 158
Camuzzini G, 261
Canning LR, 412
Carapella C, 403
Carey JE, 275
Caron M, 310
Carpenter AL, 249
Carpentier W, 223
Carretta R, 262
Carrió I, 236
Casas AT, 42, 157
Casas R, 118
Castaigne A, 340
Cave V, 286
Cavoretto D, 379
Cazzuola F, 162
Cerino M, 310
Chae SC, 286
Chaitman BR, 288, 304
Champagne CL, 179
Chapman JD, 409
Charlotte F, 205
Chen CC, 34
Cherqui D, 205
Chierchia SL, 339
Chierichetti F, 271
Chin JKT, 373
Chinen LK, 418
Chinol M, 418
Chipperfield P, 24
Chiu KW, 412
Chlouverakis G, 327
Choi Y, 187, 335

Chossat FM, 405
Choudhury L, 346
Chua T, 305
Cicoria AD, 139
Cioffi R, 403
Cleynhens B, 416
Cliff RO, 107
Cload P, 320
Cloninger K, 306
Cloutier DJ, 308
Coade G, 262
Coade GE, 22
Coleman RE, 8, 18, 311, 365, 426, 429
Colombo F, 339
Coma-Canella I, 301
Comazzi V, 324
Comet M, 284, 324
Comtois R, 169
Conversano A, 338, 339
Conway JJ, 186
Cooke CD, 306, 309
Cooke T, 155
Cothren CC, 146
Counsell RE, 411
Coupland DB, 24
Couson F, 71
Coutris G, 53
Crake T, 346
Crawford R, 1
Crecco M, 403
Crichton KJ, 147
Croll MN, 421
Cronan JJ, 372
Crouzel C, 344
Crozatier B, 340
Csernay L, 93
Culver CM, 437
Cuocolo A, 55, 329
Curran P, 167
Czernin J, 332

D

Dahlberg ST, 317, 319
Dalen JE, 6
Dalinka MK, 353
Dam M, 271
Daniels GH, 167
D'Aoust S, 310
Darcourt J, 235, 291
Datseris IE, 198
Davidson M, 332
Davies TF, 167
Dayanikli BF, 89
Debatin JF, 38
Degrado TR, 343
DeGroot LJ, 167
de Herder WW, 395
de Jong M, 388
De Keyzer Y, 160
de Labriolle-Vaylet C, 443
Delecluse F, 279
Delforge J, 344

Delmont J, 235
Del Sole A, 268
del Val Gómez Martínez M, 301
Del Vecchio P, 169
de Moerloose P, 4
Denis B, 284
DePuey EG, 306
Deraska DJ, 167
De Roo M, 416
De Roo MJ, 177
Desai KB, 161
De Silva R, 346
Deutsch E, 323
Deutsch EA, 418
Deutsch KF, 418
Devillers A, 228
Devous MD Sr, 259
Dewan NA, 26
Dey HM, 199
Dhumeaux D, 205
Di Carli MF, 332
Di Chiro G, 366
Dienemann D, 57
Dierckx R, 273
Diggles L, 376
Dijkstra PF, 141
Dillehay GL, 174
Dillon WA, 22
Dilsizian V, 296, 297, 299, 315
Diodati JG, 315
Divgi CR, 378
Dobbeleir A, 273
Dogan AS, 220
Dölkemeyer U, 80
Donath A, 71
Doolittle MH, 2
Duatti A, 324
du Bois RM, 36
Dudczak R, 400
Dupont M, 238
Dusold R, 223
Dussol B, 200
Dworkin HJ, 437
Dwyer AJ, 366
Dyck WP, 223

E

Eberl S, 431
Ebner SA, 167
Eckard DA, 259
Economou G, 358
Edwards B, 412
Edwards NC, 314
Eggli DF, 172
Ehman RL, 180
Eidt JF, 210
Eigler N, 287
Eisenschenk A, 57
Elder RC, 323
El-Desouki M, 243
Elgazzar AH, 323
El-Kenawy MR, 190

El-Khoury GY, 97
Ell PJ, 15, 243
Elliott CG, 2
Elmaleh DR, 337
El-Sherif A, 190
Elting JJ, 139
Emmrich F, 105
Endo K, 48, 64
Epelbaum J, 160
Epelbaum R, 61
Epstein SE, 299
Erbas B, 189
Erbengi G, 189
Esterhai JL, 353
Estorch M, 236
Ettorre F, 261
Even-Sapir E, 227, 229
Eybalin M-C, 310
Eykyn S, 111

F

Fagret D, 284, 324
Faibel M, 150
Fairbank JT, 312
Fananapazir , 299
Fancher S, 210
Faraggi M, 443
Farlow DC, 68
Farman J, 85
Fazio F, 268, 339
Fedullo PF, 1
Feinmesser R, 164
Feldman F, 349
Fenton AH, 218
Ferdeghini M, 162
Ferlin G, 271
Fernández-Nogués F, 118
Ferrari E, 291
Fessler JA, 275
Fetterman RC, 313
Fiche M, 131
Fideler BM, 50
Fig L, 316
Fink-Bennett D, 306
Firlit CF, 186
Fischman AJ, 106, 334, 337, 404
Fisher RS, 278
Fisher SJ, 411
Fleming SJ, 127
Floyd CE, 18
Floyd CE Jr, 433
Fogarasi M, 414
Folks R, 306, 309
Foo TK, 38
Forster AM, 412
Fossella FV, 441
Foult J-M, 291
Fragasso G, 339
Franceschi M, 268
Frankenschmidt A, 187
Freedman NMT, 296, 297
Freiberger RH, 359

Freund J, 214
Frey KA, 74, 275
Frick MP, 26
Friedman J, 305, 306
Friedman JD, 289
Friedmann LW, 281
Froelich JW, 8
Front D, 61
Fulham MJ, 366
Fulton RR, 431
Furudate M, 191
Futatsuya R, 239

G

Gad HM, 190
Gaitini D, 61
Gallacher SJ, 155
Garada B, 251
Garber CE, 308
Garcia EV, 306, 309
Gardin I, 443
Gelormini RG, 216
Geltman EM, 338
George CD, 374
Germano G, 287, 289, 305, 306, 309
Gerson MC, 323
Gewirtz H, 334
Gherli T, 379
Ghoneim MA, 190
Giacometti A, 183
Gibson RN, 241
Gilardi MC, 268, 339
Gildersleeve DL, 275
Gill HK, 412
Gilson M, 334
Gilula LA, 362
Gion M, 70
Giunta S, 401
Gjerris F, 279
Glover DK, 314
Goddu SM, 439
Goins B, 107
Gökçora N, 280
Golberg LE, 409
Gold WL, 117
Goldhaber SZ, 2
Goldsmith SJ, 139, 170, 378, 418
Goodman RA, 86
Gordon B, 278
Gordon DL, 174
Gordon I, 32
Gosfield E III, 355
Gosselin M, 228
Gottschalk A, 8, 10, 13
Gould KL, 333
Goumnerova LC, 44
Grafton ST, 435
Graham W, 106
Gramatzki M, 80
Grant AD, 134
Grassi F, 268

Gravelle DR, 179
Gray HW, 16
Greene DA, 342
Greenough R, 245
Greer KL, 429
Grégoire J, 310
Gribble MJ, 112
Grier D, 144
Griffeth LK, 435
Griffioen G, 225
Grimaldi C, 235
Grist TM, 38
Gropler RJ, 338
Groshar D, 409
Gross M, 316
Gross MD, 411
Grossman AB, 56
Grotta JC, 254
Gruenewald SM, 68, 125
Grunwald AM, 283
Grünwald F, 104
Gubler FM, 353
Gücüyener K, 280
Güger G, 383
Guignier A, 291
Gulec S, 170
Gullberg GT, 428, 429
Gupta NC, 26

H

Haddad MC, 114
Hademenos GJ, 422
Haire WD, 2
Hall EC, 183
Hallgring E, 251
Ham HR, 238
Hamdy RC, 99
Hammami MM, 166
Handa N, 257
Hanrath P, 293
Hansell DM, 36
Hanson MW, 311
Hanson SK, 254
Haramati N, 349
Harcke HT, 136
Harrington T, 147
Harris AG, 235
Harris B, 95
Harris EW, 63
Harris J, 245
Harrison NK, 36
Hart J Jr, 278
Hashikawa K, 257
Hashimoto S, 423
Hatakeyama R, 45
Hattner RS, 76
Hawkins L, 56
Hawkins R, 332
Hawkins RA, 187, 335, 435
Hayashida K, 37, 194
He Z-X, 291
Heller GV, 308
Heller LI, 317, 319

Hellman RS, 262
Henry JH, 146
Henry JW, 10, 13
Heo J, 286
Heresbach D, 228
Herman WH, 336
Hertel A, 70
Hicks RJ, 336
Hietala S-O, 351
Higashi S, 252
Higley B, 412
Hildingsson C, 351
Hillmann A, 364
Hilson AJW, 373
Hindricks G, 326
Hirano T, 48
Hirayama K, 270
Hirner A, 104
Hisada K, 28, 252, 328
Hittinger L, 340
Hnatowich DJ, 414
Hodge JC, 359
Hoffer PB, 199
Hoffman EJ, 435
Hoffman JM, 365
Hoffmann RG, 262
Hoffschir D, 324
Hofland LJ, 388, 395
Hoh CK, 187, 335, 435
Holman BL, 251
Hoogland D, 22
Hoogma RPLM, 397
Hopper J, 241
Hör G, 70
Horattas MC, 218
Horneff G, 105
Hoskinson M, 409
Hosono M, 64
Hotze AL, 104
Houston AS, 267
Hovi I, 101
Howell RW, 439
Howman-Giles RB, 75
Hsieh KS, 90
Hsu C-Y, 88
Huang S-C, 233, 335
Hughes JM, 86
Huitink JM, 331
Hurtig R, 276
Hurwitz GA, 179
Hutchins GD, 342
Hutton BF, 425, 431
Hyodo A, 45
Hyun M, 434

I

Ichihara T, 423
Iervasi G, 162
Iles SE, 229
Ilgin N, 280
Imanishi M, 194
Imbriaco M, 329
Inoue O, 270

Inoue T, 48
Ishida Y, 194
Ishikawa H, 45
Iskandrian AS, 286
Israel O, 61
Itoh K, 191
Itti R, 320

J

Jacobson A, 203
Jaffe BM, 153
Jain D, 322, 330, 413
Jamieson C, 155
Jaszczak RJ, 426, 428, 429
Jeekel J, 399
Jeghers O, 238
John CS, 408
Johnson KA, 251
Jones BE, 21
Jones PBB, 358
Jones RH, 311
Jones T, 346
Jordan KG, 122
Joseph K, 381
Jouanne E, 376
Juni JE, 8
Junod A, 4
Junod AF, 71
Juweid M, 209

K

Kaboli P, 15
Kageyama M, 239
Kakishita M, 239
Kalatzis Y, 98
Kalden JR, 105
Kalff V, 336
Kamada T, 257
Kamm MA, 237
Kamp O, 331
Kanegae K, 191
Kania U, 104
Kao C-H, 88, 90
Kaplan WE, 186
Karatrandou A, 185
Kasagi K, 31
Kashyap R, 133
Kasi LP, 441
Katsiyiannis PT, 315
Kauffmann P, 405
Kaul S, 294
Kavanah MT, 52
Kawamoto M, 321
Kawano Y, 194
Kaweblum M, 134
Keiser HR, 55
Kelleher A, 214
Kelly JD, 412
Kelly P, 155
Kemp PM, 267
Kempf JS, 85

Kenney IJ, 32
Kerin MJ, 240
Kerns RD, 330
Kester RC, 240
Khafagi FA, 127
Khalkhali I, 376
Khanna S, 332
Khedkar N, 174
Kiat H, 287, 289, 305, 306, 309
Kilpatrick TK, 241
Kim CK, 19, 209, 246
Kimura G, 194
Kimura RL, 232
King BF, 180
King MA, 422
Kinne RW, 105
Kinuya K, 252
Kinuya S, 28, 408
Kirchner B, 364
Kirchner PT, 97, 220, 276
Kirsch M, 343
Klein MJ, 418
Klein S, 376
Kleinhans E, 293
Kletter K, 400
Klipper R, 107
Klotter HJ, 381
Kneeland B, 355
Knight LC, 244
Kobayashi H, 64
Koeppe RA, 275
Köhler H-P, 356
Kojima S, 194
Kong M-S, 233
Konishi J, 31, 64, 321
Kooij PPM, 388, 397
Koper JW, 388
Koskinen M, 300
Koss JH, 283
Köster G, 356
Kotoura Y, 64
Koukouliou V, 98
Krajbich JI, 99
Krenning EP, 388, 393, 395, 396, 397, 399
Krohn KA, 325
Kroon D, 106
Kropp J, 104
Kubo A, 423
Kuhl DE, 275
Kuijper AFM, 292
Kwan AJ, 44
Kwekkeboom DJ, 388, 393, 395, 397

L

Labarre PG, 405
Labovitz AJ, 288
Lahiri A, 320
Lai E, 170
Laks H, 332
Lalau JD, 160

Lamberts SWJ, 388, 393, 395, 396, 397, 399
Lambrecht RM, 245
Lamers CBHW, 225
Lamki LM, 254
Lammertsma AA, 346
Landoni C, 339
Láng J, 93
Lang NP, 210
Lantto T, 101
Lapalus F, 235
Larar JN, 44
Larcos G, 125
LaRosa CA, 153
Larson SM, 170, 378
Latham IA, 412
Lawrence R, 36
Lebot E, 235
LeBrun GP, 227
Lee F-T, 245
Lee KS, 336
Lee M, 283
Lee VW, 52
Lefroy DC, 346
Le Guludec D, 291, 344
Lehman WB, 134
Lehnert M, 57
Leitha T, 400
Lemoine R, 71
Lennard-Jones JE, 237
Lenney W, 32
Lentle BC, 24
Leonetti F, 200
Leppo JA, 317, 319
Lerch H, 326
Lerner E, 199
Lesser RP, 278
Lette J, 310
Levenson D, 170
Levesseur A, 310
Levine SE, 353
Levy R, 164
Lewis C, 183
Lewis PJ, 278
Lewis RD, 218
Li DJ, 103
Li J, 426, 428, 429
Li YM, 252
Liao S-Q, 88
Lichtenstein M, 241
Liebergall M, 110
Lin J-N, 233
Lin W-Y, 88
Lindemans J, 399
Line BR, 247
Linehan WM, 55
Linnarz M, 57
Lippin Y, 150
LitteJohn JK, 1
Little JM, 68
Little R, 332
Lively RS, 446
Ljungberg M, 422
Llacer J, 435
Logue FC, 155

Lomas FE, 90
Longère P, 284
Lopez M, 401
Lottes G, 364
Louis O, 71
Lubin E, 164
Lucignani G, 268, 339
Luke DL, 362
Lukes J, 323
Lumbroso J, 171
Lusins JO, 139
Lutkin JE, 32

M

McAfee JG, 408
McAneny DB, 52
Macapinlac HA, 378
McCarthy WH, 75
McCormick PA, 373
McEllin K, 167
McEwan AJB, 409
Macey DJ, 441
MacFall JR, 38, 365
MacFarlane DJ, 127
Machecourt J, 284
McIntyre N, 373
McKearn TJ, 69
McKillop JH, 16, 155
McKusick KA, 8
Macleod MA, 267
McMahon M, 413
McNamara D, 310
MacNeily AE, 186
McPartlin M, 412
McSherry BA, 317, 319
Maddahi J, 287, 289, 306, 309, 332
Madelmont JC, 405
Madsen JR, 44
Madsen MT, 276
Magdinec M, 368
Magid SK, 359
Magill HL, 201
Maillie HD, 445
Maini CL, 401, 403
Mairal L, 118
Maizels M, 186
Malabarey T, 243
Malamitsi J, 98
Malkin RD, 308
Mañá J, 118
Mandell GA, 136
Maneval DC, 201
Mangoni di S Stefano ML, 329
Maniawski P, 313
Mannan RH, 409
Mansberger AR Jr, 42, 157
Maragoudakis P, 98
Marchandise X, 160
Mariani G, 162
Marin-Neto JA, 297, 315
Marosi C, 400
Marsh JI, 24

Marsh JL, 97
Martin FC, 111
Martin GV, 325
Martin RH, 227
Martinez CJ, 174
Martinez-Duncker D, 320
Massie JD, 130
Matan Y, 110
Mather SJ, 237
Mathews D, 259
Matsuda H, 252
Matsui Y, 31
Matsumoto M, 257
Matsuoka H, 194
Matsushima Y, 194
Mattera J, 413
Matteucci F, 162
Matzer L, 287, 289, 306
Mauclaire LP, 405
Maughan J, 240
Maurea S, 55
Maurer AH, 244
Maurer G, 305
Maurer U, 383
Mazoyer B, 340
Mazziotta JC, 435
Mechlis-Frish S, 164
Medina M, 261
Meghdadi S, 400
Mehta MN, 161
Meier CA, 167
Meignan M, 205
Meikle SR, 425, 431
Melcarne A, 261
Melisi JW, 366
Mello NK, 251
Mena I, 376
Mendelson J, 251
Menendez LR, 50
Mensch B, 53
Mensh BD, 22
Mercer JR, 409
Merlet P, 340, 344
Merli G, 246
Messa C, 268
Messinger DE, 308
Metayer S, 310
Metz CE, 435
Meyer MA, 74
Michelot JM, 405
Michigishi T, 28
Miles KA, 103
Miller DD, 288, 303, 304
Miller JH, 150
Miller TR, 76, 432
Minoshima S, 275
Mirra J, 50
Misaki T, 31
Miyamoto S, 31
Miyauchi T, 28
Mody FV, 332
Mohamadiyeh MK, 243
Moisan A, 228
Molea N, 162
Mondal A, 133

Monés J, 236
Monsein LH, 278
Montravers F, 53
Morabia A, 4
Morady F, 343
Morand P, 291
Moreau MFC, 405
Moreno AJ, 249
Moretti J-L, 291, 443
Moriwaki H, 257
Morrell NW, 21
Morris GP, 237
Morrison JC, 216
Moser EA, 187
Moser KM, 1
Mosheiff R, 110
Motomura N, 423
Mouratidis B, 90
Mozley DP, 209
Muls V, 238
Mungovan JA, 372
Munz DL, 356
Muradali D, 117
Muramori A, 328
Murray P, 245
Musso C, 261
Mutairi MA, 114
Muzik O, 316, 343

N

Nagao K, 191
Nagle KR, 412
Nagy F, 93
Nakada K, 191
Nakajima K, 328
Nappi A, 329
Neagle CE, 353
Neerhut P, 241
Nepola JV, 97
Neuhaus C, 381
Neuman A, 291
Neumann M, 400
Neumann RD, 55, 408
Newberg AB, 265
Newman GE, 38
Nicod L, 71
Nicolai E, 329
Nicoletti R, 383
Nicolino F, 200
Niggel JB, 312
Nightingale JMD, 237
Nihoyannopoulos P, 346
Nijran KS, 21, 198
Nikiforidis G, 185
Nishihara M, 253
Nishimiya J, 366
Nishimura T, 37, 257
Nitzsche EU, 187
Nocaudie M, 160
Nohara R, 321
Nonomura A, 28
Norton JA, 55
Nose T, 45

Noujaim A, 70
Nunan TO, 82

O

Oakley CM, 346
Oates E, 95, 113, 221
Odano I, 253
O'Doherty MJ, 82
Oei HY, 388, 393, 396, 399
Ogawa K, 423
Ogawa Y, 37
Ohye C, 48
Okazaki Y, 257
Oku N, 257
Okuda K, 321
O'Leary DS, 276
Olken NM, 411
Omae T, 194
O'Neill P, 68
Oram E, 189
Oriuchi N, 48
Ortiz-Alonso FJ, 336
Osterholm MT, 86
Otake S, 120
Ott G, 104
O'Tuama LA, 44
Overbeck B, 104
Özdemir O, 189

P

Pace L, 329
Pacheco EJ, 249
Packard AB, 44
Padhy AK, 198
Paik CH, 408
Palevsky HI, 19
Papafragou K, 98
Papaleo A, 261
Papanicolaou M, 287
Papapoulos SE, 158
Papon JM, 405
Papós M, 93
Parisi MT, 76
Parkin A, 240
Parliament MB, 409
Parmentier C, 171
Parmett S, 61
Pasqualini R, 324
Patsalos PN, 346
Paul R, 101
Paulson OB, 279
Pauw BKH, 397
Pauwels EKJ, 158, 225, 292
Pelizzari CA, 365
Penny R, 214
Perani D, 268
Pérez JE, 338
Perrier A, 4
Perrin-Resche I, 131
Perrone-Filardi P, 296, 297
Phalen JJ, 26

Phelps ME, 332, 335
Phillips WT, 107
Philpott NJ, 374
Phlipponneau M, 160
Pickett RD, 412
Pigorini F, 401
Pike MC, 106
Pitts NL, 216
Pizzolato G, 271
Plagne RJ, 405
Plotzke KP, 411
PMcL Black , 44
Pocock N, 214
Polidori C, 284
Politoske EJ, 215
Pollack S, 52
Polvani GL, 379
Pompilio G, 379
Porat S, 110
Porqueddu M, 379
Postema PTE, 388
Powe JE, 179
Powers ER, 294
Poznanski AK, 144
Prigent FM, 434
Proukakis C, 98
Prpic H, 158
Pruitt DL, 362
Puma J, 311
Purdy PD, 259

Q

Quinn BR, 445
Quinn D, 214
Quyyumi AA, 296, 315

R

Radcliffe R, 244
Ragosta M, 294
Rahmouni A, 205
Rakow JI, 63
Ramos-Gabatin A, 216
Rand N, 110
Randé JLD, 340
Rao DV, 439
Raoul J-L, 228
Rasey JS, 325
Reba RC, 408
Rechtman D, 291
Redepenning LS, 26
Reijs AEM, 388
Remes K, 101
Reub JC, 388
Reubi JC, 393, 395, 396, 399
Revillon Y, 171
Reynolds J, 167
Reynolds JC, 55
Rezai K, 276
Rhoades H, 254
Rhodes CG, 346
Ricard M, 171

Riccabona M, 383
Rigo P, 320
Ring E, 383
Rizzo G, 268
Robbins J, 167
Robertson JS, 440
Robinson PJ, 240
Rodman JH, 201
Rodrigo F, 301
Rodriguez AA, 249
Rodwell JD, 244
Rogers M, 276
Rokhsar S, 332
Roos JC, 66
Ross DS, 167
Rossato A, 271
Rossetti C, 339
Rothmund M, 381
Rowen M, 298, 302
Rozanski A, 434
Rubin RH, 106
Rudolph AS, 107
Ruiz M, 314
Rusckowski M, 414

S

Sääf J, 370
Saal JP, 340
Sabia PJ, 294
Saga T, 408
Sainz S, 236
Saitta B, 271
Sakahara H, 64
Sakai K, 253
Sala A, 379
Sallan SE, 44
Saltzberg MT, 322
Saltzman HA, 38
Salvatore M, 329
Sammak BM, 114
Sampathkumaran K, 338
Sampson CB, 103
Samuel AM, 161
Sandler ED, 76
Sarda L, 53
Sarwark J, 144
Sasayama S, 321
Sathyanarayana, 157
Satou M, 45
Sawada SG, 316
Sawroop K, 133
Sax EJ, 52
Sayli A, 280
Schechtman KB, 338
Scheele J, 80
Schelbert HR, 332, 335
Schiffman FJ, 60
Schifter T, 365
Schlick W, 400
Schlumberger M, 171
Schmidt JF, 279
Schmidt P, 245
Schneider JA, 378

Schneider MU, 80
Schneider R, 359
Schober O, 326, 364
Schroeder EV, 232
Schubert A, 368
Schwab J, 105
Schwaiger M, 74, 316, 336, 342, 343
Schwartz M, 70
Schwarz A, 105
Schwerdt P, 278
Sciuk J, 364
Sciuto R, 401, 403
Scott AM, 378
Scott RM, 44
Seabold JE, 97
Sebes J, 130
Seder JS, 232
Seed WA, 21
Segal K, 164
Segarra MI, 118
Seike Y, 257
Semprebene A, 401
Senekowitsch R, 70
Setaro JF, 199
Seto H, 239
Shaaban AA, 190
Shaban AA, 243
Shaha AR, 153
Shahabpour M, 128
Shamaa MA, 190
Shand J, 155
Shapiro M, 110
Sharif HS, 114
Shaw HM, 75
Shaw LJ, 288
Shelhamer J, 34
Shi Q, 322
Shi QX, 313
Shibazaki T, 48
Shih WJ, 104
Shimizu M, 239, 328
Shimonagata T, 37
Shimoni A, 164
Shinotoh H, 270
Shirato M, 64
Shivkumar K, 10
Shokeir AA, 190
Shuke N, 28
Shvoron A, 150
Siegel BA, 338
Sigmund G, 187
Silagan G, 287, 306, 309
Siles S, 200
Silvestri JH, 232
Simanis JP, 314
Simon W, 445
Simons GR, 2
Sinusas AJ, 313, 322, 413
Siproudhis L, 228
Siraj QH, 198
Sketch MH Jr, 311
Skinner S, 411
Slama M, 344
Slosman D, 4

Slosman DO, 71
Smith CC, 100
Smith FJ, 179
Smith FW, 100
Smith WH, 294
Sobel BE, 338
Sochor H, 320
Solanki C, 103
Solomon H, 106
Solomon SL, 86
Sonenberg M, 170, 378
Sorenson MK, 210
Sostman HD, 8, 18, 38
Souder E, 265
Soufer R, 330
Souteyrand PA, 405
Spaeth J, 122
Spieth ME, 232
Spiliopoulos A, 71
Spritzer CE, 38
Sridhara B, 320
Stack R, 311
Stanberry CD, 286
Stapp J, 381
Staron RB, 349
Steck DJ, 446
Stein PD, 10, 13
Steinberg EH, 283
Stevens MJ, 342
Stevenson LW, 332
Storey AE, 412
Stöver B, 187
Strand S-E, 422
Stratmann HG, 303, 304
Strauss HW, 334, 337, 404
Striano G, 339
Strongwater A, 134
Studnicka M, 400
Sturgess I, 111
Suhara T, 270
Sumiya H, 252
Sunderland M, 201
Supino PG, 327
Syrota A, 340, 344

T

Taavitsainen M, 101
Tadamura E, 321
Takahashi N, 321
Takamiya M, 194
Takase B, 288
Takashima T, 28
Takeuchi R, 31
Taki J, 28, 328
Talbot J-N, 53
Tamaki N, 321
Tamesis BR, 303
Tamgac F, 291
Tamura M, 48
Tan P, 431
Tanaka R, 253
Tapson V, 38
Tarbell NJ, 44

Tateno M, 48
Tateno Y, 270
Taylor A, 183
Taylor WJ, 254
Telepak RJ, 122
Tenenbaum F, 171
Teoh SK, 251
Ter S-E, 246
Teule GJJ, 66, 331
Thacker SB, 86
Thériault C, 169
Thompson JF, 75
Thrall J, 8
Thys O, 238
Tiel-van Buul MMC, 141, 353
Tien RD, 365
Tikofsky RS, 262
Tischler MD, 312
Tofani A, 401, 403
Tofe AJ, 418
Toltzis R, 2
Tomiyoshi K, 48
Tompkins RG, 106
Tonami N, 28
Toni MG, 162
Toolanen G, 351
Torizuka T, 321
Torres VE, 180
Tourassi GD, 18, 433
Tran HD, 254
Trautmann ME, 381
Travagli J-P, 171
Travin MI, 308
Treves ST, 44
Trimarco B, 329
Tsapakos MJ, 247
Tse KMK, 209
Tsuchiya T, 253
Tsuji S, 252
Tsukamoto E, 191
Tsur H, 150
Tulchinsky M, 172
Tumeh SS, 55
Turchi S, 162
Turjanmaa V, 300
Turkington TG, 365
Turnbull GL, 249
Tzen K-Y, 233

U

Uebis R, 293
Uehara T, 37, 257
Ugur Ö, 189
Unger P-F, 4
Ur E, 56
Urbain D, 238
Uren NG, 346
Uren RF, 75
Urtasun RC, 409
Uszler JM, 203
Uusitalo A, 300

V

Vacarro J, 372
Valentine M, 167
Valette H, 340
Valkema R, 158
Vallabhajosula S, 418
van Beek EJR, 141
Van Beek EJR, 353
van der Sijp JRM, 237
van der Sluys Veer A, 225
van der Wall EE, 292
van Eck-Smit BLF, 292
van Eijck CHJ, 393, 399
van Eyck CHJ, 396
van Hagen M, 388
van Hagen PM, 393
Van Heertum R, 262
Van Heertum RL, 85
van Leeuwen GR, 331
van Lingen A, 331
Van Nerom CG, 177
van Pel R, 399
Van Royen EA, 353
van Train K, 289, 305
Van Train K, 287
Van Train KF, 306, 309
van Urk H, 397
Vanzetto G, 284
Varma VM, 408
Varoglu E, 189
Vassilakos P, 185
Veklerov E, 435
Vellend H, 117
Venegas R, 376
Venturo I, 401
Verbruggen A, 416
Verbruggen AM, 177
Verbruggen LA, 128
Veronikis I, 167
Verspaget HW, 225
Veyre AJ, 405
Vilardell F, 236
Villegas BJ, 317, 319
Vilner BJ, 408
Virzi F, 414
Visser CA, 331
Visser FC, 331
Visser GWM, 331
Visser TJ, 388
Vitols P, 322
Vitols PJ, 313
vom Dahl J, 293, 336
von Kleist S, 70
Vorne M, 101

W

Wackers FJT, 322, 413
Wackers FJTH, 313
Wagner R, 174
Wahl RL, 89, 411
Wahlund L-O, 370

Wakasugi S, 337
Walamies M, 300
Waldemar G, 279
Walker BS, 259
Wallis JB, 327
Wallis JW, 432
Walsh RA, 323
Walther MM, 55
Wang FP, 289
Wang H, 426, 429
Wang S-J, 88, 90
Wang YL, 90
Ward RJ, 52
Wardell S, 144
Washburn LC, 323
Wasserleben V, 286
Watanabe N, 48, 239
Watanabe Y, 28
Watson BA, 418
Watson DD, 294, 314
Watts RJ, 445
Waugh R, 245
Webbon PM, 412
Wei JP, 42, 157
Weinberg DS, 2
Weinel RJ, 381
Weiner BH, 317, 319
Weiner M, 63
Weinmann P, 291
Weintraub BD, 167
Weiss J, 281
Weiss L, 281
Weissman AF, 89
Wells AU, 36
Wetterberg L, 370
Wichter T, 326
Wiege LI, 409
Wieland D, 343
Wieland DM, 275, 342, 343
Wilkinson D, 240
Wilkinson R, 337
Williams GA, 304
Wilson AG, 374
Wilson DM, 180
Winkelmann W, 364
Winnard P Jr, 414
Wittekind C, 70
Wittry MD, 303, 304
Witty L, 38
Woda A, 209
Wolf F, 80, 105
Wolf JE, 284
Wolf RL, 180
Wolfe ER, 342
Wolfe ER Jr, 316, 336, 343
Wolzt M, 400
Wong A, 103
Worsley DF, 19, 24
Wright DG, 353
Wu Y, 239

Y

Yamada Y, 45

Yamamoto T, 45
Yamamuro T, 64
Yamashita J, 252
Yamazaki T, 270
Yano M, 194
Yao M, 155
Yeh SH, 90
Yeung DW, 22
Yokoyama K, 28
Yonekura Y, 321
Yoshida K, 333

Yoshii Y, 45
Yoshio H, 328
Younis LT, 288, 303
Yudd AP, 85
Yuja RE, 232

Z

Zafrani ES, 205

Zalutsky MR, 426
Zanco P, 271
Zaret BL, 313, 322, 330, 413
Zatz S, 164
Zeng GL, 428
Zenorini A, 268
Ziffer J, 306
Zimmerhackl LB, 187
Zito F, 268
Zubal IG, 199
Zwinderman AH, 292